# Advanced Principles and Applications of Anesthesiology

# Advanced Principles and Applications of Anesthesiology

Editor: Dennis Hanks

AMERICAN
MEDICAL PUBLISHERS
www.americanmedicalpublishers.com

AMERICAN
MEDICAL PUBLISHERS
www.americanmedicalpublishers.com

**Cataloging-in-Publication Data**

Advanced principles and applications of anesthesiology / edited by Dennis Hanks.
p. cm.
Includes bibliographical references and index.
ISBN 978-1-63927-532-8
1. Anesthesiology. 2. Anesthesiology--Apparatus and instruments. 3. Anesthesia. I. Hanks, Dennis.
RD81 .A38 2022
617.96--dc23



American Medical Publishers,
41 Flatbush Avenue,
1st Floor, New York,
NY 11217, USA

ISBN 978-1-63927-532-8 (Hardback)

# Contents

# Preface

This book aims to highlight the current researches and provides a platform to further the scope of innovations in this area. This book is a product of the combined efforts of many researchers and scientists, after going through thorough studies and analysis from different parts of the world. The objective of this book is to provide the readers with the latest information of the field.

Anesthesiology refers to the perioperative care of patients before, during and after the surgery. It also includes intensive care medicine, pain medicine and critical emergency medicine. Its primary principle includes the use of anesthesia and anesthetics for safely supporting a patient's vital functions during surgery. An understanding of operative risk and complications, the methods to mitigate such risks and the management of the illness is crucial to the practice of anesthesiology. Active airway management, ultrasonography, echocardiography imaging and hemodynamic monitoring are also performed within this discipline. In recent years, the scope of anesthesiology has extended to the identification of high-risk patients and optimization of their fitness, improvement of safety during the surgery and promotion of recovery. This book traces the progress of this field and highlights some of its key concepts and applications. The topics covered herein offer the readers new insights in the field of anesthesiology. This book explores all the important aspects of anesthesiology in the present day scenario.

I would like to express my sincere thanks to the authors for their dedicated efforts in the completion of this book. I acknowledge the efforts of the publisher for providing constant support. Lastly, I would like to thank my family for their support in all academic endeavors.

**Editor**

1

# Attenuation of Hemodynamic Responses to Laryngoscopy and Tracheal Intubation: Propacetamol versus Lidocaine

**Ali Kord Valeshabad,[1] Omid Nabavian,[2] Keramat Nourijelyani,[3] Hadi Kord,[4] Hossein Vafainejad,[2] Reza Kord Valeshabad,[5] Ali Reza Feili,[6] Mehdi Rezaei,[2] Hamed Darabi,[2] Mohammad Koohkan,[2] Poorya Golbinimofrad,[2] and Samira Jafari[2]**

[1] *Department of Ophthalmology and Visual Sciences, University of Illinois at Chicago, IL 60612, USA*
[2] *Department of Anaesthesiology, Tehran University of Medical Sciences, P.O. Box 14155-6447, Tehran, Iran*
[3] *Department of Epidemiology of Biostatistics, Tehran University of Medical Sciences, P.O. Box 14155-6447, Tehran, Iran*
[4] *Department of Dermatology, Golestan University of Medical Sciences, Gorgan 4934174515, Iran*
[5] *Zainaldin Martyr Research Center, Gorgan University of Agricultural Sciences and Natural Resources, P.O. Box 15739-49138, Gorgan, Iran*
[6] *Center for Cardiovascular Research, University of Illinois at Chicago, 835 S. Wolcott Avenue, Chicago, IL 60612, USA*

Correspondence should be addressed to Omid Nabavian; omidnab@hotmail.com

Academic Editor: D. John Doyle

The purpose of this study is to assess the effects of propacetamol on attenuating hemodynamic responses subsequent laryngoscopy and tracheal intubation compared to lidocaine. In this randomized clinical trial, 62 patients with the American Anesthesiologists Society (ASA) class I/II who required laryngoscopy and tracheal intubation for elective surgery were assigned to receive propacetamol 2 g/I.V./infusion (group P) or lidocaine 1.5 mg/kg (group L) prior to laryngoscopy. Systolic and diastolic blood pressures (SBP, DBP), mean arterial pressure (MAP), and heart rate (HR) were recorded at baseline, before laryngoscopy and within nine minutes after intubation. In both groups P and L, MAP increased after laryngoscopy and the changes were statistically significant ($P < 0.001$). There were significant changes of HR in both groups after intubation ($P < 0.02$), but the trend of changes was different between two groups ($P < 0.001$). In group L, HR increased after intubation and its change was statistically significant within 9 minutes after intubation ($P < 0.001$), while in group P, HR remained stable after intubation ($P = 0.8$). Propacetamol 2 gr one hour prior intubation attenuates heart rate responses after laryngoscopy but is not effective to prevent acute alterations in blood pressure after intubation.

## 1. Introduction

Propacetamol [4-(acetamido)phenyl N,N-diethylglycinate] is a prodrug, which is quickly hydrolyzed by plasma esterase to vigorous paracetamol; 1 gr propacetamol metabolized to 500 mg paracetamol [1]. It has an onset of about half an hour to an hour, has a half-life of one to four hours, and has duration effect of six to eight hours. Its optimal effects appear about one hour after injection and its maximum recommended dose in adults is 4 grams per day. This drug inhibits prostaglandins synthesis in the central nervous system and also blocks pain impulses peripherally and has antipyretic effects through hypothalamus [2]. This drug is safe, cost effective and its beneficial effects for pain management and reducing opioids amounts have been confirmed in patients who underwent dental, orthopaedic and gynaecologic surgeries [3–8].

Laryngoscopy and tracheal intubation are among the most painful processes carried out on the human body which are associated with acute hemodynamic responses, lasting for at least ten minutes [3–9]. Sympathoadrenal stimulation and subsequent catecholamine release may partially contribute to this hemodynamic instability, which is typically signified by an increase in heart rate (HR) and blood pressure (BP) [10];

however, the main mechanism is not clearly defined. These acute changes in hemodynamic status are particularly significant in patients with preexisting predisposing situations like hypertension, myocardial infarction, myocardial malfunction, and cardiovascular diseases [11, 12].

Various techniques have been examined for attenuating hemodynamic responses to laryngoscopy and tracheal intubation, including deeper anaesthesia [10], and numerous drugs, such as beta blockers [13, 14], calcium channel blockers [15], opioids [16–18], sodium channel blockers [18, 19], vasodilators [20], and alpha agonists [21]. Opioids are the most commonly used drugs with satisfactory outcomes for preventing hemodynamic subsequence of intubation. These drugs are not cost effective, however, and are associated with some unfavourable complications such as nausea, vomiting, consumedly sedation, and respiratory depression [22]. Therefore, there has been a growing trend to find an effective substitute to reduce these side effects as much as possible [23, 24]. However, the beneficial effects of propacetamol have been confirmed for postoperative pain management. The purpose of this study is to assess the effects of propacetamol on attenuating hemodynamic responses subsequent laryngoscopy and tracheal intubation compared to lidocaine, which is routinely used in most of operation rooms.

## 2. Subjects and Methods

*2.1. Study Design, Inclusion and Exclusion Criteria.* This single-blind randomized clinical trial was conducted between January 2010 and September 2011. The study protocol was approved by the ethical committee of Tehran University of Medical Sciences (TUMS). The cases were selected among the patients who underwent elective gynecologic and reconstructive surgeries in two operating rooms of Imam Khomeini Hospital, in Tehran, Iran. These cases had laryngoscopy and tracheal intubation before the surgery. The inclusion criteria were patients between the ages of 20 and 60 as well as American Anesthesiologists society (ASA) classes I and II. Patients with preexisting conditions were not included, namely, hard intubation (previous history of hard intubation, laryngoscopic view >II, body mass index >30, micrognathia, and macroglossia), diabetic patients with autonomic dysfunction, patients with renal and liver dysfunction, patients with a history of cardiovascular disease, hypertension, cerebrovascular diseases, respiratory disease (e.g., asthma), pheochromocytoma, cushing's syndrome, opium addiction, propacetamol or lidocaine contraindications, and hypersensitivity, and patients who needed emergent surgery.

*2.2. Randomization and Study Protocol.* The study protocol was explained in detail for those who met the inclusion criteria. Those who agreed and filled informed consent were enrolled in the study. A specific code was considered for each patient, and they were randomly allocated to two study groups, propacetamol (P) and lidocaine (L).

In the operating room setting, a peripheral I.V. line was drawn from the patient's hand, and a ringer lactate (2 cc/kg) was administered. A standard monitoring system, including electrocardiogram and noninvasive blood pressure and pulse oximetry, was set for each participant. One hour preceding anaesthesia induction, patients in group P received propacetamol 2 g/IV/infusion diluted in 100 cc of normal saline (N.S). Patients in group L received lidocaine (1.5 mg/kg) two minutes before anesthesia. The grouping was concealed from anesthesiologist performed intubation and also from patients who participated in the study. Only the researcher who recorded hemodynamic variables at studied time points was aware of the grouping that was different from the person who analyzed the data.

The routine protocol for anaesthesia induction was similarly applied for both groups using I.V. administration of midazolam 0.02 mg/kg, fentanyl 2 $\mu$g/kg, sodium thiopental 5 mg/kg, and atracurium 0.5 mg/kg. Three minutes afterwards, laryngoscopy and tracheal intubation were performed by two anesthesiologists, using tracheal tubes number 7–7.5 for men and number 6.5–7 for women. Anesthesia was maintained based on the operation by means of isoflurane with or without $N_2O$ and fentanyl 50 $\mu$g each 30 minutes.

Hemodynamic status, including systolic and diastolic blood pressures (SBP, DBP), mean arterial pressure (MAP), and heart rate were recorded in a prepared check list for each individual in six time points, before drug administration (as baseline), after drug administration (before laryngoscopy), and at 1, 3, 6, and 9 minutes after tracheal intubation.

*2.3. Primary and Secondary Outcomes.* The primary outcome was to determine the effects of groups (L versus P) and time (before intubation and at 1, 3, 6, and 9 minutes after intubation) on MAP and HR. Secondary outcomes were assessment of changes in SBP, DBP, MAP, and HR before and after drug administration, and also their changes within the 9 minutes after laryngoscopy. The incidence rates of tachycardia (HR > 120 beat/min) and bradycardia (HR < 60 beat/min), hypertension (MAP > 120 mmHg), and hypotension (MAP < 70 mmHg) were assessed and compared between two groups.

*2.4. Statistical Analysis.* Results were reported as mean ± standard deviation (SD) for quantitative variables and percentages for categorical variables. SBP, DBP, MAP, and HR were compared using the unpaired $t$-test between two studied groups. The changes of these variables after drug administration were compared assessed using a paired test. A two-way analysis of variance (ANOVA) with repeated measures was conducted to determine the effects of groups (L versus P) and time (before intubation and at 1, 3, 6, and 9 minutes after intubation) on MAP and HR. In addition, a repeated measures one-way ANOVA was performed in each group to determine the effects of time on MAP and HR. Statistical analysis was performed using SPSS version 21 (SPSS Inc, Chicago, IL, USA) and statistical significance was accepted at $P \leq 0.05$.

## 3. Results

Of 89 initial patients, 66 patients (Male 32) with the mean age of 41 ± 12 years (range: 20–60 years), who met inclusion criteria, were selected for study procedure and equally divided into two groups L and P. In total, four patients were removed

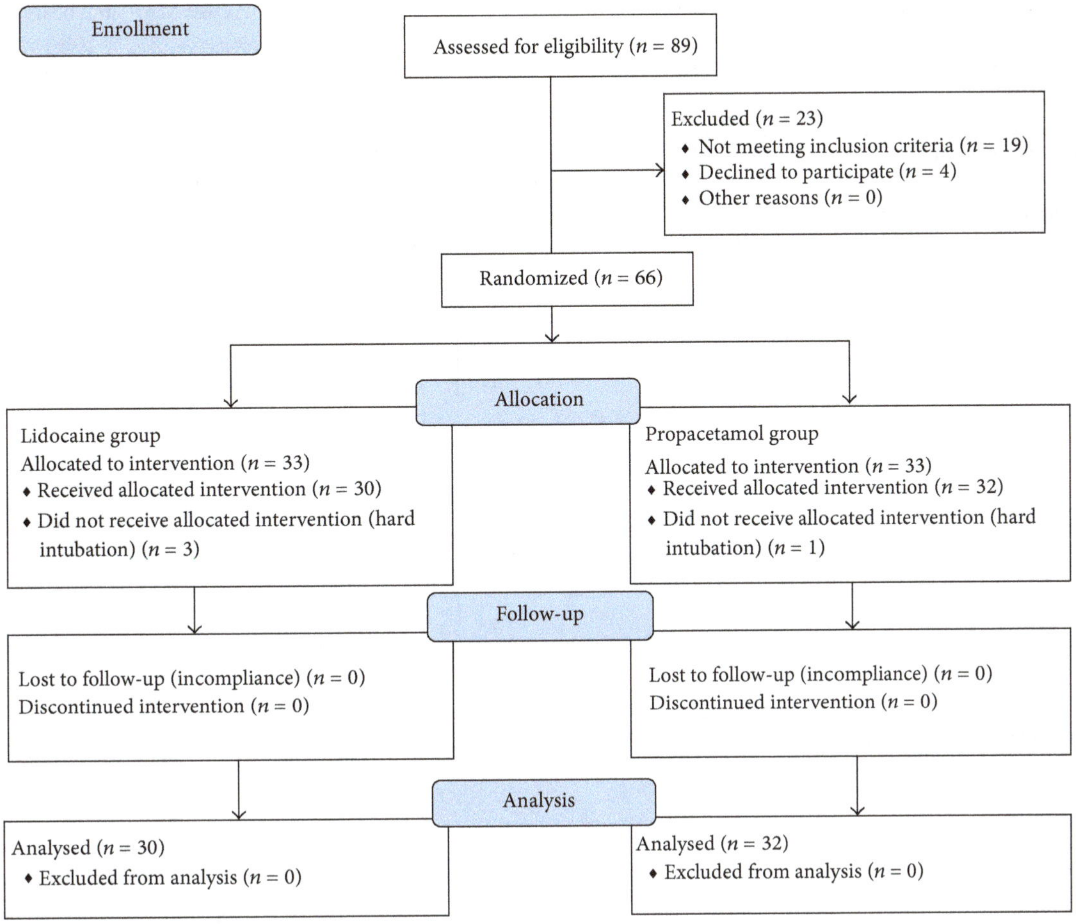


FIGURE 1: Study diagram.

from the study due to hard intubation (3 patients in group L and 1 patient in placebo group). Figure 1 shows study fellow diagram.

Patients' demographic data in each group is shown in Table 1. Two groups did not have significant difference for age, sex, weight, height, ASA class, and endoscopic view ($P \geq 0.2$). Hemodynamic status including SBP, DBP, MAP, and HR before and after drug administration (before laryngoscopy) has been summarized in Table 2. SBP, DBP, MAP, and HR were similar between two groups before drug administration ($P \geq 0.2$). In both groups SBP, DBP, and MAP decreased after drug administration ($P < 0.001$). In group P HR decreased after drug administration ($P < 0.001$), while in group L it did not change significantly ($P = 0.2$).

The trend of SBP, DBP, MAP, and HR changes in each group has been shown in Figure 2. There was a significant effect of time on MAP ($P < 0.001$), but there was not a significant difference between two groups over the time points after intubation ($P = 0.8$). In both groups P and L, MAP increased after laryngoscopy and the changes were statistically significant ($P < 0.001$). There were significant effects of groups (P versus L) and time on HR after intubation ($P \leq 0.02$). There were significant changes of HR in both groups after intubation, but the trend of changes was not the same between two groups. In group L, HR increased after intubation and its change was statistically significant within 9 minutes after intubation ($P < 0.001$). In group P, HR remained stable within the 9 minutes after intubation ($P = 0.8$).

TABLE 1: Patients' baseline data in each group.

| Variables | Propacetamol ($n = 32$) | Lidocaine ($n = 30$) | $P$ value |
|---|---|---|---|
| Age (year) | 43 ± 12 | 39 ± 11 | 0.2 |
| ASA (I/II) | 1/31 | 2/28 | 0.6 |
| Sex (M/F) | 15/17 | 13/17 | 0.8 |
| Weight (kg) | 74 ± 10 | 77 ± 10 | 0.3 |
| Height (cm) | 164 ± 15 | 166 ± 12 | 0.6 |
| Endoscopic view (I/II) | 20/12 | 19/11 | 0.9 |

The incidence rates of hypertension (3.0% versus 20.0%, $P = 0.034$), hypotension (0.0% versus 20%, $P = 0.007$), and tachycardia (3.0% versus 20.0%, $P = 0.034$) were significantly lower in group P as compared to group L ($P < 0.05$).

## 4. Discussion

In the present study, our findings showed beneficial effects of preoperative administration of propacetamol on attenuation

Table 2: Hemodynamic variables including systolic, diastolic, and mean arterial blood pressures (SBP, DBP, MAP) and heart rate (HR) before and after drug in each group.

| Variables | Propacetamol ($N = 32$) | | | Lidocaine ($N = 30$) | | |
|---|---|---|---|---|---|---|
| | Before | After | $P$ value | Before | After | $P$ value |
| Systolic blood pressure (mmHg) | 125 ± 11 | 112 ± 22 | <0.001 | 126 ± 21 | 97 ± 21 | <0.001 |
| Diastolic blood pressure (mmHg) | 82 ± 10 | 72 ± 9 | <0.001 | 83 ± 14 | 65 ± 14 | <0.001 |
| Mean arterial blood pressure (mmHg) | 96 ± 9 | 86 ± 11 | <0.001 | 97 ± 15 | 75 ± 17 | <0.001 |
| Hear rate (beat/min) | 81 ± 8 | 72 ± 5 | <0.001 | 85 ± 17 | 89 ± 21 | 0.2 |

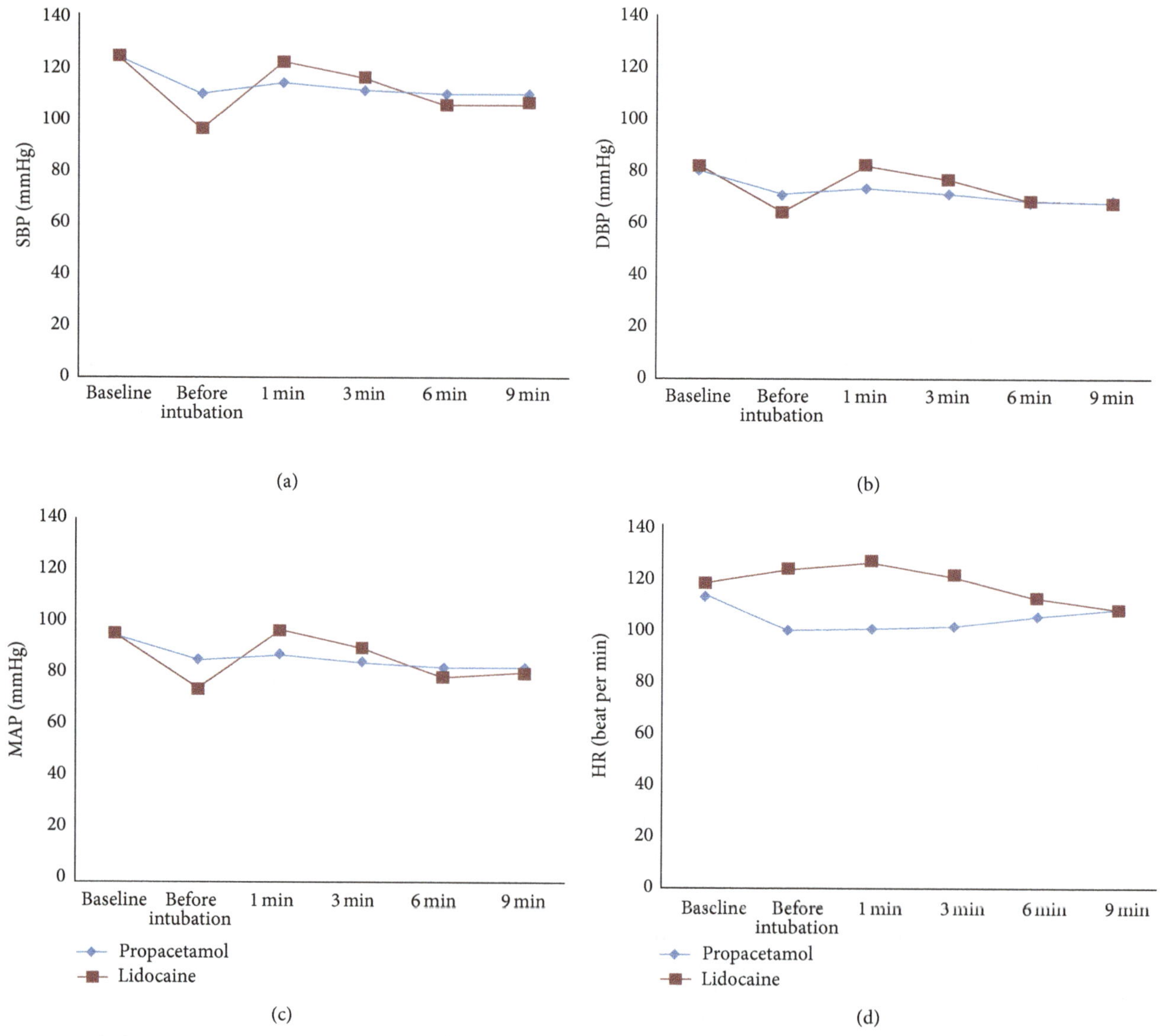


Figure 2: Hemodynamic status including systolic, diastolic, and mean arterial blood pressures (SBP, DBP, MAP) and heart rate (HR) within 9 minutes after tracheal intubation in each studied group.

of heart rate responses after tracheal intubation compared to lidocaine. None of the lidocaine or propacetamol was effective to attenuate blood pressure responses after laryngoscopy and changes of MAP after laryngoscopy were significant in both groups.

Although favorable effects of propacetamol on postoperative pain management have been well documented [3–8], there is no published evidence about its preventive effects on hemodynamic stimulations after tracheal intubation. However, there are some reports about the effects of acetaminophen on hemodynamic changes in subjects with a regular consumption of acetaminophen. These alterations include increase in blood pressure and cardiovascular events in subjects consuming acetaminophen [25–28]. In one two-week randomized crossover trial, acetaminophen (1 g three times daily) and not placebo increased systolic and diastolic blood pressure as determined by ambulatory monitoring [28]. However, other authors had reverse opinions [29, 30]. It seems that a single injection of propacetamol could not develop these side effects; however, it was not to attenuate the responses after laryngoscopy as well.

The exact underlying mechanism of the effect of propacetamol on cardiovascular responses is not clear. It might be attributed to its analgesic action mediated by the antiprostaglandin effect. Similar to NSAID and aspirin, propacetamol inhibits cyclooxygenase, prostaglandin H2 synthase in its analgesic pathway [31]. Propacetamol, however, blocks this enzyme at its peroxidase catalytic and not cyclooxygenase catalytic site and is not considered a NSAID. Riad and Moussa assessed the effects of lornoxicam on hemodynamic changes after tracheal intubation and found that administration of 8 mg of lornoxicam 30 minutes before surgery significantly decreased HR and BP subsequent laryngoscopy and tracheal intubation compared to placebo [32]. Lornoxicam, which is a novel nonsteroidal anti-inflammatory drug (NSAID), is more known for its postoperative pain reduction [33].

Lidocaine is used as a routine drug to relieve pain and cardiovascular responses to tracheal intubation in a considerable number of operating rooms. Recent studies have demonstrated that lidocaine alone or in combination with esmolol is not as effective as opioids on attenuating blood pressure and heart rate after intubation [14, 18]. Min et al., in a well-designed trial on 66 patients who underwent elective surgery, compared preventive effects of remifentanil 1 mg/kg and lidocaine 1.5 mg/kg + esmolol 1 mg/kg on hypertension and tachycardia after endotracheal intubation [14]. They revealed that remifentanil 1 mg/kg is more effective than the combination of lidocaine 1.5 mg/kg and esmolol 1 mg/kg for attenuating hemodynamic responses to rapid sequence intubation. Incidence rates of hypertension (3% versus 20%), hypotension (0.0% versus 20%), and tachycardia (3% versus 20%) were significantly lower in group P compared to group L. Feng et al. reported postintubation tachycardia (HR > 100 beat/min) and hypertension (SBP > 180 mmHg) in seventy-five percent of patients who received lidocaine [34]. In our trial, the definitions of tachycardia (HR > 120) and hypertension (MAP > 120 mmHg) were different, which might explain the observed differences. Further studies are required to assess various doses of propacetamol in order to compare it with other drugs like fentanyl, remifentanil, and esmolol or in combination with other drugs. The selected patients in our trial were between 20 and 60 years old and did not have any considerable predisposing factor, which may have affected their cardiovascular system. If potential benefits of propacetamol are confirmed, it will be possible to examine it in more specific cases, including patients with hypertension, cardiovascular diseases, the elderly, pregnant patients, and those with contraindication to other drugs.

## 5. Conclusion

Propacetamol 2 gr one hour prior intubation attenuates heart rate responses after laryngoscopy, but is not effective to prevent acute alterations in blood pressure after intubation.

## Conflict of Interests

The authors declare that there is no conflict of interests regarding the publication of this paper.

## References

[1] B. Flouvat, A. Leneveu, S. Fitoussi, B. Delhotal-Landes, and A. Gendron, "Bioequivalence study comparing a new paracetamol solution for injection and propacetamol after single intravenous infusion in healthy subjects," *International Journal of Clinical Pharmacology and Therapeutics*, vol. 42, no. 1, pp. 50–57, 2004.

[2] M. Depre, A. van Hecken, R. Verbesselt, T. B. Tjandra-Maga, M. Gerin, and P. J. de Schepper, "Tolerance and pharmacokinetics of propacetamol, a paracetamol formulation for intravenous use," *Fundamental & Clinical Pharmacology*, vol. 6, no. 6, pp. 259–262, 1992.

[3] E. D. McNicol, A. Tzortzopoulou, M. S. Cepeda, M. B. D. Francia, T. Farhat, and R. Schumann, "Single-dose intravenous paracetamol or propacetamol for prevention or treatment of postoperative pain: a systematic review and meta-analysis," *British Journal of Anaesthesia*, vol. 106, no. 6, pp. 764–775, 2011.

[4] D. Memis, M. T. Inal, G. Kavalci, A. Sezer, and N. Sut, "Intravenous paracetamol reduced the use of opioids, extubation time, and opioid-related adverse effects after major surgery in intensive care unit," *Journal of Critical Care*, vol. 25, no. 3, pp. 458–462, 2010.

[5] J. A. Alhashemi, Q. A. Alotaibi, M. S. Mashaat, T. M. Kaid, R. H. Mujallid, and A. M. Kaki, "Intravenous acetaminophen vs oral ibuprofen in combination with morphine PCIA after Cesarean delivery," *Canadian Journal of Anesthesia*, vol. 53, no. 12, pp. 1200–1206, 2006.

[6] A. A. Eremenko and E. V. Kuslieva, "Analgesic and opioid-sparing effects of intravenous paracetamol in the early period after aortocoronary bypass surgery," *Anesteziologiia i Reanimatologiia*, no. 5, pp. 11–14, 2008.

[7] G. Varrassi, F. Marinangeli, F. Agrò et al., "A double-blinded evaluation of propacetamol versus ketorolac in combination with patient-controlled analgesia morphine: analgesic efficacy and tolerability after gynecologic surgery," *Anesthesia & Analgesia*, vol. 88, no. 3, pp. 611–616, 1999.

[8] H. van Aken, L. Thys, L. Veekman, and H. Buerkle, "Assessing analgesia in single and repeated administrations of propacetamol for postoperative pain: comparison with morphine after dental surgery," *Anesthesia & Analgesia*, vol. 98, no. 1, pp. 159–165, 2004.

[9] N. Bruder, D. Ortega, and C. Granthil, "Consequences and prevention methods of hemodynamic changes during laryngoscopy and intratracheal intubation," *Annales Françaises d'Anesthèsie et de Rèanimation*, vol. 11, no. 1, pp. 57–71, 1992.

[10] M. S. Rao, "Airway management," in *Clinical Anesthesia*, P. G. Barash, B. F. Cullen, and R. K. Stoelting, Eds., pp. 586–587, Lippincott-Raven, Philadelphia, Pa, USA, 3rd edition, 1997.

[11] A. L. Kovac, "Controlling the hemodynamic response to laryngoscopy and endotracheal intubation," *Journal of Clinical Anesthesia*, vol. 8, no. 1, pp. 63–79, 1996.

[12] N. D. Edwards, A. M. Alford, P. M. S. Dobson, J. E. Peacock, and C. S. Reilly, "Myocardial ischaemia during tracheal intubation and extubation," *British Journal of Anaesthesia*, vol. 73, no. 4, pp. 537–539, 1994.

[13] S. Sugiura, S. Seki, K. Hidaka, M. Masuoka, and H. Tsuchida, "The hemodynamic effects of landiolol, an ultra-short-acting

$\beta$1-selective blocker, on endotracheal intubation in patients with and without hypertension," *Anesthesia & Analgesia*, vol. 104, no. 1, pp. 124–129, 2007.

[14] J.-H. Min, H.-S. Chai, Y.-H. Kim et al., "Attenuation of hemodynamic responses to laryngoscopy and tracheal intubation during rapid sequence induction: remifentanil vs. lidocaine with esmolol," *Minerva Anestesiologica*, vol. 76, no. 3, pp. 188–192, 2010.

[15] K. Mikawa, K. Nishina, N. Maekawa, and H. Obara, "Comparison of nicardipine, diltiazem and verapamil for controlling the cardiovascular responses to tracheal intubation," *British Journal of Anaesthesia*, vol. 76, no. 2, pp. 221–226, 1996.

[16] A. A. van den Berg, E. M. Halliday, N. A. Soomro, A. Rasheed, and M. Baloch, "Reducing cardiovascular responses to laryngoscopy and tracheal intubation: a comparison of equipotent doses of tramadol, nalbuphine and pethidine, with placebo," *Middle East Journal of Anesthesiology*, vol. 17, no. 6, pp. 1023–1036, 2004.

[17] A. Casati, G. Fanelli, A. Albertin et al., "Small doses of remifentanil or sufentanil for blunting cardiovascular changes induced by tracheal intubation: a double-blind comparison," *European Journal of Anaesthesiology*, vol. 18, no. 2, pp. 108–112, 2001.

[18] J. H. Lee, B.-N. Koo, J.-J. Jeong, H.-S. Kim, and J.-R. Lee, "Differential effects of lidocaine and remifentanil on response to the tracheal tube during emergence from general anaesthesia," *British Journal of Anaesthesia*, vol. 106, no. 3, pp. 410–415, 2011.

[19] K. Takita, Y. Morimoto, and O. Kemmotsu, "Tracheal lidocaine attenuates the cardiovascular response to endotracheal intubation," *Canadian Journal of Anesthesia*, vol. 48, no. 8, pp. 732–736, 2001.

[20] A. A. van den Berg, D. Savva, and N. M. Honjol, "Attenuation of the haemodynamic responses to noxious stimuli in patients undergoing cataract surgery. A comparison of magnesium sulphate, esmolol, lignocaine, nitroglycerine and placebo given i.v. with induction of anaesthesia," *European Journal of Anaesthesiology*, vol. 14, no. 2, pp. 134–147, 1997.

[21] T. Ishiyama, S. Kashimoto, T. Oguchi, A. Furuya, H. Fukushima, and T. Kumazawa, "Clonidine-ephedrine combination reduces pain on injection of propofol and blunts hemodynamic stress responses during the induction sequence," *Journal of Clinical Anesthesia*, vol. 18, no. 3, pp. 211–215, 2006.

[22] E. Freye and J. V. Levy, "Reflex activity caused by laryngoscopy and intubation is obtunded differently by meptazinol, nalbuphine and fentanyl," *European Journal of Anaesthesiology*, vol. 24, no. 1, pp. 53–58, 2007.

[23] R. D. Miller, *Anesthesia*, Churchill Livingstone, Philadelphia, Pa, USA, 6th edition, 2005.

[24] S. Mackanes and J. L. Spendlove, "Acetaminophen as an adjunct to morphine by patient-controlled analgesia in the management of acute post operative pain," *Anesthesia & Analgesia*, vol. 87, no. 2, pp. 368–371, 1998.

[25] A. T. Chan, J. E. Manson, C. M. Albert et al., "Nonsteroidal antiinflammatory drugs, acetaminophen, and the risk of cardiovascular events," *Circulation*, vol. 113, no. 12, pp. 1578–1587, 2006.

[26] J. P. Forman, E. B. Rimm, and G. C. Curhan, "Frequency of analgesic use and risk of hypertension among men," *Archives of Internal Medicine*, vol. 167, no. 4, pp. 394–399, 2007.

[27] J. Dedier, M. J. Stampfer, S. E. Hankinson, W. C. Willett, F. E. Speizer, and G. C. Curhan, "Nonnarcotic analgesic use and the risk of hypertension in US women," *Hypertension*, vol. 40, no. 5, pp. 604–608, 2002.

[28] I. Sudano, A. J. Flammer, D. Périat et al., "Acetaminophen increases blood pressure in patients with coronary artery disease," *Circulation*, vol. 122, pp. 1789–1796, 2010.

[29] M. Hersch, D. Raveh, and G. Izbicki, "Effect of intravenous propacetamol on blood pressure in febrile critically ill patients," *Pharmacotherapy*, vol. 28, no. 10, pp. 1205–1210, 2008.

[30] K. L. Radack, C. C. Deck, and S. S. Bloomfield, "Ibuprofen interferes with the efficacy of antihypertensive drugs. A randomized, double-blind, placebo-controlled trial of ibuprofen compared with acetaminophen," *Annals of Internal Medicine*, vol. 107, no. 5, pp. 628–635, 1987.

[31] D. M. Aronoff, J. A. Oates, and O. Boutaud, "New insights into the mechanism of action of acetaminophen: its clinical pharmacologic characteristics reflect its inhibition of the two prostaglandin $H_2$ synthases," *Clinical Pharmacology & Therapeutics*, vol. 79, no. 1, pp. 9–19, 2006.

[32] W. Riad and A. Moussa, "Lornoxicam attenuates the haemodynamic responses to laryngoscopy and tracheal intubation in the elderly," *European Journal of Anaesthesiology*, vol. 25, no. 9, pp. 732–736, 2008.

[33] D. E. Rosenow, M. Albrechtsen, and D. Stolke, "A comparison of patient-controlled analgesia with lornoxicam versus morphine in patients undergoing lumbar disk surgery," *Anesthesia & Analgesia*, vol. 86, no. 5, pp. 1045–1050, 1998.

[34] C. K. Feng, K. H. Chan, K. N. Liu, C. H. Or, and T. Y. Lee, "A comparison of lidocaine, fentanyl, and esmolol for attenuation of cardiovascular response to laryngoscopy and tracheal intubation," *Acta Anaesthesiologica Sinica*, vol. 34, no. 2, pp. 61–67, 1996.

2

# Analgesic Techniques in Hip and Knee Arthroplasty: From the Daily Practice to Evidence-Based Medicine


**Denisa Madalina Anastase,[1] Simona Cionac Florescu,[1] Ana Maria Munteanu,[1] Traian Ursu,[2] and Cristian Ioan Stoica[2]**

[1] *Department of Anesthesiology, Clinical Hospital of Orthopedy Foisor, Bulevardul Ferdinand, No. 35-37, 021382 Bucharest, Romania*
[2] *Department of Orthopedics, Foisor Clinical Orthopedics Hospital and "Carol Davila" University of Medicine and Pharmacy, 020022 Bucharest, Romania*

Correspondence should be addressed to Denisa Madalina Anastase; danastasel@gmail.com



Academic Editor: Enrico Camporesi



Total hip arthroplasty (THA) and total knee arthroplasty (TKA) are major orthopedic surgery models, addressing mainly ageing populations with multiple comorbidities and treatments, ASA II–IV, which may complicate the perioperative period. Therefore effective management of postoperative pain should allow rapid mobilization of the patient with shortening of hospitalization and social reintegration. In our review we propose an evaluation of the main analgesics models used today in the postoperative period. Their comparative analysis shows the benefits and side effects of each of these methods and guides us to how to use evidence-based medicine in our daily practice.


## 1. Background

Primary total arthroplasty of the hip or knee is a common surgery today with an increasing incidence related to age. The mean age at surgery for TKA is 70 years, but there is a tendency worldwide to increase the proportion of younger patients (the age interval between 55 and 64 years) [1–3]. To allow comparison between data from different arthroplasty national registers, the term "age-standardised" was introduced as a statistically corrected result for age structure of the population [4] and the "rate" as the number of the knee TKA per 100.000 inhabitants is used. The leaders are USA (221,5) and Austria (186,3), Switzerland (173,6) [5], Germany (132,5) [6]. TKA data from Registers Nordic Association (including the 4 countries Sweden, Norway, Denmark, and Finland) show 151 814 knee prostheses till 2011 [7] with a higher incidence in Denmark (123) in 2007 than in Sweden (115) and Norway (75) [1].

Besides increasing the number and the age of patients receiving prosthetic joint, a number of comorbidities are associated with increasing age. According to a national cohort report from 2009, 32,6% of the patients with TKA had three comorbidities or more and the most common ones are hypertension (67,8%), diabetes (20%), and obesity (19,8%) [8]. Therefore, there was an almost parallel evolution of surgical techniques and methods of analgesia, allowing effective pain control, rapid mobilization of patients with reduced side effects and no damage to existing comorbidities.

Effective treatment of postoperative pain continues to be a challenge because it influences the surgical outcome [9] and for prosthetic joints pain management is a must for early mobilization and functionality of the new joints.

Relationship between analgesic technique and the immediate and remote postoperative outcome and success of surgery is not new, and postoperative pain assessment using visual analogue scale (VAS) and opioid requirements is the primary outcome variable in most studies.

That is why, since 1996, the pain was declared the fifth vital sign by the American Pain Society [10] (http://www.americanpainsociety.org/uploads/pdfs/npc/section_2.pdf).

Moreover, effective treatment of postoperative pain was the most important factor for early mobilization, shortened hospital stay, and discharge [11].

## 2. Comparative Analgesia Techniques

Epidural analgesia offers advantages over systemic opioid administration by patient controlled analgesia (PCA) and has been the gold-standard for a long time in postoperative pain control in THA.

Regarding TKA, Mahoney et al. administered bupivacaine and morphine continuously on epidural catheter and reported good-to-excellent analgesia but with a high incidence of adverse effects related to epidural catheter and opioids [12]. The necessity for other solutions with a lower incidence of opioid-associated side effects was obvious.

Moiniche et al. study the effect of pain relief with balanced analgesia on postoperative convalescence parameters in 20 patients scheduled for TKA [13]. At 48 hours the epidural analgesia group had significantly lower pain scores, but no important differences were observed between groups related to ambulation, daily patient activity, or hospital stay [13].

Opioid dose reduction is one of the important goals of postoperative analgesia, to reduce both side effects (nausea, itching, vomiting, respiratory depression, and ileus) and consecutive sedation, leading to a delay in patient mobilization. In addition to careful monitoring, symptomatic management is required for each type of secondary reaction that occurred, leading to a higher consumption of drugs and therefore higher costs of hospitalization.

Understanding the mechanisms involved in nociceptive acute pain, identifying the effect of opioid-induced hyperalgesia and persistent postsurgical pain by regional anesthesia, directs the development of new drugs or different analgesia regimens for improving postprosthetic outcome [14].

Therefore, epidural technique has quickly gained popularity compared to intravenous opioid analgesia. Several studies have shown that epidural analgesia may reduce the risk of myocardial ischemia and tachyarrhythmia in coronary high-risk patients proposed for elective noncardiac surgery [15] and even to those proposed for cardiac surgery [16], as well as in major abdominal and thoracic surgery [17].

Besides the protective effect in high-risk cardiac patient, epidural analgesia has a beneficial effect on lung function with decreased incidence of postoperative pulmonary morbidity as shown by meta-analysis of Ballantyne et al. [18]. All these positive effects may become important in the elderly patient with comorbidities.

Cochrane data of evidence-based medicine led a study in 2003, trying to answer the question, "Is the lumbar epidural analgesia more efficient than the systemic analgesia or spinal analgesia for pain relief after elective primary hip or knee arthroplasty?" [19]. Their conclusion was unequivocal: there is not enough evidence to draw conclusions about the efficiency of epidural analgesia compared with systemic analgesia, epidural analgesia effect on postoperative serious complications, the functional outcome, or length of hospital stay. The benefit of epidural analgesia on pain is limited to the first 4–6 postoperative hours and epidural administration of local anesthetic or a local anesthetic and opioid combination may be more effective than the epidural opioid administration only.

In the same year, a study compared the analgesic effectiveness and side effects of intrathecal morphine sulphate in small doses, between 0.0 and 0.3 mg, on 40 patients with THA and 40 patients with TKA [20]. The conclusion was consistent with other studies: analgesic needs are higher in total knee replacement than in THA where the pain is moderate [21], and the combination of low-dose intrathecal morphine 0.2 mg with standard dose of morphine administered on the PCA provides good-to-excellent analgesia in most patients with THA but not in those with TKA, thereby reducing the consumption of morphine administered systemically.

Peripheral nerves blocks (PNB) offer advantages over epidural analgesia for the TKA patients. Ganapathy as well as Capdevilla used a modified 3-in-1 Winnie continuous femoral block [22, 23] with local anesthetic, compared to continuous epidural. The results were a lower quantity of opioid required to control pain at rest and during passive mobilization and a better articular mobility in the immediate postoperative period [22]. The epidural group had significantly elevated incidence of urinary retention, dysesthesia, and arterial hypotension [23]. Singelyn et al. showed 4 times less incidence of secondary effects with a femoral catheter compared to an epidural one [24] and Chelly et al. showed more cardiovascular stability and less nausea and vomiting [25].

Some of these better results may be due to the new mixture used by Capdevilla with the femoral catheter: lidocaine 1% and clonidine plus morphine. The usefulness of these adjuvants in brachial plexus block had been demonstrated by Singelyn et al. [26] and Bernard and Macaire [27].

Continuous administration using a femoral catheter is more useful than single shot but with minimal impact on hospital length of stay and long-term functional recovery [28].

Among local anesthetics, lidocaine 1% performs a better motor block than bupivacaine 0.25% and seems to be more efficient in alleviating quadriceps muscle spasm [29]; this spasm is the main effect of postoperative TKA pain that impairs early articular mobilization; at the same time a good quality femoral block may be associated with weakness of the muscle and risk of falling during the postoperative recuperation [30].

Fowler's meta-analysis from 2008 undertook a systematic review of all randomized trials comparing epidural analgesia with peripheral PNB for TKA. There was an evaluation on 464 patients of morphine consumption, epidural and PNB side effects, and the patient satisfaction [31]. The conclusions are as follows: (1) there was no significant difference in pain VAS scores between epidural and PNB for the first 24 hours; (2) patient satisfaction was higher with PNB in only two studies [32, 33]; (3) the addition of sciatic nerve block improves the quality of analgesia by reducing posterior knee and calf pain, corresponding to the area innervated by the sciatic nerve [34–38]. Fowler's analysis failed to demonstrate inferior analgesia for patients without sciatic block between

0 and 24 h after operation; (4) neurological complications referred to sphincteric disturbance in approximately 250 patients who received an epidural analgesia whereas no neurological complications were reported in the 766 patients from the PNB group. Hypotension associated with epidural analgesia occurred more frequently among the peridural patients and may contribute to end organ ischaemia or infarction if left untreated. This is the reason why epidural analgesia is not appropriate in the ward setting in every institution. If general anaesthesia is not indicated, spinal anesthesia combined with PNB provides a good analgesia with a lower incidence of neurological complications than epidural analgesia in this risk patients group (older age, degenerative spinal disorders, and chronic anticoagulation) [31, 39, 40].

Advantageous for femoral nerve block (FNB) is pain reduction related to significant reduction of quadriceps spasm, secondary after TKA and therefore it improves toleration of passive motion [41]. The FNB critics reproach quadriceps weakness on the operative side compared to the controlateral side, but in the Fowler's analysis this is unclear [31].

Ilfeld et al.'s study in 2010 introduces the concept of continuous ambulatory FNB for 4 days after a TKA discharge [42]. Beaupre et al.'s study brings back in 2012 the idea of a preemptive multimodal analgesia plus FNB protocol on rehabilitation, hospital length of stay, and postoperative analgesia after TKA [43]. In the study a combination of Oxycodone controlled release and celecoxib is used as a preemptive analgesia before the surgery. The study reflects the FNB efficacy in standard clinical conditions, although it was not randomised. There are more quadriceps motor blocks reported in the FNB group; however, no patient experienced any falls, and there were no delays in rehabilitation program secondary to FNB and no significant differences between groups in terms of pain scores, knee flexion, or hospital stay. The only restriction to use widely FNB is the accidental fall secondary to quadriceps weakness limiting an aggressive postoperative rehabilitation [30].

Regarding the quadriceps weakness secondary to FNB, Wasserstein concluded that single-shot FNB did not increase the fall's risk. Advanced age, obesity, and continuous femoral nerve blockade are independent risk factors for inpatient falls after primary total knee arthroplasty [44].

The evidence-based data regarding FNB are as follows: continuous FNB provides better pain relief than that attained with single-injection FNB and information was insufficient for review authors to conclude on the comparison of FNB with local infiltration analgesia or oral analgesia or on the safety of the various analgesic techniques [45].

A modern and easy identification method of the femoral nerve is the ultrasound. For experienced hands, the femoral nerve block under the echographic guidance has a fast installation with a high success rate [46]. The use of ultrasound in regional anaesthesia for femoral nerve is not a new idea [47, 48].

The sciatic nerve block contribution is still controversial. Pros are Cappelleri et al. who concluded that continuous sciatic nerve block improves analgesia, decreases morphine request, and improves early rehabilitation compared with single-injection sciatic nerve block [49], in contrast with Abdallah and Brulls' review, who cannot define the effect of adding sciatic nerve block to FNB on acute pain [50].

The knee innervation is mainly covered by the femoral, sciatic, and obturatorius nerves, excepting few areas of the classical incision that are innervated by the lateral cutaneous femoral nerve. The injection of the femoral nerve catheter even on a large volume of local anesthetic or the distribution of the solution more cranially does not cover the obturatorius nerve in terms of analgesia [35, 51, 52]. So the idea arose to add the analgesia in the territory of the obturatorius nerve to the combination of the femoral/sciatic nerve blocks; 2 studies confirmed hypothesis [53, 54].

Adductor canal block is a sensory blockade that provides analgesia in the territory of obturatorius nerve and saphenous nerve. There are only two studies related to the efficiency of adductor canal block analgesia compared with other established techniques in TKA, FNB. Adductor canal block preserved quadriceps muscle strength better than FNB and therefore promotes early ambulation, without a significant difference in postoperative pain [55, 56].

The psoas block analgesia should be theoretically superior to that of the femoral nerve block in TKA. Paradoxically, Morin found that the analgesia via femoral/sciatic nerves blocks combination is superior to the psoas block with decreased need for opioid [35].

Decreasing opioid consumption can be achieved by using a combination of analgesics belonging to different pharmacological classes. The multimodal analgesia is actually a balanced analgesia through a multimodal approach to postoperative pain, with synergistic effect of various analgesics and consecutive reduction of side effects associated with them by lowering doses [33].

This synergistic analgesic effect can be achieved by the following: (1) peripheral techniques using local anesthetics, nonsteroidal anti-inflammatory agents, opioids, and other analgesics or (2) peripheral nerves blocks with the use of local anesthetics and $\alpha$-2 adrenergic agonists or (3) subarachnoid or epidural administration of local anesthetics, opioids, and $\alpha$-2 adrenergic agonists or (4) combinations thereof.

In a systematic review of analgesics and anesthetics interventions dedicated to optimal pain influencing primary hip arthroplasty, Fischer et al. use in their analysis the Cochrane protocol and evidence-based recommendations are the following: PROSPECT group recommended for postoperative analgesia general anesthesia combined with peripheral nerve block or intrathecal administration of local anesthetic and opioid [40]. Moreover, the primary anesthetic technique must be combined with paracetamol and nonsteroidal anti-inflammatory agent, opioid stronger or weaker depending on needs, including gabapentin [57].

There is evidence of multimodal approach to pain, suggesting that that the use of analgesics in different pharmacological classes improves postoperative pain control in patients with arthroplasty.

Nonsteroidal anti-inflammatory drugs and cyclooxygenase-2 inhibitors added systemic route have a synergistic effect with local anesthetic in most cases and a safety profile regarding side effects [31]. Regarding nonspecific nonsteroidal anti-inflammatory drugs, there is evidence of a clinically relevant local effect in peripheral administration of intra-articular administration [32].

Several studies are dedicated to the adding of gabapentin to the multimodal analgesia in arthroplasty. Mathiesen starts from the evidence that gabapentin is effective in reducing postoperative pain and opioid consumption [58]. He studied the effect of administration of pregabalin 300 mg p.o. and dexamethasone 8 mg i.v. on postoperative pain control; preoperatively patients received also paracetamol 1 g and postoperative paracetamol and morphine on PCA. The study concludes that pregabalin reduced to half postoperative morphine requirements, but this reduction was not accompanied by a decrease in the incidence of nausea and vomiting; pregabalin administration was accompanied by an increased level of sedation and in combination with dexamethasone did not provide an additional effect on the score of pain or opioid requirements [58]. Although gabapentin does not have its own analgesic action, it reduces hyperexcitability in neurons of the posterior horn caused by tissue damage.

Clarke et al. study the effect of a single dose of pregabalin 600 mg administered preoperatively or postoperatively with spinal regional anesthesia and multimodal analgesia in THA. Multimodal regimen includes preoperative administration of acetaminophen p.o., celecoxib p.o., and dexamethasone i.v. The study concludes that gabapentin added to a multimodal regimen does not reduce acute pain, opioid consumption, or chronic pain after total hip arthroplasty [59].

Over the last decade, technological progress of the types of prostheses and minimally invasive surgical approaches have resulted in a faster recovery, decreased length of stay and lower costs. Parallel analgesic techniques migrate from the central (epidural or spinal analgesia) to periphery (nerve blocks and local intra-articular injection-LIA).

Soon, the concept of intra-articular local infiltration of the wound developed by Kerr and Kohan is picked up by a lot of clinics and schools, especially Scandinavia, UK, and Australia. Kerr and Kohan have developed the type of technique "local infiltration analgesia (LIA)" for pain control after total knee and hip arthroplasty. This requires systematic infiltration of a mixture of ropivacaine, ketorolac, and adrenaline in the tissues surrounding the surgical wound to achieve satisfactory analgesia with minimal discomfort [60].

The technique is revolutionary because it allows virtually immediate mobilization; most of the 325 patients included in the study can walk with assistance in 5-6 hours after surgery and regain independent mobility in 13 to 22 hours of surgery. Pain score was satisfactory, between 0 and 3 on the VAS, and side effects were infrequent; 71% of the patients were directly discharged home after one night spent in the hospital. The study's conclusion was that "LIA is simple, practical, safe and effective pain control after THA/TKA."

Study of Andersen et al. in 2007 starts from preliminary experience using intra-articular ropivacaine in the shoulder surgery by Gottschalk and Horn [61, 62] and also from a combination of morphine and intra-articular local anesthetic in total knee prosthesis by Mauerhan and Rasmunssen [63, 64]. Andersen et al. compare prospectively randomized effectiveness LIA (with a mixture of ropivacaine, ketorolac, and adrenaline) with epidural analgesia in THA and recommend this type of analgesia [65].

Thorsell et al.'s study, also a prospective randomized trial, found no clinically important effect of LIA on the catheter compared to peridural analgesia, although patients with LIA were mobilized faster and had a higher degree of satisfaction, but there was no reduction in the consumption of morphine [66].

In the same way the prospective randomized study of Specht finds no statistically significant analgesic differences between LIA administered on catheter and placebo administered into intra-articular space in THA [67].

The prospective, randomized Lunn et al.'s study on a larger number of patients, 120, compares the analgesic efficiency between LIA with large volumes, 150 mL, and placebo in the presence of a multimodal analgesia system composed of acetaminophen, celecoxib, and gabapentin preoperatively and analyzes the first variable pain to walk from a distance of 5 m 8 hours after the surgery. The study concludes that the administration of high-volume LIA does not reduce acute pain compared to placebo in the presence of a multimodal system that combines the three drugs in total hip prosthesis [68].

The administration of local anesthetic in the surgical wound is a reasonable approach to reduce nociceptive transmission from the source [69]. Development of LIA with multimodal analgesia regimen has allowed the extension fast-track prosthetic surgery and the appearance of specialized centers in this kind of surgery and recovery.

The Swedish National Arthroplasty Registry data show for THA a steady increase in the number of replacements under the LIA in fast-track mode, as well as for TKA, the percentage being 75%. None of the studies published till 2011 could reproduce the short duration of hospitalization reported by Kerr and Kohan original study, but the average time of hospitalization decreased from 6–10 days to 3–5 days [69].

Kehlet and Andersen create a review of randomized clinical trials on the basis of existing data at the level of the year 2011 related to efficiency of LIA with large volumes in the THA and TKA. At that time, there was little evidence to recommend in both intraoperative and postoperative THA technique of letting the catheter in the wound when given nonopioid oral multimodal analgesia; regarding TKA, evidence supported the intraoperative analgesic effectiveness of LIA but not the use of the catheter for postoperative analgesia [70].

Moreover, for TKA there are sufficient data to sustain that the compressive bandage may prolong analgesia after administration of high-volume LIA intraoperative [71]. As with the length of hospitalization, lower duration was made possible by administering an oral multimodal nonopioid medication with an optimization of care in fast-track methodology.

Another recent study dedicated to the effectiveness of LIA in the THA is Solovyova et al.'s study who come into contradiction with Andersen: LIA "per se" or followed by continuous administration of ropivacaine as part of multimodal analgesia with acetaminophen, celecoxib, and pregabalin does not bring additional benefit or reduction of the opioid consumption compared to placebo [72].

If THA has not demonstrated the effectiveness of LIA in managing conditions of multimodal analgesia, for TKA there are multiple studies that compare LIA with different analgesic techniques that demonstrate the superiority of LIA on evidence-based grounds.

Thus, Toftdahl et al. by comparing the intraoperative and perioperative analgesia of LIA with continuous femoral nerve block in TKA show a superiority of the LIA and early mobilization, without influencing the duration of hospitalization [73].

Essving et al. found the same positive analgesic LIA effect and a reduction of the postoperative morphine consumption, comparing the intraoperative versus postoperative administration only, with a high degree of patient satisfaction [74].

Spreng et al. compare epidural analgesia with large volumes LIA and local adjuvants combined such as ketorolac and morphine (or administered systemically). The study concludes that the LIA with local adjuvants reduces opioid consumption, allow a faster mobilization and a reduction in length of stay; ketorolac and morphine were more effective locally than systemically administered [75].

Dillon's study starts from the Kerr and Kohan technique and presents in a review several changes related to evidence-based data that they use in patients proposed for joint replacement: add dexamethasone to the initial mixture and use minimally invasive surgical approaches, give up the use of intraoperative tourniquet limiting edema and allowing reducing of pain associated with edema, and use bandage from toe to thigh also involved in improving analgesia associated with LIA [60].

Their experience shows that LIA is well tolerated by patients allowing early walking on the day of surgery for both THA and TKA with a good pain control and decreasing the duration of hospitalization [76].

Perlas retrospective study of 298 patients analyzed analgesia and recovery at 48 hours in patients with TKA and LIA versus continuous femoral nerve block or LIA plus adductor canal block. LIA was associated with improved early analgesia and walking in the first postoperative day; the adding of the adductor canal block allowed a faster gait with the increased incidence of discharge to home [77].

Fowler explores in a recent review the LIA with large volume in THA/TKA versus peripheral nerves blocks in terms of functional outcome, persistent postoperative pain, costs, and the revision rate. Despite the growing popularity and good postoperative analgesia the role of LIA in the context of a recovery program, the persistent postoperative pain, or efficiency compared with peripheral nerves blocks is not clear [78].

The most recent review is from 2014, analyzing 27 randomized controlled studies including 756 patients operated on with THA and 888 patients with TKA. Andersen and Kehlet explore the effectiveness of LIA in early treatment of postoperative pain, the analgesic efficiency of the surgical wound catheter in postoperative period, and if there is any impact on the duration of hospitalization. As shown earlier, LIA has similar analgesic effectiveness with administration of intrathecal morphine and epidural analgesia in THA. For TKA, most trials provide a reduction of pain with LIA and also a reduction in the amount of opioids compared to placebo. LIA is similar to continuous femoral nerve, intrathecal morphine analgesia, or epidural analgesia for early postoperative period, with a high risk of error due to different systemic analgesia between groups. Using the wound catheters for postoperative analgesia does not bring additional benefits; length of hospital stay is not related to analgesic effectiveness [79].

## 3. Conclusion

THA and TKA are surgical procedures for removal of pain and restoration of mobility to patients with gonarthrosis and coxarthrosis, which are associated with moderate to severe postoperative pain. If former analgesic approaches addressed first the postoperative pain, appearance of new operative techniques, like minimally invasive surgical approaches, has led to an adaptation of postoperative analgesia methods with the aim of more early mobilization, even on the day of surgery, and a shorter hospital stay with home discharge directly without the need for an intermediary rehabilitation center. Each of these new models has its adepts and the choice of one or another belongs to the anesthetic-surgical team according to the surgeon technique and has a single aim: a better prognosis for the patient.

## Conflict of Interests

The authors declare that there is no conflict of interests regarding the publication of this paper.

## References

[1] O. Robertsson, S. Bizjajeva, A. M. Fenstad et al., "Knee arthroplasty in Denmark, Norway and Sweden: a pilot study from the Nordic Arthroplasty Register Association," *Acta Orthopaedica*, vol. 81, no. 1, pp. 82–89, 2010.

[2] S. G. Memtsoudis, A. G. Della Valle, M. C. Besculides, L. Gaber, and R. Laskin, "Trends in demographics, comorbidity profiles, in-hospital complications and mortality associated with primary knee arthroplasty," *The Journal of Arthroplasty*, vol. 24, no. 4, pp. 518–527, 2009.

[3] CIHI (Canadian Institute for Health Information), *Canadian Joint Replacement Registry (CJRR) 2006 Annual Report Hip and Knee Replacements in Canada*, 2006, https://secure.cihi.ca/free_products/CJRR_Annual_Report_Hip_Knee_Replacements_2006_e.pdf.

[4] J. A. H. Waterhouse, S. C. Muir, P. Correa, and J. Powell, Eds., *Cancer Incidence in Five Continents*, vol. 3 of *IARC Scientific Publications No. 15*, IARC, Lyon, France, 1976.

[5] M. de Fatima Pina, A. I. Ribeiro, and C. Santos, "Epidemiology and variability of orthopaedic procedures worldwide," in *European Instructional Lectures: 12th EFORT Congress, Copenhagen, Denmark*, G. Bentley, Ed., vol. 11 of *European Instructional Lectures*, pp. 9–19, Springer, Berlin, Germany, 2011.

[6] T. Schäfer, R. Pritzkuleit, C. Jeszenszky et al., "Trends and geographical variation of primary hip and knee joint replacement in Germany," *Osteoarthritis and Cartilage*, vol. 21, no. 2, pp. 279–288, 2013.

[7] L. I. Havelin, O. Robertsson, A. M. Fenstad, S. Overgaard, G. Garellick, and O. Furnes, "A Scandinavian experience of register collaboration: the Nordic Arthroplasty Register Association (NARA)," *The Journal of Bone and Joint Surgery A*, vol. 93, supplement 3, pp. 13–19, 2011.

[8] A. J. Pugely, C. T. Martin, Y. Gao, D. A. Belatti, and J. J. Callaghan, "Comorbidities in patients undergoing total knee arthroplasty: do they influence hospital costs and length of stay?" *Clinical Orthopaedics and Related Research*, 2014.

[9] H. Kehlet, "Surgical stress: the role of pain and analgesia," *British Journal of Anaesthesia*, vol. 63, no. 2, pp. 189–195, 1989.

[10] H. Merskey and N. Bogduk, "Part III: pain terms, a current list with definitions and notes on usage," in *Classification of Chronic Pain*, IASP Task Force on Taxonomy, pp. 209–214, IASP Press, Seattle, Wash, USA, 2nd edition, 1994.

[11] H. Kehlet and J. B. Dahl, "Anaesthesia, surgery, and challenges in postoperative recovery," *The Lancet*, vol. 362, no. 9399, pp. 1921–1928, 2003.

[12] O. M. Mahoney, P. C. Noble, J. Davidson, and H. S. Tullos, "The effect of continuous epidural analgesia on postoperative pain, rehabilitation, and duration of hospitalization in total knee arthroplasty," *Clinical Orthopaedics and Related Research*, no. 260, pp. 30–37, 1990.

[13] S. Moiniche, N.-C. Hjortso, B. L. Hansen et al., "The effect of balanced analgesia on early convalescence after major orthopaedic surgery," *Acta Anaesthesiologica Scandinavica*, vol. 38, no. 4, pp. 328–335, 1994.

[14] C. L. Wu and S. N. Raja, "Treatment of acute postoperative pain," *The Lancet*, vol. 377, no. 9784, pp. 2215–2225, 2011.

[15] W. S. Beattie, D. N. Buckley, and J. B. Forrest, "Epidural morphine reduces the risk of post-operative myocardial ischaemia in patients with cardiac risk factors," *Canadian Journal of Anaesthesia*, vol. 40, no. 6, pp. 532–541, 1993.

[16] D. T. Mangano, D. Siliciano, M. Hollenberg et al., "Postoperative myocardial ischemia: therapeutic trials using intensive analgesia following surgery," *Anesthesiology*, vol. 76, no. 3, pp. 342–353, 1992.

[17] M. P. Yeager, D. D. Glass, R. K. Neff, and T. Brinck-Johnsen, "Epidural anesthesia and analgesia in high-risk surgical patients," *Anesthesiology*, vol. 66, no. 6, pp. 729–736, 1987.

[18] J. C. Ballantyne, D. B. Carr, S. DeFerranti et al., "The comparative effects of postoperative analgesic therapies on pulmonary outcome: cumulative meta-analyses of randomized, controlled trials," *Anesthesia and Analgesia*, vol. 86, no. 3, pp. 598–612, 1998.

[19] P. T. Choi, M. Bhandari, J. Scott, and J. Douketis, "Epidural analgesia for pain relief following hip or knee replacement," *Cochrane Database of Systematic Reviews*, no. 3, Article ID CD003071, 2003.

[20] J. P. Rathmell, C. A. Pino, R. Taylor, T. Patrin, and B. A. Viani, "Intrathecal morphine for postoperative analgesia: a randomized, controlled, dose-ranging study after hip and knee arthroplasty," *Anesthesia & Analgesia*, vol. 97, no. 5, pp. 1452–1457, 2003.

[21] L. Nikolajsen, B. Brandsborg, U. Lucht, T. S. Jensen, and H. Kehlet, "Chronic pain following total hip arthroplasty: a nationwide questionnaire study," *Acta Anaesthesiologica Scandinavica*, vol. 50, no. 4, pp. 495–500, 2006.

[22] S. Ganapathy, R. A. Wasserman, J. T. Watson et al., "Modified continuous femoral three-in-one block for postoperative pain after total knee arthroplasty," *Anesthesia and Analgesia*, vol. 89, no. 5, pp. 1197–1202, 1999.

[23] X. Capdevila, Y. Barthelet, P. Biboulet, Y. Ryckwaert, J. Rubenovitch, and F. d'Athis, "Effects of perioperative analgesic technique on the surgical outcome and duration of rehabilitation after major knee surgery," *Anesthesiology*, vol. 91, no. 1, pp. 8–15, 1999.

[24] F. J. Singelyn, M. Deyaert, D. Joris, E. Pendeville, and J. M. Gouverneur, "Effects of intravenous patient-controlled analgesia with morphine, continuous epidural analgesia, and continuous three-in-one block on postoperative pain and knee rehabilitation after unilateral total knee arthroplasty," *Anesthesia & Analgesia*, vol. 87, no. 1, pp. 88–92, 1998.

[25] J. E. Chelly, J. Greger, R. Gebhard et al., "Continuous femoral blocks improve recovery and outcome of patients undergoing total knee arthroplasty," *Journal of Arthroplasty*, vol. 16, no. 4, pp. 436–445, 2001.

[26] F. J. Singelyn, J.-M. Gouverneur, and A. Robert, "A minimum dose of clonidine added to mepivacaine prolongs the duration of anesthesia and analgesia after axillary brachial plexus block," *Anesthesia and Analgesia*, vol. 83, no. 5, pp. 1046–1050, 1996.

[27] J.-M. Bernard and P. Macaire, "Dose-range effects of clonidine added to lidocaine for brachial plexus block," *Anesthesiology*, vol. 87, no. 2, pp. 277–284, 1997.

[28] F. V. Salinas, S. S. Liu, and M. F. Mulroy, "The effect of single-injection femoral nerve block versus continuous femoral nerve block after total knee arthroplasty on hospital length of stay and long-term functional recovery within an established clinical pathway," *Anesthesia and Analgesia*, vol. 102, no. 4, pp. 1234–1239, 2006.

[29] J. J. Bonica, "Current status of postoperative pain therapy," in *Current Topics in Pain Research and Therapy*, R. Dubnet, Ed., pp. 169–189, Yokota, Tokyo, Japan, 1983.

[30] B. M. Ilfeld, K. B. Duke, and M. C. Donohue, "The association between lower extremity continuous peripheral nerve blocks and patient falls after knee and hip arthroplasty," *Anesthesia & Analgesia*, vol. 111, no. 6, pp. 1552–1554, 2010.

[31] S. J. Fowler, J. Symons, S. Sabato, and P. S. Myles, "Epidural analgesia compared with peripheral nerve blockade after major knee surgery: a systematic review and meta-analysis of randomized trials," *British Journal of Anaesthesia*, vol. 100, no. 2, pp. 154–164, 2008.

[32] A. F. Davies, E. P. Segar, J. Murdoch, D. E. Wright, and I. H. Wilson, "Epidural infusion or combined femoral and sciatic nerve blocks as perioperative analgesia for knee arthroplasty," *The British Journal of Anaesthesia*, vol. 93, no. 3, pp. 368–374, 2004.

[33] W. T. Long, S. R. Ward, L. D. Dorr, J. Raya, M. Boutary, and L. E. Sirianni, "Postoperative pain management following total knee arthroplasty: a randomized comparison of continuous epidural versus femoral nerve infusion," *The Journal of Knee Surgery*, vol. 19, no. 2, pp. 137–143, 2006.

[34] A. Weber, R. Fournier, E. Van Gessel, and Z. Gamulin, "Sciatic nerve block and the improvement of femoral nerve block analgesia after total knee replacement," *European Journal of Anaesthesiology*, vol. 19, no. 11, pp. 834–836, 2002.

[35] A. M. Morin, C. D. Kratz, L. H. J. Eberhart et al., "Postoperative analgesia and functional recovery after total-knee replacement: comparison of a continuous posterior lumbar plexus (psoas compartment) block, a continuous femoral nerve block, and the

combination of a continuous femoral and sciatic nerve block," *Regional Anesthesia and Pain Medicine*, vol. 30, no. 5, pp. 434–445, 2005.

[36] B. Ben-David, K. Schmalenberger, and J. E. Chelly, "Analgesia after total knee arthroplasty: is continuous sciatic blockade needed in addition to continuous, femoral blockade?" *Anesthesia & Analgesia*, vol. 98, no. 3, pp. 747–749, 2004.

[37] P. Cook, J. Stevens, and C. Gaudron, "Comparing the effects of femoral nerve block versus femoral and sciatic nerve block on pain and opiate consumption after total knee arthroplasty," *Journal of Arthroplasty*, vol. 18, no. 5, pp. 583–586, 2003.

[38] C. P. Dang, E. Gautheron, J. Guilley et al., "The value of adding sciatic block to continuous femoral block for analgesia after total knee replacement," *Regional Anesthesia and Pain Medicine*, vol. 30, no. 2, pp. 128–133, 2005.

[39] C. Simanski and B. Fischer, "Procedure specific postoperative pain management (PROSPECT) recommendations for total knee arthroplasty," 2007, http://www.postoppain.org.

[40] H. B. J. Fischer, C. J. P. Simanski, C. Sharp et al., "A procedure-specific systematic review and consensus recommendations for postoperative analgesia following total knee arthroplasty," *Anaesthesia*, vol. 63, no. 10, pp. 1105–1123, 2008.

[41] A. P. Winnie, S. Ramamurthy, and Z. Durrani, "The inguinal paravascular technic of lumbar plexus anesthesia: the '3 in 1 block'," *Anesthesia and Analgesia*, vol. 52, no. 6, pp. 989–996, 1973.

[42] B. M. Ilfeld, E. R. Mariano, P. J. Girard et al., "A multicenter, randomized, triple-masked, placebo-controlled trial of the effect of ambulatory continuous femoral nerve blocks on discharge-readiness following total knee arthroplasty in patients on general orthopaedic wards," *Pain*, vol. 150, no. 3, pp. 477–484, 2010.

[43] L. A. Beaupre, D. B. C. Johnston, S. Dieleman, and B. Tsui, "Impact of a preemptive multimodal analgesia plus femoral nerve blockade protocol on rehabilitation, hospital length of stay, and postoperative analgesia after primary total knee arthroplasty: a controlled clinical pilot study," *The Scientific World Journal*, vol. 2012, Article ID 273821, 6 pages, 2012.

[44] D. Wasserstein, C. Farlinger, R. Brull, N. Mahomed, and R. Gandhi, "Advanced age, obesity and continuous femoral nerve blockade are independent risk factors for inpatient falls after primary total knee arthroplasty," *Journal of Arthroplasty*, vol. 28, no. 7, pp. 1121–1124, 2013.

[45] E. Chan, M. Fransen, D. A. Parker, P. N. Assam, and N. Chua, "Femoral nerve blocks for acute postoperative pain after knee replacement surgery," *The Cochrane Database of Systematic Reviews*, 2014.

[46] P. Marhofer, M. Greher, and S. Kapral, "Ultrasound guidance in regional anaesthesia," *British Journal of Anaesthesia*, vol. 94, no. 1, pp. 7–17, 2005.

[47] H. Evans, S. M. Steele, K. C. Nielsen, M. S. Tucker, and S. M. Klein, "Peripheral nerve blocks and continuous catheter techniques," *Anesthesiology Clinics of North America*, vol. 23, no. 1, pp. 141–162, 2005.

[48] F. K. Enneking, V. Chan, J. Greger, A. Hadžić, S. A. Lang, and T. T. Horlocker, "Lower-extremity peripheral nerve blockade: essentials of our current understanding," *Regional Anesthesia and Pain Medicine*, vol. 30, no. 1, pp. 4–35, 2005.

[49] G. Cappelleri, D. Ghisi, A. Fanelli, A. Albertin, F. Somalvico, and G. Aldegheri, "Does continuous sciatic nerve block improve postoperative analgesia and early rehabilitation after total knee arthroplasty? A prospective, randomized, double-blinded study," *Regional Anesthesia and Pain Medicine*, vol. 36, no. 5, pp. 489–492, 2011.

[50] F. W. Abdallah and R. Brull, "Is sciatic nerve block advantageous when combined with femoral nerve block for postoperative analgesia following total knee arthroplasty? A systematic review," *Regional Anesthesia and Pain Medicine*, vol. 36, no. 5, pp. 493–498, 2011.

[51] P. Marhofer, C. Našel, C. Sitzwohl, and S. Kapral, "Magnetic resonance imaging of the distribution of local anesthetic during the three-in-one block," *Anesthesia and Analgesia*, vol. 90, no. 1, pp. 119–124, 2000.

[52] S. K. Parkinson, J. B. Mueller, W. L. Little, and S. L. Bailey, "Extent of blockade with various approaches to the lumbar plexus," *Anesthesia & Analgesia*, vol. 68, no. 3, pp. 243–248, 1989.

[53] D. Macalou, S. Trueck, P. Meuret et al., "Postoperative analgesia after total knee replacement: the effect of an obturator nerve block added to the femoral 3-in-1 nerve block," *Anesthesia and Analgesia*, vol. 99, no. 1, pp. 251–254, 2004.

[54] D. A. McNamee, L. Parks, and K. R. Milligan, "Post-operative analgesia following total knee replacement: an evaluation of the addition of an obturator nerve block to combined femoral and sciatic nerve block," *Acta Anaesthesiologica Scandinavica*, vol. 46, no. 1, pp. 95–99, 2002.

[55] S. C. Mudumbai, T. E. Kim, S. K. Howard et al., "Continuous adductor canal blocks are superior to continuous femoral nerve blocks in promoting early ambulation after TKA," *Clinical Orthopaedics and Related Research*, vol. 472, no. 5, pp. 1377–1383, 2014.

[56] P. Jæger, D. Zaric, J. S. Fomsgaard et al., "Adductor canal block versus femoral nerve block for analgesia after total knee arthroplasty: a randomized, double-blind study," *Regional Anesthesia and Pain Medicine*, vol. 38, no. 6, pp. 526–532, 2013.

[57] L. Nikolajsen, B. Brandsborg, U. Lucht, T. S. Jensen, and H. Kehlet, "Chronic pain following total hip arthroplasty: a nation-wide questionnaire study," *Acta Anaesthesiologica Scandinavica*, vol. 50, no. 4, pp. 495–500, 2006.

[58] O. Mathiesen, L. S. Jacobsen, H. E. Holm et al., "Pregabalin and dexamethasone for postoperative pain control: a randomized controlled study in hip arthroplasty," *British Journal of Anaesthesia*, vol. 101, no. 4, pp. 535–541, 2008.

[59] H. Clarke, S. Pereira, D. Kennedy et al., "Adding Gabapentin to a multimodal regimen does not reduce acute pain, opioid consumption or chronic pain after total hip arthroplasty," *Acta Anaesthesiologica Scandinavica*, vol. 53, no. 8, pp. 1073–1083, 2009.

[60] D. R. Kerr and L. Kohan, "Local infiltration analgesia: a technique for the control of acute postoperative pain following knee and hip surgery—a case study of 325 patients," *Acta Orthopaedica*, vol. 79, no. 2, pp. 174–183, 2008.

[61] A. Gottschalk, M.-A. Burmeister, P. Radtke et al., "Continuous wound infiltration with ropivacaine reduces pain and analgesic requirement after shoulder surgery," *Anesthesia and Analgesia*, vol. 97, no. 4, pp. 1086–1091, 2003.

[62] E.-P. Horn, F. Schroeder, S. Wilhelm et al., "Wound infiltration and drain lavage with ropivacaine after major shoulder surgery," *Anesthesia & Analgesia*, vol. 89, no. 6, pp. 1461–1466, 1999.

[63] D. R. Mauerhan, M. Campbell, J. S. Miller, J. G. Mokris, A. Gregory, and G. M. Kiebzak, "Intra-articular morphine and/or bupivacaine in the management of pain after total knee arthroplasty," *Journal of Arthroplasty*, vol. 12, no. 5, pp. 546–552, 1997.

[64] S. Rasmussen, M. U. Kramhøft, K. P. Sperling, and J. H. L. Pedersen, "Increased flexion and reduced hospital stay with continuous intraarticular morphine and ropivacaine after primary total knee replacement: open intervention study of efficacy and safety in 154 patients," *Acta Orthopaedica Scandinavica*, vol. 75, no. 5, pp. 606–609, 2004.

[65] K. V. Andersen, M. Pfeiffer-Jensen, V. Haraldsted, and K. Søballe, "Reduced hospital stay and narcotic consumption, and improved mobilization with local and intraarticular infiltration after hip arthroplasty: a randomized clinical trial of an intraarticular technique versus epidural infusion in 80 patients," *Acta Orthopaedica*, vol. 78, no. 2, pp. 180–186, 2007.

[66] M. Thorsell, P. Holst, H. C. Hyldahl, and L. Weidenhielm, "Pain control after total knee arthroplasty: a prospective study comparing local infiltration anesthesia and epidural anesthesia," *Orthopedics*, vol. 33, no. 2, pp. 75–78, 2010.

[67] K. Specht, J. S. Leonhardt, P. Revald et al., "No evidence of a clinically important effect of adding local infusion analgesia administrated through a catheter in pain treatment after total hip arthroplasty," *Acta Orthopaedica*, vol. 82, no. 3, pp. 315–320, 2011.

[68] T. H. Lunn, H. Husted, S. Solgaard et al., "Intraoperative local infiltration analgesia for early analgesia after total hip arthroplasty: a randomized, double-blind, placebo-controlled trial," *Regional Anesthesia and Pain Medicine*, vol. 36, no. 5, pp. 424–429, 2011.

[69] N. Rawal, "Local infiltration analgesia and other multicomponent techniques to improve postoperative outcome—are we comparing oranges and apples?" *Regional Anesthesia and Pain Medicine*, vol. 36, no. 5, pp. 417–420, 2011.

[70] H. Kehlet and L. Ø. Andersen, "Local infiltration analgesia in joint replacement: the evidence and recommendations for clinical practice," *Acta Anaesthesiologica Scandinavica*, vol. 55, no. 7, pp. 778–784, 2011.

[71] L. Ø. Andersen, H. Husted, K. S. Otte, B. B. Kristensen, and H. Kehlet, "A compression bandage improves local infiltration analgesia in total knee arthroplasty," *Acta Orthopaedica*, vol. 79, no. 6, pp. 806–811, 2008.

[72] O. Solovyova, C. G. Lewis, J. H. Abrams et al., "Local infiltration analgesia followed by continuous infusion of local anesthetic solution for total hip arthroplasty: a prospective, randomized, double-blind, placebo-controlled study," *Journal of Bone and Joint Surgery A*, vol. 95, no. 21, pp. 1935–1941, 2013.

[73] K. Toftdahl, L. Nikolajsen, V. Haraldsted, F. Madsen, E. K. Tönnesen, and K. Søballe, "Comparison of peri- and intraarticular analgesia with femoral nerve block after total knee arthroplasty: a randomized clinical trial," *Acta Orthopaedica*, vol. 78, no. 2, pp. 172–179, 2007.

[74] P. Essving, K. Axelsson, J. Kjellberg, Ö. Wallgren, A. Gupta, and A. Lundin, "Reduced morphine consumption and pain intensity with local infiltration analgesia (LIA) following total knee arthroplasty: a randomized double-blind study involving 48 patients," *Acta Orthopaedica*, vol. 81, no. 3, pp. 354–360, 2010.

[75] U. J. Spreng, V. Dahl, A. Hjall, M. W. Fagerland, and J. Ræder, "High-volume local infiltration analgesia combined with intravenous or local ketorolac + morphine compared with epidural analgesia after total knee arthroplasty," *British Journal of Anaesthesia*, vol. 105, no. 5, pp. 675–682, 2010.

[76] J. P. Dillon, L. Brennan, and D. Mitchell, "Local infiltration analgesia in hip and knee arthroplasty: an emerging technique," *Acta Orthopaedica Belgica*, vol. 78, no. 2, pp. 158–163, 2012.

[77] A. Perlas, K. R. Kirkham, R. Billing et al., "The impact of analgesic modality on early ambulation following total knee arthroplasty," *Regional Anesthesia and Pain Medicine*, vol. 38, no. 4, pp. 334–339, 2013.

[78] S. J. Fowler and N. Christelis, "High volume local infiltration analgesia compared to peripheral nerve block for hip and knee arthroplasty—what is the evidence?" *Anaesthesia and Intensive Care*, vol. 41, no. 4, pp. 458–462, 2013.

[79] L. O. Andersen and H. Kehlet, "Analgesic efficacy of local infiltration analgesia in hip and knee arthroplasty: a systematic review," *British Journal of Anaesthesia*, 2014.

3

# The Impact of a Dedicated Research Education Month for Anesthesiology Residents

**Robert E. Freundlich,[1] Jessica W. Newman,[1] Kevin K. Tremper,[1] Jill M. Mhyre,[2] Sachin Kheterpal,[1] Theodore J. Sanford Jr.,[1] and Alan R. Tait[1]**

[1] *Department of Anesthesiology, University of Michigan Medical School, Ann Arbor, MI 48105, USA*
[2] *Department of Anesthesiology, University of Arkansas, Little Rock, AR 72205, USA*

Correspondence should be addressed to Robert E. Freundlich; freundli@med.umich.edu

Academic Editor: Steven K. Howard

An educational intervention was implemented at the University of Michigan starting in 2008, in which anesthesiology interns complete a dedicated month-long didactic rotation in evidence-based medicine (EBM) and research methodology. We sought to assess its utility. Scores on a validated EBM test before and after the rotation were compared and assessed for significance of improvement. A survey was also given to gauge satisfaction with the quality of the rotation and self-reported improvement in understanding of EBM topics. Fourteen consecutive interns completed the research rotation during the study period. One hundred percent completed both the pre- and postrotation test. The mean pretest score was 7.78 ± 2.46 (median = 7.5, 0–15 scale, and interquartile range 7.0–10.0) and the mean posttest score was 10.00 ± 2.35 (median = 9.5, interquartile range 8.0–12.3), which represented a statistically significant increase ($P = 0.011$, Wilcoxon signed-rank test). All fourteen of the residents "agreed" or "strongly agreed" that they would recommend the course to future interns and that the course increased their ability to critically review the literature. Our findings demonstrate that this can be an effective means of improving understanding of EBM topics and anesthesiology research.

## 1. Introduction

While most medical schools teach EBM in one form or another, it has been our experience that the quality of this preparation varies between residents. Furthermore, the relevance to anesthesiology practice may be limited, since most examples from medical school courses are drawn from the general medical disciplines. A 2004 meta-analysis comparing various studies reporting EBM learning in medical education suggested that postgraduate medical education in EBM topics may be particularly useful in teaching critical appraisal skills. The authors attributed this value to a general desire among medical postgraduates to learn for the sake of improved patient care, as opposed to the undergraduate motivation of higher test scores [1].

There have been several reports of successful teaching methods, such as regular journal clubs [2], in anesthesiology residency programs to increase critical thinking and appraisal of anesthesiology research. Other fields have also reported the successful adoption of dedicated research rotations in their residencies, notably internal medicine [3] and pediatrics [4]. In addition, residency programs have reported regularly setting aside dedicated time for EBM teaching [5–7].

To the best of our knowledge, we have implemented the first dedicated month-long EBM course in an anesthesiology residency program. We sought to assess whether participation in the research rotation would lead to quantitative and self-reported improved understanding of EBM topics among our intern class and whether residents were satisfied with their experience.

## 2. Materials and Methods

*Informed Consent.* This study was granted a waiver of informed consent under the educational exemption by the

TABLE 1: Didactic topics in the intern research rotation.

| | |
|---|---|
| 1 | Research committee and ongoing research |
| 2 | Descriptive statistics |
| 3 | Selecting a statistical test |
| 4 | Hypothesis testing |
| 5 | Measures of association and effect size and logistic regression |
| 6 | Cohort and observational studies |
| 7 | Designing and evaluating randomized controlled trials |
| 8 | Assessing randomized controlled trials |
| 9 | Diagnosis and screening |
| 10 | Meta-analysis and systemic review |
| 11 | The manuscript process |
| 12 | Evidence-based practice |
| 13 | Reading and presenting a research study |
| 14 | Introduction to the institutional review board (IRB) |

University of Michigan Institutional Review Board (Ann Arbor, Michigan).

*2.1. Prospective Cohort and Questionnaire.* In 2008, due to a perceived weakness in resident understanding and appreciation of evidence-based medicine (EBM) topics and as a vehicle to offer early research exposure to residents, a month-long dedicated research rotation was implemented at the University of Michigan. All categorical anesthesiology Postgraduate Year-1 (PGY-1) residents now take the course as a required part of their intern curriculum. During this month, participants complete reading assignments in preparation for small group discussions on various EBM topics (Table 1). Residents also review an assigned journal article and present it during a departmental journal club. Lastly, under the guidance of a research mentor, residents design and present an original research proposal. In preparing the proposal, they must develop an answerable research question, devise a hypothesis, and perform a focused literature review. The resulting proposal is presented to the Department Chair for review. To evaluate the impact of the research rotation, a prospective cohort study was conducted on a consecutive group of PGY-1 interns during the 2011-12 academic year. This present study was the result of a research rotation proposal from two of the rotation's participants (Robert E. Freundlich and Jessica W. Newman). All interns who participated in the research rotation were eligible for inclusion. The English version of the Berlin EBM Questionnaire was used to assess the value of the rotation [3, 8, 9]. The Berlin Questionnaire consists of two distinct sets (A and B) of 15 multiple-choice questions, in which participants apply statistical concepts to resolve theoretical patient care issues. Each participant completed one of the sets (set A or set B) before and the other after the intervention. All questions were weighted equally when determining the score and for statistical analysis.

The Berlin Questionnaire focuses on the following domains of EBM: ability to understand and critically appraise evidence, relating a clinical problem to a clinical question, identifying relevant study design, and using basic statistics to solve specific patient issues [10]. Furthermore, the Berlin Questionnaire has proven content validity and internal consistency. The Berlin Questionnaire has been used in prior studies involving medical students [11], internal medicine residents [3], and other health care professionals [8] to evaluate the impact of educational interventions on EBM knowledge and skills.

A research assistant distributed the questionnaire on the first and last day of the course. Faculty lecturers did not have access to the questionnaire and the results were not used in the residents' course evaluation. The primary outcome measure was the mean change in scores on the Berlin Questionnaire before and after the research month.

*2.2. Survey.* At the conclusion of the research rotation residents were required to fill out a survey to evaluate the course (Table 2). The survey included ten questions with a five-point Likert response scale and a narrative comments' section. Questions covered the organization of the course, lecture topics, and perceived increase in knowledge.

*2.3. Statistical Analysis.* A pilot study was performed in 2011 to calculate statistical power and for sample size determination. Five residents enrolled in the research rotation took the Berlin Questionnaire before and after the course.

Residents' scores on the Berlin Questionnaire before and after the course were recorded. The Wilcoxon signed-rank test was used to analyze paired data. The mean and standard deviations for the answers to the survey were analyzed and the statistical difference of the mean was calculated from a neutral response using the one-sample $t$-test. Data are presented as mean, standard deviation, median, and interquartile range (IQR). Statistical significance was accepted at $P < 0.05$.

The mean initial score during the pilot study was 8.0/15 ($\sigma = 1.2$) and the mean final score during the pilot study was 10.8/15 ($\sigma = 2.3$). Based on these findings, we estimated that we would need 9 residents to participate in order to generate a power of 0.9 to detect a difference in scores of at least this large with an alpha of 0.05 (2-sided).

## 3. Results

Fourteen consecutive participants completed the pre- and postcourse test during the 2011-12 academic year, including the five included in the pilot study. All participants completed both the pre- and postcourse test. The mean baseline score was 7.78/15 ($\sigma = 2.46$, median 7.5, and IQR 7.0–10.0) and the mean postcourse score was 10.0/15 ($\sigma = 2.35$, median 9.5, and IQR 8.0–12.3), which represented a statistically significant increase ($P = 0.011$).

Results from the survey are described in Table 2. The response rate for the survey was 100%. All of the residents stated that they either "agree" or "strongly agree" that they would recommend the course to future interns and that the course increased their ability to critically review the literature.

Residents have actively pursued their intern research projects and seen them through to completion. To date, several of these projects have been published [12, 13] and others are currently under journal review.

TABLE 2: Resident final course evaluation survey.

| | Strongly disagree | Disagree | Neither agree nor disagree | Agree | Strongly agree |
|---|---|---|---|---|---|
| (1) The research rotation was well organized | 0/14 | 0/14 | 0/14 | 7/14 | 7/14 |
| (2) The goals/objectives of the rotation were met | 0/14 | 0/14 | 0/14 | 4/14 | 10/14 |
| (3) The instructors demonstrated a thorough grasp of the material | 0/14 | 0/14 | 0/14 | 3/14 | 11/14 |
| (4) The lecture topics were comprehensive | 0/14 | 0/14 | 0/14 | 5/14 | 9/14 |
| (5) The lecture topics were relevant | 0/14 | 0/14 | 0/14 | 3/14 | 11/14 |
| (6) The course increased my understanding of research | 0/14 | 0/14 | 0/14 | 2/14 | 12/14 |
| (7) The course increased my interest in pursuing research | 0/14 | 0/14 | 3/14 | 1/14 | 10/14 |
| (8) The course increased my ability to critically review the literature | 0/14 | 0/14 | 0/14 | 4/14 | 10/14 |
| (9) I would recommend this course to future interns | 0/14 | 0/14 | 0/14 | 3/14 | 11/14 |
| (10) I would have preferred a clinical rotation | 6/14 | 6/14 | 0/14 | 0/14 | 2/14 |
| (11) Suggestions for improvement | | | | | |
| (12) Additional comments | | | | | |

## 4. Discussion

We sought to prospectively evaluate the impact of a dedicated, month-long research rotation in an anesthesiology residency program. This educational intervention successfully improved resident performance on a standardized metric and resulted in high self-reported improvement in comprehension of EBM topics. We anticipate that the skills and knowledge obtained in this course will advance our residents' abilities to critically review the literature and use EBM in their own practice and in their clinical decision-making.

The research rotation was implemented using existing resources. Certain aspects of its structure may have influenced its success. An intern class at the University of Michigan has 24 residents. To ensure high faculty-to-participant ratios, the course is offered eight times per year to only three residents at a time. Didactic topics (Table 1) are generally presented in a discussion-based format, although some topics are also reviewed in supplemental online lectures. We believe that this could serve as a model for teaching EBM at other anesthesiology residency programs. Furthermore, the program could be applied to other specialties, medical students, or other health professionals, such as nurse anesthetists and anesthesiology assistants.

Although this was not our primary aim in implementing the research rotation, it is interesting to note that 11 participants felt that the course increased their interest in pursuing research. As has been discussed elsewhere, there is considerable appeal in finding successful means of increasing resident training and interest in anesthesiology research [14–16].

There are several limitations to our intervention that deserve further discussion. Although we found an increased score on a validated EBM questionnaire, we are unable, at this time, to determine if this increase will ultimately translate into improved patient outcomes, better utilization of the literature, and long-term understanding of EBM topics. Given that this test was administered immediately after the end of the course's completion, we were unable to assess long-term retention of knowledge gained. In addition, given the relatively small sample size, we were also unable to conduct analyses to determine if improvement on the test was global or limited to certain EBM topics. It is possible that some programs may find it difficult to place residents in a nonclinical rotation, given patient care needs at their institution. Finally, the single center nature of this intervention may limit the generalizability of our findings. Future studies will seek to address many of these issues.

## 5. Conclusions

In conclusion, results of this study suggest that implementation of a month-long, dedicated intern research rotation successfully increased understanding of EBM topics in a cohort of anesthesiology residents. Future work will seek to better refine how we can improve resident understanding of topical areas as we continue to offer the course to our residents and track their performance using the Berlin Questionnaire. We believe that this course has had a significant impact on our resident education and could be successfully applied elsewhere.

## Conflict of Interests

The authors declare that there is no conflict of interests regarding the publication of this paper.

## Acknowledgments

Dr. Regina Kunz, Professor, Institut für Versicherungsmedizin, Universitätsspital, Basel, Switzerland, graciously provided the Berlin Questionnaire for our study. Susan V. Stokes assisted with the preparation and administration of the test.

## References

[1] A. Coomarasamy and K. S. Khan, "What is the evidence that postgraduate teaching in evidence based medicine changes

anything? A systematic review," *British Medical Journal*, vol. 329, no. 7473, pp. 1017–1019, 2004.

[2] R. S. Moharari, E. Rahimi, A. Najafi, P. Khashayar, M. R. Khajavi, and A. P. Meysamie, "Teaching critical appraisal and statistics in anesthesia journal club," *QJM*, vol. 102, no. 2, pp. 139–141, 2009.

[3] E. A. Akl, I. S. Izuchukwu, S. El-Dika, L. Fritsche, R. Kunz, and H. J. Schünemann, "Integrating an evidence-based medicine rotation into an internal medicine residency program," *Academic Medicine*, vol. 79, no. 9, pp. 897–904, 2004.

[4] E. Dinkevich, A. Markinson, S. Ahsan, and B. Lawrence, "Effect of a brief intervention on evidence-based medicine skills of pediatric residents," *BMC Medical Education*, vol. 6, article 1, 2006.

[5] S. J. Haines and J. S. Nicholas, "Teaching evidence-based medicine to surgical subspecialty residents," *Journal of the American College of Surgeons*, vol. 197, no. 2, pp. 285–289, 2003.

[6] C. L. F. Temple and D. C. Ross, "Acquisition of evidence-based surgery skills in plastic surgery residency training," *Journal of Surgical Education*, vol. 68, no. 3, pp. 167–171, 2011.

[7] H. B. Kersten, T. M. Randis, and A. P. Giardino, "Evidence-based medicine in pediatric residency programs: where are we now?" *Ambulatory Pediatrics*, vol. 5, no. 5, pp. 302–305, 2005.

[8] R. Kunz, K. Wegscheider, L. Fritsche et al., "Determinants of knowledge gain in evidence-based medicine short courses: an international assessment," *Open Medicine*, vol. 4, no. 1, pp. e3–e10, 2010.

[9] L. Fritsche, T. Greenhalgh, Y. Falck-Ytter, H.-H. Neumayer, and R. Kunz, "Do short courses in evidence based medicine improve knowledge and skills? Validation of Berlin questionnaire and before and after study of courses in evidence based medicine," *British Medical Journal*, vol. 325, no. 7376, pp. 1338–1341, 2002.

[10] T. Shaneyfelt, K. D. Baum, D. Bell et al., "Instruments for evaluating education in evidence-based practice: a systematic review," *The Journal of the American Medical Association*, vol. 296, no. 9, pp. 1116–1127, 2006.

[11] C. P. West, T. M. Jaeger, and F. S. McDonald, "Extended evaluation of a longitudinal medical school evidence-based medicine curriculum," *Journal of General Internal Medicine*, vol. 26, no. 6, pp. 611–615, 2011.

[12] J. Newman, K. Blake, J. Fennema et al., "Incidence, predictors and outcomes of postoperative coma: an observational study of 858 606 patients," *European Journal of Anaesthesiology*, vol. 30, no. 8, pp. 476–482, 2013.

[13] M. R. Mathis, N. N. Naughton, A. M. Shanks et al., "Patient selection for day case-eligible surgery: identifying those at high risk for major complications.," *Anesthesiology*, vol. 119, no. 6, pp. 1310–1321, 2013.

[14] D. A. Schwinn and J. R. Balser, "Anesthesiology physician scientists in academic medicine: a wake-up call," *Anesthesiology*, vol. 104, no. 1, pp. 170–178, 2006.

[15] M. A. Warner, "Who better than anesthesiologists? The 44th Rovenstine lecture," *Anesthesiology*, vol. 104, no. 5, pp. 1094–1101, 2006.

[16] A. M. Juve, J. R. Kirsch, and C. Swide, "Training intensivists and clinician-scientists for the 21st century: the Oregon scholars program," *Journal of Graduate Medical Education*, vol. 2, no. 4, pp. 585–588, 2010.

4

# Local Infiltration Analgesia for Postoperative Pain Control following Total Hip Arthroplasty

**Denise McCarthy and Gabriella Iohom**

*Department of Anaesthesia and Intensive Care Medicine, Cork University Hospital, Cork, Ireland*

Correspondence should be addressed to Denise McCarthy, dmc_btown@yahoo.co.uk

Academic Editor: Attila Bondar

Local infiltration analgesia (LIA) is an analgesic technique that has gained popularity since it was first brought to widespread attention by Kerr and Kohan in 2008. The technique involves the infiltration of a large volume dilute solution of a long-acting local anesthetic agent, often with adjuvants (e.g., epinephrine, ketorolac, an opioid), throughout the wound at the time of surgery. The analgesic effect duration can then be prolonged by the placement of a catheter to the surgical site for postoperative administration of further local anesthetic. The technique has been adopted for use for postoperative analgesia following a range of surgical procedures (orthopedic, general, gynecological, and breast surgeries). The primary objective of this paper was to determine, based on the current evidence, if LIA is superior when compared to no intervention, placebo, and alternative analgesic methods in patients following total hip arthroplasty, in terms of certain outcome measures. The outcomes considered were postoperative analgesia scores, joint function/rehabilitation, and length of hospital stay. Secondary objectives were to review available evidence and current knowledge regarding the pharmacokinetics of local anesthetic and adjuvant drugs when administered in this way and the occurrence of adverse events.

## 1. Methods

*1.1. Literature Search.* The National Library of Medicine's Medline database and the Cochrane Central Register of Controlled Trials were searched for the time period January 1, 1966 to present (last search performed 21st January 2012). The search terms used were local infiltration analgesia, joint infiltration, joint infusion, wound infiltration, continuous wound infusion and local anesthetic infusion, local anesthetic infiltration. These search terms were then combined with the term total hip arthroplasty/replacement and searched again. Searches were restricted to adults (older than 18 years of age) and clinical trials or randomized controlled trials. Abstracts in English only were specified.

*1.2. Inclusion Criteria.* Studies were selected for inclusion if they had investigated the use of intraoperative local anesthetic infiltration for postoperative pain management following total hip arthroplasty (THA).

*1.3. Exclusion Criteria.* Studies that did not record either pain scores or analgesic consumption were excluded. Studies that used solely an intra-articular injection (as opposed to a tissue infiltration technique) or a postoperative infusion alone (not preceded by tissue infiltration) were excluded.

*1.4. Data Extraction and Analysis.* Each study's methodology and results were recorded. Randomized controlled trials (RCTs) were assessed using the Jadad criteria and scored on the 0–5 scale [1]. The Jadad score is based on a three-point questionnaire that asks the following questions: was the study described as randomized, as double blind, and was there a description of withdrawals and dropouts? A point is awarded for each affirmative answer. Additional points are given one, if the method of randomization was described in the paper, and that method was appropriate, and two, if the method of blinding was described, and it was appropriate. Points are deducted if the method of randomization was described but was inappropriate and/or the method of blinding was described but was inappropriate. By these criteria a maximum score of 5 points is possible. A Jadad score (where applicable) of ≥3 was considered acceptable for inclusion. No studies required exclusion based on this criterion. The outcomes (pain scores at rest and on movement, ambulation, length of hospital stay, adverse events) were recorded as defined by the original studies.

## 2. Results

Ten studies (a total of 893 patients) were identified as pertinent and included for analysis—eight RCTs and two case series. It should be noted that four of these studies looked at a mixt population of patients undergoing hip resurfacing arthroplasty and total knee arthroplasty. The exclusions are outlined in Figure 1. The study characteristics of all articles included are detailed in Table 1.

## 3. Discussion

*3.1. Introduction.* Established methods of postoperative analgesia for total hip arthroplasty are central neuraxial opioids, epidural analgesia, intravenous patient-controlled opioid analgesia (PCA), and peripheral nerve blocks [2]. The prospect collaboration, which aims to provide evidence-based recommendations on a procedure-specific basis, issued guidelines for THA anesthetic management in 2005. The group concluded that there are "various clinical pathways with which to manage pain effectively after THA" and, in summary, recommended use of either general anesthesia plus strong opioids or general anesthesia plus peripheral nerve blockade (femoral or posterior lumber plexus block) or spinal local anesthetic (single shot) plus morphine or epidural local anesthetic plus/minus opioid.

Peripheral nerve blockade (PNB) has been shown to provide equivalent analgesia compared to epidural analgesia with the benefit of a lesser incidence of hypotension and urinary retention [3], however PNB requires a high level of expertise to perform [4]. Recently, in a "pooled data" report of the combined findings of three separate studies of continuous peripheral nerve blockade (CPNB) following total hip (and knee) arthroplasty, a possible causal relationship was suggested between CPNB affecting quadriceps strength and the risk of falling [5]. Choi et al. reviewed the use of epidural analgesia for pain relief following hip (and knee) replacement in a Cochrane review in 2003 and concluded that the beneficial effect of epidural analgesia was limited to 4–6 hours postoperatively, and side effects (hypotension, pruritus, urinary retention) were more frequent with epidural analgesia compared to systemic analgesia [3].

With a move towards earlier ambulation of patients following joint replacement surgery, comprehensive analgesia regimes that provide excellent pain relief both at rest and on movement, without reduction in motor function/power and with minimal side effects, are desirable. A number of investigators have found LIA to be superior to placebo/no infiltration and epidural analgesia in terms of postoperative analgesia scores, joint function/rehabilitation, and length of hospital stay. This may explain the increased number of trials investigating the LIA technique in recent years.

*3.2. Review of the Evidence-Published Trials.* Kerr and Kohan published a case series of 325 patients who were given intra- and periarticular infiltration for postoperative analgesia following total hip or knee arthroplasty [6]. The injectate mixture consisted of ropivacaine 2 mg/mL, ketorolac 30 mg, epinephrine 10 mcg/mL. The volume used for THA and hip resurfacing arthroplasty (HRA) was 150–200 mL. The maximum dose of ropivacaine was limited to 300 mg (or 250 mg in some cases). If volumes over 150 mL were required, the injectate was diluted with saline. The mixture was injected into all the tissues of the surgical field in a systematic fashion during surgery. They termed this local infiltration analgesia. The patients were subsequently given a bolus of 50 mL of the mixture (100 mg ropivacaine) at 15 to 20 hours postoperatively via an intra-articular catheter that was sited during the surgery. The authors reported that pain scores were generally satisfactory (0–3/10) and that two thirds of patients did not require morphine during the postoperative period. Most patients were able to walk with assistance between 5 and 6 hours postoperatively. The exact infiltration method as described by Kerr and Kohan was used in a subsequent series of 24 patients undergoing elective HRA and TKA by Otte et al. with similar postoperative analgesic efficacy [7].

Parvataneni et al. investigated the use of local anesthetic infiltration as part of a multimodal pain protocol following THA (and TKA) [8]. A mixture containing bupivacaine 40–80 mg and epinephrine (plus morphine, methylprednisolone, and cefuroxime) in a volume of 75–115 mL was used for infiltration. The control patients received intravenous PCA morphine (plus femoral nerve block for TKA patients). Lower pain scores and a shorter length of stay (3.2 versus 4.2 days, $P < 0.05$) were reported in the THA patients who received infiltration.

Two studies [9, 10] have compared LIA with placebo saline. Bianconi used ropivacaine 200 mg (40 mL) for infiltration and followed it with an extra-articular infusion of ropivacaine 10 mg/hr for 35 hours [9]. The control group received an extra-articular saline infusion. The LIA group reported lower pain scores at rest and on movement up to 72 hours postoperatively and had lesser opioid consumption. There was a shorter length of stay in the LIA group (6.34 (0.67) versus 8.79 (1.39) days, $P < 0.05$). Andersen et al. used ropivacaine 300 mg (150 mL) plus ketorolac 30 mg plus epinephrine 0.5 mg for infiltration and followed by, on the first postoperative morning, an intra-articular bolus of ropivacaine 150 mg (20 mL) plus ketorolac 30 mg plus epinephrine 0.5 mg [10]. The LIA group reported lower pain scores from 4 hours up to two weeks postoperatively and lower opioid consumption. Joint function was better in the LIA group at one week but not thereafter.

One study was published comparing LIA with no infiltration [11]. Busch et al. infiltrated ropivacaine 400 mg (100 mL) plus ketorolac 30 mg plus epinephrine 0.6 mg plus morphine 5 mg [11]. Further infiltration was not given in the

Table 1: Published trials examining use of local infiltration analgesia following total hip arthroplasty.

| Author, year | Type of surgery | Study design | Intervention | Control | Pain scores | Opioid consumption | Function | Length of stay | comment |
|---|---|---|---|---|---|---|---|---|---|
| Andersen et al. [12] 2007 | THA | RCT $n = 80$ | LIA 100 mL: ropivacaine 200 mg + epi 0.5 mg + ketorolac 30 mg IA bolus 20 mL (ropivacaine 150 mg + epinephrine 0.5 mg + ketorolac 30 mg at 8 hrs) | Epidural to 20 hours | Lower VAS LIA group from 20 to 96 hours $P < 0.001$ to $P = 0.04$ (variable with time) | Reduced in LIA group $P = 0.04$ for first 20 hrs, $P = 0.05$ for total study period up to 96 hrs | More patients able to walk at 8 hours in LIA group $P < 0.001$ | Reduced LIA group 4.5 (3–6) versus 7 (5.5–7) days (mean, range), $P < 0.001$ | Jadad score = 3 96 hour follow-up |
| Andersen et al. [10] 2007 | THA | RCT $n = 40$ | LIA 150 mL: ropivacaine 300 mg + ketorolac 30 mg + epinephrine 0.5 mg IA bolus next morning 20 mL of mixture | Saline infiltration and injection | Lower in LIA group from 4 hours up to 2 weeks $P < 0.001$ to $P = 0.04$ (variable with time) | Lower in LIA group $P < 0.001$ to $P = 0.01$ (variable with time) | Better at 1 week with LIA ($P = 0.02$), no difference after | No difference | Jadad score = 4 6-week followup |
| Andersen et al. [14] 2011 | Bilateral THA | RCT $n = 12$ | LIA: ropivacaine 340 mg + epinephrine 1.7 mg to one hip | Saline to control hip | Low, similar between hips | | N/R | 4 days median | Jadad score = 4 48-hour followup |
| Bianconi et al. [9] 2003 | TKA and THA Results pertain to THA ($n = 29$) | RCT $n = 37$ | LIA 40 mL: ropivacaine 200 mg Extra-articular infusion ropivacaine 10 mg/hr for 55 hrs | Extra-articular saline infusion | Lower scores in LIA group at rest and on movement up to 72 hours $P < 0.05$ | Lower in LIA group $P < 0.05$ | | Reduction in length of hospital stay in LIA group 6.34 (0.67) versus 8.79 (1.39) days (mean, SD) $P < 0.05$ | Jadad score = 4 72-hour followup |
| Busch et al. [11] 2010 | THA | RCT $n = 64$ | LIA 100 mL: ropivacaine 400 mg + epinephrine 0.6 mg + ketorolac 30 mg + morphine 5 mg | Nil | Lower VAS on movement in PACU in LIA group $P = 0.0019$ | Lower PCA use first 24 hours in LIA group $P = 0.0093$ | | | Jadad score = 5 6-week followup |
| Kerr and Kohan [6] 2008 | TKA THA HRA Results pertain to all surgery types not only THA ($n = 54$) | Series $n = 325$ | LIA 150 mL: ropivacaine 300 mg + epinephrine 1.5 mg + ketorolac 30 mg IA bolus 50 mL of mixture at 15–20 hours | No control | Pain control satisfactory with NRS of 0–3/10 | 2/3 of patients did not require opioid analgesia | | | |

Table 1: Continued.

| Author, year | Type of surgery | Study design | Intervention | Control | Pain scores | Opioid consumption | Function | Length of stay | comment |
|---|---|---|---|---|---|---|---|---|---|
| Lunn et al. [15] 2011 | THA | RCT $n = 120$ | LIA: ropivacaine 300 mg + epinephrine 1.5 mg Multimodal analgesic regime | Saline infiltration multimodal analgesic regime | No difference between groups $P = 0.71$ | No difference between groups $P = 0.45$ | N/R | N/R | Jadad score = 5 8-hour followup |
| Otte et al. [7] 2008 | TKA HR Results pertain to HRA group | Series $n = 24$ | LIA150 mL: ropivacaine 300 mg + epinephrine 1.5 mg | No control | VAS scores at rest: HRA $\leq 33$ | | | | Replication of Kerr and Kohan technique |
| Parvata-neni et al. [8] 2007 | THA and TKA Results pertain to THA group ($n = 60$) | RCT $n = 131$ | LIA: bupivacaine 200–400 mg + morphine 4–10 mg + epinephrine 0.3 mg + methylprednisolone 40 mg + cefuroxime 750 mg + saline 22 mL | TKA: FNB + PCA THA: PCA No infiltration | Lower pain scores in THA patients in LIA group $P < 0.05$ | | More patients able to SLR on POD 1 in LIA group 52% versus 15%, $P < 0.05$ | THA patients in LIA group had reduced length of stay 3.2 versus 4.2 days (mean), $P < 0.05$ | Jadad score = 3 3-month followup |
| Specht et al. [13] 2011 | THA | RCT $n = 60$ | LIA: ropivacaine 200 mg + ketorolac 30 mL + epinephrine 1 mg (102 mL) 51 mL of the solution via IA catheter at 10 and 22 hrs multimodal analgesic regime | Also LIA. Saline via catheter at 10 and 22 hrs multimodal analgesic regime | No difference between groups $P = 0.04$ to $P = 0.1$ Further statistical analysis meant that this result "should be regarded as insignificant" as per authors | Similar between groups $P = 0.5$ | N/R | Trend to shorter in intervention group, NS 3 (2–6) versus 3 (2–7) days (mean, range) $P = 0.09$ | Jadad score = 5 Followup 3 days |

THA: total hip arthroplasty, HRA: hip resurfacing arthroplasty, TKA: total knee arthroplasty, NRS: numerical rating scale, POD: postoperative day, RCT: randomized controlled trial, N/R: not reported, NS: not statistically significant.

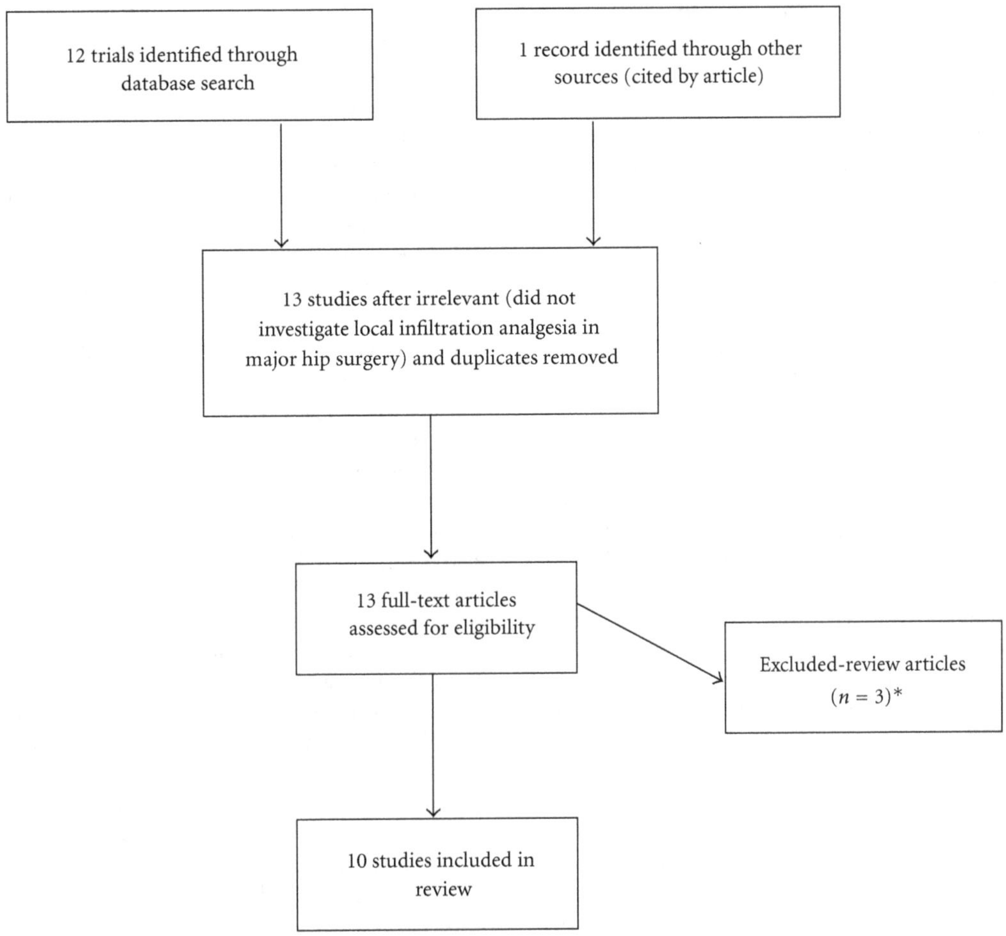


FIGURE 1: Flow diagram of exclusion of clinical trials for review [40–42].

postoperative period. The control group received standard care with no infiltration. The LIA group reported lower pain scores in the PACU on movement and lower opioid consumption in the first 24 hours.

Andersen et al. [12] investigated the analgesic effect of wound infiltration (intraoperative bolus plus top-up via catheter at 8 hours postoperatively) versus epidural analgesia in patients undergoing THA. The patients who received LIA had reduced opioid consumption and length of hospital stay and improved mobilization. Interestingly the LIA group reported significantly lower VAS for pain at both rest and movement from 20 to 96 hours postoperatively, after active pain treatment had ended (20 hours postoperatively).

Specht et al. [13] compared an LIA regimen of intra-operative ropivacaine, epinephrine, and ketorolac infiltration followed by an intra-articular bolus at 10 and 22 hours postoperatively versus a regimen of intra-operative LIA as above followed by a postoperative intra-articular saline bolus in 60 patients undergoing THA. They found no difference in pain scores or opioid consumption between the two groups and a non-significant trend to shorter hospital stay in the intervention group. It should be pointed out that in this study both groups received intra-operative LIA, the difference being in the postoperative bolus drug (LIA mixture or saline). The conclusion from this study was that a postoperative bolus did not seem to offer an additional benefit to intra-operative LIA.

The studies outlined above all found that the LIA technique was an effective analgesic method following THA (superior to placebo/no infiltration or epidural analgesia) and that opioid consumption could be reduced with its use. Three of the studies reported that hospital length of stay could be shortened with the use of the LIA technique [8, 9, 12] and three found a difference in the postoperative functional assessment of the operative hip in favor of the LIA technique [8, 10, 12].

Whilst recommended by a number of studies, two recent trials do not advocate the use of the LIA technique in addition to a multimodal analgesic regimen. In a study published in 2011, Andersen et al. investigated the analgesic efficacy of the LIA technique by comparing its use versus placebo in 12 patients undergoing bilateral THA [14]. In this study all patients received intra-operative infiltration of a ropivacaine-epinephrine solution to one hip and 0.9% saline to the other. Supplementary boluses of the solutions used were administered at 8 and 24 hours postoperatively. All patients had a multimodal analgesic regimen (gabapentin, celecoxib, and acetaminophen) commenced preoperatively. The authors reported that postoperative pain scores were low and similar between the hip given ropivacaine and that given saline. They concluded that they could not therefore recommend the LIA technique in addition to the multi-modal approach.

Also published in 2011, Lunn et al. compared the use of LIA (ropivacaine with epinephrine) versus placebo infiltration with saline in 120 patients undergoing unilateral THA, again in the setting of using a preoperatively instituted multimodal analgesic regime of gabapentin, celecoxib, and acetaminophen [15]. The postoperative pain scores in both groups were low (20 (14–38) versus 22 (10–40), ropivacaine versus placebo) and there was no significant difference between the groups ($P = 0.71$). Here again, the authors concluded that they could not recommend LIA as being superior to a multimodal approach. These two studies used only local anesthetic with epinephrine for the LIA. Therefore the possibly confounding effect of ketorolac or another NSAID in the infiltration mixture being responsible for the analgesic benefit with LIA was removed. In both of these studies the authors asserted that the LIA technique may not have a clinically relevant effect when combined with a multimodal analgesic approach and therefore was not recommended. The difference in outcome between the aforementioned trials advocating LIA and these two appears to be related to the use of a comprehensive multimodal analgesic regimen which seems to be as effective as the LIA technique. The LIA technique has been reported to be easy to perform effectively and appears to be safe. Whether or not it provides the most effective analgesia following THA has been questioned however it may have a role in certain subsets of patients such as those who are intolerant of or unsuitable for the multimodal regimen referred to above. Patients who have chronic pain conditions or are habitual opioid users may benefit from the administration of LIA; however these patients are generally not included in studies of postoperative analgesia, and therefore data is lacking.

*3.3. LIA Regimens.* The systematic infiltration of all tissues in the wound in a staged fashion as the surgery progresses as described by Kerr and Kohan has been widely adopted as the preferred method of infiltration analgesia. The local anesthetic used most often in published work so far is ropivacaine, likely chosen for its reduced cardiotoxicity in comparison to bupivacaine as well as for its intrinsic vasoconstrictor properties [16, 17]. The optimal total dose for maximal analgesic effect and safety has not been determined. Practitioners have reported using doses of 200 mg [9, 12], 300 mg [6, 7, 10], and 400 mg [11] of ropivacaine for infiltration. The use of a fixed recipe or dose is common; the introduction of a dose based on patient weight may be a future consideration.

The postoperative management also has a number of permutations. Most investigators site a catheter for postoperative local anesthetic administration but whether it is better to administer a postoperative bolus dose at a fixed time or a continuous postoperative infusion of local anesthetic is unclear. Bolus intra-articular doses [6, 7, 10, 15] and continuous extra-articular [9] infusions have been used. The timing of administration of the bolus dose, if used, varies. One group gave the bolus at 8 hours [12] while the others waited until the first postoperative day [6, 7, 10]. However, in a study carried out to investigate the effect of adding a local anesthetic infusion via an intra-articular catheter to an intra-operative LIA regime, the authors found no evidence of an improvement in pain scores in the group who received the ropivacaine/ketorolac/epinephrine infusion versus the placebo group and concluded that the catheter delivered infusion could not be recommended [13].

While the placement of a catheter for further administration of local anesthetic is favored, there is no definitive evidence regarding the optimal catheter placement site. Both intra-articular and extra-articular catheters have been used.

The use of adjuvants in the infiltration mixture varies. Nonsteroidal anti-inflammatory drugs (NSAIDs)—mostly ketorolac 30 mg [6, 10–12] which is a directly acting injectable formulation and morphine [8]—have been used, in addition to epinephrine. Steroid (methylprednisolone) has also been used in the infiltration mixture [8]. The contribution these agents make to the analgesic effect of LIA is difficult to determine. Little data exists directly comparing local administration of NSAIDs and opioids with enteral/parenteral administration, and no trial has compared LIA with adjuvants versus LIA without adjuvants.

The use of a multimodal analgesic approach is an important factor in the successful early mobilization and rehabilitation of patients following THA. It is likely that the success seen with tailored perioperative programmes in shortening time to mobilization and hospital length of stay is due to the comprehensive approach taken to achieve these aims [8, 14, 15].

In studies of patients undergoing THA where a comprehensive multimodal analgesic regimen was not used, LIA has been shown to be superior to placebo both in terms of postoperative pain scores and postoperative functional ability [10]. It has not, however, been conclusively proven to be superior to epidural analgesia. In addition, it does not appear to be of value when used in addition to a perioperative multimodal analgesia regime of gabapentin, celecoxib, and acetaminophen. The superior analgesia provided by LIA when compared to placebo has led to secondary benefits, namely, reduction in opioid consumption [9–12], and earlier hospital discharge [8, 9, 12]. Although a number of investigators have examined the use of the LIA technique, most of the studies are small and have not been powered to detect complications such as infection or local anesthetic toxicity.

*3.4. Pharmacology of Analgesic Agents Used for Local Infiltration Analgesia.* The analgesic effect derived from the local anesthetic can be ascribed to the direct actions of the constituent drug (blockage of ion-gated Na channels on A-delta and C-type nerves and therefore nociceptive nerve endings). However in a number of studies the beneficial effect (both in terms of pain scores and mobility) of the local infiltration analgesia seems to extend well beyond the expected duration of effect of the local anesthetic itself. The anti-inflammatory effect that local anesthetic drugs have been shown to exert may be a factor [18–20]. Local anesthetics reduce the release of inflammatory mediators from neutrophils, reduce neutrophil adhesion to the endothelium, reduce formation of free oxygen radicals, and decrease edema formation [21, 22]. However, a recent study designed to examine the effects of the instillation of the local anesthetic bupivacaine to the surgical wound following Caesarean section found rather unexpectedly that the instillation markedly decreased IL-10 and increased substance P in wound exudates [23]. This may indicate an overall proinflammatory wound response caused by bupivacaine. It would appear that further research in the area is necessary to fully elucidate the effects of local anesthetics agents on the local and systemic inflammatory response.

*3.5. Epinephrine.* Epinephrine is added for its vasoconstrictor properties which may decrease the systemic absorption of the local anesthetic and also aid in reducing perioperative blood loss. The administration of epinephrine by this technique will result in systemic absorption with resultant alpha- and beta-agonist effects. No deleterious effects have been reported in the literature on LIA in relation to this. The potential for elderly patients or patients with ischemic heart disease to tolerate these systemic effects poorly should, however, not be underestimated.

*3.6. Nonsteroidal Anti-Inflammatory Drugs.* Nonsteroidal anti-inflammatory drugs (NSAIDs) reduce prostaglandin formation. Prostaglandins sensitize nociceptive fibers and lead to amplification and sustaining of pain. However, there is no rigorous data to support a direct peripheral anti-inflammatory effect of NSAIDs. The use of these drugs in the LIA solution may actually be conferring a systemic rather than a local effect.

*3.7. Opioids.* It has been shown that opioids can produce potent analgesia by activating opioid receptors on peripheral sensory neurons [24]. Inflammation causes a number of cellular processes that result in a higher density of opioid receptors at peripheral nerve terminals [25, 26], and this as well as other alterations in intra- and extracellular mechanisms leads to the increased antinociceptive efficacy of peripherally administered opioids in inflamed tissue [27].

*3.8. Pharmacokinetics and Safety Profile.* Total hip arthroplasty creates a large incision area with exposed tissue, blood vessels, and bone into which a large volume of local anesthetic is injected with the LIA technique. Such high-dose administration of local anesthetic raises the potential concern of the occurrence of local anesthetic systemic toxicity, a potentially lethal complication.

Only a small number of studies have undertaken blood sampling for serum local anesthetic levels at various time points after the intraoperative infiltration and during subsequent intra- and periarticular joint infusions in an attempt to clarify the pharmacokinetics of local anesthetics administered in this way [9, 11, 28]. Highest total plasma concentrations of ropivacaine seen with the infiltration of ropivacaine 200 mg followed by an infusion at 10 mg/hr were between 0.30 and 1.28 mcg/mL, with a mean of 0.71 mcg/mL [9]. Stringer and colleagues carried out a study to investigate the pharmacokinetic and safety profile of ropivacaine 360–400 mg given via wound infiltration followed by a continuous wound infusion of 300 mg over 48 hours (6.25 mg/hr) started 12 hours postoperatively in patients undergoing THA (and TKA) [28]. The bolus infiltration resulted in peak plasma levels below 2 mcg/mL until the infusion was commenced which increased levels to up to 4.36 mcg/mL (range of peak 0.65 to 4.36 mcg/mL). Although the peak levels during the infusion were in excess of previously reported safe thresholds, there was no clinical evidence of toxicity.

The question of safe plasma levels of the various local anesthetic agents arises. One study on volunteers reported the toxic level of ropivacaine to be 0.6 mcg/mL (range 0.3–0.9 mcg/mL) [29]. Other investigators have found no systemic toxic effects with peak plasma levels, in patients receiving ropivacaine infusion, of up to 3.70, 6.08, and 7.1 mcg/mL [30–32]. The reported toxic level of bupivacaine is 0.3 mcg/mL (range 0.1–0.5 mcg/mL) [29].

*3.9. Complications.* Information on the incidence of potential complications is lacking due to the comparatively recent introduction of the technique and the small numbers of patients enrolled in published trials.

*3.10. Infection.* Concerns have been raised about the potential for infection in the presence of an indwelling catheter [33]. In a published collection of case reports, 34 reports describing adverse events in 40 patients during the use of continuous infusion pumps delivering local anesthetic were documented. Eighteen of these patients (45%) had undergone orthopedic surgery. The most commonly reported complication was tissue necrosis ($n = 17$, 42.5%) followed by surgical wound infection ($n = 15$, 37.5%). The addition of epinephrine to the local anesthetic infusion was postulated as a potential cause. The nature of the reports, however, does not allow definitive conclusions regarding a causal link between the presence of the infusion device and the complication. A number of authors using the LIA technique describe using an epinephrine-containing solution for the deep tissue infiltration and a solution without epinephrine for the subcutaneous tissue infiltration.

In a review of continuous wound catheters for all types of surgery, the overall incidence of infection was reported as 0.7% in active group catheters and 1.2% in the nonactive or control group catheters [34]. Nearly all patients had a catheter placed; therefore comparison with noncatheter groups was not possible in this review. In the study by Bianconi et al. the catheter tips underwent microbiological analysis after removal at 55 hours, and the results were negative for growth in the two groups (ropivacaine and saline infusions) [9].

A study of patients receiving postoperative wound infusion following total knee arthroplasty reported one deep wound infection in the series of 154 patients [35].

The published work investigating the use of indwelling catheters for administration of local anesthetic so far has not been powered to detect if the catheters pose an added infection risk. It would seem prudent to be cognizant of the fact that they represent a potential source of infection and as such should be inserted under sterile conditions and any boluses given using aseptic technique. How long it is safe to leave a catheter in situ postoperatively remains unclear.

*3.11. Local Anesthetic Systemic Toxicity.* The studies that investigating the LIA technique have not reported any instances of local anesthetic toxicity despite the infiltration of large doses of local anesthetic. However, these are small studies on a limited number of patients, and consequently this cannot be extrapolated to mean that there is no risk of local anesthetic systemic toxicity.

*3.12. Chondro- and Myotoxicity.* Local anesthetic agents can be directly toxic to tissues. Continuous infusion of local anesthetic agents into joint cavities has been linked with subsequent chondrolysis [36–38]. It has been postulated that this direct toxic effect may be related to the modulation of the local inflammatory response by local anesthetic agents [23]. Chondrotoxicity has not been reported following the use of LIA for THA. Patients undergoing this surgery usually have preexisting severe degeneration of the joint with associated loss of cartilage, hence the need for joint replacement. Myotoxicity—in the form of myopathy—has been reported with local anesthetic use [38, 39]. It is a rare but sometimes serious side effect of local anesthetic application. In comparison with ropivacaine, the extent of bupivacaine-induced muscle lesions was significantly larger in one experimental study [38].

*3.13. Limitations.* The limitations of this paper should be noted. The RCTs investigating LIA to date are small single-centre studies. Other studies may have recruited larger numbers, but these were in the form of retrospective series. The RCTs detailed in this paper vary in their design and quality. Only a proportion of these studies were double-blinded therefore the risk of bias in the outcome reporting of the other studies cannot be excluded. This paper only included studies published in English introducing an inherent publication bias.

## 4. Conclusion

In conclusion, the existing data regarding the use of local infiltration analgesia following total hip arthroplasty consists of the results from a relatively small number of small-moderate-sized clinical trials. The LIA technique has been shown to be an effective analgesic method. It has been proven to be superior to no infiltration, placebo saline infiltration and, in one study, epidural analgesia. It has not been shown to provide additional analgesic or outcome benefit in the setting of a comprehensive multimodal analgesic approach but can be regarded as an effective analgesic method following THA, and consideration should be given to its use by the surgeon and the anesthetist in the planning of the analgesic management strategy for this surgical procedure.

## References


[1] A. R. Jadad, R. A. Moore, D. Carroll et al., "Assessing the quality of reports of randomized clinical trials: is blinding necessary?" *Controlled Clinical Trials*, vol. 17, no. 1, pp. 1–12, 1996.

[2] H. B. J. Fischer and C. J. P. Simanski, "A procedure-specific systematic review and consensus recommendations for analgesia after total hip replacement," *Anaesthesia*, vol. 60, no. 12, pp. 1189–1202, 2005.

[3] P. T. Choi, M. Bhandari, J. Scott, and J. Douketis, "Epidural analgesia for pain relief following hip or knee replacement," *Cochrane Database of Systematic Reviews*, no. 3, p. CD003071, 2003.

[4] A. P. Boezaart, "Perineural infusion of local anesthetics," *Anesthesiology*, vol. 104, no. 4, pp. 872–880, 2006.

[5] B. M. Ilfeld, K. B. Duke, and M. C. Donohue, "The association between lower extremity continuous peripheral nerve blocks and patient falls after knee and hip arthroplasty," *Anesthesia and Analgesia*, vol. 111, no. 6, pp. 1552–1554, 2010.

[6] D. R. Kerr and L. Kohan, "Local infiltration analgesia: a technique for the control of acute postoperative pain following knee and hip surgery: a case study of 325 patients," *Acta Orthopaedica*, vol. 79, no. 2, pp. 174–183, 2008.

[7] K. S. Otte, H. Husted, L. Ø. Andersen, B. B. Kristensen, and H. Kehlet, "Local infiltration analgesia in total knee arthroplasty and hip resurfacing: a methodological study," *Acute Pain*, vol. 10, no. 3-4, pp. 111–116, 2008.

[8] H. K. Parvataneni, V. P. Shah, H. Howard, N. Cole, A. S. Ranawat, and C. S. Ranawat, "Controlling pain after total hip and knee arthroplasty using a multimodal protocol with local periarticular injections. A prospective randomized study," *Journal of Arthroplasty*, vol. 22, no. 6, pp. 33–38, 2007.

[9] M. Bianconi, L. Ferraro, G. C. Traina et al., "Pharmacokinetics and efficacy of ropivacaine continuous wound instillation after joint replacement surgery," *British Journal of Anaesthesia*, vol. 91, no. 6, pp. 830–835, 2003.

[10] L. J. Andersen, T. Poulsen, B. Krogh, and T. Nielsen, "Postoperative analgesia in total hip arthroplasty: a randomized double-blinded, placebo-controlled study on peroperative and postoperative ropivacaine, ketorolac, and adrenaline wound infiltration," *Acta Orthopaedica*, vol. 78, no. 2, pp. 187–192, 2007.

[11] C. A. Busch, M. R. Whitehouse, B. J. Shore, S. J. MacDonald, R. W. McCalden, and R. B. Bourne, "The efficacy of periarticular multimodal drug infiltration in total hip arthroplasty," *Clinical Orthopaedics and Related Research*, vol. 468, no. 8, pp. 2152–2159, 2010.

[12] K. V. Andersen, M. Pfeiffer-Jensen, V. Haraldsted, and K. Søballe, "Reduced hospital stay and narcotic consumption, and improved mobilization with local and intraarticular infiltration after hip arthroplasty: a randomized clinical trial of an intraarticular technique versus epidural infusion in 80 patients," *Acta Orthopaedica*, vol. 78, no. 2, pp. 180–186, 2007.

[13] K. Specht, J. S. Leonhardt, P. Revald et al., "No evidence of a clinically important effect of adding local infusion analgesia administrated through a catheter in pain treatment after total hip arthroplasty," *Acta Orthopaedica*, vol. 82, no. 3, pp. 315–320, 2011.

[14] L. Ø. Andersen, K. S. Otte, H. Husted, L. Gaarn-Larsen, B. Kristensen, and H. Kehlet, "High-volume infiltration analgesia in bilateral hip arthroplasty," *Acta Orthopaedica*, vol. 82, no. 4, pp. 423–426, 2011.

[15] T. H. Lunn, H. Husted, S. Solgaard et al., "Intraoperative local infiltration analgesia for early analgesia after total hip arthroplasty: a randomized, double-blind, placebo-controlled trial," *Regional Anesthesia and Pain Medicine*, vol. 36, no. 5, pp. 424–429, 2011.

[16] D. J. Kopacz, R. L. Carpenter, and D. C. Mackey, "Effect of ropivacaine on cutaneous capillary blood flow in pigs," *Anesthesiology*, vol. 71, no. 1, pp. 69–74, 1989.

[17] D. B. Scott, A. Lee, D. Fagan, G. M. R. Bowler, P. Bloomfield, and R. Lundh, "Acute toxicity of ropivacaine compared with that of bupivacaine," *Anesthesia and Analgesia*, vol. 69, no. 5, pp. 563–569, 1989.

[18] B. J. Swanton and G. D. Shorten, "Anti-inflammatory effects of local anesthetic agents," *International Anesthesiology Clinics*, vol. 41, no. 1, pp. 1–19, 2003.

[19] S. Herroeder, S. Pecher, M. E. Schönherr et al., "Systemic lidocaine shortens length of hospital stay after colorectal surgery: a double-blinded, randomized, placebo-controlled trial," *Annals of Surgery*, vol. 246, no. 2, pp. 192–200, 2007.

[20] J. Cassuto, R. Sinclair, and M. Bonderovic, "Anti-inflammatory properties of local anesthetics and their present and potential clinical implications," *Acta Anaesthesiologica Scandinavica*, vol. 50, no. 3, pp. 265–282, 2006.

[21] M. W. Hollmann and M. E. Durieux, "Local anesthetics and the inflammatory response: a new therapeutic indication?" *Anesthesiology*, vol. 93, no. 3, pp. 858–875, 2000.

[22] K. Hahnenkamp, G. Theilmeier, H. K. van Aken, and C. W. Hoenemann, "The effects of local anesthetics on perioperative coagulation, inflammation, and microcirculation," *Anesthesia and Analgesia*, vol. 94, no. 6, pp. 1441–1447, 2002.

[23] B. Carvalho, D. J. Clark, D. C. Yeomans, and M. S. Angst, "Continuous subcutaneous instillation of bupivacaine compared to saline reduces interleukin 10 and increases substance p in surgical wounds after cesarean delivery," *Anesthesia and Analgesia*, vol. 111, no. 6, pp. 1452–1459, 2010.

[24] C. Stein and C. Zöllner, "Opioids and sensory nerves," in *Handbook of Experimental Pharmacology*, B. J. Canning and D. Spina, Eds., vol. 194 of *Sensory Nerves*, Springer, Heidelberg, Germany, 2009.

[25] C. Stein, M. Schäfer, and H. Machelska, "Attacking pain at its source: new perspectives on opioids," *Nature Medicine*, vol. 9, no. 8, pp. 1003–1008, 2003.

[26] S. A. Mousa, B. P. Cheppudira, M. Shaqura et al., "Nerve growth factor governs the enhanced ability of opioids to suppress inflammatory pain," *Brain*, vol. 130, no. 2, pp. 502–513, 2007.

[27] C. Stein and L. J. Lang, "Peripheral mechanisms of opioid analgesia," *Current Opinion in Pharmacology*, vol. 9, no. 1, pp. 3–8, 2009.

[28] B. W. Stringer, A. K. Singhania, J. E. Sudhakar, and R. B. Brink, "Serum and wound drain ropivacaine concentrations after wound infiltration in joint arthroplasty," *Journal of Arthroplasty*, vol. 22, no. 6, pp. 884–892, 2007.

[29] K. Knudsen, M. Beckman Suurküla, S. Blomberg, J. Sjövall, and N. Edvardsson, "Central nervous and cardiovascular effects of i.v. infusions of ropivacaine, bupivacaine and placebo in volunteers," *British Journal of Anaesthesia*, vol. 78, no. 5, pp. 507–514, 1997.

[30] H. Wulf, F. Worthmann, H. Behnke, and A. S. Bohle, "Pharmacokinetics and pharmacodynamics of ropivacaine 2 mg/ml, 5 mg/ml, or 7.5 mg/ml after ilioinguinal blockade for ilioinguinal hernia repair in adults," *Anesthesia & Analgesia*, vol. 89, pp. 1471–1474, 1999.

[31] D. Wiedemann, B. Mühlnickel, E. Staroske, W. Neumann, and W. Röse, "Ropivacaine plasma concentrations during 120-hour epidural infusion," *British Journal of Anaesthesia*, vol. 85, no. 6, pp. 830–835, 2000.

[32] A. G. L. Burm, R. Stienstra, R. P. Brouwer, B. M. Emanuelsson, and J. W. van Kleef, "Epidural infusion of ropivacaine for postoperative analgesia after major orthopedic surgery: pharmacokinetic evaluation," *Anesthesiology*, vol. 93, no. 2, pp. 395–403, 2000.

[33] S. L. Brown and A. E. Morrison, "Local anesthetic infusion pump systems adverse events reported to the food and drug administration," *Anesthesiology*, vol. 100, no. 5, pp. 1305–1306, 2004.

[34] S. S. Liu, J. M. Richman, R. C. Thirlby, and C. L. Wu, "Efficacy of continuous wound catheters delivering local anesthetic for postoperative analgesia: a quantitative and qualitative systematic review of randomized controlled trials," *Journal of the American College of Surgeons*, vol. 203, no. 6, pp. 914–932, 2006.

[35] S. Rasmussen, M. U. Kramhøft, K. P. Sperling, and J. H. L. Pedersen, "Increased flexion and reduced hospital stay with continuous intraarticular morphine and ropivacaine after primary total knee replacement: open intervention study of efficacy and safety in 154 patients," *Acta Orthopaedica Scandinavica*, vol. 75, no. 5, pp. 606–609, 2004.

[36] B. T. Busfield and D. M. Romero, "Pain pump use after shoulder arthroscopy as a cause of glenohumeral chondrolysis," *Arthroscopy*, vol. 25, no. 6, pp. 647–652, 2009.

[37] S. T. Webb and S. Ghosh, "Intra-articular bupivacaine: potentially chondrotoxic?" *British Journal of Anaesthesia*, vol. 102, no. 4, pp. 439–441, 2009.

[38] W. Zink and B. M. Graf, "Local anesthetic myotoxicity," *Regional Anesthesia and Pain Medicine*, vol. 29, no. 4, pp. 333–340, 2004.

[39] A. Borgeat and J. Aguirre, "Update on local anesthetics," *Current Opinion in Anaesthesiology*, vol. 23, no. 4, pp. 466–471, 2010.

[40] S. Ganapathy, J. Brookes, and R. Bourne, "Local infiltration analgesia," *Journal of Anaesthesiology Clinical Pharmacology*, vol. 29, pp. 329–342, 2011.

[41] H. Kehlet and L. O. Andersen, "Local infiltration analgesia in joint replacement: the evidence and recommendations for clinical practice," *Acta Anaesthesiologica Scandinavica*, vol. 55, no. 7, pp. 778–784, 2011.

[42] R. Tang, H. Evans, A. Chaput, and C. Kim, "Multimodal analgesia for hip arthroplasty," *Orthopedic Clinics of North America*, vol. 40, pp. 377–387, 2009.

5

# Designing and Implementing a Competency-Based Training Program for Anesthesiology Residents at the University of Ottawa

**Emma J. Stodel,[1] Anna Wyand,[2] Simone Crooks,[2] Stéphane Moffett,[2] Michelle Chiu,[2] and Christopher C. C. Hudson[3]**

[1]*Learning 4 Excellence, 749 Long Point Circle, Ottawa, ON, Canada K1T 4H5*
[2]*Department of Anesthesiology, The Ottawa Hospital, 1053 Carling Avenue, Ottawa, ON, Canada K1Y 4E9*
[3]*University of Ottawa Heart Institute, 40 Ruskin Street, Ottawa, ON, Canada K1Y 4W7*

Correspondence should be addressed to Emma J. Stodel; estodel@learning4excellence.com

Academic Editor: Pedro Tanaka

Competency-based medical education is gaining traction as a solution to address the challenges associated with the current time-based models of physician training. Competency-based medical education is an outcomes-based approach that involves identifying the abilities required of physicians and then designing the curriculum to support the achievement and assessment of these competencies. This paradigm defies the assumption that competence is achieved based on time spent on rotations and instead requires residents to demonstrate competence. The Royal College of Physicians and Surgeons of Canada (RCPSC) has launched Competence by Design (CBD), a competency-based approach for residency training and specialty practice. The first residents to be trained within this model will be those in medical oncology and otolaryngology-head and neck surgery in July, 2016. However, with approval from the RCPSC, the Department of Anesthesiology, University of Ottawa, launched an innovative competency-based residency training program July 1, 2015. The purpose of this paper is to provide an overview of the program and offer a blueprint for other programs planning similar curricular reform. The program is structured according to the RCPSC CBD stages and addresses all CanMEDS roles. While our program retains some aspects of the traditional design, we have made many transformational changes.

## 1. Introduction

Around the world, medical education is undergoing a major transformation. Calls for reform in how physicians are trained are longstanding [1]. In many of the current systems, programs define the successful completion of training based on the length of time a trainee is in a program, assuming that trainees will develop the required competencies to practice after a predetermined amount of time. However, factors such as the restrictions around resident duty hours [2], pressure to reduce costs associated with resident training [3], and the need for improved accountability for patient safety [4] have led many countries to consider a competency-based approach to medical education. Competency-based medical education is an outcomes-based approach that involves identifying the abilities required of the physician and then designing the curriculum to support the achievement of these predefined competencies. This paradigm defies the assumption that competence to practice as a fully rounded physician is achieved based on time spent on rotations, that is, through an on-the-job training and/or apprenticeship model [5], and instead requires residents to demonstrate the competencies deemed necessary for patient care. For some trainees, this may require more time than the typical programs, while others may be able to accelerate their training and enter the workforce earlier and/or engage in further specialized training.

By definition, competency-based medical education needs a robust and multifaceted assessment system. Multiple data points are needed to make judgments about residents' competence. Assessments need to occur in a combination of classroom, clinical, and simulated environments and be criterion based. Frequent assessment enables the provision of high quality feedback to guide development of competence and facilitates the early identification of both residents in difficulty and those who may benefit from focused training for rapid advancement.

The Royal College of Physicians and Surgeons of Canada (RCPSC) has launched a multiyear initiative to implement a competency-based medical education approach to residency training in Canada called Competence by Design (CBD) [6]. The RCPSC's CBD program focuses on physicians' lifelong learning from the time they graduate from medical school to retirement. The CBD Competence Continuum [7] breaks down physician education into a series of stages: Transition to Discipline, Foundations of Discipline, Core of Discipline, Transition to Practice, Continuing Professional Development, and Transition out of Professional Practice.

Within each stage of resident training (from Transition to Discipline to Transition to Practice) there are a series of Entrustable Professional Activities (EPAs) and milestones. According to the RCPSC, an EPA "is a task in the clinical setting that may be delegated to a resident by their supervisor once sufficient competence has been demonstrated" [8]. Each EPA typically includes several milestones. Milestones are "observable marker[s] of an individual's ability along a developmental continuum" [8]. So, while an EPA may be considered an end task or activity (e.g., management of cardiac surgery using cardiopulmonary bypass), the milestones are the abilities of the individual needed to be able to complete the task (e.g., place and interpret a pulmonary artery catheter). The expectation from the RCPSC is that milestones will be used to design curriculum and then EPAs used to assess resident competence [8]. If a resident is struggling with an EPA, the milestones can be examined to see which individual abilities the resident is lacking and thus determine where focused training and support are needed.

The first two specialties to implement the RCPSC's CBD program will be medical oncology and otolaryngology-head and neck surgery in 2016. However, following the successful application for a Fundamental Innovations in Residency Education (FIRE) project (http://www.royalcollege.ca/portal/page/portal/rc/resources/publications/oe_news/vol6_1/fire_project) from the RCPSC, the Department of Anesthesiology, University of Ottawa, launched a competency-based residency training program on July 1, 2015, two years ahead of the RCPSC schedule for national implementation of CBD for anesthesiology. This is the second program in Canada to make this transformational change (following the orthopedic surgery residency program in Toronto). The purpose of this paper is to provide an overview of the University of Ottawa anesthesiology competency-based residency program and to offer a blueprint for other programs that plan to reform their training to meet 21st century healthcare needs.

## 2. Methods

While the entire faculty of the Department of Anesthesiology is involved in this initiative, a smaller Education Design Steering Group guided the conceptual design of the program and submitted the FIRE project application to the RCPSC. The FIRE proposal described the EPAs and milestones for the program based on the National Curriculum for Canadian Anesthesia Residency [9], as well as innovative and nontraditional approaches for teaching and assessment designed to support and evaluate residents' achievement of the EPAs and milestones. The Education Design Steering Group defined EPAs that are to be achieved by the end of the program, with milestones for each stage of training. This is in contrast to the RCPSC that has defined EPAs for each stage of training. The proposed program also eliminates curricula that do not contribute to the achievement of the defined EPAs and milestones, thus maximizing clinical exposure to include only those critical elements for the practice of anesthesia. As a result, residents who demonstrate all required competencies without the need for remediation will be able to complete their training in four years instead of the current five-year minimum as per the RCPSC specialty training requirements in anesthesiology [10]. With the FIRE project approved by the RCPSC, the Department of Anesthesiology started work on further developing the new curriculum. The objectives for the new competency-based program were as follows:

(1) To adopt an outcomes-based approach to program and curriculum design by

   (a) using an evidence-based approach to develop EPAs and milestones to shape a modular curriculum;
   (b) leveraging faculty expertise in the development of EPAs and milestones.

(2) To develop a curriculum that cultivates and assesses competency in all seven CanMEDS roles equally [11].

(3) To use a learner-centered approach that emphasizes active learning processes and recognizes that trainees learn differently and at different speeds.

(4) To build in opportunities to encourage resident self-reflection as a means of learning and self-assessment [12].

(5) To create a modular-based spiral curriculum that revisits and reinforces core and subspecialty competencies of anesthesia.

(6) To develop a robust formative and summative assessment approach.

(7) To control progression through the program based on achievement of milestones through formative and summative assessments and thus identify residents in difficulty early and establish appropriate supports.

(8) To establish a faculty development program to support the implementation of the new program.

(9) To support change management as appropriate for faculty and residents.

(10) To disseminate best practices for teaching and assessment nationally and internationally.

(11) To engage in continuous evaluation of the program both internally and externally during both the development and implementation stages.

(12) To identify economies of scale and economies of scope as appropriate in the development of learning and assessment strategies.

## 3. Program Description

The new competency-based anesthesiology residency program at the University of Ottawa is structured according to the RCPSC CBD stages [7]: Transition to Discipline, Foundations of Discipline, Core of Discipline, and Transition to Practice. The instructional design of the residency training stages is geared towards the assessment and achievement of the EPAs and milestones and is described in the following sections.

*3.1. Transition to Discipline.* Transition to Discipline comprises one four-week rotation (one block) on general adult anesthesia that serves as an introduction and orientation to the specialty, the university, and the Department of Anesthesiology. Further, it provides an opportunity to assess residents' clinical skills and knowledge and to orient them to on-call activities through a "buddy call" system. "Buddy call" involves pairing the novice resident with a more senior resident deemed competent for independent call. Two faculty member leads (Anna Wyand and Stéphane Moffett) were recruited and, in consultation with an educational expert (Emma J. Stodel), were responsible for designing the curriculum and assessment approaches for this stage of training.

Residents are provided with an orientation package and required reading two weeks prior to the start of the program. Transition to Discipline starts with an orientation day where residents are oriented to both the physical locations within which they will practice and logistical resources they will require during residency. They are introduced to the process for setting up invasive hemodynamic monitors and point-of-care testing systems.

Following orientation, residents engage in daily elective and on-call clinical anesthesia. Clinical exposure is standardized for all residents. Residents are responsible for completing a number of tasks described on the Anesthesia Resident Checklist. This checklist serves as a guide to continue to orient residents to the locations, equipment, and on-call responsibilities they will be working towards achieving over the course of Transition to Discipline. Residents are also required to seek feedback on seven supervised clinical skills including endotracheal intubation, intravenous cannulation, and postanesthesia care unit (PACU) handover to a registered nurse. A mandatory lecture series provides introductions to the CanMEDS framework [13], the preoperative and intraoperative patient management software, and how to safely check the anesthesia machines.

During Transition to Discipline, residents are assessed on their clinical competence using the Clinical Case Assessment Tool (CCAT), an online daily assessment tool used to assess competence in all CanMEDS roles (see full description in Section 3.6). Knowledge is assessed using the Anesthesia Knowledge Test 1 (AKT-1 pretest) (http://www.metricsinc.org/akt-testing.html), which assesses their incoming knowledge, and the AKT-1 posttest administered one month later (at the start of Foundations of Discipline). Residents who fail to complete the educational requirements within the four weeks of Transition to Discipline must remediate during the following two weeks in order to be permitted to continue in the Foundations of Discipline stage.

*3.2. Foundations of Discipline.* Foundations of Discipline comprises a 12-week (three-block) Boot Camp followed by a 12-week (three-block) clinical component. One faculty member was recruited to design Boot Camp (Simone Crooks) and two were recruited to design the clinical component of the stage (Anna Wyand and Stéphane Moffett).

The Foundations Boot Camp is designed to accelerate the development of junior residents' technical and nontechnical skills in a safe learning environment so they are at a relatively advanced level when in the clinical environment providing patient care. The Boot Camp approach has gained a lot of attention recently, especially in the surgical fields [14–18]. Boot Camps enable residents to develop clinical skills in a lower stress environment with less time pressure than they would face in a clinical setting, and they let residents self-reflect and receive feedback in a nonthreatening environment. Further, deficiencies in skills and knowledge can be identified early and remediated.

A typical Boot Camp week in our new competency-based anesthesiology program comprises two days of clinical work; two days of instructional sessions that include partial task training, workshops, lectures, and problem-based learning; and one day of high fidelity simulation. Residents complete 18 high fidelity simulation scenarios geared towards a junior level of training. Simulation sessions are formatively assessed and residents engage in a formal debriefing with faculty simulation instructors. Lectures in Boot Camp cover both clinical topics and the intrinsic CanMEDS roles. In addition, residents complete the following courses: Advanced Trauma Life Support (ATLS), Advanced Cardiac Life Support (ACLS), and Acute Critical Events Simulation (ACES) (an interactive course on the acute resuscitation of critically ill patients and the management of crisis situations).

Following successful completion of Boot Camp, residents progress to the clinical component of Foundations. This provides them with the opportunity to consolidate their knowledge of basic anesthesiology and refine their technical skills in the clinical setting. Over the course of the 12-week clinical component, the residents are scheduled in the main operating room, the obstetrical operating room, and the preoperative assessment unit and acute pain service. Similar to Transition to Discipline, residents are given a checklist of tasks they must complete. During this part of their training, residents transition from "buddy call" to solo call responsibilities.

Assessment is multifaceted. Formative assessment of simulated crisis management in Boot Camp involves the use of checklists following partial task training workshops, online modules, and postcrisis management reflective exercises. As with Transition to Discipline, clinical competence is assessed using the CCAT. In addition, attending staff use checklists to assess the residents' skills with epidural and spinal techniques. Summative assessment includes the AKT-6 six months into the program and an eight-station Objective Structured Clinical Examination (OSCE) designed to assess the Foundations of Discipline milestones. Two expert raters judge residents' performance on the OSCE at each station using modified Delphi-derived checklists and the Managing Emergencies in Pediatric Anesthesia Global Rating Scale (MEPA GRS) [19]. Residents who fail to meet the milestones of Foundations of Discipline do not progress to the next stage of training.

*3.3. Core of Discipline.* Core of Discipline comprises 13 subspecialty-specific modules based on the National Curriculum for Canadian Anesthesia Residency [9]: acute pain, airway, cardiac anesthesia, chronic pain, clinical pharmacology and complex surgery, neuroanesthesia, obstetrical anesthesia, pediatric anesthesia, perioperative medicine, regional anesthesia, remote location anesthesia, thoracic anesthesia, and vascular anesthesia. The Core of Discipline stage is divided into Core I and Core II, equivalent to junior and senior residency, respectively, over 40 four-week blocks. Core II revisits and reinforces more advanced core and subspecialty competencies of anesthesia first addressed in Core I. Subspecialty experts were recruited as Module Leads and were responsible for designing the curriculum and assessment approaches for their module with the support of an educational expert (Emma J. Stodel).

Each module has predefined educational requirements designed to help residents achieve the defined milestones and EPAs. Educational activities include presenting rounds; partial task training; participating in required clinical case experiences, procedures, and techniques; preparing for and writing case summaries; and completing learning cases specific to each module. The learning cases are designed to replace the RCPSC mandated core academic half-days, which usually comprise expert-led lectures that are typically not synchronized with relevant clinical experiences. Our learning cases are linked to the module the resident is in so residents learn topics relevant to their current clinical context. For example, if they are in the pediatrics module they only complete pediatric learning cases.

The learning cases are based on the format of the RCPSC oral examinations. Residents are provided with a case scenario followed by questions to direct their learning, as well as selected resources (e.g., journal articles, textbook chapters, videos, and learning activities). Residents are expected to spend one to one-and-a-half hours engaged in self-directed learning for each case. They then meet with a staff anesthesiologist to discuss the case and are assessed against the expected level of competence defined in the case. This design enables residents to complete the cases when and where they choose and spend as long on each case as required. By reviewing the topic before interacting with staff, the staff-resident discussions can be at a more advanced level, mirroring a "flipped classroom" [20]. The content of the learning cases is resource based and curated by subject matter experts, thus minimizing demands on staff time for case creation. Staff have also shown interest in using these cases for their own Continuing Professional Development.

Learning cases are delivered through a custom-built electronic system that stores and manages access to cases, tracks completion, and documents assessment. Permission settings restrict access to the staff versions of the cases that list the critical features that residents need to cover to demonstrate understanding and determine who can assess residents on the cases. Data from this system will be automatically fed into in-training evaluation reports (ITERs) so evaluators know whether module requirements have been satisfied, as well as to a central dashboard that will provide a summary of resident progress. An overview of the learning case platform can be found at https://www.youtube.com/watch?v=OLirP-QjFQA.

Simulation-based education continues through this and the next stage of training with a four-year rotation of core topics via the Global Simulation Curriculum. Delivery of this curriculum is coordinated by the Department of Anesthesiology Simulation Director (Michelle Chiu). In Core of Discipline and Transition to Practice, residents complete 33 high fidelity simulation scenarios of higher complexity than those experienced in Foundations of Discipline. The scenarios are designed to reflect rare, but important, clinical situations that residents may never be exposed to in residency and/or clinical situations that are critical to competency as an anesthesiologist. Fifty percent of all simulation scenarios are interprofessional and this proportion is growing. All the simulation scenarios focus on the intrinsic CanMEDS roles, as well as the role of Medical Expert. Objectives come from the Association of Canadian University Departments of Anesthesia (ACUDA) National Curriculum for Canadian Anesthesia Residency document [9]. During Core of Discipline and Transition to Practice, residents also participate in several interdisciplinary high fidelity simulation sessions with other specialties, such as obstetrics/gynecology, surgery, and emergency medicine.

Module Leads determined how competency is assessed in their module. Assessment tools include the CCAT, checklists, multiple-choice examinations, short answer questions, and case summaries where residents are required to reflect on the case and make links to best practices and the literature. Residents are formatively assessed following simulation scenarios and summatively assessed against the ACLS and Canadian National Anesthesiology Simulation Curriculum (CanNASC) Simulation Milestones. Assessment of a resident's management of a perioperative cardiac arrest (ACLS Simulation Milestone) occurs midway through the training program using high fidelity simulation. The CanNASC Simulation Milestone is assessed at the end of Core of Discipline using nationally developed and standardized high fidelity simulation scenarios and accompanying rubrics.

If residents fail to meet the required competencies by the end of Core I and Core II they complete supplemental blocks focusing on remediating gaps in their knowledge and skills before progressing to the next stage of training (i.e., Core II or Transition to Practice).

*3.4. Transition to Practice.* Transition to Practice is the final stage of CBD and is designed to prepare residents for autonomous practice. Residents engage in independent practice across a wide scope of subspecialties, working, in effect, as junior staff members. Staff anesthesiologists are immediately available to assess, guide reflection, and provide support as needed. As in the earlier stages of training, residents are required to complete a checklist of tasks and complete simulation scenarios and continue to be assessed using the CCAT. Further, they are encouraged to complete oral examination questions daily. The RCPSC specialty examination is a milestone in the Transition to Practice stage and one of a number of requirements for certification. Passing the examination will not lead to certification. The RCPSC will only grant certification when the resident has successfully completed the Transition to Practice stage and received sign-off (using the MAINPORT ePortfolio) from the Program Director. Allowing the resident to practice autonomously while continuing to evaluate competence ensures that we prepare physicians for practice in a way that is fundamentally oriented to graduate success and patient safety.

*3.5. Intrinsic CanMEDS Roles.* The teaching and assessment of the intrinsic CanMEDS roles (Communicator, Collaborator, Leader, Health Advocate, Scholar, and Professional) occurs throughout the program. Faculty member Role Leads are assigned to each role to support the teaching and assessment of the role. The roles are first introduced during Transition to Discipline through a session on the CanMEDS framework [13]. In Foundations of Discipline, each role is addressed through an interactive session involving small group discussions, case-based learning, educational "games" (e.g., scratch card quizzes), role playing, reflections, online modules, self-assessments, and small assignments. For example, for the Collaborator role, residents interview other members of the healthcare team to develop an understanding of their role, responsibilities, skill set, and training. Throughout Core of Discipline and Transition to Practice there are three sessions a year, organized by themes (e.g., ethics in anesthesia practice, safety, and quality improvement in anesthesiology practice), which specifically address the intrinsic roles using similar approaches to those described for Foundations.

The CCAT is used on a daily basis to document competence in the intrinsic roles. Residents are responsible for soliciting feedback on all of the CanMEDS competencies over the course of the block. A counter displays the number of CCATs completed for each role during the current block. Residents and staff are responsible for ensuring that all roles have been assessed and documented before the end of the block.

Competency within the intrinsic CanMEDS roles is further developed through an online coaching platform by encouraging reflection on practice in each of the roles. Residents are expected to post at least one reflection related to each role each year of their training (i.e., at least six posts a year) but are encouraged to post more. Every two months, residents receive an automated email prompting them to reflect on a specific role and post their reflection on the coaching platform within two weeks. Guidelines are provided to assist residents as they reflect. Role Leads support the residents through online coaching to deepen their reflections and develop competence in the intrinsic CanMEDS roles.

*3.6. Clinical Case Assessment Tool (CCAT).* As multiple data points are needed to make judgments about residents' competence, frequent resident assessments are essential to the program's success. We needed a new assessment tool that would be intuitive to use, engage both staff and residents in the assessment process, and assess competence in all CanMEDS roles. We therefore developed the CCAT; an online resident-driven assessment tool that capitalizes on faculty's ability to judge competent clinical performance. The CCAT is designed to increase both face-to-face feedback to residents and resident self-assessment. Residents are required to complete at least 12 CCATs every four-week block throughout the program.

The CCAT was adapted from the validated Ottawa Surgical Competency Operating Room Evaluation (O-SCORE) [21] and is completed electronically on a computer or tablet. The CCAT is initiated by the resident who is required to reflect on his/her performance and assess him/herself prior to receiving assessment and face-to-face feedback from the supervising staff anesthesiologist. Residents enter identifying data about the case and then reflect on what they did well, what they would do differently next time, and the next steps in their learning plan. Responses are organized by CanMEDS role. The resident's self-assessment is then shared with the staff who assesses resident performance on a three-item, five-response option behaviorally anchored scale ranging from "Staff had to do" to "Staff did not need to be there" and documents their assessment of what was done well, what needs to be improved, and next steps for learning. Staff use the resident's device to do this, thus promoting timely face-to-face feedback.

The electronic format of the tool allows data to be easily analyzed and interpreted for evaluation, learning, research, and quality improvement purposes. A video tutorial demonstrating the CCAT can be found at https://www.youtube.com/watch?v=k6-Gj8ZDjhs.

## 4. Conclusion

A paradigm shift is occurring in the way in which physicians are trained. Globally, regulatory bodies are considering a shift to competency-based medical education as an answer to the mounting barriers and challenges of time-based models of training. The RCPSC is in the early stages of implementing the CBD program to all specialty training, with the first programs starting July 1, 2016. The Department of Anesthesiology at the University of Ottawa was granted permission from the RCPSC to pilot a competency-based medical education anesthesiology program two years ahead of the rest of the country. While our program retains some aspects of the traditional design, we made many key changes. First, our program offers the potential for residents to complete the program in four years instead of five if they demonstrate the required competence. The possible reduction in training time represents potential savings to the healthcare system through the provincial government subsidy for residency training. Second, the replacement of academic half-days with learning cases ensures that residents' learning outside the clinical setting is coordinated with their clinical experience and is focused on the subspecialty of the module they are in. Third, assessment is more robust and more frequent. This enables early identification of residents' strengths and weaknesses so remediation and/or tailored learning experiences can be implemented to accelerate learning and progression to new skills and knowledge. Further, the electronic nature of many of the assessments used facilitates tracking and reporting. Fourth, our program clearly defines the educational requirements for each stage of training and module. These must be completed before residents can progress to the next stage of training. Lastly, we have introduced a new, comprehensive curriculum for the teaching and assessment of the intrinsic CanMEDS roles.

This paper provides a comprehensive overview of our implementation of a competency-based approach to resident education and offers a blueprint for other programs planning a similar curricular reform. An in-depth evaluation of the program is underway, guided by a logic model and evaluation framework. Findings from the evaluation will be disseminated as they become available.

## Conflict of Interests

The authors declare that there is no conflict of interests regarding the publication of this paper.

## Acknowledgments

The authors would like to recognize the work of the Education Design Steering Group in the development of this program: (i) Viren Naik, M.D., MEd, F.R.C.P.C., MBA: Professor, Department of Anesthesiology, uOttawa, and Vice-President of Education, The Ottawa Hospital; (ii) Rob Anderson, M.D., F.R.C.P.C.: Assistant Professor and Program Director, Department of Anesthesiology, Northern Ontario School of Medicine; (iii) Sylvain Boet, M.D., MEd, Ph.D.: Assistant Professor, Department of Anesthesiology, uOttawa; (iv) M. Dylan Bould, MBChB, FRCA, MEd: Associate Professor, Department of Anesthesiology, uOttawa; (v) Alan Chaput, BScPhm, D.pharm., M.D., M.S., F.R.C.P.C.: Associate Professor, Department of Anesthesiology, uOttawa, Vice-Chair of Education, Department of Anesthesiology, uOttawa, and Assistant Dean, Postgraduate Medical Education, uOttawa; (vi) Stéphane Moffett, M.D., F.R.C.P.C.: Assistant Professor, Department of Anesthesiology, uOttawa. The authors are also indebted to Dr. Alan Chaput and Dr. Daniel Dubois for their comments on earlier drafts of this paper, as well as to Heather Kelly for her editorial expertise. This program was funded by the Office of Postgraduate Medical Education, the Department of Anesthesiology, and the Faculty of Medicine at the University of Ottawa.

## References

[1] J. R. Frank, L. S. Snell, O. Ten Cate et al., "Competency-based medical education: theory to practice," *Medical Teacher*, vol. 32, no. 8, pp. 638–645, 2010.

[2] Canadian Association of Internes & Residents, "Position Paper on Resident Duty Hours. Canadian Patient and Physician Safety and Wellbeing: Resident Duty Hours," 2012, http://residentdoctors.ca/wp-content/uploads/2015/09/POSITION-PAPER-Resident-Duty-Hours-EN.pdf.

[3] Canadian Federation of Medical Students, "Debt Repayment and Interest Deferral on Canada Student Loans Until the Completion of Medical Training," 2009, http://www.cfms.org/downloads/LobbyDay2009english.pdf.

[4] Royal College of Physicians and Surgeons of Canada, "Competence by Design: Reshaping Canadian Medical Education," 2014, http://www.royalcollege.ca/portal/page/portal/rc/common/documents/educational_initiatives/rc_competency-by-design_ebook_e.pdf.

[5] T. Dornan, "Osler, Flexner, apprenticeship and 'the new medical education,'" *Journal of the Royal Society of Medicine*, vol. 98, no. 3, pp. 91–95, 2005.

[6] Royal College of Physicians and Surgeons of Canada, "Competence by Design (CBD): Moving towards competency-based medical education," http://www.royalcollege.ca/portal/page/portal/rc/resources/cbme.

[7] Royal College of Physicians and Surgeons of Canada, "The CBD Competence Continuum," 2015, http://www.royalcollege.ca/portal/page/portal/rc/common/documents/canmeds/framework/competence_continuum_diagram_e.pdf.

[8] Royal College of Physicians and Surgeons of Canada, "Milestones and EPAs: practical and manageable teaching and assessment in residency training," http://www.royalcollege.ca/portal/page/portal/rc/canmeds/canmeds2015/milestones.

[9] M. Levine, P. Murphy, J. Stewart, and D. Pierce, Eds., *National Curriculum for Canadian Anesthesiology Residency*, 1st edition, 2014, https://www.mcgill.ca/anesthesia/files/anesthesia/national_curriculum_2014_8.pdf.

[10] Royal College of Physicians and Surgeons of Canada, "Specialty Training Requirements in Anesthesiology," 2006, https://www.medicine.mcgill.ca/postgrad/accreditation_2013/PSQs/1_Anesthesiology/06_STR_Anesthesiology_2006.pdf.

[11] J. R. Frank and D. Danoff, "The CanMEDS initiative: implementing an outcomes-based framework of physician competencies," *Medical Teacher*, vol. 29, no. 7, pp. 642–647, 2007.

[12] D. Schön, *The Reflective Practitioner*, Jossey-Bass, San Francisco, Calif, USA, 1983.

[13] J. R. Frank, L. Snell, and J. Sherbino, *Draft CanMEDS 2015 Physician Competency Framework—Series IV*, The Royal College of Physicians and Surgeons of Canada, Ottawa, Canada, 2015, http://www.royalcollege.ca/portal/page/portal/rc/common/documents/canmeds/framework/canmeds2015_framework_series_IV_e.pdf.

[14] R. R. Sonnadara, A. Van Vliet, O. Safir et al., "Orthopedic boot camp: examining the effectiveness of an intensive surgical skills course," *Surgery*, vol. 149, no. 6, pp. 745–749, 2011.

[15] R. M. Esterl Jr., D. L. Henzi, and S. M. Cohn, "Senior medical student 'Boot Camp': can result in increased self-confidence before starting surgery internships," *Current Surgery*, vol. 63, no. 4, pp. 264–268, 2006.

[16] E. R. Cohen, J. H. Barsuk, F. Moazed et al., "Making july safer: simulation-based mastery learning during intern boot camp," *Academic Medicine*, vol. 88, no. 2, pp. 233–239, 2013.

[17] A. A. Min, L. R. Stoneking, K. H. Grall, and K. Spear-Ellinwood, "Implementation of the introductory clinician development series: an optional boot camp for emergency medicine interns," in *Advances in Medical Education and Practice*, vol. 5, pp. 275–279, Dove Medical Press, Auckland, New Zealand, 2014.

[18] A. Nishisaki, R. Hales, K. Biagas et al., "A multi-institutional high-fidelity simulation 'boot camp' orientation and training program for first year pediatric critical care fellows," *Pediatric Critical Care Medicine*, vol. 10, no. 2, pp. 157–281, 2009.

[19] T. C. Everett, E. Ng, D. Power et al., "The Managing Emergencies in Paediatric Anaesthesia global rating scale is a reliable tool for simulation-based assessment in pediatric anesthesia crisis management," *Paediatric Anaesthesia*, vol. 23, no. 12, pp. 1117–1123, 2013.

[20] E. Mazur, *Peer Instruction: A User's Manual*, Prentice-Hall, Upper Saddle River, NJ, USA, 1997.

[21] W. T. Gofton, N. L. Dudek, T. J. Wood, F. Balaa, and S. J. Hamstra, "The Ottawa Surgical Competency Operating Room Evaluation (O-SCORE): a tool to assess surgical competence," *Academic Medicine*, vol. 87, no. 10, pp. 1401–1407, 2012.

6

# Anesthesia with Propofol versus Sevoflurane: Does the Longer Neuromuscular Block under Sevoflurane Anesthesia Reduce Laryngeal Injuries?

**Thomas Mencke,[1] Amelie Zitzmann,[1] Susann Machmueller,[1] Arne Boettcher,[2] Martin Sauer,[1] Hans-Wilhelm Pau,[2] Gabriele Noeldge-Schomburg,[1] and Steffen Dommerich[2]**

[1] *Department of Anesthesia and Intensive Care Medicine, University of Rostock, Schillingallee 35, 18057 Rostock, Germany*
[2] *Department of Otorhinolaryngology, University of Rostock, 18057 Rostock, Germany*

Correspondence should be addressed to Thomas Mencke; thomas.mencke@googlemail.com

Academic Editor: Kouichiro Minami

Anesthesia can be maintained with propofol or sevoflurane. Volatile anesthetics increase neuromuscular block of muscle relaxants. We tested the hypothesis, that sevoflurane would cause less vocal cord injuries than an intravenous anesthesia with propofol. In this prospective trial, 65 patients were randomized in 2 groups: SEVO group, anesthesia with sevoflurane, and TIVA group, total intravenous anesthesia with propofol. Intubating and extubating conditions were evaluated. Vocal cord injuries were examined by stroboscopy before and 24 and 72 h after surgery; hoarseness and sore throat were assessed up to 72 h after surgery. Hoarseness and sore throat were comparable between both groups (not significant). Similar findings were observed for vocal cord injuries: 9 (SEVO) versus 5 (TIVA) patients; $P = 0.36$; the overall incidence was 24%. Type of vocal cord injuries: 9 erythema and 5 edema of the vocal folds. Neuromuscular block was significantly longer in the SEVO group compared with the TIVA group: 71 (range: 38–148) min versus 52 (range: 21–74) min; $P < 0.001$. Five patients (TIVA group) versus 11 patients (SEVO group) needed neostigmine to achieve a TOF ratio of 1.0 ($P = 0.14$). Under anesthesia with propofol laryngeal injuries were not increased; the risk for residual curarization, however, was lower compared with sevoflurane.

## 1. Introduction

We showed that tracheal intubation with atracurium significantly decreased vocal cord injuries compared with tracheal intubation without muscle relaxants (8% versus 42%) [1]. Tracheal intubation with atracurium at maximum neuromuscular block, however, did not decrease vocal cord injuries compared with tracheal intubation two minutes after injection of atracurium; the overall incidence was 27%, that is, higher than described in the literature (up to 12%) [2]. Maybe vocal cord injuries did not only occur during tracheal intubation but also during surgery and during removal of the tracheal tube.

Volatile anesthetics increase neuromuscular block of muscle relaxants; anesthesia induction with desflurane increased neuromuscular block compared with a total intravenous anesthesia [3]. Thus, sevoflurane as part of the anesthesia would increase neuromuscular block; moreover, sevoflurane would lengthen neuromuscular block; vocal cords, therefore, would be longer relaxed. We speculated that sevoflurane would cause less vocal cord injuries than propofol during surgery and after removal of the tracheal tube.

After surgery, we assessed hoarseness, sore throat, and vocal cord injuries—by stroboscopy—up to 72 hours. We expected that the patients receiving sevoflurane would have had a lower incidence and severity of hoarseness and vocal cord injuries than the patients receiving an intravenous anesthesia with propofol.

## 2. Methods

The study was performed at the University Hospital of Rostock, Germany, between August 2010 and October 2011. Ethical approval for this study (registration number: A 2010 29) was provided by the Institutional Review Committee (Ethikkommission der Universitat Rostock, Rostock, Germany) on 10 May 2010. The study was registrated at ClinicalTrialsGov under number NCT01616966.

After obtaining written informed consent, we studied 65 adult patients, aged 18–80 yr, ASA I–III, undergoing orotracheal intubation for surgery of the ear. All patients were examined by stroboscopy one day before surgery and were excluded from the study when preexisting pathologies of the vocal cords were found. Exclusion criteria were obesity (defined as body mass index (BMI) > 40 kg/m$^2$), an allergy against the study drugs, and patients with a known or suspected difficult airway (Mallampati score 3 or 4 and a mouth opening < 3.5 cm).

*2.1. Randomization and Monitoring.* Patients were randomized—by a study nurse—in two groups, according to the randomization list, which was prepared via a computer-generated randomization program, as follows [4]: SEVO group, receiving sevoflurane during anesthesia, or TIVA group, receiving an intravenous anesthesia with propofol. We used neuromuscular monitoring to have comparable muscular block at time of intubation in both groups; neuromuscular monitoring was performed with the TOF Watch SX device (Organon Teknika, Eppelheim, Germany). We used neuromonitoring to have comparable depth of anesthesia between the study groups; neuromonitoring was performed with the BIS Vista brain monitoring system (Aspect Medical Systems, Norwood, MA, USA).

The acceleromyographic measurements were done according to the guidelines of Good clinical research practice in pharmacodynamic studies of neuromuscular blocking agents from 2007 [5]. We used a calibrated TOF watch SX. After recalibration of the acceleromyography, rocuronium 0.45 mg/kg was injected over 5 s. Time to a train-of-four (TOF) ratio of 1.0 (defined as the time from start of injection of rocuronium until the TOF ratio reached 1.0) was measured.

The bispectral index (BIS) monitoring was applied according to the manufacturer's guidelines; BIS Quatro sensor electrodes were placed on the patient's forehead. The BIS values were noted continuously every minute during surgery. The target BIS was between 40 and 50. In the TIVA group, propofol infusion was increased from 4.0 mg/kg/h by 1.0 mg/kg/h than the BIS value was above 50; propofol infusion was decreased by 1.0 mg/kg/h than the BIS value was under 40 (minimum dosage was 4.0 mg/kg/h). In the SEVO group, sevoflurane was increased by 0.1 vol.% than the BIS value was above 50; sevoflurane was decreased by 0.1 vol.% than the BIS value was under 40 (minimum concentration was 1.0 vol.%).

*2.2. Induction and Maintenance of Anesthesia.* One hour before the beginning of surgery, the patients received midazolam 7.5 mg orally. Induction was standardized for both groups. Remifentanil 0.4 $\mu$g/kg/min was applied continuously for 2 min; afterwards, propofol 2.0 mg/kg was administered. After calibration of the TOF Watch SX, rocuronium 0.45 mg/kg was given. If the neuromuscular block was incomplete, rocuronium 0.15 mg/kg was added. Tracheal intubation was performed, when maximum block was achieved. All tracheal intubations were performed by the same anesthesiologist to control interindividual differences.

Maintenance of anesthesia was standardized; TIVA group: propofol 4.0 mg/kg/h and remifentanil 0.25–0.35 $\mu$g/kg/min; SEVO group: sevoflurane 1.0 vol.% in a 50% oxygen-air mixture and remifentanil 0.25–0.35 $\mu$g/kg/min. Fifteen minutes before the expected end of surgery, all patients received piritramide 0.05–0.1 mg/kg i.v. The patient's tracheas were extubated, when the TOF ratio was 1.0 and patients opened their eyes or began to cough; afterwards, the patients were moved to the postanesthesia care unit (PACU).

*2.3. Assessment of Hoarseness, Sore Throat, and Vocal Cord Injuries.* Hoarseness was defined as an acoustic quality that was different than the previous voice quality of the patient [6]. Sore throat was defined as continuous throat pain [7]. In the PACU and 24 h, 48 h, and 72 h after surgery, an investigator blinded to the group assignment of the patients assessed the incidence and severity of hoarseness and sore throat (see Appendix). If hoarseness or sore throat persisted over 72 h, a daily follow-up examination was performed until complete restitution. Vocal cord injuries were assessed by laryngostroboscopy by an ear-nose-throat physician who was unaware of the patient's group assignment (see Appendix); all examinations were performed by the same ear-nose-throat physician.

Compared to indirect laryngoscopy, laryngostroboscopy can detect functional disorders of the vocal cords, such as dysfunction of the mucosal wave. All patients were examined by stroboscopy 24 h after surgery. When hoarseness was lasting longer than 48 h, a second stroboscopy was performed 72 h after surgery.

*2.4. Assessment of Intubating Conditions, Intubating Variables, and Extubating Conditions.* The intubating conditions were assessed according to the consensus conference on Good Clinical Research Practice (GCRP) in Pharmacodynamic Studies of Neuromuscular Blocking Agents [5]. In addition, the following variables were assessed: Cormack's grades, time for intubation, the number of intubation attempts (see Appendix), and the extubating conditions—excellent = no coughing, good = slight coughing, and poor = sustained coughing during removing of the tracheal tube. The following factors were standardized: tube size (men: ID = 8.0 mm; women: ID = 7.0 mm), type of tube, and cuff inflation with air (cuff pressure was ≤25 mmHg) [1, 8].

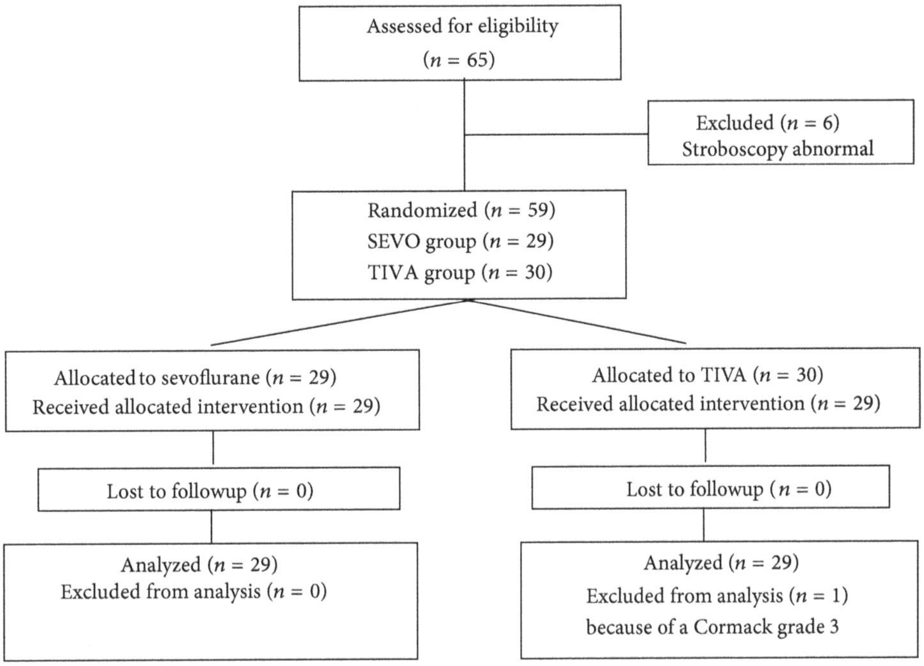


FIGURE 1: Flow diagram of patient distribution. Sevoflurane = anesthesia with sevoflurane and remifentanil. TIVA = anesthesia with propofol and remifentanil.

TABLE 1: Demographic data, duration of surgery, and anesthesia.

| | SEVO group ($n$ = 29) | TIVA group ($n$ = 29) | $P$ value |
|---|---|---|---|
| Age (yr) | 47 (17) | 49 (15) | 0.76 |
| Weight (kg) | 75.0 (14.2) | 81.2 (16.8) | 0.13 |
| Height (cm) | 172.2 (8.9) | 173.5 (9.8) | 0.61 |
| Body mass index (kg/m$^2$) | 25.2 (4.1) | 26.7 (3.1) | 0.13 |
| Gender ratio (female/male) | 15/14 | 11/18 | 0.43 |
| Smoking | 10 (34%) | 12 (41%) | 0.78 |
| Reflux | 3 (10%) | 4 (14%) | 1.00 |
| Duration of surgery (min) | 75 (37) | 73 (33) | 0.87 |
| Duration of anesthesia (min) | 102 (36) | 94 (34) | 0.33 |

Values are mean (SD) or numbers (%). SEVO group: anesthesia with sevoflurane and remifentanil. TIVA group: anesthesia with propofol and remifentanil.

*2.5. Statistical Analysis.* Statistical analysis was performed using the SigmaStat for Windows Version 3.5, (Systat Sotware Inc., San Jose, California, USA). Demographic data were analyzed using Mann-Whitney $U$-test or $t$-test; results are presented as mean (SD) or as median (range). Comparisons between groups were performed using the $\chi^2$ test, Fisher's exact test, or Kruskal-Wallis' ANOVA test. Results were considered statistically significant, when $P < 0.05$.

The sample size calculation was based on the study by Maruyama et al. [9]. The required number of patients for our study groups was calculated on the assumption that 55% of the patients suffered from hoarseness after a total intravenous anesthesia [9] and 16% after an anesthesia with desflurane [1]. For an 80% power and an $\alpha = 0.05$, 52 patients (26 patients in each group) were needed. To compensate for possible drop-outs, we enrolled 59 patients (10% more than needed).

## 3. Results

Six patients (10%) had preexisting pathologies at the vocal folds; consequently, these patients were excluded from the study. 59 patients were randomized for the study, 30 patients in the TIVA group, and 29 patients in the SEVO group. One patient—from the TIVA group—was excluded because of a Cormack grade 3 (Figure 1). There were no significant differences in the patient's characteristics (Table 1). Dosages of propofol, remifentanil, and rocuronium and end-tidal concentrations of sevoflurane are shown in Table 2.

*3.1. Intubating Conditions, Intubating Variables, and Extubating Conditions.* The patient's tracheas were extubated at a TOF ratio of 1.0. Patients in the SEVO group had a significantly longer neuromuscular block compared with the

Table 2: Doses of rocuronium, propofol, remifentanil, and end-tidal concentrations of sevoflurane and administration of neostigmine.

| | SEVO group ($n$ = 29) | TIVA group ($n$ = 29) | $P$ value |
|---|---|---|---|
| Propofol for induction of anesthesia (mg) | 150 (100–280) | 170 (90–260) | 0.37 |
| Remifentanil ($\mu$g/kg/min)* | 0.256 (0.015) | 0.259 (0.026) | 0.98 |
| Propofol (mg/kg/h)* | — | 4.9 (0.8) | |
| Sevoflurane (vol.%)† | 1.3 (0.3) | — | |
| Rocuronium (mg) | 30 (25–55) | 40 (25–70) | 0.17 |
| Administration of neostigmine ($n$) | 11 | 5 | 0.14 |

Values are mean (SD), median (range), or numbers. SEVO group: anesthesia with sevoflurane and remifentanil. TIVA group: anesthesia with propofol and remifentanil. *Mean dosage during maintenance of anesthesia. †Mean end-tidal concentration of sevoflurane during anesthesia.

Table 3: Neuromuscular measurements, intubating variables, and coughing during removal of the tracheal tube.

| | SEVO group ($n$ = 29) | TIVA group ($n$ = 29) | $P$ value |
|---|---|---|---|
| Neuromuscular measurements | | | |
| Time till TOF ratio = 1.0 (min) | 71 (38–148) | 52 (21–74) | <0.001 |
| Time without relaxation (min) | 14 (2–151) | 34 (0–118) | 0.03 |
| Intubating variables | | | |
| Cormack grades 1/2 | 17/12 | 19/10 | 0.78 |
| Time for intubation (s) | 16 (9–170) | 16 (9–26) | 0.49 |
| Attempts ($n$) 1/2/3 | 25/3/1 | 29/0/0 | 0.12 |
| Extubating conditions | | | |
| Coughing | 17 (59%) | 22 (76%) | 0.26 |

Values are median (range) or numbers (%). Time till TOF ratio = 1.0 (min) = time from start of injection of rocuronium until the TOF ratio reached 1.0. Time without relaxation = time from TOF ratio of 1.0 till tracheal extubation. SEVO group = anesthesia with sevoflurane and remifentanil. TIVA group = anesthesia with propofol and remifentanil.

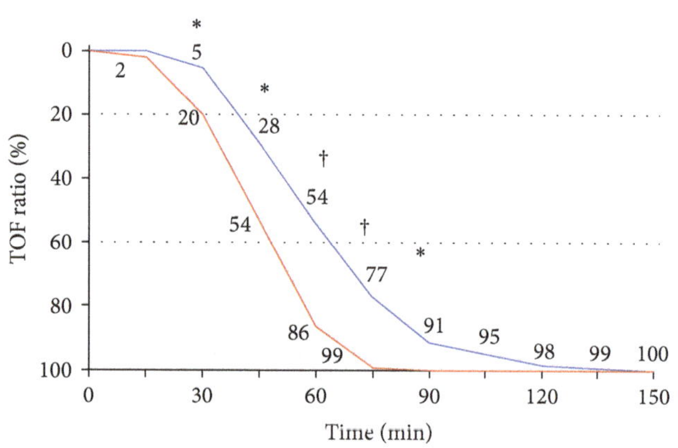


Figure 2: Mean TOF ratio values during surgery in patients receiving sevoflurane (SEVO group; upper blue line) or propofol (TIVA group; lower red line). *$P$ = 0.003 SEVO group versus TIVA group. †$P$ < 0.001 SEVO group versus TIVA group.

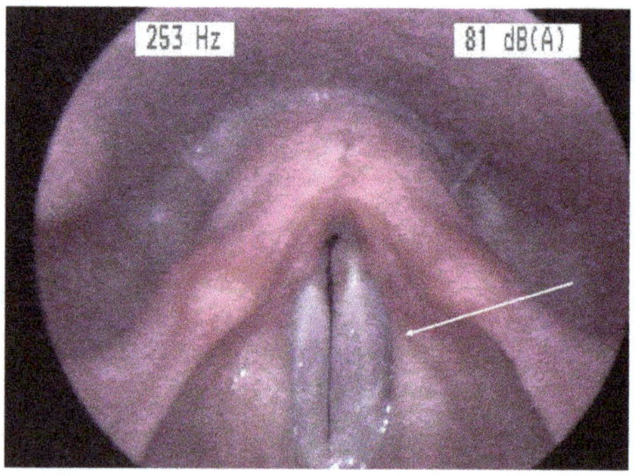


Figure 3: Edema of the left vocal cord (arrow) at 24 h after surgery (sevoflurane group).

TIVA group (Table 3; Figure 2). Tracheal intubation was successful in all patients of both groups. Intubating variables and intubating conditions were comparable (not significant). Overall 39 patients (67%) had coughing during removal of tracheal tubes; 17 (59%) patients in the SEVO group versus 22 (76%) patients in the TIVA group; $P$ = 0.26 (Table 3).

*3.2. Hoarseness, Sore Throat and Vocal Cord Injuries.* The overall incidence (TIVA and SEVO groups together) of hoarseness was 10% (6 patients); the overall incidence of sore throat was 15% (9 patients). The incidence was comparable between groups (Table 4); the severity was comparable, too (data not shown). The overall incidence of vocal cord injuries after surgery was 24% (14 patients). There was no significant difference between the TIVA and SEVO groups: 5 versus 9 patients ($P$ = 0.36). No patient suffered from hoarseness or had vocal cord injuries longer than 3 days. Vocal cord injuries were edema in 7 patients and erythema in 7 patients (Figure 3); there were no hematoma and no granuloma. The majority of vocal cord injuries were unilateral (left: 3; right: 6 patients); 5 patients had bilateral vocal cord injuries (1 patient;

Table 4: Incidence of hoarseness, sore throat, and vocal cord injuries.

| | Hoarseness | | | Sore throat | | | Vocal cord injuries | | |
|---|---|---|---|---|---|---|---|---|---|
| | SEVO ($n = 29$) | TIVA ($n = 29$) | $P$ value | SEVO ($n = 29$) | TIVA ($n = 29$) | $P$ value | SEVO ($n = 29$) | TIVA ($n = 29$) | $P$ value |
| PACU | 2 | 2 | 1.00 | 2 | 1 | 1.00 | — | — | — |
| At 24 h | 1 | 1 | 1.00 | 5 | 2 | 0.42 | 9 | 5 | 0.36 |
| At 48 h | 0 | 0 | — | 2 | 1 | 1.00 | — | — | — |
| At 72 h | 0 | 0 | — | 1 | 1 | 1.00 | 0 | 0 | 1.00 |
| >72 h | 0 | 0 | — | 0 | 1 | 1.00 | — | — | — |
| Patients* | 3 (10%) | 3 (10%) | 1.00 | 6 (21%) | 3 (10%) | 0.47 | 9 (31%) | 5 (17%) | 0.36 |

Values are shown as numbers of patients (%).* Patients = number of patients with hoarseness, sore throat, or vocal cord injuries (without dysfunction of mucosal wave). PACU: postanesthesia care unit. SEVO group: anesthesia with sevoflurane and remifentanil. TIVA group: anesthesia with propofol and remifentanil.

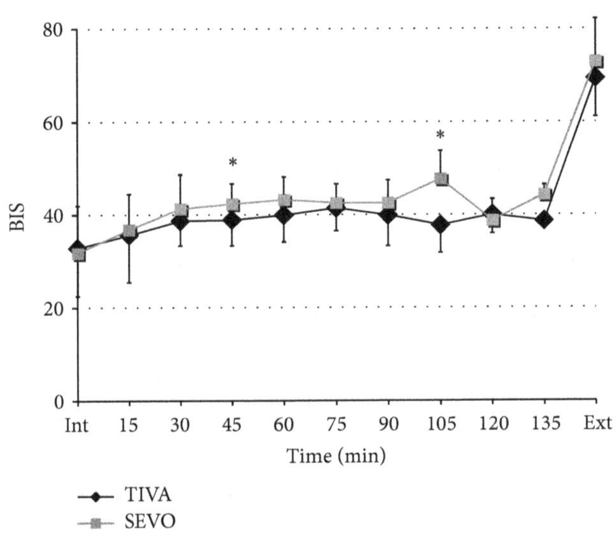


Figure 4: BIS values during surgery in patients receiving sevoflurane (gray square) or propofol (black diamond) (mean and SD). $^*P < 0.05$ SEVO group versus TIVA group. BIS = bispectral index.

SEVO group versus 4; TIVA group; $P = 0.35$). A dysfunction of the mucosal wave was found in 20 patients: 8 patients in the SEVO group and 12 patients in the TIVA group.

Postoperative nausea and vomiting (PONV) were not observed in the PACU. The BIS values are shown in Figure 4.

## 4. Discussion

We showed that both anesthesia techniques—anesthesia with sevoflurane and intravenous anesthesia with propofol—may be used. The rate of vocal cord injuries was comparable between the two anesthetics. The risk for postoperative residual curarization, however, was higher in the sevoflurane group.

The incidence of hoarseness and sore throat was 10% in the TIVA group; this is lower than reported by Maruyama et al. [9]. He found hoarseness in 55% and sore throat in 50% of patients after a total intravenous anesthesia. The reason is, in our opinion, that the general anesthesia was maintained with propofol, fentanyl, and ketamine in his study. In our study, general anesthesia was maintained with propofol and remifentanil—a potent ultra short-acting synthetic opioid drug—which was applied continuously. Therefore, the depth of anesthesia, measured by BIS monitoring, was stable during surgery (between 29 and 42). BIS values between 45 and 60 are recommended for a balanced anesthesia [10]. An anesthesia with fentanyl as a bolus technique provides unstable consciousness states during surgery compared with remifentanil.

The trauma causing laryngeal injury can occur on several occasions [11]: during tracheal intubation, during surgery, and during tracheal extubation. We standardized the anesthesia induction and tracheal intubation to control the risk factors for laryngeal injury.

During surgery, the head was moved only slightly by the surgeon. The incidence of vocal cord injuries was 24% in the present study. Laryngeal injuries following tracheal intubation vary between 4% and 12% [12–14]; without muscle relaxant it was 42% [1]; with double-lumen tube it was 44% [15]; with intravenous anesthesia it was 27% [2]. We found only minor injuries such as erythema and edema at the vocal folds. The majority of the vocal cord injuries were unilateral with 65%, indicating a slight injury during tracheal intubation or resulting from the movement of the head during surgery of the ear. Bilateral vocal cord injuries—as a typical sign for an injury during removal of the tracheal tube—were observed only in 35%. It is difficult to determine, when the vocal cord injuries occurred. We performed tracheal intubation, when maximum neuromuscular block was achieved; therefore, we hope that the baseline injuries—caused by tracheal intubation—are comparable in both groups. Bilateral injuries occur when the vocal cords beat against the tracheal tube during surgery or during removal of the tracheal tube. The incidence of coughing at tracheal extubation was comparable between groups (59% SEVO group versus 76% TIVA group; $P = 0.26$); the incidence of bilateral injuries was comparable, too (1 patient SEVO group versus 4 TIVA group; $P = 0.35$).

Inhalational agents may increase the neuromuscular block by a central mechanism; [3] this may explain why the time of muscle relaxation in the SEVO group was increased compared with the TIVA group. Time to a TOF ratio of 1.0 was significantly longer in the SEVO group; doses of rocuronium were comparable between groups. Five patients in the TIVA group needed neostigmine to achieve a TOF ratio of 1.0; eleven patients in the SEVO group, however, needed neostigmine ($P = 0.14$); this is not significantly related, but this is clinically relevant. The risk for residual curarization is increased with sevoflurane. Residual curarization in the postanesthesia care unit is associated with an increased incidence of critical respiratory events, such as hypoxemia [16]. In our study, all patients were monitored with a calibrated TOF Watch SX; therefore, patient's tracheas were extubated, when the TOF ratio had reached 1.0.

We demonstrated that sevoflurane did not decrease laryngeal morbidity; the risk for residual curarization, however, was higher compared with total intravenous anesthesia. Neuromuscular monitoring is—especially under sevoflurane anesthesia—necessary to detect residual neuromuscular blockade.

## Appendix

### Assessment of Hoarseness, Sore Throat, and Vocal Cord Injuries

(A) *Hoarseness* [1][1]. Do you have any hoarseness at all since your operation?

> If the answer was no, hoarseness was graded 0 = none; if the answer was yes, hoarseness was recorded as follows: 1 = noticed by patient, 2 = obvious to observer, and 3 = aphonia.

(B) *Sore Throat* [7, 17]. Do you have any sore throat?

> If the answer was no, sore throat was graded 0 = no sore throat; if the answer was yes, sore throat was recorded as follows: 1 = mild (pain with deglutition), 2 = moderate (pain present constantly and increasing with deglutition), and 3 = severe (pain interfering with eating and requiring analgesic medication).

(C) *Vocal Cord Injuries* [1, 2, 11]. Location: unilateral (left or right vocal cord) or bilateral (both vocal cords).

Type of injury: erythema = redness of the mucosa with surrounding inflammatory swelling, edema = swollen mucosa at the vocal folds, hematoma = bleeding into vocal cord, granuloma = granulation tissue remains as chronic, localized, one rounded tissue, and dysfunction of the mucosal wave = abnormal movement of the vocal cords.

(D) *Intubating Variables*. These variables are as follows.

(i) Time for intubation = time in seconds from the initial inserting of the laryngoscope into the patient's mouth until blocking of the cuff.

(ii) Number of intubation attempts.

## References

[1] T. Mencke, M. Echternach, S. Kleinschmidt et al., "Laryngeal morbidity and quality of tracheal intubation: a randomized controlled trial," *Anesthesiology*, vol. 98, no. 5, pp. 1049–1056, 2003.

[2] T. Mencke, M. Echternach, P. K. Plinkert et al., "Does the timing of tracheal intubation based on neuromuscular monitoring decrease laryngeal injury? A randomized, prospective, controlled trial," *Anesthesia and Analgesia*, vol. 102, no. 1, pp. 306–312, 2006.

[3] U. Grundmann, T. Mencke, S. Soltesz, and T. Fuchs-Buder, "Onset properties of rocuronium during co-induction of anaesthesia with desflurane and isoflurane or total intravenous anaesthesia: a randomised, controlled clinical trial," *Clinical Drug Investigation*, vol. 20, no. 5, pp. 351–355, 2000.

[4] G. C. Urbaniak and S. Plous, "Research Randomizier," http:/www.randomizer.org, 2007.

[5] T. Fuchs-Buder, C. Claudius, L. T. Skovgaard, L. I. Eriksson, R. K. Mirakhur, and J. Viby-Mogensen, "Good clinical research practice in pharmacodynamic studies of neuromuscular blocking agents II: the Stockholm revision," *Acta Anaesthesiologica Scandinavica*, vol. 51, no. 7, pp. 789–808, 2007.

[6] P. Woo, R. Colton, J. Casper, and D. Brewer, "Diagnostic value of stroboscopic examination in hoarse patients," *Journal of Voice*, vol. 5, no. 3, pp. 231–238, 1991.

[7] F. E. McHardy and F. Chung, "Postoperative sore throat: cause, prevention and treatment," *Anaesthesia*, vol. 54, no. 5, pp. 444–453, 1999.

[8] M. Echternach, T. Mencke, B. Richter, and A. Reber, "Laryngeal alterations following endotracheal intubation and use of larynx masks," *HNO*, vol. 59, no. 5, pp. 485–498, 2011.

[9] K. Maruyama, H. Sakai, H. Miyazawa et al., "Sore throat and hoarseness after total intravenous anaesthesia," *British Journal of Anaesthesia*, vol. 92, no. 4, pp. 541–543, 2004.

[10] T. J. Gan, P. S. Glass, A. Windsor et al., "Bispectral index monitoring allows faster emergence and improved recovery from propofol, alfentanil and nitrous oxide anesthesia," *Anesthesiology*, vol. 87, no. 4, pp. 808–815, 1997.

[11] B. Benjamin, "Laryngeal trauma from intubation: endoscopic evaluation and classification," in *Otolaryngology & Head & Neck Surgery*, C. W. Cummings and J. M. Frederickson, Eds., pp. 2013–2035, Mosby, St. Louis, Mo, USA, 2001.

[12] S. B. Peppard and J. H. Dickens, "Laryngeal injury following short-term intubation," *Annals of Otology, Rhinology and Laryngology*, vol. 92, no. 4 I, pp. 327–330, 1983.

[13] V. Kambic and Z. Radsel, "Intubation lesions of the larynx," *British Journal of Anaesthesia*, vol. 50, no. 6, pp. 587–590, 1978.

[14] M. A. Grzonka and O. Kleinsasser, "Laryngeal lesions due to intubation—manifestations, notes on pathogenesis, treatment and prevention," *Laryngo-Rhino-Otologie*, vol. 75, no. 2, pp. 70–76, 1996.

[15] H. Knoll, S. Ziegeler, J. U. Schreiber et al., "Airway injuries after one-lung ventilation: a comparison between double-lumen tube and endobronchial blocker—a randomized, prospective, controlled trial," *Anesthesiology*, vol. 105, no. 3, pp. 471–477, 2006.

[16] M. Sauer, A. Stahn, S. Soltesz, G. Noeldge-Schomburg, and T. Mencke, "The influence of residual neuromuscular block on the incidence of critical respiratory events. A randomised, prospective, placebo-controlled trial," *European Journal of Anaesthesiology*, vol. 28, no. 12, pp. 842–848, 2011.

[17] L. M. Capan, D. L. Bruce, and K. P. Patel, "Succinylcholine-induced postoperative sore throat," *Anesthesiology*, vol. 59, no. 3, pp. 202–206, 1983.

# 7

# Prediction of Optimal Reversal Dose of Sugammadex after Rocuronium Administration in Adult Surgical Patients

**Shigeaki Otomo, Hajime Iwasaki, Kenichi Takahoko, Yoshiko Onodera, Tomoki Sasakawa, Takayuki Kunisawa, and Hiroshi Iwasaki**

*Department of Anesthesiology and Critical Care, Asahikawa Medical University, 2-1-1-1 Midorigaoka-higashi, Asahikawa, Hokkaido 078-8510, Japan*

Correspondence should be addressed to Shigeaki Otomo; s1631@asahikawa-med.ac.jp

Academic Editor: D. John Doyle

The objective of this study was to determine the point after sugammadex administration at which sufficient or insufficient dose could be determined, using first twitch height of train-of-four (T1 height) or train-of-four ratio (TOFR) as indicators. Groups A and B received 1 mg/kg and 0.5 mg/kg of sugammadex, respectively, as a first dose when the second twitch reappeared in train-of-four stimulation, and Groups C and D received 1 mg/kg and 0.5 mg/kg of sugammadex, respectively, as the first dose at posttetanic counts 1–3. Five minutes after the first dose, an additional 1 mg/kg of sugammadex was administered and changes in T1 height and TOFR were observed. Patients were divided into a recovered group and a partly recovered group, based on percentage changes in T1 height after additional dosing. T1 height and TOFR during the 5 min after first dose were then compared. In the recovered group, TOFR exceeded 90% in all patients at 3 min after sugammadex administration. In the partly recovered group, none of the patients had a TOFR above 90% at 3 min after sugammadex administration. An additional dose of sugammadex can be considered unnecessary if the train-of-four ratio is ≥90% at 3 min after sugammadex administration. This trial is registered with UMIN000007245.

## 1. Introduction

The recommended dose of sugammadex is determined based on the body weight of the patient and is set at 2 mg/kg of patient body weight for reversal of moderate neuromuscular block (NMB), that is, upon reappearance of the second twitch (T2) in train-of-four (TOF) stimulation, and at 4 mg/kg of patient body weight for reversal of deep NMB, that is, posttetanic count (PTC) 1-2. These recommendations have been defined by clinical consensus as the dose capable of exerting a reversal effect on NMB based on patient body weight, irrespective of individual differences. As a result, some patients administered the recommended dose receive more sugammadex than necessary. For example, moderate NMB is sufficiently reversed by 1 mg/kg sugammadex in some patients [1], and the recommended dose of 2 mg/kg sugammadex would constitute an overdose in such patients. An insufficient dose can lead to a return to NMB after temporary block reversal [2, 3], and avoiding underdosing is therefore essential. However, if it were possible to ascertain shortly after sugammadex administration that a patient required less than the recommended dose, adjustments could be made. Safe reduction of the sugammadex dose in individual patients would also contribute to reducing drug costs. In addition, if NMB is required again for reoperation after sugammadex administration, a dose of the blocking agent rocuronium or vecuronium sufficient to overcome the reversal effect of sugammadex must be administered to reinstigate blocking. In such situations, the amount of blocking agent required to reinstigate blocking could potentially be minimized if the appropriate sugammadex dose has been used. Recent research suggests that sugammadex, 1.0 mg/kg, rapidly and effectively reverses rocuronium-induced neuromuscular block which has recovered spontaneously to four twitches of TOF stimulation [4]. However, there is little research that considers the possibilities of safe reduction of the sugammadex dose for reversal of moderate or deep NMB. Against this background, we investigated the possibility of predicting whether the administered dose of sugammadex would be sufficient or insufficient by monitoring first twitch height of TOF (T1 height) and TOF ratio (TOFR) during recovery in adult patients receiving sugammadex. The primary objective of this study was thus to determine the point shortly after sugammadex administration at which sufficient or insufficient dose could be determined, using T1 height or TOFR as indicators.

## 2. Materials and Methods

The study was conducted at Asahikawa Medical University Hospital, Japan. The study protocol was approved by the ethics committee at the university and informed consent was obtained from all patients prior to enrolment. The protocol was reported to the UMIN clinical trials registry and given the code number UMIN000007245.

Subjects comprised 32 patients (18 male, 14 female) scheduled to undergo general anesthesia with tracheal intubation. ASA physical status was I-II, and patients with diabetes and neuromuscular disorders were excluded. Patients ranged in age from 20 to 82 years. Anesthesia was induced without premedication, using 1.5–2 mg/kg propofol, 0.3 $\mu$g/kg/min remifentanil, and oxygen, and was maintained with 1.5–2% sevoflurane, 0.1–0.25 $\mu$g/kg/min remifentanil, oxygen, and air. Rocuronium was administered at 0.6 mg/kg before tracheal intubation, then subsequently at 0.2-0.3 mg/kg when T2 reappeared in TOF stimulation. Routine monitoring included electrocardiography, pulse oximetry, and noninvasive blood pressure monitoring. Skin temperature of the hand was measured and kept above 33°C. Central temperature was monitored at the esophagus and kept above 35°C. During maintenance of anesthesia, end-tidal Pco2 was kept between 33 and 42 mm Hg. NMB was monitored using a TOF-Watch SX (Organon Ireland, Dublin, Ireland) and the accelography of the adductor pollicis muscle response to ulnar nerve stimulation was recorded. The TOF mode of stimulation (2 Hz; 0.2 ms) was applied at 15 s intervals throughout the procedure. Stabilization was achieved with a 5 s, 50 Hz tetanic stimulation. One minute after this tetanic stimulation, the fingers were fixated and completely immobilized, except for the thumb by using hand adapter (TOF-Watch Hand Adapter, Organon). After repetitive TOF stimulation for at least 3 min, calibration occurred by pressing the CAL button. Supramaximal stimuli were applied after automatic calibration of the device after an initial tetanic stimulus (CAL 2 mode). After calibration, the TOF-Watch SX was switched to the repetitive TOF stimulation again, which lasted until the end of anesthesia. NMB agent was not to be administered until at least 3 min after calibration, to check for correct setup. No preload was used, but we fixed the patient's arm and other 4 fingers throughout the entire duration of the procedure to avoid artifacts caused by movement. All neuromuscular monitoring data were transferred to a personal computer using a fiber-optic cable (TOF-Link), and saved using TOF-Watch SX Monitor software.

In the present study, a lower dose of sugammadex than what is recommended was administered as the first dose.

Eight patients each were assigned randomly to 4 groups differentiated by extent of NMB remaining before first dose of sugammadex and size of first sugammadex dose. Groups A and B received 1 mg/kg and 0.5 mg/kg of sugammadex, respectively, as the first dose when T2 reappeared in TOF stimulation, while Groups C and D received 1 mg/kg and 0.5 mg/kg of sugammadex, respectively, as the first dose at PTC 1–3 in posttetanic stimulation. In each patient, T1 height and TOFR values were recorded every 15 s for 5 min after first dose of sugammadex. Five minutes after first dose, an additional 1 mg/kg of sugammadex was administered and changes in T1 height and TOFR were observed. Patients were divided into a recovered group and a partly recovered group based on percentage change in T1 height after the additional dose. T1 height and TOFR values every minute for 5 min after the first dose of sugammadex were then compared. The recovered group was defined as having <10% increase in T1 height after 3 min of the additional dose of sugammadex. The partly recovered group was defined as having ≥10% increase in T1 height after 3 min of the additional dose of sugammadex (Figure 1). After observations, all patients received a last additional dose of sugammadex so that the total dose matched the recommended dose stated in the product documentation, and recovery from NMB was confirmed in all patients after 30 min of the last additional dose. After recording all data, administration of sevoflurane and remifentanil was stopped and sufficient spontaneous breathing and patient response to verbal commands was confirmed. The airway tube was then removed.

The sample size was determined based on data for eight patients (two patients each for Groups A, B, C, and D) obtained from a preliminary study. There were 2 patients in the recovered group and 6 patients in the partly recovered group. T1 height at 3 min after first dose of sugammadex was 69.5 ± 10.6 in the recovered group and 40.0 ± 30.7 in the partly recovered group. Obtaining statistically significant results with $\alpha = 0.05$ and a power of 0.8 required 28 patients in total. Considering dropouts, we enrolled 32 patients in total.

T1 height and TOFR were each compared between the recovered and partly recovered groups using an unpaired $t$-test. Characteristics of patients in Groups A to D were tested using a Kruskal-Wallis test for male-female ratio and one-way analysis of variance for age, height, weight, and body mass index. A significance level of $P < 0.05$ was set for each test.

## 3. Results

All enrolled patients completed the study. The breakdown of Groups A to D is shown in Table 1. No significant differences were seen between the characteristics of patients in Groups A to D (Table 1).

The recovered group included 6 of the 8 patients in Group A. The remaining 2 patients in Group A and all patients of Groups B–D were classed as partly recovered group (Table 2). T1 height and TOFR values from 1 to 5 min after the first dose and from 1 to 3 min after the additional dose of sugammadex in the recovered and partly recovered groups are shown in Tables 3 and 4. T1 height and TOFR values differed significantly between the recovered and partly

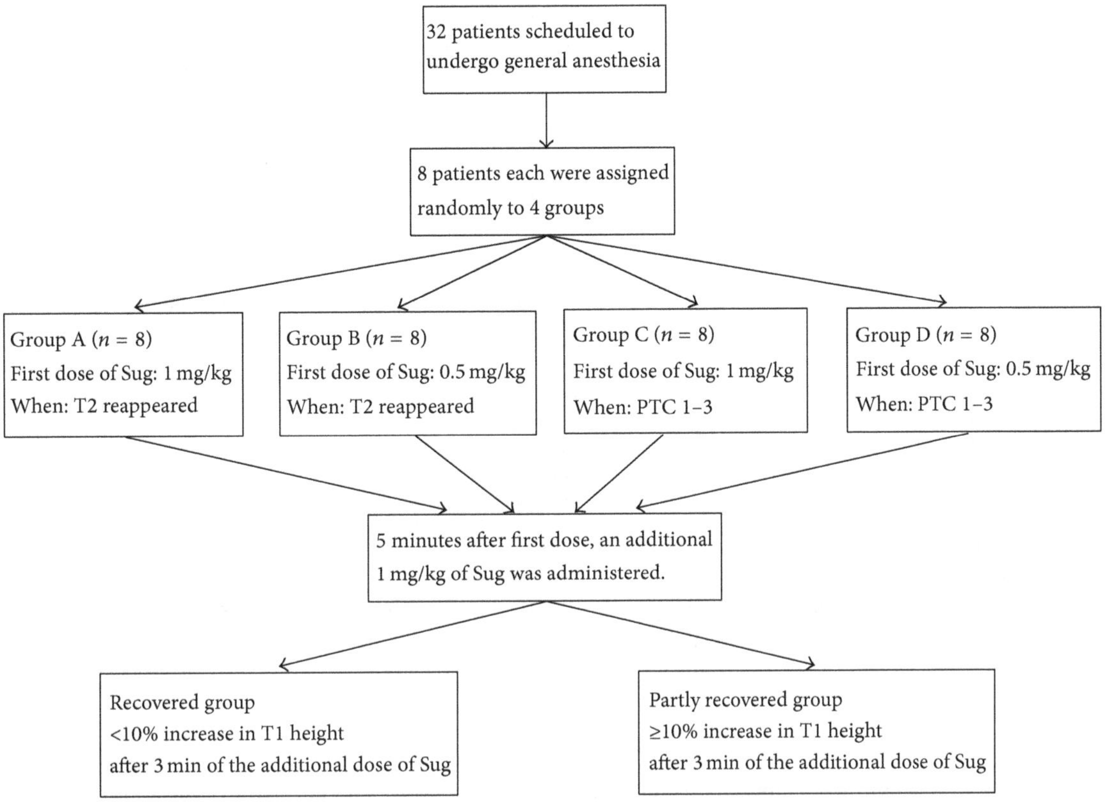


FIGURE 1: Patient flow through the study. Groups A and B received 1 mg/kg and 0.5 mg/kg of sugammadex (Sug), respectively, as a first dose when the second twitch (T2) reappeared in train-of-four stimulation (TOF), and Groups C and D received 1 mg/kg and 0.5 mg/kg of Sug, respectively, as the first dose at posttetanic counts 1–3 (PTC 1–3). Five minutes after the first dose, an additional 1 mg/kg of Sug was administered and changes in first twitch height of TOF (T1 height) and train-of-four ratio (TOFR) were observed. Patients were divided into a recovered group and a partly recovered group, based on percentage changes in T1 height after additional dosing. T1 height and TOFR during the 5 min after first dose were then compared.

TABLE 1: Patient characteristics.

| | Sex (M/F) | Age (years) | Height (cm) | Weight (kg) | BMI (kg/cm$^2$) |
|---|---|---|---|---|---|
| Group A ($n$ = 8) | 5/3 | 49.5 ± 18.9 | 167.0 ± 10.9 | 62.5 ± 8.6 | 22.4 ± 1.3 |
| Group B ($n$ = 8) | 5/3 | 66.1 ± 9.4 | 160.4 ± 10.2 | 58.9 ± 9.6 | 23.1 ± 4.2 |
| Group C ($n$ = 8) | 3/5 | 60.2 ± 19.7 | 158.3 ± 8.7 | 60.1 ± 13.3 | 24.0 ± 5.0 |
| Group D ($n$ = 8) | 5/3 | 52.5 ± 23.0 | 163.0 ± 12.2 | 66.4 ± 12.5 | 25.0 ± 4.0 |

Values are given as mean ± SD or number. No significant differences are seen between groups.
Sug: sugammadex; BMI: body mass index.

recovered groups at all time points from 1 to 5 min after the first dose and from 1 to 3 min after the additional dose of sugammadex. In the recovered group, TOFR exceeded 90% in all patients at 3 min after the first dose of sugammadex administration. In the partly recovered group, none of the patients had a TOFR above 90% at 3 min after the first dose of sugammadex administration.

## 4. Discussion

Recovered group patients only came from Group A, and all patients of Groups B–D were in the partly recovered group. Six of the 8 patients in Group A were in the recovered group and 2 were in the partly recovered group, a finding in line with other studies on the optimum dose of sugammadex [2, 5]. Although some patients given 1 mg/kg sugammadex while in moderate NMB (when T2 reappeared in TOF) recovered to the same extent as those given 2 mg/kg, a large variation existed between patients and some only showed partial recovery.

Also this result was consistent with the findings of Duvaldestin et al. that sugammadex, 0.5 mg/kg and 1.0 mg/kg, could not provide rapid reversal of deep rocuronium-induced NMB under sevoflurane maintenance anesthesia [6]. T1 height and TOFR both differed significantly between the recovered and partly recovered groups at all time points from 1 to 5 min after the first dose of sugammadex administration.

TABLE 2: Breakdown of recovered group and partly recovered group.

| | Sug dose timing | Sug first dose (mg/kg) | Recovered group/partly recovered group |
|---|---|---|---|
| Group A ($n$ = 8) | T2 | 1 | 6/2 |
| Group B ($n$ = 8) | T2 | 0.5 | 0/8 |
| Group C ($n$ = 8) | PTC1-3 | 1 | 0/8 |
| Group D ($n$ = 8) | PTC1-3 | 0.5 | 0/8 |

Sug: sugammadex.

TABLE 3: T1 height at 1–5 min after first dose and at 1–3 min after the additional dose of sugammadex.

| | T1 height 1 min after first dose | T1 height 2 min after first dose | T1 height 3 min after first dose | T1 height 4 min after first dose | T1 height 5 min after first dose | T1 height 1 min after additional dose | T1 height 2 min after additional dose | T1 height 3 min after additional dose |
|---|---|---|---|---|---|---|---|---|
| Partly recovered group ($n$ = 26) | 11.00 (0–43) | 22.12 (0–68) | 32.27 (0–75) | 41.08 (0–94) | 46.54 (0–92) | 60.04 (0–109) | 77.27 (14–125) | 84.73 (37–133) |
| Recovered group ($n$ = 6) | 49.17 (29–75) | 77.33 (50–99) | 86.17 (62–108) | 94.17 (70–116) | 99.0 (86–115) | 100.5 (85–115) | 102.3 (86–115) | 103.7 (88–117) |
| $P$ values | <0.0001 | <0.0001 | 0.0001 | 0.0008 | 0.0018 | 0.0085 | 0.0272 | 0.0438 |

Values are given as mean (min–max). T1 height values differed significantly between the recovered and partly recovered groups at all time points ($P < 0.05$).
T1: height first twitch height of TOF.

TABLE 4: TOF ratio at 1–5 min after first dose and at 1–3 min after the additional dose of sugammadex.

| | TOF ratio 1 min after first dose | TOF ratio 2 min after first dose | TOF ratio 3 min after first dose | TOF ratio 4 min after first dose | TOF ratio 5 min after first dose | TOF ratio 1 min after additional dose | TOF ratio 2 min after additional dose | TOF ratio 3 min after additional dose |
|---|---|---|---|---|---|---|---|---|
| Partly recovered group ($n$ = 26) | 4.154 (0–30) | 17.73 (0–63) | 30.58 (0–83) | 38.31 (0–89) | 43.62 (0–90) | 59.08 (0–102) | 78.58 (0–109) | 89.04 (23–116) |
| Recovered group ($n$ = 6) | 50.17 (28–64) | 84.83 (70–97) | 98.67 (92–110) | 103.2 (94–116) | 103.3 (98–115) | 104.5 (100–117) | 105.8 (102–116) | 105.2 (101–118) |
| $P$ values | <0.0001 | <0.0001 | <0.0001 | 0.0001 | 0.0009 | 0.0049 | 0.0244 | 0.0479 |

Values are given as mean (min–max). TOF ratio values differed significantly between the recovered and partly recovered groups at all time points ($P < 0.05$).
TOF ratio: train-of-four ratio.

TOFR ≥ 90% is used as a clinical indicator of recovery from NMB after NMB reversal [7]. TOFR exceeded 90% in all patients in the recovered group at 3 min after the first dose of sugammadex administration. In the partly recovered group, no patients showed TOFR above 90% at 3 min after the first dose of sugammadex administration. We therefore concluded that an additional dose of sugammadex can be considered unnecessary if TOFR is ≥90% at 3 min after sugammadex administration.

We used TOFR as the optimum indicator of recovery from NMB after sugammadex administration for the following two reasons. When evaluating recovery from NMB after sugammadex administration with reference to T1 height, comparisons must be made with control values taken before administration of the neuromuscular blocking agent. This control value is taken before surgery and is thus susceptible to the influence of slight positional changes and so forth during surgery. We therefore considered that T1 height would be much more susceptible to measurement errors than TOFR. Also, TOFR is known to recover more quickly than T1 height with sugammadex-induced NMB reversal [8, 9], unlike in neostigmine-induced NMB reversal or spontaneous recovery. We therefore considered TOFR as a more suitable indicator for quickly determining the need for additional administration of sugammadex after the first dose.

Recurarization after insufficient doses of sugammadex has been reported in adults at around 20 min after sugammadex administration [3]. When postoperative NMB reversal is insufficient, the risk of postoperative respiratory complications such as aspiration is increased, potentially compromising airway maintenance [10]. The ability to determine the necessity for additional sugammadex doses at 3 min after first dose would largely remove the dangers of recurarization and contribute to cutting the risks of postoperative respiratory complications. The ability to determine at an early stage the suitability of additional sugammadex doses and NMB recovery could also lead to shorter times in the operating theatre and reductions in overall costs.

Sugammadex is a highly safe drug with few serious side effects. In phase I clinical trials, human subjects receiving a high intravenous dose of 96 mg/kg only showed taste disturbance as a characteristic adverse reaction [11]. Overdose in itself is thus not particularly problematic, and the risks of underdose would not seem to warrant a deliberate reduction in dose. However, if the sugammadex dose can be appropriately reduced, it may contribute to reductions in drug costs. For example, the recommended dose of sugammadex for reversal of moderate NMB in a patient weighing 120 kg is 240 mg (2 mg/kg). In this case, it would be necessary to use either two vials of 200 mg preparation or one vial of 500 mg preparation. If, however, it could be determined in a short period of time that a dose of 200 mg (1.67 mg/kg) was sufficient for the patient, only one 200 mg vial would be needed, thus reducing the drug cost.

Suitable reductions in sugammadex dose would also likely prove advantageous in the following situations.

Where reoperation requiring tracheal intubation and NMB is performed shortly after sugammadex administration, the benzylisoquinoline-based agents mivacurium and cisatracurium are suitable alternatives in some countries, as they do not bind to sugammadex. However, these agents are unapproved and therefore unavailable in other countries, including Japan. If suxamethonium is used, tracheal intubation can be performed rapidly, but subsequent maintenance of NMB is difficult. In these situations, the only alternative is to readminister rocuronium while remaining mindful of the fact that NMB reversal has been induced by sugammadex. At these times, keeping the sugammadex dose as low as possible becomes advantageous. According to Cammu et al. [12], when administering 0.6 mg/kg rocuronium, followed by the recommended dose of 4 mg/kg sugammadex during deep NMB of PTC 1-2, and then readministering rocuronium at 1.2 mg/kg at 5 min after sugammadex, the time for rocuronium to exert its action was 3.06 min (range, 1.92–4.72 min), notably slower than the original time for rocuronium to take effect when administered at 1.2 mg/kg. As sugammadex and rocuronium molecules normally bind in a 1:1 ratio, a lower amount of sugammadex in the body would be more conducive to reoccurrence of NMB when rocuronium is readministered.

The present study targeted patients ≥20 years old, and we do not know if similar results would be seen in children. Results might also differ in patients susceptible to peripheral nerve damage, such as diabetic patients. Sugammadex dose reduction in these patients is a topic for further research.

## 5. Conclusion

In adult patients with ASA physical status I-II, an additional dose of sugammadex appears unnecessary if TOFR is ≥90% at 3 min after initial administration. This suggests that safe and suitable reductions in sugammadex dose may be possible.

## Conflict of Interests

The authors declare that there is no conflict of interests regarding the publication of this paper.

## References

[1] K. Suy, K. Morias, G. Cammu et al., "Effective reversal of moderate rocuronium- or vecuronium-induced neuromuscular block with sugammadex, a selective relaxant binding agent," *Anesthesiology*, vol. 106, no. 2, pp. 283–288, 2007.

[2] S. B. Groudine, R. Soto, C. Lien, D. Drover, and K. Roberts, "A randomized, dose-finding, phase II study of the selective relaxant binding drug, sugammadex, capable of safely reversing profound rocuronium-induced neuromuscular block," *Anesthesia and Analgesia*, vol. 104, no. 3, pp. 555–562, 2007.

[3] D. J. Eleveld, K. Kuizenga, J. H. Proost, and J. M. K. H. Wierda, "A temporary decrease in twitch response during reversal of rocuronium-induced muscle relaxation with a small dose of sugammadex," *Anesthesia and Analgesia*, vol. 104, no. 3, pp. 582–584, 2007.

[4] A. Pongrácz, S. Szatmári, R. Nemes et al., "Reversal of neuromuscular blockade with sugammadex at the reappearance of four twitches train-of-four stimulation," *Anesthesiology*, vol. 119, pp. 36–42, 2013.

[5] I. F. Sorgenfrei, K. Norrild, P. B. Larsen et al., "Reversal of rocuronium-induced neuromuscular block by the selective relaxant binding agent sugammadex: a dose-finding and safety study," *Anesthesiology*, vol. 104, no. 4, pp. 667–674, 2006.

[6] P. Duvaldestin, K. Kuizenga, V. Saldien et al., "A randomized, dose-response study of sugammadex given for the reversal of deep rocuronium- or vecuronium-induced neuromuscular blockade under sevoflurane anesthesia," *Anesthesia and Analgesia*, vol. 110, no. 1, pp. 74–82, 2010.

[7] L. I. Eriksson, M. Sato, and J. W. Severinghaus, "Effect of a vecuronium-induced partial neuromuscular block on hypoxic ventilatory response," *Anesthesiology*, vol. 78, no. 4, pp. 693–699, 1993.

[8] T. Suzuki, "A train-of-four ratio of 0.9 may not certify adequate recovery after sugammadex," *Acta Anaesthesiologica Scandinavica*, vol. 55, no. 3, pp. 368–369, 2011.

[9] M. Mosing, U. Auer, D. Bardell, R. S. Jones, and J. M. Hunter, "Reversal of profound rocuronium block monitored in three muscle groups with sugammadex in ponies," *British Journal of Anaesthesia*, vol. 105, no. 4, pp. 480–486, 2010.

[10] M. S. Arbous, A. E. E. Meursing, J. W. van Kleef et al., "Impact of anesthesia management characteristics on severe morbidity and mortality," *Anesthesiology*, vol. 102, no. 2, pp. 257–268, 2005.

[11] P. A. M. Peeters, M. W. van den Heuvel, E. van Heumen et al., "Safety, tolerability and pharmacokinetics of sugammadex using single high doses (Up to 96 mg/kg) in healthy adult subjects: a randomized, double-blind, crossover, placebo-controlled, single-centre study," *Clinical Drug Investigation*, vol. 30, no. 12, pp. 867–874, 2010.

[12] G. Cammu, P.-J. De Kam, K. De Graeve et al., "Repeat dosing of rocuronium 1.2 mg $kg^{-1}$ after reversal of neuromuscular block by sugammadex 4.0 mg $kg^{-1}$ in anaesthetized healthy volunteers: a modelling-based pilot study," *British Journal of Anaesthesia*, vol. 105, no. 4, pp. 487–492, 2010.

8

# Pre-Emptive Treatment of Lidocaine Attenuates Neuropathic Pain and Reduces Pain-Related Biochemical Markers in the Rat Cuneate Nucleus in Median Nerve Chronic Constriction Injury Model

**Chi-Te Lin,[1] Yi-Ju Tsai,[2] Hsin-Ying Wang,[1] Seu-Hwa Chen,[1,3] Tzu-Yu Lin,[1] and June-Horng Lue[1]**

[1] *Department of Anatomy and Cell Biology, College of Medicine, National Taiwan University, Taipei 10018, Taiwan*
[2] *School of Medicine, College of Medicine, Fu Jen Catholic University, Taipei 24205, Taiwan*
[3] *Department of Anatomy, Taipei Medical College, Taipei 100, Taiwan*

Correspondence should be addressed to June-Horng Lue, thomas@ntu.edu.tw

Academic Editor: Jacques E. Chelly

This study investigates the effects of lidocaine pre-emptive treatment on neuropathic pain behavior, injury discharges of nerves, neuropeptide Y (NPY) and c-Fos expression in the cuneate nucleus (CN) after median nerve chronic constriction injury (CCI). Behavior tests demonstrated that the pre-emptive lidocaine treatment dose dependently delayed and attenuated the development of mechanical allodynia within a 28-day period. Electrophysiological recording was used to examine the changes in injury discharges of the nerves. An increase in frequency of injury discharges was observed and peaked at postelectrical stimulation stage in the presaline group, which was suppressed by lidocaine pre-emptive treatment in a dose-dependent manner. Lidocaine pretreatment also reduced the number of injury-induced NPY-like immunoreactive (NPY-LI) fibers and c-Fos-LI neurons within the CN in a dose-dependent manner. Furthermore, the mean number of c-Fos-LI neurons in the CN was significantly correlated to the NPY reduction level and the sign of mechanical allodynia following CCI.

## 1. Introduction

Pre-emptive analgesia is broadly used in clinical practice for relieving postoperation pain and preventing the subsequent development of chronic neuropathic pain after surgery [1, 2]. In chronic constriction injuries (CCIs) of rat sciatic nerves [3], neuropathic pain behavior was also relieved by pre-emptive treatment of MK-801 [4], nociceptin [5], or lidocaine [6], but little is known about the effect of pre-emptive analgesia on neuropathic pain behavior after median nerve CCI. Attenuating ectopic discharges, originating from the damaged nerves [7, 8] and/or their dorsal root ganglia (DRG) [9], were considered to be one of the pre-emptive analgesia mechanisms to relieve neuropathic pain. Topical or systemic application of local anesthetics has been reported to attenuate ectopic discharges [9, 10]. Clinical studies have also indicated that neuropathic pain is alleviated by application of local anesthetics to the painful target areas [11, 12]. Lidocaine is a local anesthetic that produces a transient analgesic effect in humans affected by neuropathic and postoperative pain [13, 14]. Local pretreatment of lidocaine effectively suppresses injury discharges induced by median nerve transection (MNT) [15], but lack of evidence regarding the median nerve CCI model.

Injury to median nerve, neuropeptide Y-like immunoreactive (NPY-LI) fibers are dramatically induced in the lesion side cuneate nucleus (CN), but not detected in the intact side [16]. Furthermore, given an electrical stimulation to the injured median nerve, c-Fos-like immunoreactive (c-Fos-LI) cells are detected only in the ipsilateral CN [17, 18]. The expression of Fos, which is the protein product of the immediate-early proto-oncogene c-fos, has been accepted as a neural marker of pain [19, 20]. Pre-emptive analgesia treatment with lidocaine [21] effectively suppresses c-Fos expression in the spinal cord after peripheral nerve injury. Furthermore, the expression of c-Fos is modulated by NPY and is considered to be involved in neuropathic pain [22]. We previously demonstrated that lidocaine pre-treatment dose-dependently suppressed injury discharges to reduce NPY expression in the CN, which in turn significantly attenuated c-Fos expression after MNT along with electrical stimulation [15]. However, there is still only very little of behavioral evidence to support the effect of pre-emptive treatment on neuropathic pain relief after median nerve CCI.

In this study, we wanted to examine whether a single topical application of lidocaine prior to median nerves undergoing CCI would influence the development of neuropathic pain and ectopic discharges after CCI. Furthermore, morphological changes in NPY and c-Fos expression in the CN were examined to evaluate whether their expression levels correlated with the degree of mechanical allodynia.

## 2. Materials and Methods

The experiments were inspected and approved by the National Science Council Committee and the Animal Center Committee, College of Medicine, National Taiwan University, Taiwan (IACUCA Approval no. 20030114 and no. 20080267). Ethical guidelines from the International Association for the Study of Pain [23] were followed in the use of animals. Animals were housed under approved circumstances with a 12/12 h light/dark cycle with food and water available *ad libitum*.

*2.1. Chronic Constriction Injury (CCI) Operation.* Thirty-three male Sprague-Dawley rats (175–200 g) purchased from BioLASCO (Taiwan) were randomly divided into a control group (sham operation, median nerve exposure without injury, $n = 3$), and pretreated with saline (presaline, $n = 10$), 1% lidocaine (pre-1% lido, $n = 10$) and 5% lidocaine (pre-5% lido, $n = 10$) groups along with CCI. Under chloral hydrate anesthesia (31.5 mg/100 g body weight, i.p.), the above-mentioned pretreated groups alternatively underwent unilateral ($n = 5$) or bilateral ($n = 5$) median nerve CCI operations, the nerves were carefully separated from the surrounding tissue at the level of the elbow immediately proximal to entering between the two heads of the pronator teres muscle. Saline and various concentrations of lidocaine (Sigma, St. Louis, Mo, USA) were applied topically to the exposed median nerves (100 $\mu$L) at 15 min prior to CCI. Fifteen minutes after the application of the saline or lidocaine, four ligatures of 4.0 chromic gut were tied loosely around the nerves [3, 17, 22]. After the operation, the wound was subsequently sutured.

*2.2. Behavior Assessment.* We examined the behavioral signs with mechanical stimulation between 09:00 and 17:00 at one day before (−1) and at 3, 7, 14, 21, and 28 days after CCI to the median nerves of the pre-treatment groups, controls, or uninjured contralateral forepaw. All behavioral measurements were obtained by an investigator blind to the treatment groups.

Mechanical allodynia was estimated by means of Von Frey filaments [24]. Von Frey filaments (Somedic Sales AB, Hörby, Sweden) of different bending forces including 0.145, 0.32, 0.39, 1.1, 1.7, 3.3, 5.1, 8.3, 17, and 24 g were used to test the mechanical threshold of the rat forepaws [17, 22]. Briefly, tests were started with the smallest bending force and continued in increasing order. Each filament was applied five times in the medial surface of a forepaw; the first filament in the series that elicited withdraw three times was regarded as the paw withdrawal threshold. The thresholds of individual rats in each group were averaged and presented as mean and the standard error of the mean (mean ± SEM).

*2.3. Electrical Stimulation and Electrophysiological Recording.* On the 29th day post-CCI operation, the right nerves of the control and CCI rats were reexposed under anesthesia and at least a 12 mm segment proximal to the CCI ligature or on the same level in the control group were isolated. Then, two pairs of platinum hook electrodes were placed on the nerve; the distal pair of the hook electrodes were connected to a Grass S88 stimulator (Grass, Quincy, Mass, USA) for electrical stimulation, and the proximal pair of hook electrodes were connected to an Xction View Data Acquisition System (Model XD-04; Singa, Tao Yuan, Taiwan) for recording. Warm paraffin oil was applied around the exposed nerves to prevent them from drying out. The discharges in the median nerve at pre-electrical stimulation (pre-ES, a 5-min interval just prior to electrical stimulation) and post-ES (a 5-min interval immediately after stimulation) stages were also collected, transformed into frequency histogram (Figure 3), and analyzed by Xction view software (Figure 4) [15]. For electrical stimulation, a 10-min electric square wave pulse current with 0.1 ms duration, 10 Hz frequency, 0.1 mA intensity [15, 17, 22, 25] was applied through a constant current unit.

*2.4. Tissue Preparation and Immunohistochemistry.* Two hours after electrical stimulation (or, in the control group, 2 h after nerve exposure), the rats were reanesthetized and perfused with 500 mL 4% paraformaldehyde in 0.1 M phosphate buffer (PB) at pH 7.4. The brain stems containing the CN were removed, postfixed with the same fixative for 2 hr and stored in PB containing 30% sucrose. The tissue blocks were cut transversely into 30-$\mu$m-thick serial sections and orderly divided them into four sets. Two of the four serial sections were treated with 1% $H_2O_2$ and blocked with 5% normal goat serum in 0.1 M PB containing 0.2% Triton X-100 for 2 hr. They were incubated alternatively in rabbit polyclonal anti-NPY (1 : 2000; DiaSorin, Stillwater, Mont, USA) [16, 22, 26] or anti-c-Fos (1 : 2000, Calbiochem, San Diego, Calif, USA) antibodies at 4°C for 48 hr. After several washing with phosphate buffered saline (PBS), the sections were processed with biotinylated anti-rabbit IgG secondary antiserum (Vector, Burlingame, Calif, USA) at room temperature for 2 hr, treated with avidin-biotin-HRP complex (ABC kit, Vector) for 1 hr, and visualized with a Vector SG Substrate Kit. Finally, they were mounted onto gelatinized slides and their images were captured with a digital camera (Nikon, D1X, Tokyo, Japan) through a light microscope (Zeiss, Axiophot, Goettingen, Germany) to measure the NPY-LI fibers or c-Fos-LI cells in the CN.

Table 1: Statistical comparison of mean values of the nerve discharges.

| Group | Pre-ES | Post-ES |
|---|---|---|
| Control | 8.21 ± 0.48 Hz | 7.65 ± 0.95 Hz |
| Presaline | 91.86 ± 4.39 Hz | 137.39 ± 23.90 Hz* |
| Pre-1% lido | 50.31 ± 2.90 Hz | 56.86 ± 2.97 Hz* |
| Pre-5% lido | 23.76 ± 0.57 Hz | 32.86 ± 2.10 Hz* |

Control: sham operation with electrophysiological recording at the corresponding stages. ES: electrical stimulation. Data are presented as mean ± standard error of the mean (SEM) and $^*P < 0.05$ compared with the pre-ES stage.

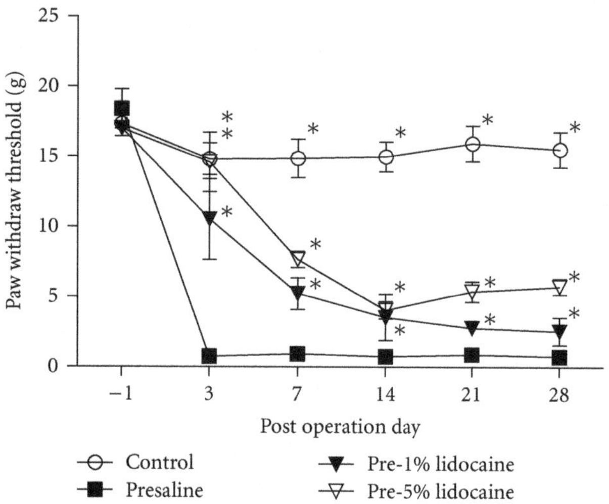


Figure 1: Effects of pre-emptive treatment of saline or various concentrations of lidocaine on paw withdrawal threshold in CCI rats. Pre-treatment of lidocaine increased paw withdrawal threshold and attenuated the TH in CCI rats. $^*P < 0.05$ compared to the presaline group.

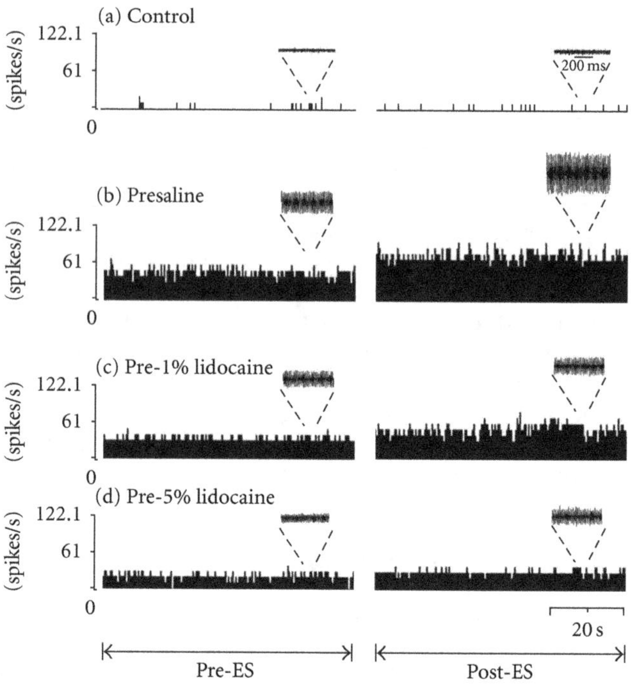


Figure 2: Electrophysiological recording of chronic constricted median nerves at pre- and postelectrical stimulation, (pre-ES and post-ES) stages. Data were collected and transformed into frequency histogram for control (a), presaline (b), pre-1% lido (c), and pre-5% lido (d) groups. Original recordings presented above the histogram, respectively. Note that the rates of discharges were significantly reduced with increasing concentrations of lidocaine pre-treatment.

*2.5. Data Presentation and Statistical Analysis.* All measurements of the behavior tests, rates of injury discharges, NPY-LI fibers, and c-Fos-LI cells in the CN were performed blind to drug treatments. The behavior test of the Von Frey filaments was compared between groups at each time point and statistical analysis was performed with the Student's *t*-test. $P < 0.05$ was considered as significant.

The rate of nerve discharges was presented as the number of discharges divided by the time period of the respective stages and presented as mean ± SEM. In order to investigate the inter-pre-treatment group (Figure 3) and interstage (Table 1) differences, the rates of discharges were compared with two-way ANOVA with a Newman-Keuls posthoc test. $P < 0.05$ was considered statistically significant.

For quantitative analysis, the sections of middle CN, which was defined as an area 0.3–0.7 mm caudal to the obex [16–18, 27], were collected from the entire rostrocaudal extent of the CN. Four sections were collected from the middle region of each animal. To assess the changes in NPY and c-Fos immunoreactivity in the CN, sections were investigated with a Zeiss light microscope and images were captured with a Nikon digital camera at a magnification of 200X. Pictures were processed and evaluated with a computer-based image analysis system (MGDS) and Image Pro-Plus software (Media Cybernetics, Md, USA). The area occupied by NPY-LI fibers and the area of outlined CN were measured [15, 16, 22]. The former divided by the latter was defined as the percentage of area occupied by NPY-LI fibers in the ipsilateral CN and were compared statistically, using two-way ANOVA, with the Newman-Keuls post-test between pretreatment groups (electrically stimulated and nonelectrically stimulated) (Figure 5). The mean number of c-Fos-LI cells in the CN was defined as the number of the surveyed c-Fos-LI cells divided by the number of tissue sections and were calculated and statistically compared with one-way ANOVA and posthoc with the Newman-Keuls test in the respective groups (Figure 7). In order to clarify the relationship between c-Fos-LI cells and the NPY reduction level caused by electrical stimulation (defined as the ratio of the NPY-LI fibers occupied area in the nonstimulated rat minus that in the stimulated rats in different treatment groups), the mean number of c-Fos-LI cells and NPY reduction level of the individual rats were collected and analyzed by linear regression (Figure 8). In order to examine the relationship between c-Fos-LI cells and mechanical allodynia, the mean number of c-Fos-LI cells in the CN and mechanical withdrawal scale (defined as the

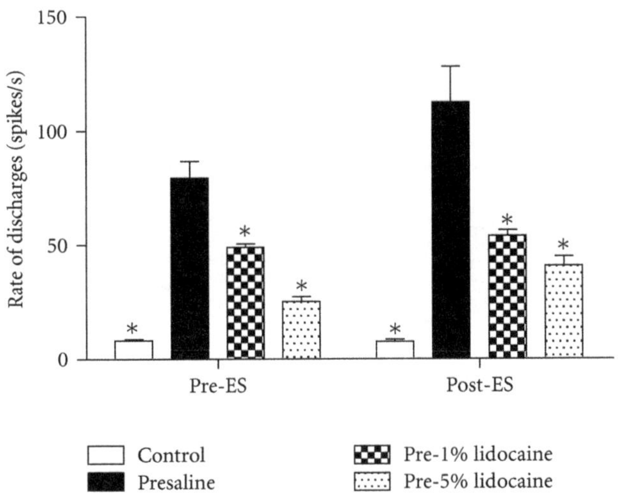


FIGURE 3: Average rate of discharges (spikes/sec) in different treatment groups at pre-electrical stimulation (pre-ES), and postelectrical stimulation (post-ES) stages. The rates of discharges decreased with increasing doses of lidocaine pre-treatment compared with the presaline group ($^*P < 0.05$ compared with the presaline group).

logarithm of paw withdraw threshold to the base 10 and presented as $\log_{10}$-gram) of the individual rats were analyzed by linear regression (Figure 9).

## 3. Results

*3.1. Effect of Lidocaine Pretreatment on Mechanical Allodynia of the CCI Rats.* Von Frey filament assessment demonstrated that there were no significant differences between bilateral-CCI and unilateral-CCI in mechanical allodynia throughout the experiment period. Von Frey filament tests also showed that in CCI rats, paw withdrawal thresholds decreased from a control of 14.83 ± 1.14 g to 0.75 ± 0.20 g at three days after CCI in the presaline group. Rats established mechanical allodynia three day after CCI, and throughout the 28-day experiment period (control: 15.53 ± 1.26 g, presaline: 0.75 ± 0.20 g, Figure 1). However, pretreatment of lidocaine to CCI increased paw withdrawal threshold and attenuated the tactile hypersensitivity (TH) (Figure 1).

*3.2. Effect of Lidocaine Pretreatment on Injury Discharges of the Chronic Constriction Injured Median Nerves.* At 29 days after CCI, electrophysiological recording was used to examine the changes in discharges of the median nerves before and after electrical stimulation (pre-ES and post-ES stages) in all groups (Figure 2). The nerves in the control group displayed a few spikes at pre-ES and post-ES stages (Figure 2(a)). Following median nerve CCI, the rates of discharges at both pre-ES and post-ES stages in all CCI groups increased on the injured nerves (Figures 2(b)–2(d)). Two-way ANOVA of the rate of discharges displayed significant differences between different stages ($F = 15.09$, $P < 0.05$) and between the pretreatment groups ($F = 47.98$, $P < 0.0001$). The rates of discharges at the post-ES stage were significantly higher than that at the pre-ES stage in all CCI groups, respectively (Table 1). Of note, the rates of discharges at both pre-ES and post-ES stages in presaline and pre-1% lido CCI groups were dramatically higher than those in the control group (Figure 3). Furthermore, the rates of discharges in all the lidocaine pretreatment groups at pre-ES (pre-1% lido: 50.31 ± 2.90 Hz, pre-5% lido: 23.76 ± 0.57 Hz) and post-ES (pre-1% lido: 56.86 ± 2.97 Hz, pre-5% lido: 32.86 ± 2.10 Hz) stages were significantly lower than those in the presaline group (pre-ES: 91.86 ± 4.39 Hz; post-ES: 137.39 ± 23.90 Hz), and revealed a dose-dependent suppression manner (Figure 3).

*3.3. Effect of Lidocaine Pretreatment on NPY and c-Fos Expression in the Cuneate Nucleus.* There were little to no NPY-LI fibers in the CN of uninjured control rats, with or without electrical stimulation (control, 0.13 ± 0.01%; control + ES, 0.14 ± 0.03%; Figures 4(a), 4(b), and 5). However, in the presaline group, numerous NPY-LI fibers were detected in the middle CN four weeks after CCI in both the unstimulated (30.62±1.21%) and stimulated (22.53±4.44%) sides (Figures 4(c), 4(d), and 5). The percentage of NPY-LI fibers in the lidocaine pretreatment CCI groups in both the unstimulated (pre-1% lido, 19.81 ± 2.03%; pre-5% lido, 6.04 ± 1.63%) and stimulated (pre-1% lido, 12.12 ± 4.07%; pre-5% lido, 4.26 ± 0.78%) sides of the CN were significantly decreased in a dose-dependent manner compared with those in the presaline group (Figures 4(c)–4(h) and 5). Furthermore, in all CCI groups the amount of NPY-LI fibers in the unstimulated side of the CN (Figures 4(c), 4(e), 4(g), and 5) was significantly higher than that in the stimulated side of the CN (Figures 4(d), 4(f), 4(h), and 5), respectively, except for the pre-5% lido group.

No, or only very few, c-Fos-LI cells were found in the CN of the control rats, the median nerves with or without electrical stimulation, or in CCI rats without electrical stimulation (Figure 6(a)). However, numerous c-Fos-LI cells were detected when injured median nerves treated with electrical stimulation in all CCI groups and predominantly distributed in the ventral portion of the middle CN (Figure 6). Furthermore, quantitative analysis showed that the mean number of c-Fos-LI cells in the presaline group (42.9 ± 2.8 cells) was significantly greater than that in other groups (Figures 7(b) and 8). The mean number of c-Fos-LI cells in the CN was also reduced by lidocaine pretreatment in a dose-dependent manner (pre-1% lido, 26.6 ± 1.6 cells; pre-5% lido, 18.5 ± 1.4 cells) (Figures 6(c), 6(d), and 7).

In addition, the NPY reduction level was assessed by the percentage of NPY-LI fibers in the stimulated side of the CN subtracted from that in the unstimulated side of the CN, regarded as an index of the extent of NPY release by electrical stimulation. Statistical analysis by linear regression demonstrated that the mean number of c-Fos-LI cells in the stimulated side of the CN was significantly correlated to the NPY reduction level (Figure 8, $r = 0.64$, $P < 0.01$). Finally, linear regression manifested that the mean number of c-Fos-LI cells in the CN was negatively proportional to the mechanical withdrawal scale (Figure 9, $r = -0.80$, $P < 0.005$).

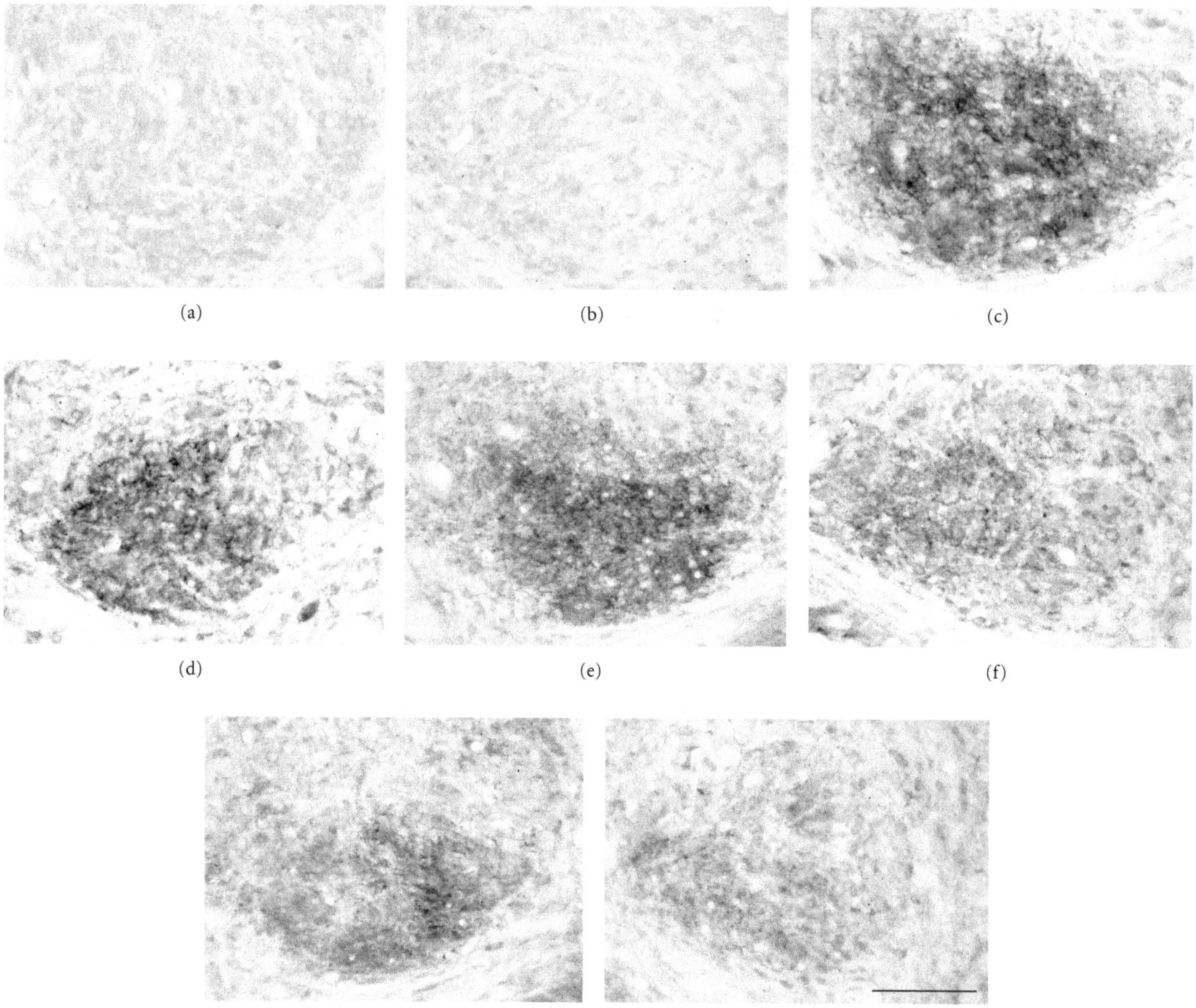

(a) (b) (c) (d) (e) (f) (g) (h)

FIGURE 4: Photomicrographs showing NPY-LI fibers in the middle region of the ipsilateral CN four weeks after chronic constriction injury in control (a, b) or four weeks after CCI without (left panel) or with (right panel) electrical stimulation in presaline (c, d), 1% (e, f), and 5% (g, h) lidocaine pre-treatment groups. Bar = 100 $\mu$m.

## 4. Discussion

The results of the present study demonstrate the attenuation of TH and reduction of injury discharges following CCI on median nerves by lidocaine pretreatment. Correspondingly, both the level of the injury-induced NPY fibers and the number of injury-induced c-Fos-LI cells in the CN at four weeks after medina nerve CCI were also dose-dependently reduced by lidocaine pretreatment. These results provide a possible mechanism in that the suppression of injury discharges by lidocaine pretreatment not only relieves neuropathic pain but also attenuates the NPY and c-Fos expressions in the CN after CCI.

Following median nerve CCI, signs of mechanical allodynia were detected three days after CCI and lasted throughout the experiment period of 28 days in the present study. Similar results have been reported, where hyperalgesia responses to noxious radiant heat were observed on the second postoperative day and lasted for over two months after sciatic nerve CCI [3]. Another study also indicated that mechanical allodynia was found three to five days following CCI [28], whereas this neuropathic sign was detected one day after CCI in our recent study [22]. There are discrepancies in the time points of neuropathic pain initiating after CCI between various studies. The reason for these discrepancies may be simply due to different time points being examined. We focused on the role of lidocaine pretreatment in the paw withdrawal threshold of the CCI rats. The reductions in the paw withdrawal threshold after median nerve CCI were reversed by lidocaine pretreatment in a dose-dependent manner.

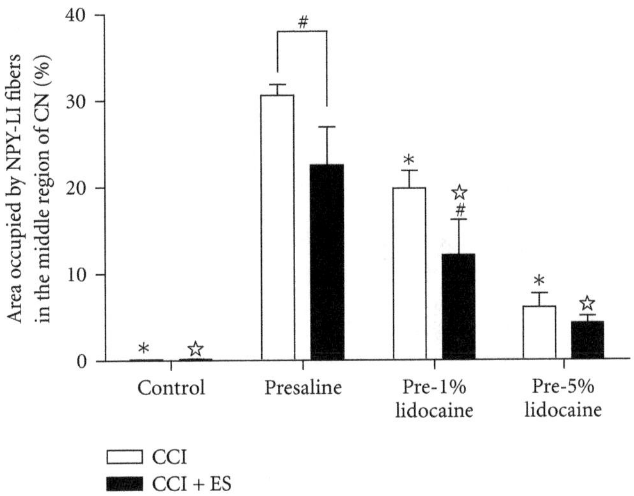


FIGURE 5: Histograms showing morphometric assessments used to quantify intensity of NPY-LI fibers in the middle CN at four weeks after chronic constriction injury without (CCI) or with electrical stimulation (CCI + ES). It is notable that the intensities of NPY-LI fibers in the CN were significantly lower in rats with electrical stimulation than those without stimulation in the presaline and pre-1% lidocaine groups ($^{\#}P < 0.05$ compared with unstimulated side in respective group). The intensity of NPY-LI fibers in the CN was also reduced by lidocaine pretreatment in a dose-dependent manner (☆, $^{*}P < 0.05$ compared with the stimulated and unstimulated side of the presaline group, resp.).

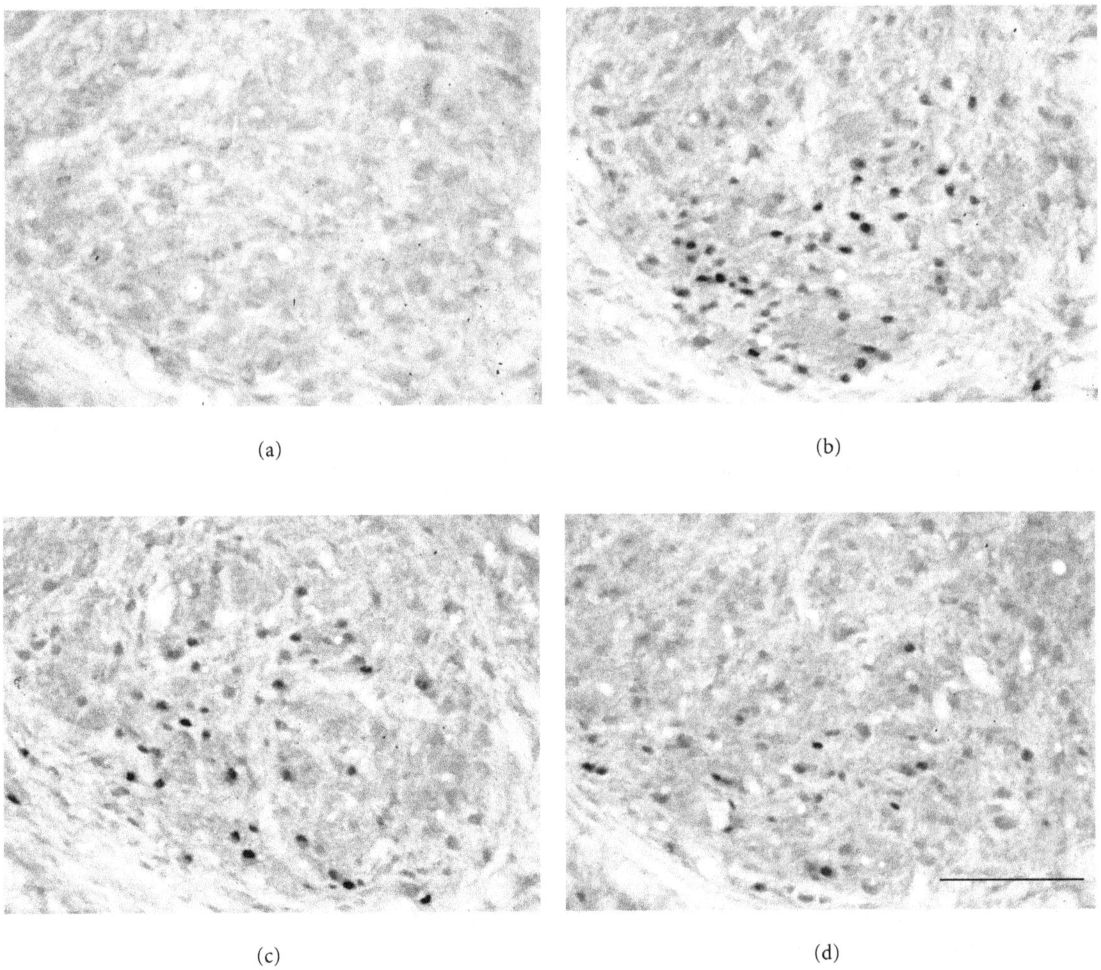


FIGURE 6: Photomicrographs showing c-Fos-LI cells in the middle region of the CN ipsilateral to electrical stimulation four weeks after chronic constriction injury in control (a), presaline (b), pre-1% lido (c) and pre-5% lido (d) groups. Bar = 100 $\mu$m.

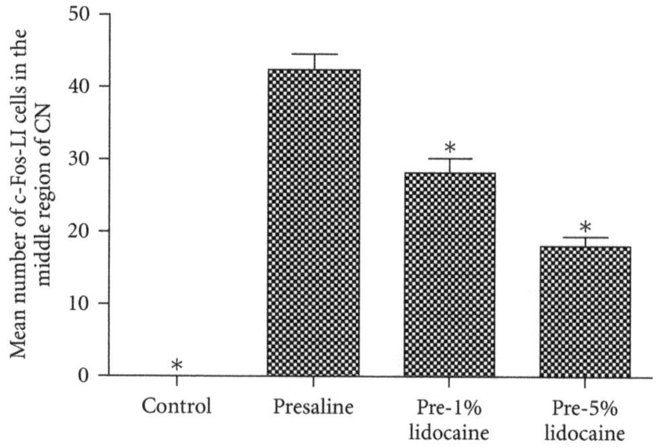


FIGURE 7: Histograms showing the mean number of c-Fos-LI cells in the middle region of the CN following electrical stimulation in control (a), presaline (b), pre-1% lido (c), and pre-5% lido (d) groups. Note that the mean numbers of c-Fos-LI cells in the pre-1% lido and pre-5% lido groups were significantly less than that in the presaline group (*$P < 0.05$ compared with the presaline group).

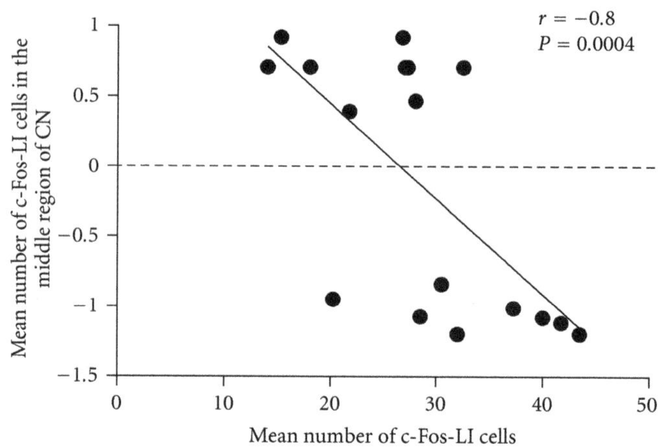


FIGURE 9: Linear regression of the mean number of c-Fos-LI cells and mechanical withdrawal scale (presented as $\log_{10}$-gram) four weeks after chronic constriction injury (each point represents an individual animal; $r = -0.80$, $P < 0.005$).

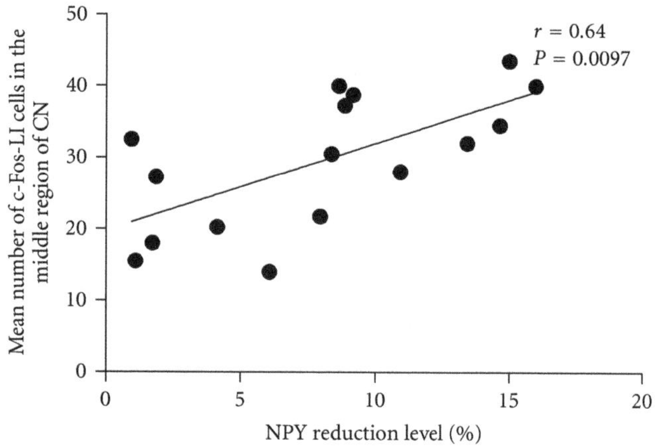


FIGURE 8: Linear regression of the mean number of c-Fos-LI cells and NPY reduction level in the CN four weeks after chronic constriction injury (each point represents an individual animal; $r = 0.64$, $P < 0.01$).

A previous study [6] reported that lidocaine pretreatment relieved thermal hyperalgesia for a long postoperative period (up to three weeks) after sciatic nerve CCI. However, another study showed that prior to spinal nerve ligation (SNL), lignocaine pretreatment increased the paw withdrawal threshold for only 24 h [29]. These discrepancies may be related to differences in the injury models used in the above-mentioned studies (CCI versus SNL). The lesion site to the DRG in the CCI model was more distal than that in the SNL model. The injury level caused by the former was less severe than that by the latter, so the neuropathic pain induced by the CCI model could be prevented by lidocaine pre-treatment.

Furthermore, four weeks after CCI (29 days postinjury), a significant increase in the number of spikes in all CCI groups, which was regarded as ectopic discharges induced after nerve injury. Then, our results also demonstrated that the ectopic discharges were suppressed by lidocaine pre-treatment in a dose-dependent manner. The suppression in ectopic discharges was considered as one of the contributing factors in relieving neuropathic pain induced by median nerve CCI. Our recent study reported that ectopic discharges evoked by median nerve transection (MNT) were suppressed by pre-treatment with 5% and 10% lidocaine, but not 1% lidocaine [15]. However, in the present study, ectopic discharges induced by CCI were significantly attenuated by 1% lidocaine pre-treatment. This discrepancy may also be explained by the difference in injury model employed between these two studies. The injury severity induced by CCI was milder than that by MNT. For this reason, the rate of injury discharges in the CCI rats, but not MNT, could be significantly reduced by low-dose (1%) lidocaine pre-treatment.

The present study further demonstrated that a significant increase in NPY in the CN at four weeks (29 days) post-CCI was also dose-dependently reduced by lidocaine pre-treatment. Previous studies have reported that intense afferent discharges and depolarization enhanced NPY induction [30, 31]. Furthermore, the NPY induction in the CN exclusively originated from injured DRG neurons, particularly medium- and large-size neurons, via primary afferent fibers [26]. It is reasonable to infer that the reduction of NPY expression in the CN would result from the suppression in injury discharges following CCI with lidocaine pre-treatment. This is consistent with NPY reduction in the CN after MNT [15] with lidocaine pre-treatment and in the spinal cord laminae 3-4 following sciatic nerve CCI with MK-801 and clonidine pre-treatment [30]. Taken together, these findings suggest that the magnitude of nerve discharges may be one of the most important factors to induce NPY synthesis.

In the rats with bilateral median nerve CCI, c-Fos-LI cells were found only in the CN with electrical stimulation, but not in the unstimulated side of the CN; the level of

NPY-LI fibers in the stimulated side of the CN was also significantly lower than that in the unstimulated side. One possible explanation for this is that NPY is released from the injured median nerve in the stimulated side of the CN resulting in NPY reduction and induced c-Fos expression in the same region. This is compatible with previous studies where NPY reduction and c-Fos induction were detected in the stimulated side of the CN following electrical stimulation with the transected median nerve; injection of an NPY receptor antagonist into the CN coupled with electrical stimulation to the injured nerve resulted in a dramatic decrease in the number of c-Fos-LI cells in the ipsilateral CN [15, 22]. In the present study, we also found that the number of c-Fos-LI cells in the CN after electrical stimulation of the injured nerve was dose-dependently reduced by lidocaine pre-treatment. Statistical analysis further demonstrated that the number of c-Fos-LI cells in the stimulated side of the CN was significantly correlated to the level of NPY reduction. Taken together, these results suggest that the amount of NPY release (NPY reduction level), following electrical stimulation of the injured nerve, directly modulates c-Fos expression in the CN.

Although the function of c-Fos induction in the CN remains uncertain, the expression of c-Fos immunoreactivity in the spinal cord has been considered as a convincing marker of pain [19, 20]. Our results showed that the number of c-Fos-LI cells in the CN coincided with the reduction in paw withdrawal thresholds, regarded as mechanical allodynia. This is in agreement with a previous study which reported that the number of c-Fos-LI cells was positively associated with the magnitude of mechanical allodynia [22]. Earlier studies have also clarified that after electrical stimulation of the injured median nerve, about 78% of c-Fos-LI cells in the middle CN were cuneothalamic projection neurons (CTNs) [17, 18]. This study further showed that the number of c-Fos-LI cells was dose-dependently reduced by lidocaine pre-treatment. Injury discharges have been reported to be implicated in the increase of c-Fos LI cell expression in the spinal cord dorsal horn [32–34], while lidocaine pre-treatment attenuates the discharges to prevent c-Fos induction [21, 34].

## 5. Conclusions

Our results suggest that lidocaine pre-treatment dose-dependently suppressed injury discharges development to attenuate NPY expression after median nerve injury. This in turn significantly reduces the NPY release to decrease the transmitting of TH to the thalamus and c-Fos expression in the CTNs.

## Acknowledgment

This study was supported by Research Grants from the National Science Council (NSC 94-2320-B002-003; NSC 98-2320-B002-033-MY3), Taiwan.

## References

[1] D. Palmes, S. Röttgermann, C. Classen, J. Haier, and R. Horstmann, "Randomized clinical trial of the influence of intraperitoneal local anaesthesia on pain after laparoscopic surgery," *British Journal of Surgery*, vol. 94, no. 7, pp. 824–832, 2007.

[2] C. S. Wong, C. C. Lu, C. H. Cherng, and S. T. Ho, "Pre-emptive analgesia with ketamine, morphine and epidural lidocaine prior to total knee replacement," *Canadian Journal of Anaesthesia*, vol. 44, no. 1, pp. 31–37, 1997.

[3] G. J. Bennett and Y. K. Xie, "A peripheral mononeuropathy in rat that produces disorders of pain sensation like those seen in man," *Pain*, vol. 33, no. 1, pp. 87–107, 1988.

[4] R. Munglani, M. J. Hudspith, B. Fleming et al., "Effect of pre-emptive NMDA antagonist treatment on long-term Fos expression and hyperalgesia in a model of chronic neuropathic pain," *Brain Research*, vol. 822, no. 1-2, pp. 210–219, 1999.

[5] T. Yamamoto, S. Ohtori, and T. Chiba, "Effects of pre-emptively administered nociceptin on the development of thermal hyperalgesia induced by two models of experimental mononeuropathy in the rat," *Brain Research*, vol. 871, no. 2, pp. 192–200, 2000.

[6] M. L. Sotgiu, A. Castagna, M. Lacerenza, and P. Marchettini, "Pre-injury lidocaine treatment prevents thermal hyperalgesia and cutaneous thermal abnormalities in a rat model of peripheral neuropathy," *Pain*, vol. 61, no. 1, pp. 3–10, 1995.

[7] O. Matzner and M. Devor, "Hyperexcitability at sites of nerve injury depends on voltage-sensitive Na+ channels," *Journal of Neurophysiology*, vol. 72, no. 1, pp. 349–359, 1994.

[8] P. D. Wall, S. Waxman, and A. I. Basbaum, "Ongoing activity in peripheral nerve: injury discharge," *Experimental Neurology*, vol. 45, no. 3, pp. 576–589, 1974.

[9] M. Devor, P. D. Wall, and N. Catalan, "Systemic lidocaine silences ectopic neuroma and DRG discharge without blocking nerve conduction," *Pain*, vol. 48, no. 2, pp. 261–268, 1992.

[10] P. D. Wall and M. Gutnick, "Properties of afferent nerve impulses originating from a neuroma," *Nature*, vol. 248, no. 5451, pp. 740–743, 1974.

[11] A. M. Comer and H. M. Lamb, "Lidocaine patch 5%," *Drugs*, vol. 59, no. 2, pp. 245–249, 2000.

[12] R. H. Gracely, S. A. Lynch, and G. J. Bennett, "Painful neuropathy: altered central processing maintained dynamically by peripheral input," *Pain*, vol. 51, no. 2, pp. 175–194, 1992.

[13] J. Kastrup, P. Petersen, and A. Dejgard, "Intravenous lidocaine infusion—a new treatment of chronic painful diabetic neuropathy?" *Pain*, vol. 28, no. 1, pp. 69–75, 1987.

[14] P. Marchettini, M. Lacerenza, C. Marangoni, G. Pellegata, M. L. Sotgiu, and S. Smirne, "Lidocaine test in neuralgia," *Pain*, vol. 48, no. 3, pp. 377–382, 1992.

[15] C. T. Lin, H. Y. Wang, Y. J. Tsai, C. T. Huang, S. H. Chen, and J. H. Lue, "Pre-treatment with lidocaine suppresses ectopic discharges and attenuates neuropeptide Y and c-Fos expressions in the rat cuneate nucleus following median nerve transection," *Journal of Chemical Neuroanatomy*, vol. 38, no. 1, pp. 47–56, 2009.

[16] Y. J. Tsai, S. M. Leong, A. S. Day, C. Y. Wen, J. Y. Shieh, and J. H. Lue, "A time course analysis of the changes in neuropeptide Y immunoreactivity in the rat cuneate nucleus following median nerve transection," *Neuroscience Research*, vol. 48, no. 4, pp. 369–377, 2004.

[17] A. S. Day, J. H. Lue, W. Z. Sun, J. Y. Shieh, and C. Y. Wen, "A$\beta$-fiber intensity stimulation of chronically constricted median nerve induces c-fos expression in thalamic projection neurons of the cuneate nucleus in rats with behavioral signs of neuropathic pain," *Brain Research*, vol. 895, no. 1-2, pp. 194–203, 2001.

[18] J. H. Lue, S. M. Leong, A. S. Day, Y. J. Tsai, J. Y. Shieh, and C. Y. Wen, "Changes in c-Fos protein expression in the rat cuneate nucleus after electric stimulation of the transected median nerve," *Journal of Neurotrauma*, vol. 19, no. 7, pp. 897–907, 2002.

[19] J. A. Harris, "Using c-fos as a neural marker of pain," *Brain Research Bulletin*, vol. 45, no. 1, pp. 1–8, 1998.

[20] S. P. Hunt, A. Pini, and G. Evan, "Induction of c-fos-like protein in spinal cord neurons following sensory stimulation," *Nature*, vol. 328, no. 6131, pp. 632–634, 1987.

[21] S. I. Chi, J. D. Levine, and A. I. Basbaum, "Effects of injury discharge on the persistent expression of spinal cord fos-like immunoreactivity produced by sciatic nerve transection in the rat," *Brain Research*, vol. 617, no. 2, pp. 220–224, 1993.

[22] Y. J. Tsai, C. T. Lin, C. T. Huang et al., "Neuropeptide y modulates c-fos protein expression in the cuneate nucleus and contributes to mechanical hypersensitivity following rat median nerve injury," *Journal of Neurotrauma*, vol. 26, no. 9, pp. 1609–1621, 2009.

[23] M. Zimmermann, "Ethical guidelines for investigations of experimental pain in conscious animals," *Pain*, vol. 16, no. 2, pp. 109–110, 1983.

[24] M. Tal and G. J. Bennett, "Extra-territorial pain in rats with a peripheral mononeuropathy: mechano-hyperalgesia and mechano-allodynia in the territory of an uninjured nerve," *Pain*, vol. 57, no. 3, pp. 375–382, 1994.

[25] C. Molander, J. Hongpaisan, and G. Grant, "Changing pattern of c-FOS expression in spinal cord neurons after electrical stimulation of the chronically injured sciatic nerve in the rat," *Neuroscience*, vol. 50, no. 1, pp. 223–236, 1992.

[26] Y. J. Tsai, C. T. Lin, and J. H. Lue, "Characterization of the induced neuropeptide Y-like immunoreactivity in primary sensory neurons following complete median nerve transection," *Journal of Neurotrauma*, vol. 24, no. 12, pp. 1878–1888, 2007.

[27] S. Maslany, D. P. Crockett, and M. D. Egger, "Somatotopic organization of the dorsal column nuclei in the rat: transganglionic labelling with B-HRP and WGA-HRP," *Brain Research*, vol. 564, no. 1, pp. 56–65, 1991.

[28] W. Xie, J. A. Strong, J. T. A. Meij, J. M. Zhang, and L. Yu, "Neuropathic pain: early spontaneous afferent activity is the trigger," *Pain*, vol. 116, no. 3, pp. 243–256, 2005.

[29] S. Abdi, D. H. Lee, S. K. Park, and J. M. Chung, "Lack of pre-emptive analgesic effects of local anaesthetics on neuropathic pain," *British Journal of Anaesthesia*, vol. 85, no. 4, pp. 620–623, 2000.

[30] R. Munglani, A. Bond, G. D. Smith et al., "Changes in neuronal markers in a mononeuropathic rat model relationship between neuropeptide Y, pre-emptive drug treatment and long-term mechanical hyperalgesia," *Pain*, vol. 63, no. 1, pp. 21–31, 1995.

[31] M. S. Rao, S. Tyrrell, S. C. Landis, and P. H. Patterson, "Effects of ciliary neurotrophic factor (CNTF) and depolarization on neuropeptide expression in cultured sympathetic neurons," *Developmental Biology*, vol. 150, no. 2, pp. 281–293, 1992.

[32] Y. P. Feng, K. Yang, and Y. Q. Li, "Activation of capsaicin receptors on the sciatic nerve induces FOS expression in the spinal dorsal horn of adult rats," *NeuroSignals*, vol. 11, no. 3, pp. 151–157, 2002.

[33] C. Stenberg, K. Øvlisen, O. Svendsen, and B. Lauritzen, "Effect of local anaesthesia on neuronal c-fos expression in the spinal dorsal horn and hypothalamic paraventricular nucleus after surgery in rats," *Basic and Clinical Pharmacology and Toxicology*, vol. 96, no. 5, pp. 381–386, 2005.

[34] X. Sun, M. Yokoyama, S. Mizobuchi et al., "The effects of pretreatment with lidocaine or bupivacaine on the spatial and temporal expression of c-Fos protein in the spinal cord caused by plantar incision in the rat," *Anesthesia and Analgesia*, vol. 98, no. 4, pp. 1093–1098, 2004.

# 9

# Potential Risk Factors for the Onset of Complex Regional Pain Syndrome Type 1

**Tracey Pons,[1] Edward A. Shipton,[1] Jonathan Williman,[2] and Roger T. Mulder[3]**

[1]*Department of Anaesthesia, University of Otago, Christchurch, Corner of Riccarton and Hagley Avenues, Christchurch 8042, New Zealand*
[2]*Department of Population Health, University of Otago, Christchurch, Corner of Riccarton and Hagley Avenues, Christchurch 8042, New Zealand*
[3]*Department of Psychological Medicine, University of Otago, Christchurch, Corner of Riccarton and Hagley Avenues, Christchurch 8042, New Zealand*

Correspondence should be addressed to Edward A. Shipton; shiptonea@xtra.co.nz

Academic Editor: Alex Macario

Anaesthetists in the acute and chronic pain teams are often involved in treating Complex Regional Pain Syndromes. Current literature about the risk factors for the onset of Complex Regional Pain Syndrome Type 1 (CRPS 1) remains sparse. This syndrome has a low prevalence, a highly variable presentation, and no gold standard for diagnosis. In the research setting, the pathogenesis of the syndrome continues to be elusive. There is a growing body of literature that addresses efficacy of a wide range of interventions as well as the likely mechanisms that contribute to the onset of CRPS 1. The objective for this systematic search of the literature focuses on determining the potential risk factors for the onset of CRPS 1. Eligible articles were analysed, dated 1996 to April 2014, and potential risk factors for the onset of CRPS 1 were identified from 10 prospective and 6 retrospective studies. Potential risk factors for the onset of CRPS 1 were found to include being female, particularly postmenopausal female, ankle dislocation or intra-articular fracture, immobilisation, and a report of higher than usual levels of pain in the early phases of trauma. It is not possible to draw definite conclusions as this evidence is heterogeneous and of mixed quality, relevance, and weighting strength against bias and has not been confirmed across multiple trials or in homogenous studies.

## 1. Introduction

There is a growing body of literature addressing a variety of disorders known as Complex Regional Pain Syndrome (CRPS). It is a condition that presents with a pain experience that is severe and disproportionate to the inciting event and is accompanied by highly variable signs and symptoms of inflammatory, sensory, autonomic, trophic, or motor features. Anaesthetists in the acute and chronic pain teams are often involved in treating Complex Regional Pain Syndromes. The onset of CRPS can follow injuries ranging from minor injuries to fracture(s), from lesions of the central nervous system, or from surgery [1–3]. Its prevalence is low, ranging from 5.46 to 26.2 per 100 000 [4, 5]. This low prevalence has led to difficulty in research where robust statistical analysis necessitates larger sample sizes [6, 7].

Furthermore, CRPS nomenclature continues to be debated and remains controversial [8–11]. Research had shown that this condition is not wholly a problem of the sympathetic nervous system. The old terms "reflex sympathetic dystrophy" and "causalgia" needed to be changed [12]. In 1994, the committee for taxonomy of the International Association for the Study of Pain (IASP) identified specific diagnostic criteria for this syndrome that were termed the IASP criteria. This IASP committee changed the name to Complex Regional Pain Syndrome or CRPS. The term CRPS Type 1 (CRPS 1) applies, if there is no nerve damage, or CRPS Type 11, if the nerve is physically and permanently damaged, and this nomenclature replaced the terms "reflex sympathetic dystrophy" and "causalgia," respectively [13]. Other diagnostic criteria developed were the Veldman [14] and Harden/Bruehl [15] criteria that continue to be used in clinical practice and research. The Harden/Bruehl criteria became known as "The Budapest Criteria" with minor modifications. Though published in an IASP-sanctioned book, the Harden/Bruehl criteria have not been officially endorsed by the IASP. The "Budapest Criteria" are used in clinical diagnosis. Here a report of at least one symptom in 3 or 4 categories (sensory, vasomotor, sudomotor/oedema, motor/trophic) with at least one sign at time of evaluation in 2 or more of the categories (sensory, vasomotor, sudomotor/oedema, motor/trophic) confirms a clinical CRPS diagnosis. There must be no other diagnosis that better explains the signs and symptoms. Budapest Clinical Criteria have retained sensitivity almost identical to the IASP criteria but with much improved specificity.

In the "Budapest Research Criteria," diagnostic decision rule is at least one symptom in all four symptom categories and at least one sign (observed at evaluation) in two or more sign categories. The intent of the Budapest Research Criteria was to maximize specificity (minimize false positives) at the expense of sensitivity. They have a high specificity but a low sensitivity [16, 17]. This systematic review explores the literature since 1999. It therefore includes a level of variation for diagnostic criteria.

CRPS 1 is considered by most to be overdiagnosed [6, 18, 19]. There are a few, however, who still consider it underdiagnosed [20]. The precise pathophysiological mechanisms and predictive factors underlying CRPS 1 or subsets of CRPS 1 remain unknown [6, 21–23]. A standard diagnostic test is unavailable and the absence of a gold standard makes the validation of diagnostic criteria difficult [6, 24, 25]. Effective treatment strategies (in both the research and clinical fields) have moderate evidence [26–29]. A variety of medical and physiotherapy interventions and a multidisciplinary approach to the management of CRPS 1 continue to be widely used [23, 30, 31]. These factors contribute to the difficulty in determining potential risk factors for CRPS 1 in a reliable and statistically valid way.

There has been no systematic review of risk factors which may contribute to the onset of CRPS 1. This is the first systematic review to address factors posing as possible risk factors for the onset of CRPS 1. This paper selects from the current literature to systematically describe factors which expose a potential risk factor for a possible relationship to the onset of CRPS 1. This paper defines a risk factor as a factor contributing to a likely association of the onset of CRPS 1. This association is not necessarily causal.

Table 1: Search terms for Web of Science CRPS 1 risks.

| Database | Search statement (1996 to April 2014) | Results |
|---|---|---|
| Web of Science | CRPS and risks | 128 |

Table 2: Search terms for OVID Medline(R) CRPS 1 risks.

| Number | Search statement | Results |
|---|---|---|
| | OVID Medline(R) < 1996 to April 2014 | |
| 1 | Complex Regional Pain Syndromes (diagnosis, epidemiology, aetiology, genetics, history, physiopathology, and rehabilitation) | 617 |
| | OVID Medline(R) < 1996 to April 2014 | |
| 1 | *Complex Regional Pain Syndromes/ep, et (Epidemiology, Aetiology) | 104 |
| 2 | crps.tw. | 1122 |
| 3 | Complex Regional Pain Syndrome*.tw. | 1515 |
| 4 | 1 or 2 or 3 | 1823 |
| 5 | *Epidemiology/ | 2325 |
| 6 | epidemiology.tw. | 63875 |
| 7 | aetiology.tw. | 22487 |
| 8 | etiology.tw. | 75941 |
| 9 | 5 or 6 or 7 or 8 | 159810 |
| 10 | *Risk Factors/ | 592 |
| 11 | *Risk/ | 1573 |
| 12 | risk*.tw. | 990294 |
| 13 | 10 or 11 or 12 | 990691 |
| 14 | 4 and 9 and 13 | 9 |
| 15 | 4 and 9 | 80 |
| | OVID Medline(R) < 1996 to April 2014 | |
| 1 | Complex Regional Pain Syndromes/or Reflex Sympathetic Dystrophy/ | 2054 |
| 2 | Fractures, Bone/or Osteoporotic Fractures/or Ulna Fractures/or Tibial Fractures/or Radius Fractures | 31463 |
| 3 | 1 and 2 | 117 |

*Before the word indicates focussing the subject heading. This means the results that have been retrieved have that subject heading as a major topic in the article, rather than something more minor.
*After the word refers to truncation. This means searching for all words have the same start, but different endings. In this case, for search 12 e.g. risk*.tw would look for risk, risks, risky, and anything else that starts with risk.

## 2. Materials and Methods

*2.1. Study Selection.* Key words for CRPS (such as diagnosis, epidemiology, aetiology, genetics, history, pathophysiology, rehabilitation, risks, fractures, osteoporosis, or predictors) were combined in searches of Web of Science and OVID Medline for articles dated 1996 to April 2014. All abstracts were screened. Inclusion criteria for data extraction were articles written in English with reference to risks or predictors associated with the onset of CRPS 1. Exclusion criteria included articles written in other languages or no mention of CRPS 1 risks for either onset or outcomes or prognosis. A total of 969 abstracts were screened according to the study selection inclusion and exclusion criteria. Forty-one abstracts were included, and 928 abstracts were excluded. Search terms are outlined in Table 1 (Web of Science search) and Table 2 (Groups of OVID Medline searches).

*2.2. Data Extraction.* The methodology of the 41 articles included through the study selection was screened for data extraction with these inclusion criteria being randomised controlled trials, prospective and retrospective studies for

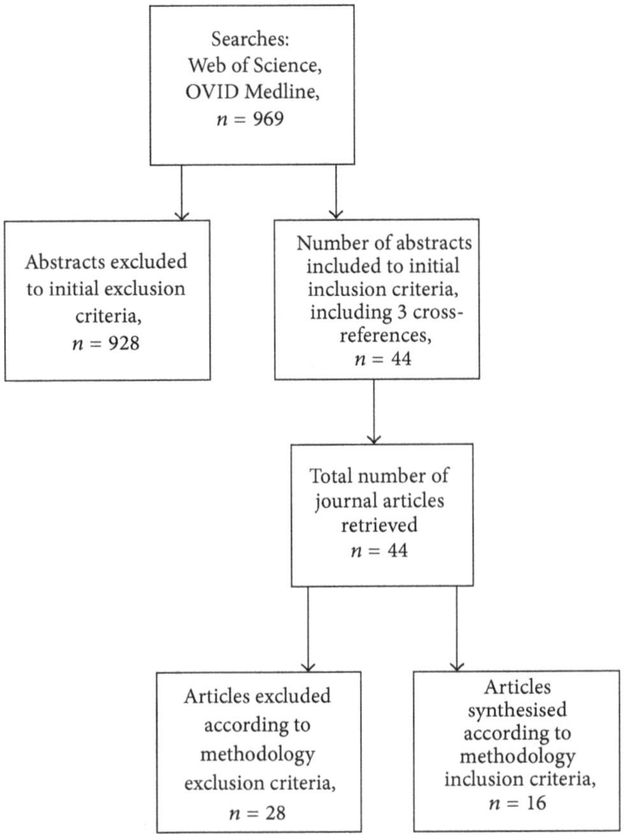


FIGURE 1: Summary of data extraction.

CRPS 1. Exclusion criteria incorporated CRPS Type 11, methodology used in animal studies, case studies, and case control studies or cross-sectional studies. Sixteen articles met these inclusion criteria (10 prospective studies, 6 retrospective studies). Twenty-five articles were excluded due to the direction of effect not being able to be determined. These inclusion and exclusion criteria were used to determine evidence for a direction of the effect specific for the likelihood or not for the potential risk for the onset of CRPS 1. A prospective or retrospective study can provide evidence for the likelihood (or not) of a risk towards the onset of a disease by determining a direction of effect. Animal studies, case studies, case control studies, and cross-sectional studies provide evidence of a relationship. They are not able to determine the direction of effect of this relationship over a period of time. Longitudinal, prospective, or retrospective studies by nature of their design are more able to determine this necessary direction of effect to reveal the potential risks for the onset of disease [7]. Figure 1 summarises the data extraction.

## 3. Results

*3.1. Data Synthesis.* No randomised controlled trials (RCTs) were found describing either possible risk or predictive factors for the onset of CRPS 1. Ten prospective studies and six retrospective studies (total of 16) were included for the data synthesis. These data were synthesised from the following patient samples: 77 patients after knee replacement surgery; 1976 patients after distal fractures of the radius; 748 patients after wrist or ankle fractures; 168 CRPS male patients from the Turkish armed forces; 1639 CRPS 1 male and female patients with duration of disease for <1 year; and 453 male and female CRPS 1 patients with duration of disease >1 year. Four hundred and sixty patients were lost to follow-up; 21 eligible fracture patients were lost due to administrative errors; 216 patients refused to participate; there were 1052 controls (male and female). The human populations from which the patient epidemiological studies were sourced consisted of a total of 297,372 people. Eight studies used the IASP criteria for diagnosis. Six studies used a variation between the Veldman and Harden/Bruehl criteria. One study did not define their criteria stating their use of "standard criteria." Criteria were not stated at all in one study. In the prospective studies, follow-up time varied from 3 months to 2 years. In the retrospective studies, follow-up time varied from 3 to 10 years. Table 3 describes the data from the literature synthesised from prospective studies. Table 4 describes the data from the literature synthesised from retrospective studies.

*3.2. Data Analysis.* The data show a high level of heterogeneity. There are no particular variables consistent across these studies with evidence strong enough to comprise a risk factor. Rating criteria for quality and relevance and weighted strength against bias were based on published recommendations [7, 62, 63]. Quality and relevance criteria used included the following: the sample had to be representative of the CRPS 1 population; an adequate control group was needed; study attrition rate was required; adequate description of study and measurements used were necessary (to identify a potential risk factor); the statistical analysis needed to be appropriate.

The data were analysed for a weighted strength against the risk of possible bias. The criteria used included bias risk in sample selection, study design, funding provision, detection, and measurement. Two authors (Tracey Pons, Roger T. Mulder) independently assessed each paper for quality, relevance, and weighted strength against potential bias. Any disagreement was discussed and resolved by consensus. Where a disagreement could not be resolved by consensus, the two other authors (Edward A. Shipton, Jonathan Williman) arbitrated disagreement and facilitated consensus amongst all four authors. Observer expectancy was considered to be reduced since 2 authors' (Roger T. Mulder, Jonathan Williman) expertise is outside the pain management field; hence, no external observer was included as they were considered objective enough with no historical or current involvement with CRPS 1 diagnosis or management.

Quality and relevance were measured against six factors. Ratings were graded as poor, adequate, or good with the following algorithm: good = five or six factors rated as yes; adequate = three or four factors rated as yes; and poor = less than two factors rated as yes. The weighting against bias was measured against five factors. Ratings were graded as weak, acceptable, or strong with the following algorithm: strong = all five factors rated as no risk; acceptable = three or four factors rated as no risk; and weak = two or less factors rated as no risk.

Table 3: Characteristics of the prospective data literature synthesized.

| Author | Number of initial sample | Outcome measure listed in italics followed by instrument used | Result for risk towards the onset of CRPS 1 | Diagnostic criteria used for CRPS 1 diagnosis | Number in sample lost to follow-up, declined to participate, or study attrition (%) | Follow-up period |
|---|---|---|---|---|---|---|
| Harden et al. 2003 [32] | 77 patients for total knee replacement | *Pain intensity*: McGill Pain Questionnaire<br>*Depression*: Beck Depressive Inventory<br>*Anxiety*: trait form of the State Trait Anxiety Inventory | CRPS 1-like symptoms following total knee replacement were not predicted by preoperative psychological distress or pain levels | IASP | 26 (33.7%) | 6 months |
| Schürmann et al. 2000 [33] | 27 distal radial fracture patients | *Oedema*: Likert scale<br>*Active ROM*: Likert scale<br>*Sympathetic function*: laser Doppler flowmetry, inspiratory gasp test, and contralateral cooling test<br>Age or gender is NOT included in analyses | Failure of the sympathetic nervous system predicted those who developed CRPS 1 in the early stages of patients who had radial fractures and also possibly suffer from a systemic sympathetic dysfunction that is not limited to the affected limb | IASP | None | 12 weeks |
| Puchalski and Zyluk 2005 [34] | 121 distal radial fractures<br>Population group: postmenopausal women, retired, or disability pensioners | *Personality traits*: Eysenck Personality Questionnaire<br>*Depression*: Beck Depressive Inventory if <60 years of age or Yesavage's Geriatric Depression Scale<br>*CRPS 1 severity*: Zyluk scoring system | In 62 patients with distal radial fractures, 18% developed CRPS 1 (8 females, one male)<br>Their psychological behaviour patterns or depression did not differ with those who had not developed CRPS 1 | Veldman and Zyluk CRPS 1 scoring system | 59 (48.7%) refuse permission for psychological examination<br>Of 62 patients included, 12 (19.4%) were lost to follow-up | 20 months |
| Beerthuizen et al. 2012 [35] | 748 wrist or ankle fractures | *Health related quality of life*: SF-36 survey<br>*Medical fracture details*: type, location of fracture with type of fracture and treatment or number of weeks in plaster | Of 596 patients with wrist or ankle fractures, 7% developed CRPS 1; wrist or ankle fracture dislocation and intra-articular fracture contributed significantly to the likelihood of the development of CRPS 1; one year following the fracture, no CRPS 1 patient was pain-free; the highest majority of patients were females (73%); the highest incidence was between 61 and 70 years of age; early reporting of high levels of pain and other musculoskeletal comorbidities made the risk of CRPS 1 more likely | 3 sets of criteria: Veldman, IASP, and Harden/Bruehl as well as confirmation with experienced clinician | 152 (20.3%) decline consent<br>46 (18.6%) are lost to follow-up | 1 year |

TABLE 3: Continued.

| Author | Number of initial sample | Outcome measure listed in italics followed by instrument used | Result for risk towards the onset of CRPS 1 | Diagnostic criteria used for CRPS 1 diagnosis | Number in sample lost to follow-up, declined to participate, or study attrition (%) | Follow-up period |
|---|---|---|---|---|---|---|
| Dijkstra et al. 2003 [36] | 91 distal radius fractures | *Pain*: Visual Analogue Scale<br>*Stressful events beforefracture*: Social Readjustment Rating Scale | Only one female patient (age 69 years) developed CRPS 1 after a follow-up of 88 patients | IASP | 3 are lost to follow-up | 1 year |
| Dilek et al. 2012 [37] | 74 with distal radius fractures treated with closed reduction and plaster casts | *Psychological assessment*: Anxiety Sensitivity Index, Toronto Alexithymia Scale-20, State Trait Anxiety Inventory, and Beck Depression Inventory | In 50 patients, a high risk for developing CRPS 1 was found in those with a high anxiety personality trait score; of the 50 patients, 26% (13/50) developed CRPS 1; 34% of the females (age 62.38 ± 10.8) developed CRPS; 11% of the males developed CRPS 1 | IASP | 13 (17.6%) refuse permission for psychological examination;<br>4 (5%) are excluded due to needing surgery;<br>7 (9%) are lost to follow-up | 16 months |
| Jellad et al. 2014 [38] | 121 consecutive patients with fractures of the distal radius treated conservatively | *Pain*: Visual Analogue Scale<br>*Active rangeof motion*: Goniometer and Kapandji distance<br>*Hand and wrist function*: Patient Related Wrist Evaluation<br>*Depression or Anxiety*: Arabic adaption of Hospital Anxiety and Depression scale<br>*Quality of Life*: Arabic adaption of SF-36 | CRPS 1 occurred in 32.2% of patients, mostly females (age 52.9. ± 13.2) [odds ratio 5.774 95% CI 1.391–23.966]; these also reported severe pain and impairment of quality of life where the CRPS 1 onset occurred in the third and fourth week after cast removal | Veldman | 31 (25.6%) excluded as treated operatively or other problems | 9 months |
| Goris et al. 2007 [39] | 114 distal radius fractures<br>95 females, 19 males, mean age of 62 years (range 22–82 years) | *Medical fracture details*: type, location of fracture with type of fracture and treatment or number of weeks in plaster<br>*Skin temperature*: infrared ear thermometer and ThermaCAM E2 infrared camera<br>*Oedema*: custom made device for measuring accurate finger circumference<br>*Active range of motion*: Goniometer<br>*Skin colour*: subjective Likert scale<br>*Grip strength*: dynamometer<br>*Blood analysis*: venous blood samples for lactate and oxygen saturation | CRPS 1 onset was associated with an increased regional inflammatory score (sensitivity 100%, specificity 16%); it was not associated with raised inflammatory markers in the blood; age and gender not included in published analyses | IASP and Harden/Bruehl criteria | 25 (21.9%) are lost to follow-up | 1 year |

Table 3: Continued.

| Author | Number of initial sample | Outcome measure listed in italics followed by instrument used | Result for risk towards the onset of CRPS 1 | Diagnostic criteria used for CRPS 1 diagnosis | Number in sample lost to follow-up, declined to participate, or study attrition (%) | Follow-up period |
|---|---|---|---|---|---|---|
| Gradl and Schürmann 2005 [40] | 10 CRPS patients, 4 males and 6 females, age 53–79 years with average age of 62 years | *Sympathetic function*: laser Doppler flowmetry, inspiratory gasp test, and contralateral cooling test | Dysfunction of the sympathetic nervous system evident in the early stage of CRPS 1 was measured in this German study; this dysfunction was transitory; it normalised over the course of the syndrome; the diagnosis of CRPS 1 was able to be made 46 to 72 days following an injury | Harden/Bruehl | None | 3 months |
| Moseley et al. 2014 [41] | 1549 near consecutive patients with radial fractures across 3 hospital out-patients | *Pain*: NRS<br>*Reaction time*: seconds<br>*Dysynchiria*: absent or present<br>*Swelling*: affected thumb and first 3 fingers' circumference as a proportion of unaffected hand<br>*Catastrophising*: Pain Catastrophising Scale | A pain score of ≥5 in the first week of fracture is shown to be predictive and should be considered a "red flag" risk for the likely onset of CRPS 1; 55 patients have developed CRPS 1 at evaluation 112 days after fracture; age and gender were not predictive of CRPS 1 onset | Referred to as "established criteria" without formal reference | 21 likely CRPS 1 patients lost due to administrative error; 93.3.% of all fractures eligible for inclusion and 94.5% agree to participate; 97.2% contacted for follow-up; no numbers of patients given, only percentages | Sequential cohort over 2 years |

Table 4: Characteristics of the retrospective data literature synthesized.

| Author | Number of initial sample | Outcome measure listed other than age and gender | Risk factor towards the onset of CRPS 1 | Diagnostic criteria used for CRPS 1 diagnosis | Period time for inspection |
|---|---|---|---|---|---|
| Allen et al. 1999 [42] | 134 CRPS patients; 70% female, 30% male<br>Mean group age at evaluation 41.8 (18–71) years | Inciting injury<br>Location<br>Job related occupation<br>Legal and worker compensation issues<br>Season<br>Bone scans<br>Treatment, medical and allied<br>Immobilisation<br>Myofascial component | A diagnostic bone scan was not predictive of a CRPS 1 diagnosis<br>The inciting event was sprains in 29%, surgical procedures in 24%, and fractures in 16%; since physician imposed immobilisation in either a cast or splint involved 47% of the sample, the possibility of immobilisation is raised as a possible risk factor as well | IASP | 1992–1997 [5 years] |
| de Mos et al. 2007 [5] | Source population 190 902 assessed from 46 general medical practices | Sensory<br>Vasomotor<br>Sudomotor<br>Motor/trophic<br>Neurologic<br>Complaints<br>Alternative diagnoses | Postmenopausal female gender and having a fracture; upper limb affected more frequently than the lower limb | 3 sets of criteria Veldman, IASP, and Harden/Bruehl | 1996–2005 [9 years] |
| Sandroni et al. 2003 [4] | Source population 106 470 with unified access to all patient records | Clinical characteristics<br>Signs and symptoms<br>Laboratory tests<br>Response to treatment | Risks for onset of CRPS 1 were identified as female gender or suffering an upper limb fracture | IASP | 1989–1999 [10 years] |
| Duman et al. 2007 [43] | 168 males in Turkish military hospitals | Inciting injury<br>Location<br>Hospitalisation | Inciting event for onset of RSD was fracture in 55.3%, incisive trauma in 16.7%, and soft tissue sprains/strains in 28% | IASP and three-phase bone scan | 2003–2006 [3 years] |
| van Rijn et al. 2007 [22] | Neurology outpatient clinic study of 185 patients with CRPS 1, 86.5% females, mean age at onset of CRPS 37.5 ± 15.4 years, 91% of whom developed dystonia | Clinical and temporal characteristics | Earlier onset of dystonia (<1 year) to be possibly related to the same mechanism and that delayed onset dystonia was related to another mechanism; 86.5% of participants were female; the inciting injury for CRPS 1 was soft tissue in 49.7%, fracture in 25.9%, and surgery in 24.3 | IASP | 1998–2004 [6 years] |
| Anderson and Fallat 1999 [44] | 33 patients with lower limb CRPS 1 or sympathetically maintained pain; 60% were female; group average age 43.5 ± 12.6 years) | Clinical characteristics<br>Type of injury or surgery<br>Time to diagnosis<br>Signs and symptoms<br>Treatment | Fracture was the most common cause for injury (45%); trauma accounted for 73% | Not given other than being confirmed by an anaesthesiologist at the pain management centre | 1990–1997 [7 years] |

Table 5: Results presenting quality and relevance of data extraction for onset of CRPS 1 from prospective studies.

| Prospective studies | Population sample representative | Adequate control group | Study attrition described | Risk/predictor outcome adequately defined | Risk/predictor outcome adequately measured | Analysis statistically appropriate | Quality |
|---|---|---|---|---|---|---|---|
| Harden et al. 2003 [32] | No | No | Yes | Yes | Yes | Yes | Adequate |
| Schürmann et al. 2000 [33] | No | No | No | Yes | Yes | No | Poor |
| Puchalski and Zyluk. 2005 [34] | No | No | Yes | Partly | Yes | Yes | Poor |
| Beerthuizen et al. 2012 [35] | Yes | Yes | Yes | Yes | Yes | Yes | Good |
| Dijkstra et al. 2003 [36, 46] | No | Yes | Yes | Partly | No | No | Poor |
| Dilek et al. 2012 [37] | No | No | Yes | Yes | Yes | No | Adequate |
| Jellad et al. 2014 [38] | No | Yes | Yes | Yes | No | Yes | Adequate |
| Goris et al. 2007 [39] | No | Yes | Yes | Yes | Yes | Yes | Good |
| Gradl and Schürmann 2005 [40] | Partly | No | No | Yes | Yes | No | Poor |
| Moseley et al. 2014 [41] | Yes | Yes | Partly | Yes | No | Yes | Adequate |

Table 6: Results presenting quality and relevance of data extraction for onset of CRPS 1 from retrospective studies.

| Retrospective studies | Population sample representative | Adequate control group | Study attrition described | Risk/predictor outcome adequately defined | Risk/predictor outcome adequately measured | Analysis statistically appropriate | Quality |
|---|---|---|---|---|---|---|---|
| Allen et al. 1999 [42] | No | No | No | Yes | Yes | Yes | Adequate |
| de Mos et al. 2007 [5] | Yes | Yes | No | Yes | Yes | Yes | Good |
| Sandroni et al. 2003 [4] | Yes | No | Yes | Yes | Yes | Yes | Good |
| Duman et al. 2007 [43] | No | No | No | Yes | No | No | Poor |
| van Rijn et al. 2007 [22] | Yes | No | No | Yes | Yes | Yes | Good |
| Anderson and Fallat 1999 [44] | Yes | No | No | No | Yes | Yes | Poor |

These data provide a broad and heterogeneous research platform towards probing for possible risk factors for the onset of CRPS 1. In this systematic review, 2 prospective studies and 3 retrospective studies were rated as good (total of 5). Four prospective studies and 1 retrospective study were rated as adequate (total of 5). Four prospective studies and 2 retrospective studies were rated as poor (total of 6). For the weighted strength against bias, 7 prospective studies were weak, 2 were acceptable, and 1 was strong. In the retrospective studies, 3 were weak, 2 were acceptable, and 1 was strong. In summary for the weighted strength against bias, 10 were weak, 4 were acceptable, and 2 were strong. However, these findings should be treated with caution as their statistical reliability and consistency have not been established across multiple or homogeneous studies.

The quality and relevance data are outlined in Table 5 for prospective studies and in Table 6 for retrospective studies. The weighting strength against bias data is illustrated in Table 7 for prospective studies and in Table 8 for retrospective studies.

The following are shown *not* to be risk factors for the onset of CRPS 1: namely, preoperative psychological distress; preoperative pain levels (with poor quality, poor relevance, and weak weighting against bias); psychological behaviour and depression (with adequate quality and relevance but with weak weighting against bias); and a diagnostic bone scan (with adequate quality and relevance but with weak weighting against bias). The factors not considered to be risk factors for the onset of CRPS 1 are summarised in Table 9.

The potential risk factors identified with a strong weighting against bias as well as good quality and relevance are being female (particularly postmenopausal), a fracture of the distal radius, and dislocation or an intra-articular fracture of the ankle. The factors presenting as possible risks for the onset of CRPS 1 are summarised in Table 10.

## 4. Discussion

Potential risk factors identified (strong weighting against bias, good quality, and relevance) across the 16 papers

TABLE 7: Results showing weighted strength against possible bias risk for prospective studies' analyses with risk rating in bold italics.

| Authors | Population sample selection bias risk | Study design bias risk | Funding provision bias risk | Detection bias risk | Measurement bias risk | Weighted strength across the five factors |
|---|---|---|---|---|---|---|
| Harden et al. 2003 [32] | 77 participants, 61.6% female, awaiting TKR in single centre setting<br>***Yes*** | 16 develop CRPS 1 by 1 month and 7 by 6 months after TKR<br>Mixed within/between designs<br>***Yes*** | No mention of funding or conflict of interests<br>***Yes*** | All samples assessed by the same physician<br>***Yes*** | Point-biserial correlations due to small sample of CRPS<br>***Yes*** | ***Weak*** |
| Schürmann et al. 2000 [33] | 27 participants, gender percentages not given, all with distal radial fractures in single centre setting<br>***Yes*** | 4 out of 27 develop CRPS 1 and two are identified as borderline<br>***Yes*** | Acknowledgment is given to funder support, potential conflict of interests is not mentioned<br>***Yes*** | Consensus between examiners only for oedema, reliable Doppler perfusion monitor<br>***Yes*** | Regression analysis<br>***No*** | ***Weak*** |
| Puchalski and Zyluk 2005 [34] | 121 patients, gender percentages not given, approached with distal displaced radial fractures, the day after fixation of the fracture in single centre setting<br>***Yes*** | 59 refuse to participate in psychological examination; 49.5% of the sample group is available for analysis<br>***Yes*** | No mention of funding or conflict of interests<br>***Yes*** | Sample assessed by "we," but clarity about authors assessment for agreement is not mentioned<br>***Yes*** | A Mann-Whitney $U$-test for determining statistical relationships<br>***No*** | ***Weak*** |
| Beerthuizen et al. 2012 [35] | Multicentre setting of 3 hospitals in single city, telephonic interview of 748 patients, 63.6% female, with single fracture of wrist, scaphoid, ankle, or metatarsal<br>***No*** | 596 participate (80%) and 18.1% of those who developed possible CRPS signs refused or were unable to attend<br>***Yes*** | Acknowledgment is given to 2 sources of funding and neither funders are involved with design, conduct, preparation, review, or approval of the manuscript<br>***No*** | Routine examination followed up by single experienced pain specialist clinician to confirm CRPS 1 diagnosis<br>***Yes*** | A Mann-Whitney $U$-test due to skewed distribution of variables, binary logistic regression analysis using SPSS<br>***No*** | ***Acceptable*** |
| Dijkstra et al. 2003 [36] | All patients, gender percentages not given, with fracture of distal radius who visit a single setting approached the day after the fracture<br>***Yes*** | 91 participants, 3 drop-outs; only 1 female develops CRPS 1<br>***Yes*** | No funding acknowledged and hospital staff thanked for cooperation<br>***Yes*** | Only researchers given as assessors for CRPS 1, no other confirmation of diagnosis<br>***Yes*** | Descriptive statistics used and analysis not possible with only one CRPS 1 subject<br>***Yes*** | ***Weak*** |
| Dilek et al. 2012 [37] | All patients, 64% female, presenting to single setting with fractures of distal radius asked to participate in psychological assessment 2 days after cast application<br>***No*** | 74 participants with 24 drop-outs<br>***Yes*** | No conflict of interests identified and no funders acknowledged, thanks given to patients who participated<br>***Yes*** | No confirmation validation given for CRPS 1 diagnosis other than fulfillment of IASP criteria<br>***Yes*** | Comparative statistics described with $P$ value for significance but no statistical approach described<br>***Yes*** | ***Weak*** |

Table 7: Continued.

| Authors | Population sample selection bias risk | Study design bias risk | Funding provision bias risk | Detection bias risk | Measurement bias risk | Weighted strength across the five factors |
|---|---|---|---|---|---|---|
| Jellad et al. 2014 [38] | All patients, 62.2% female, presenting to single setting with closed fractures of distal radius referred by orthopaedic surgeons for rehabilitation<br>***Yes*** | 90 participants with zero drop-outs.<br>***Yes*** | No mention of funding or conflict of interests<br>***Yes*** | No confirmation validation given for CRPS 1 diagnosis other than fulfillment of Veldman criteria<br>***Yes*** | Logistic regression analysis using SPSS<br>***No*** | ***Weak*** |
| Goris et al. 2007 [39] | Multicentre setting of 3 hospitals in 2 cities, 83.3% female<br>***No*** | 114 participants with 6 drop-outs 1 year later<br>***No*** | No benefit of any form is declared<br>***No*** | Confirmation of diagnosis using 2 criteria as well as assessment by 2 investigators and blinding to results at a year's follow-up<br>***No*** | Mann-Whitney $U$-test for paired data, Kruskal-Wallis test for nonparametric data, Gunn's multiple comparison test with regression coefficient for change of regional inflammation score<br>***No*** | ***Strong*** |
| Gradl and Schürmann 2005 [40] | All consecutive patients, 60% female, who develop CRPS 1 following trauma in single centre setting<br>***Yes*** | 10 participants<br>***Yes*** | No mention of funding or conflict of interests<br>***Yes*** | Confirmation of diagnosis using Harden/Bruehl criteria by 2 independent surgeons and pain specialist investigators and blinding to results at a year's follow-up<br>***No*** | Repeated measures every 10 days for 3 months with result of measures graphically presented but no statistical approach described<br>***Yes*** | ***Weak*** |
| Moseley et al. 2014 [41] | 1661 patients, 51.5% female presenting to multicentre (3) hospital settings with fractures of distal radius not needing surgical fixation; no city(s) mentioned<br>***No*** | 1549 participants, 21 drop-outs due to administrative error, only mentioned as percentages<br>***No*** | No mention of funding or conflict of interests<br>***Yes*** | Routine examination by single experienced pain specialist clinician to confirm CRPS 1 diagnosis made by "standard criteria" listed in an appendix<br>***Yes*** | A predictive model was developed using logistic regression, likelihood ratio test, with bootstrap sampling and goodness of fit with Hosmer-Lemeshow test<br>***No*** | ***Acceptable*** |

Table 8: Results showing weighted strength against possible bias risk for retrospective studies' analyses with risk rating in bold italics.

| Authors | Population sample selection bias risk | Study design bias risk | Funding provision bias risk | Detection bias risk | Measurement bias risk | Weighted strength |
|---|---|---|---|---|---|---|
| Allen et al. 1999 [42] | Medical records of all consecutive CRPS 1 patients, 70% female, who were referred to a single setting multidiscipline pain centre ***No*** | 134 consecutive CRPS 1 patients ***Yes*** | No mention of funding or conflict of interests ***Yes*** | Independent review of medical records ***No*** | Result of measures listed with $P$ values for significance but no statistical approach described ***Yes*** | ***Weak*** |
| de Mos et al. 2007 [5] | Electronic medical records of one country, population gender mix not given ***No*** | Estimation of CRPS 1 incidence from data of 600 000 patients; control groups are those who do not develop CRPS 1 ***No*** | Acknowledgment of funding provided through TREND, a Dutch government research grant; no mention of conflict of interests ***No*** | Potentially overstrict retrospective application of 3 sets of criteria: Veldman, IASP, and Harden/Bruehl, to electronic records by independent reviewers with $k$ statistics for agreement ***No*** | Poisson distribution, logistic regression, chi-square, and Student's $t$-tests using SPSS software ***No*** | ***Strong*** |
| Sandroni et al. 2003 [4] | Electronic medical records of one region, population gender mix not given ***No*** | Estimation of CRPS 1 incidence from data of 70 745 patients ***No*** | Acknowledgment of funding provided through two sources, no conflict of interests mentioned ***No*** | Potentially lenient retrospective application of IASP criteria to electronic records by one reviewer with 10% random independent assessment and 93.4% agreement ***Yes*** | Chi-square, Fisher's exact, and Wilcoxon rank sum tests with no software described ***No*** | ***Acceptable*** |
| Duman et al. 2007 [43] | Medical records of two tertiary military hospitals in one country, all male ***Yes*** | 168 CRPS 1 patients ***Yes*** | No mention of funding or conflict of interests ***Yes*** | Author review with no independent assessment using IASP criteria and three-phase bone scan ***Yes*** | Descriptive statistics only using SPSS ***Yes*** | ***Weak*** |
| van Rijn et al. 2007 [22] | Medical records of all CRPS patients, 86.5% female, who were referred to a single setting movement disorder centre ***No*** | 121 CRPS 1 patients ***Yes*** | Acknowledgment of funding provided through TREND, a Dutch government research grant; no mention of conflict of interests ***No*** | Author review with no independent assessment using IASP criteria ***Yes*** | A multivariate analysis using Cox's proportional hazards model, Mann-Whitney $U$-test, chi-square tests, and Student's $t$-tests using SPSS software ***No*** | ***Acceptable*** |
| Anderson and Fallat 1999 [44] | Medical records of all CRPS patients, 61% female, seen in a single setting foot and ankle trauma clinic ***Yes*** | 33 CRPS 1 patients ***Yes*** | No funding mentioned and acknowledgment of assistance with statistical analysis and illustrations ***Yes*** | CRPS 1 diagnosis confirmed in records by medical specialist at pain management centre ***Yes*** | Regression analysis, unpaired $t$-test, paired $t$-test, and Pearson's correlation using SPSS ***No*** | ***Weak*** |

TABLE 9: Results summary showing factors examined and not found to be risk factors for the onset of CRPS 1 with weighting bias strength and quality and relevance.

| Not a risk factor for CRPS onset | Evidence source | Weighting bias strength | Quality and relevance of data extraction |
|---|---|---|---|
| Preoperative psychological distress or pain levels | Puchalski and Zyluk 2005 [34] | Weak | Poor |
| Diagnostic bone scan | Allen et al. 1999 [42] | Weak | Adequate |
| Psychological behaviour: depression | Harden et al. 2003 [32] | Weak | Adequate |

TABLE 10: Results summary showing possible risk factors for the onset of CRPS 1 with weighting bias strength and quality and relevance.

| Risk factors for CRPS onset | Evidence source | Weighting strength against bias | Quality and relevance of data extraction |
|---|---|---|---|
| Female gender | Puchalski and Zyluk 2005 [34] | Weak | Poor |
| | Dijkstra et al. 2003 [36, 46] | Weak | Poor |
| | Dilek et al. 2012 [37] | Weak | Adequate |
| | Sandroni et al. 2003 [4] | Acceptable | Good |
| | Allen et al. 1999 [42] | Weak | Adequate |
| | van Rijn et al. 2007 [22] | Acceptable | Good |
| Postmenopausal female gender | Beerthuizen et al. 2012 [35] | Acceptable | Good |
| | Jellad et al. 2014 [38] | Weak | Adequate |
| | de Mos et al. 2007 [5] | Strong | Good |
| | Sandroni et al. 2003 [4] | Acceptable | Good |
| Fracture of distal radius or an ankle dislocation or intra-articular fracture | Beerthuizen et al. 2012 [35] | Acceptable | Good |
| | Sandroni et al. 2003 [4] | Acceptable | Good |
| | de Mos et al. 2007 [5] | Strong | Good |
| | Duman et al. 2007 [43] | Weak | Poor |
| | Anderson and Fallat 1999 [44] | Weak | Poor |
| Immobilisation | Allen et al. 1999 [42] | Weak | Adequate |
| Report of higher than usual levels of pain in early phase of trauma | Beerthuizen et al. 2012 [35] | Acceptable | Good |
| | Jellad et al. 2014 [38] | Weak | Adequate |
| | Moseley et al. 2014 [41] | Acceptable | Adequate |

are as follows: being female (particularly postmenopausal); obtaining a fracture of the distal radius; suffering an ankle dislocation or intra-articular fracture; and reports of higher than usual levels of pain in the early phases after trauma. The findings of this systematic review should be treated with caution as their statistical reliability and consistency have not yet been established across multiple or homogeneous studies and diagnostic criteria were mixed with Budapest Criteria not being used.

Age was accounted for in most studies. Age as a consistent potential risk factor for the onset of CRPS 1 could not be identified. This is shown in the population studies by Sandroni et al. [4], Moseley et al. [41], and de Mos et al. [5], as well as in the study by van Rijn et al. [22]. Although most of these data show that the risk increases in postmenopausal women [5, 34–38, 40], the retrospective studies by Allen et al. [42] and by Anderson and Fallat [44] show a lower age. This might be due to average age of the group sample with the inclusion of both genders. The average age of the female sample groups is, unfortunately, not provided in either of these studies. Females at any age pose a higher risk for the onset of CRPS 1. However, the study of males in the armed forces by Duman et al. [43] shows that males are vulnerable as well. This systematic review shows that the onset of CRPS Type 1 is higher in females than in males in the mixed gender studies.

The data show the cause of the inciting event to be mixed. It can be related to surgery, fractures, or soft tissue injuries. The presence of other comorbidities is neither predictive nor a risk factor for the onset of CRPS 1. Reports of higher than usual levels of pain in early phase of trauma were cited as strong evidence of a risk factor by Beerthuizen et al. [35] but as weak evidence by Jellad et al. [38].

Psychosocial factors are weakly weighted as a risk factor for the onset of CRPS 1. Moseley et al. find catastrophising not to be predictive for the onset of CRPS [41]. This is confirmed by other reviews and studies investigating psychological influences on the onset and progression of CRPS [58, 59, 64–66]. Psychological behaviour, depression, and preoperative psychological distress or pain levels are not predictive of the onset of CRPS. The earlier literature described the "Sudeck A personality," a personality of high anxiety, as a likely risk factor towards the onset of CRPS 1 [61]. A high anxiety personality trait was identified by this systematic review as only a weak potential risk [37]. In other persistent pain conditions, these complex interactions between the onset of the pathogenesis of CRPS 1 and psychological factors are predictive of level of function [45, 60]. Their interaction in CRPS 1 continues to be investigated by clinicians and researchers [5, 64].

These data show that a positive diagnostic bone scan is not a risk factor for the onset of CRPS 1 [46] and has been confirmed by other studies [42, 47, 48]. Interobserver consistency with interpretation of bone scans appears to be variable [49]. However, a diagnostic bone scan has been found to be helpful towards a diagnosis of CRPS 1 in some observations [50, 51], but since recovery of bone mass following ankle fractures remains variable, it is not necessarily indicative of CRPS 1 [52].

Two recent systematic reviews have collated the prognostic findings about CRPS 1 [53, 67]. Both agreed that the quality of evidence is poor. Our systematic review has confirmed this regarding the risks of onset of CRPS 1. One review retrieved 1648 relevant papers of which twelve were robust enough for qualitative analysis [53]. Prognostic factors for poor outcomes were grouped within 7 clinical clusters as follows: (1) gender, where two studies show the male gender and one study shows the female gender; (2) age, where there is a high variation in age of onset affecting prognosis; (3) inciting event, such as polytrauma, inciting event other than fracture, severe initial injury, and distal articular location; (4) localisation site, either upper or lower extremity; (5) clinical features, such as exercised induced pain, sensory disturbances, initial cold skin temperature, complications of infection, skin ulcers, chronic oedema, dystonia or myoclonus, algodystrophy score > 7 out to 10, low SF-36 general health score, disease duration > 1 year, and coexistence of misdiagnosed nerve injury and compression; (6) associated comorbidities included alcoholism and psychological background in nontraumatic CRPS 1; and (7) diagnosis where a delay of >2 months after inciting event was shown to be associated with poorer outcomes. The other review found that many CRPS 1 patients recover in 6–13 months but that a significant number continue to experience persistent pain and disability [67].

*4.1. Implications for Research.* This systematic review highlights potential risk factors that will contribute to future exploration about the onset of CRPS 1. Identifying risk factors associated with a poor prognosis is important as well. Risk factors for the onset of CRPS 1 identified in this systematic review may or may not be associated with a poor prognosis. The low prevalence of CRPS 1, its heterogeneous presentation, and its lack of highly specific or sensitive diagnostic criteria as well as the lack of clarity around consensus for these criteria create challenges in carrying out research [4, 6, 21, 42, 54, 55]. In CRPS 1, more trials across different settings are needed. The cross-sectional and case control studies excluded from this systematic review may still offer insight into the development of future longitudinal studies to determine direction and strength of the effects.

*4.2. Implications for Clinical Practice.* No specific or sensitive clinical sign or clinical symptom was shown in this review to pose a risk factor for the onset of CRPS 1. Clarity around the sensitivity and specificity of laboratory and imaging testing is needed [42, 47, 48, 51, 52]. This review confirms the importance of maintaining clinician awareness and of being aware of potential risk factors to enable the early diagnosis of CRPS 1 [56]. Evaluation by experienced clinicians hastens the diagnosis [36, 57]. Early diagnosis and referral to pain management specialists and physiotherapists are related to better outcomes [53, 68, 69]. Moseley et al. [41] suggested that a pain score of ≥5 in the first week of fracture could be considered a "red flag" risk for the likely onset of CRPS 1.

## 5. Conclusion

This systematic review shows that the accurate potential risk factors for the onset of CRPS 1 remain elusive. Studies remain heterogeneous, of mixed quality and relevance, and with varied weighting against the risks of bias. The low prevalence of CRPS 1 accompanied by a lack of a gold standard for diagnosis contributes to the difficulties around determining potential risk factors for the onset of CRPS 1.

Potential risk factors identified with strong weighting against bias and good quality and relevance are summarised as follows: being female (particularly postmenopausal); obtaining a fracture of the distal radius; suffering an ankle dislocation or intra-articular fracture; and reports of higher than usual levels of pain in the early phases after trauma. Potential risk factors with much weaker weighting against bias and poorer quality and relevance include immobilisation, psychosocial barriers, and a positive diagnostic bone scan. Definite conclusions cannot be drawn as evidence remains inconsistent across multiple trials or in homogenous studies.

## Conflict of Interests

The authors declare no conflict of interests regarding the publication of this paper.

## References

[1] M. de Mos, M. C. Sturkenboom, and F. J. Huygen, "Current understandings on complex regional pain syndrome," *Pain Practice*, vol. 9, no. 2, pp. 86–99, 2009.

[2] C. Maihöfner, F. Seifert, and K. Markovic, "Complex regional pain syndromes: new pathophysiological concepts and therapies," *European Journal of Neurology*, vol. 17, no. 5, pp. 649–660, 2010.

[3] S. Pertoldi and P. Di Benedetto, "Shoulder-hand syndrome after stroke. A complex regional pain syndrome," *Europa Medicophysica*, vol. 41, no. 4, pp. 283–292, 2005.

[4] P. Sandroni, L. M. Benrud-Larson, R. L. McClelland, and P. A. Low, "Complex regional pain syndrome type I: incidence and prevalence in Olmsted county, a population-based study," *Pain*, vol. 103, no. 1-2, pp. 199–207, 2003.

[5] M. de Mos, A. G. J. de Bruijn, F. J. P. M. Huygen, J. P. Dieleman, B. H. C. Stricker, and M. C. J. M. Sturkenboom, "The incidence

of complex regional pain syndrome: a population-based study," *Pain*, vol. 129, no. 1-2, pp. 12–20, 2007.

[6] A. T. Borchers and M. E. Gershwin, "Complex regional pain syndrome: a comprehensive and critical review," *Autoimmunity Reviews*, vol. 13, no. 3, pp. 242–265, 2014.

[7] D. F. Stroup, J. A. Berlin, S. C. Morton et al., "Meta-analysis of observational studies in epidemiology: a proposal for reporting," *Journal of the American Medical Association*, vol. 283, no. 15, pp. 2008–2012, 2000.

[8] M. Stanton-Hicks, "Complex regional pain syndrome (type I, RSD; type II, causalgia): controversies," *Clinical Journal of Pain*, vol. 16, supplement, no. 2, pp. S33–S40, 2000.

[9] A. W. Burton, S. Bruehl, R. N. Harden et al., "Current diagnosis and therapy of complex regional pain syndrome: refining diagnostic criteria and therapeutic options," *Expert Review of Neurotherapeutics*, vol. 5, no. 5, pp. 643–651, 2005.

[10] T. J. Coderre, "Complex regional pain syndrome: what's in a name?" *Journal of Pain*, vol. 12, no. 1, pp. 2–12, 2011.

[11] M. Sumitani, M. Shibata, G. Sakaue, and T. Mashimo, "Development of comprehensive diagnostic criteria for complex regional pain syndrome in the Japanese population," *Pain*, vol. 150, no. 2, pp. 243–249, 2010.

[12] M. Stanton-Hicks, "Reflex sympathetic dystrophy: a sympathetically mediated pain syndrome or not?" *Current Review of Pain*, vol. 4, no. 4, pp. 268–275, 2000.

[13] S. Bruehl, R. N. Harden, B. S. Galer et al., "External validation of IASP diagnostic criteria for complex regional pain syndrome and proposed research diagnostic criteria," *Pain*, vol. 81, no. 1-2, pp. 147–154, 1999.

[14] P. H. J. M. Veldman, H. M. Reynen, I. E. Arntz, and R. J. A. Goris, "Signs and symptoms of reflex sympathetic dystrophy: prospective study of 829 patients," *The Lancet*, vol. 342, no. 8878, pp. 1012–1016, 1993.

[15] R. N. Harden, S. Bruehl, B. S. Galer et al., "Complex regional pain syndrome: are the IASP diagnostic criteria valid and sufficiently comprehensive?" *Pain*, vol. 83, no. 2, pp. 211–219, 1999.

[16] R. N. Harden, S. Bruehl, M. Stanton-Hicks, and P. R. Wilson, "Proposed new diagnostic criteria for complex regional pain syndrome," *Pain Medicine*, vol. 8, no. 4, pp. 326–331, 2007.

[17] R. N. Harden, S. Bruehl, R. S. G. M. Perez et al., "Validation of proposed diagnostic criteria (the 'Budapest Criteria') for Complex Regional Pain Syndrome," *Pain*, vol. 150, no. 2, pp. 268–274, 2010.

[18] W. Jänig and R. Baron, "Complex regional pain syndrome: mystery explained?" *Lancet Neurology*, vol. 2, no. 11, pp. 687–697, 2003.

[19] A. L. Oaklander and H. L. Fields, "Is reflex sympathetic dystrophy/complex regional pain syndrome type I a small-fiber neuropathy?" *Annals of Neurology*, vol. 65, no. 6, pp. 629–638, 2009.

[20] A. Quisel, J. M. Gill, and P. Witherell, "Complex regional pain syndrome underdiagnosed," *Journal of Family Practice*, vol. 54, no. 6, pp. 524–532, 2005.

[21] N. Harden, "The diagnosis of CRPS: are we there yet?" *Pain*, vol. 153, no. 6, pp. 1142–1143, 2012.

[22] M. A. van Rijn, J. Marinus, H. Putter, and J. J. van Hilten, "Onset and progression of dystonia in complex regional pain syndrome," *Pain*, vol. 130, no. 3, pp. 287–293, 2007.

[23] M. D. Stanton-Hicks, A. W. Burton, S. P. Bruehl et al., "An updated interdisciplinary clinical pathway for CRPS: report of an expert panel," *Pain Practice*, vol. 2, no. 1, pp. 1–16, 2002.

[24] F. Brunner, L. M. Bachmann, U. Weber et al., "Complex regional pain syndrome 1—the Swiss cohort study," *BMC Musculoskeletal Disorders*, vol. 9, article 92, 2008.

[25] D. Q. H. Tran, S. Duong, P. Bertini, and R. J. Finlayson, "Treatment of complex regional pain syndrome: a review of the evidence," *Canadian Journal of Anesthesia*, vol. 57, no. 2, pp. 149–166, 2010.

[26] W. S. Kingery, "A critical review of controlled clinical trials for peripheral neuropathic pain and complex regional pain syndromes," *Pain*, vol. 73, no. 2, pp. 123–139, 1997.

[27] R. S. Perez, G. Kwakkel, W. W. Zuurmond, and J. J. de Lange, "Treatment of reflex sympathetic dystrophy (CRPS Type 1): a research synthesis of 21 randomized clinical trials," *Journal of Pain and Symptom Management*, vol. 21, no. 6, pp. 511–526, 2001.

[28] T. Forouzanfar, A. J. A. Köke, M. van Kleef, and W. E. J. Weber, "Treatment of complex regional pain syndrome type I," *European Journal of Pain*, vol. 6, no. 2, pp. 105–122, 2002.

[29] W. H. Merritt, "The challenge to manage reflex sympathetic dystrophy/complex regional pain syndrome," *Clinics in Plastic Surgery*, vol. 32, no. 4, pp. 575–604, 2005.

[30] R. S. Perez, P. E. Zollinger, P. U. Dijkstra et al., "Evidence based guidelines for complex regional pain syndrome type 1," *BMC Neurology*, vol. 10, article 20, 2010.

[31] F. van Eijs, M. Stanton-Hicks, J. van Zundert et al., "Evidence-based interventional pain medicine according to clinical diagnoses. 16. Complex regional pain syndrome," *Pain Practice*, vol. 11, no. 1, pp. 70–87, 2011.

[32] R. N. Harden, S. Bruehl, S. Stanos et al., "Prospective examination of pain-related and psychological predictors of CRPS-like phenomena following total knee arthroplasty: a preliminary study," *Pain*, vol. 106, no. 3, pp. 393–400, 2003.

[33] M. Schürmann, G. Gradl, J. Zaspel, M. Kayser, P. Löhr, and H.-J. Andress, "Peripheral sympathetic function as a predictor of complex regional pain syndrome type I (CRPS I) in patients with radial fracture," *Autonomic Neuroscience: Basic and Clinical*, vol. 86, no. 1-2, pp. 127–134, 2000.

[34] P. Puchalski and A. Zyluk, "Complex regional pain syndrome type 1 after fractures of the distal radius: a prospective study of the role of psychological factors," *Journal of Hand Surgery—British Volume*, vol. 30, no. 6, pp. 574–580, 2005.

[35] A. Beerthuizen, D. L. Stronks, A. V. Spijker et al., "Demographic and medical parameters in the development of complex regional pain syndrome type 1 (CRPS1): prospective study on 596 patients with a fracture," *Pain*, vol. 153, no. 6, pp. 1187–1192, 2012.

[36] P. U. Dijkstra, J. W. Groothoff, H. J. Ten Duis, and J. H. B. Geertzen, "Incidence of complex regional pain syndrome type I after fractures of the distal radius," *European Journal of Pain*, vol. 7, no. 5, pp. 457–462, 2003.

[37] B. Dilek, B. Yemez, R. Kizil et al., "Anxious personality is a risk factor for developing complex regional pain syndrome type I," *Rheumatology International*, vol. 32, no. 4, pp. 915–920, 2012.

[38] A. Jellad, S. Salah, and Z. Ben Salah Frih, "Complex regional pain syndrome type I: incidence and risk factors in patients with fracture of the distal radius," *Archives of Physical Medicine & Rehabilitation*, vol. 95, no. 3, pp. 487–492, 2014.

[39] R. J. A. Goris, M. Leixnering, W. Huber, M. Figl, M. Jaindl, and H. Redl, "Delayed recovery and late development of complex regional pain syndrome in patients with an isolated fracture of the distal radius: prediction of a regional inflammatory response by early signs," *Journal of Bone and Joint Surgery—Series B*, vol. 89, no. 8, pp. 1069–1076, 2007.

# 10

# Phenoxybenzamine in Complex Regional Pain Syndrome: Potential Role and Novel Mechanisms

**Mario A. Inchiosa Jr.**

*Departments of Pharmacology and Anesthesiology, New York Medical College, Basic Sciences Building, Valhalla, NY 10595, USA*

Correspondence should be addressed to Mario A. Inchiosa Jr.; mario_inchiosa@nymc.edu

Academic Editor: Haibo Zhang

There is a relatively long history of the use of the $\alpha$-adrenergic antagonist, phenoxybenzamine, for the treatment of complex regional pain syndrome (CRPS). One form of this syndrome, CRPS I, was originally termed reflex sympathetic dystrophy (RSD) because of an apparent dysregulation of the sympathetic nervous system in the region of an extremity that had been subjected to an injury or surgical procedure. The syndrome develops in the absence of any apparent continuation of the inciting trauma. Hallmarks of the condition are allodynia (pain perceived from a nonpainful stimulus) and hyperalgesia (exaggerated pain response to a painful stimulus). In addition to severe, unremitting burning pain, the affected limb is typically warm and edematous in the early weeks after trauma but then progresses to a primarily cold, dry limb in later weeks and months. The later stages are frequently characterized by changes to skin texture and nail deformities, hypertrichosis, muscle atrophy, and bone demineralization. Earlier treatments of CRPS syndromes were primarily focused on blocking sympathetic outflow to an affected extremity. The use of an $\alpha$-adrenergic antagonist such as phenoxybenzamine followed from this perspective. However, the current consensus on the etiology of CRPS favors an interpretation of the symptomatology as an evidence of decreased sympathetic activity to the injured limb and a resulting upregulation of adrenergic sensitivity. The clinical use of phenoxybenzamine for the treatment of CRPS is reviewed, and mechanisms of action that include potential immunomodulatory/anti-inflammatory effects are presented. Also, a recent study identified phenoxybenzamine as a potential intervention for pain mediation from its effects on gene expression in human cell lines; on this basis, it was tested and found to be capable of reducing pain behavior in a classical animal model of chronic pain.

## 1. Introduction

Complex regional pain syndrome (CRPS), types I and II, is the current accepted nomenclature for related neuropathic pain syndromes that typically develop following injury or surgery to an extremity [1]. Type I designation originally referred to conditions that were not believed to have been associated with nerve injury; this condition was previously called reflex sympathetic dystrophy (RSD). Type II CRPS was earlier termed causalgia and was associated with clear evidence of nerve damage [2]. In view of evidence that small nociceptive fibers may be damaged in CRPS I, the validity of an important distinction between type I and type II syndromes, in terms of etiology, symptomatology, and therapeutic approaches, is controversial [3–5]. No effort will be made to address this controversy, since it may not be relevant to the possible value of phenoxybenzamine for the treatment of CRPS.

Phenoxybenzamine is a noncompetitive (irreversible) antagonist of $\alpha_1$- and $\alpha_2$-adrenergic receptors [6]. It forms covalent bonds with these receptors, which results in a duration of blockade of 8 days or longer for full recovery of adrenergic effects on blood pressure (animal experiments) [7]. The irreversible action is the basis for its use in the control of hypertensive crises in patients with pheochromocytomas, tumors of the adrenal medulla that secrete massive amounts of catecholamines [8].

## 2. Current Therapy for CRPS

Although numerous drugs and interventions have been tried in attempts to treat CRPS, reliable relief of pain, restoration of function, and a "cure" remain difficult challenges. Two analyses have attempted to develop evidence-based guidelines for the treatment of CRPS. One covers trials in the period between 1980 and June 2005 [9]; the second covers the period from June 2000 to February 2012 [10]. The earlier review identified the following treatments that had varying degrees of positive therapeutic effect: subanesthetic ketamine intravenous infusion (10 to 50 mg/hr, usually over several days); gabapentin (600 to 1800 mg daily); dimethyl sulphoxide (50% cream applied to an affected area); N-acetylcysteine (600 mg three times daily); oral corticosteroids; bisphosphonates (e.g., alendronate 40 mg/day); nifedipine (20 mg/day); spinal cord stimulation (in selected patients); and various physiotherapy regimens.

Positive findings to varying degrees in the more recent analysis were as follows [10]: low-dose ketamine infusions (continuous for 4.5 days or as outpatient for 10 consecutive working days); bisphosphonates; oral tadalafil (20 mg per day, 12 weeks); intravenous regional block with a mixture of 5 mg parecoxib, 1 mg/kg lidocaine, and 30 $\mu$g/kg clonidine; intravenous immunoglobulin (0.5 mg/kg); memantine (n-methyl-d-aspartate antagonist) 40 mg per day (with morphine); and physiotherapy. Spinal cord stimulation and transcranial magnetic stimulation improved symptoms, but only transiently.

Phenoxybenzamine has been studied in CRPS because of its potential to modify sympathetic nerve effects, perhaps, particularly, for its capacity to possibly improve blood perfusion in the cold limb of the chronic CRPS patient. The drug is not labeled by the United States Food and Drug Administration (FDA) for treatment of CRPS. However, in relation to its vasodilating effects, there is an off-label indication for phenoxybenzamine in the treatment of peripheral vascular diseases (e.g., Raynaud's disease) in the official American Hospital Formulary Service Compendium [11].

## 3. Clinical Experiences with Phenoxybenzamine in CRPS

Bennett and Brookoff [12] have traced the recognition of posttraumatic neuropathic pain syndromes to antiquity and have compiled the record of reports of such syndromes during the United States Civil War and the First and Second World Wars. It is of interest that probably the first detailed report of the clinical use of phenoxybenzamine for the treatment of CRPS (designated causalgia, type II, in this case) was from Walter Reed Army Hospital; all of the pain syndromes followed injuries, some of which occurred in armed conflict [13]. Eleven of 15 patients that were treated with phenoxybenzamine appeared to obtain temporary or permanent relief of their symptoms to varying extents. A more recent report on the use of phenoxybenzamine by Ghostine et al. [14] was also for treatment of causalgia associated with battlefield wounds to soldiers. The Ghostine study included a total of 40 consecutive patients over a period of 7 years who presented with neuropathic pain resulting from missile or shrapnel wounds. Dosage escalations were used to obtain pain relief and then continued for a period of usually 6 to 8 weeks. The oral daily dose ranged from 40 to 120 mg per day, which is a large dose in terms of expected occurrence of postural hypotension. This side effect occurred in 17 of the patients but resolved after approximately one week or was controlled with vascular support wrappings. In no case was it necessary to stop the treatment. The authors reported a complete resolution of the pain syndrome in all of the cases [14].

Muizelaar et al. [15] reported their retrospective experience for the treatment of CRPS (both type I and type II) with phenoxybenzamine over an 8-year period. Of a total of 33 patients that received phenoxybenzamine, 17 (52%) improved to the point where they were able to return to their former employment or resume social activities and were no longer using any narcotic medications. The success rate was higher (8 of 9; 89%) in the early and intermediate stages of the syndrome (2–7 months) than in the later chronic stages (9 of 24; 38%). Large doses were again used in this study. The dose was escalated, as tolerated, over a period of 8 to 11 days to a maximum daily oral dose of 120 mg, taken in 3 divided doses. The side effects included, to varying degrees, symptoms of orthostatic hypotension and general malaise in almost all of the cases, and impotence in males. Treatment was usually continued for 8 to 12 weeks. Seven of the 33 patients withdrew from treatment because of the side effects.

Phenoxybenzamine was used in the treatment of a case of CRPS (RSD) of the lower extremity in a patient with long-standing tetraplegia who sustained an apparent ankle injury during a transfer maneuver [16]. The lower limb became markedly edematous, warm, and painful. The diagnosis of CRPS was made on the basis of bone scintigraphic techniques that have high sensitivities and specificities for a neuropathic syndrome. Initial treatment with indomethacin was replaced with oral phenoxybenzamine at 10 mg per day for 4 days, followed by 10 mg twice a day. Both the edema and the pain in the lower extremity resolved within a few days of treatment. The phenoxybenzamine was continued for 3 months and was then tapered off with no recurrence of symptoms. Scintigraphic scans that were repeated after 30 months showed no differences between the previously involved limb and the contralateral limb.

In view of the presumed involvement of the sympathetic nervous system in CRPS, we initiated a clinical trial to use phenoxybenzamine as part of an intravenous regional block of an affected extremity [17]. Since there was no FDA-approved intravenous preparation of phenoxybenzamine or an approved use for CRPS, we conducted our study under an FDA-approved Investigational New Drug (IND) Application. We studied 5 patients with diagnoses of CRPS of an upper extremity that had not responded to conventional therapeutic approaches. The duration of their illnesses before our intervention had ranged from 2 to 60 months. All of the patients entered our study after failures with extensive drug treatments, mostly nonsteroidal anti-inflammatory drugs (NSAIDs) and opioids, and physical therapy. In addition, the patient with the longest disease history had received multiple stellate ganglion blocks, intravenous regional lidocaine blockade, trigger point injections, and cervical epidural steroids.

Partial exsanguination of the limb was accomplished with the aid of a tourniquet proximal to the pathologically involved area, elevation of the limb, and application of an Esmarch bandage to facilitate venous drainage. The tourniquet pressure was set at 100 mmHg above systolic pressure of the extremity. The block solution consisted of 15 mL of 0.5% lidocaine HCl, 5 mg of phenoxybenzamine HCl (from sterile solution, 50 mg/mL; SmithKline-Beecham Pharmaceuticals, King of Prussia, PA), plus isotonic saline to a total volume of 30 mL. The solution was infiltrated over a period of 4 min; the tourniquet was deflated after a minimum period of 15 min. Each of the patients responded favorably to a single intravenous block containing phenoxybenzamine in the affected extremity. Visual analog pain (VAS) scores were considerably reduced one week after the block and remained close to complete reversal of pain at early (6 to 27 days) and late (5 to 17 months) follow-up evaluations (Figure 1). Skin temperature was increased by an average of 2.6 deg C in the treated arm over the pretreatment reading at the early follow-up evaluation but did not reach statistical significance. Hand-grip strength was significantly increased ($P < 0.05$) by an average of 9.9 kg over the pretreatment measurement at the early follow-up, as well. (Late follow-up measurements of skin temperature and hand-grip strength were not obtained; VAS scores were collected by telephone interview.) The experimental design might be criticized in that a local anesthetic was part of the block and that this could account for the apparent success that was seen. But a recent review on evidence-based treatment of CRPS I drew the strong conclusion that there is no evidence of therapeutic efficacy for intravenous sympathetic blockade [9]. However, it might still be allowed that there was some possible synergism elicited by the mixture of local anesthetic and phenoxybenzamine in our treatments. In fact, the need for a multimodal approach may prove to be optimal in the treatment of a syndrome that has such a complex mediation [18].

Soon after the report of our study with phenoxybenzamine as part of a regional sympathetic block, we lost complete availability of a source of phenoxybenzamine for intravenous administration. There is still no preparation of the drug at this time for intravenous injection in the United States. In an effort to be responsive to inquiries from patients with CRPS, we suggested oral treatment with phenoxybenzamine; this preparation is readily available. We have reported the experience with 4 patients that were treated with oral phenoxybenzamine and followed up for many months [19]. Since all the patients had long-standing disease before starting phenoxybenzamine treatment (13 and 20 months, and 5 and 6 years), they had received multiple drug treatments and interventions. These included oral and spinal opioids, antidepressants, multiple intravenous regional blocks with guanethidine, ankle blocks, and acupuncture. Two of the patients continued some medications in conjunction with phenoxybenzamine; more complete histories, treatments, and responses are detailed in the original report [19]. Three of the patients fulfilled classic International Association for the Study of Pain (IASP) criteria for diagnosis of CRPS type I [1, 20]. One patient did not demonstrate the classic syndrome, and we were not involved with the decision by the patient and her physician to test a course of treatment with the drug. This patient was the only one who did not have an apparent therapeutic response to the drug. The two patients who were the most severely incapacitated by disease at an advanced stage essentially returned to their predisease states. One patient had a partial, substantial improvement. She continues to take the drug at 10 mg every third day; at the time of this writing, it represents a treatment period of more than 12 years.

In comparison with the large doses of phenoxybenzamine that were used in studies noted above [14, 15], the apparent therapeutic benefit in our study was obtained with doses that did not exceed 10 mg/day, initially, and finally tapered to as low as 10 mg every third day for two of the patients. The one patient who did not have a diagnosis of CRPS and did not have a positive response eventually increased her dose to 30 mg/day before discontinuing treatment after 6 weeks. It is of interest that she did not report side effects during the treatment.

The advantage of maintenance with low doses was the avoidance of the side effects that may accompany treatment with an $\alpha$-adrenergic antagonist, in particular, orthostatic hypotension. Some symptoms of light-headedness and nausea were recorded with the first initial doses of 10 mg/day, but tolerance soon developed to these effects.

The results from the several clinical trials for treatment of CRPS with phenoxybenzamine are summarized in Table 1.

## 4. Potential Mechanisms of Action in CRPS

We have attempted to suggest a rationale for the efficacy of phenoxybenzamine in the treatment of CRPS that includes its noncompetitive (irreversible) block of both $\alpha_1$- and $\alpha_2$-adrenergic receptors [6]. The long duration of blockade of receptor access may facilitate a reversal of central nervous system sensitization, which is an accepted component of the syndrome [2]. Even in the study where the drug was administered intravenously at a total dose of 5 mg [17], the drug would have continued to be effective in the limb where it was infused (and perhaps in a wider distribution after release of the tourniquet) for many days.

We have suggested a possible multimodal mechanism of action for phenoxybenzamine in CRPS. The drug may be capable of acutely diminishing the $\alpha_1$-adrenergic-mediated vasoconstriction that is seen in the later stages of the syndrome and the hyperalgesic state, both of which are generally attributed to receptor upregulation on the vasculature and afferent sensory fibers, respectively [21, 22]. It is generally considered that the supersensitivity in CRPS is a compensatory consequence of decreased sympathetic outflow to the traumatized extremity [2, 23, 24]. The early responses to phenoxybenzamine that we observed are consistent with relatively prompt evidence of improved vascular perfusion of the limb (increased skin temperature and reduction of edema) and diminution in pain [17, 25]. In addition to these early effects, we have suggested that phenoxybenzamine may

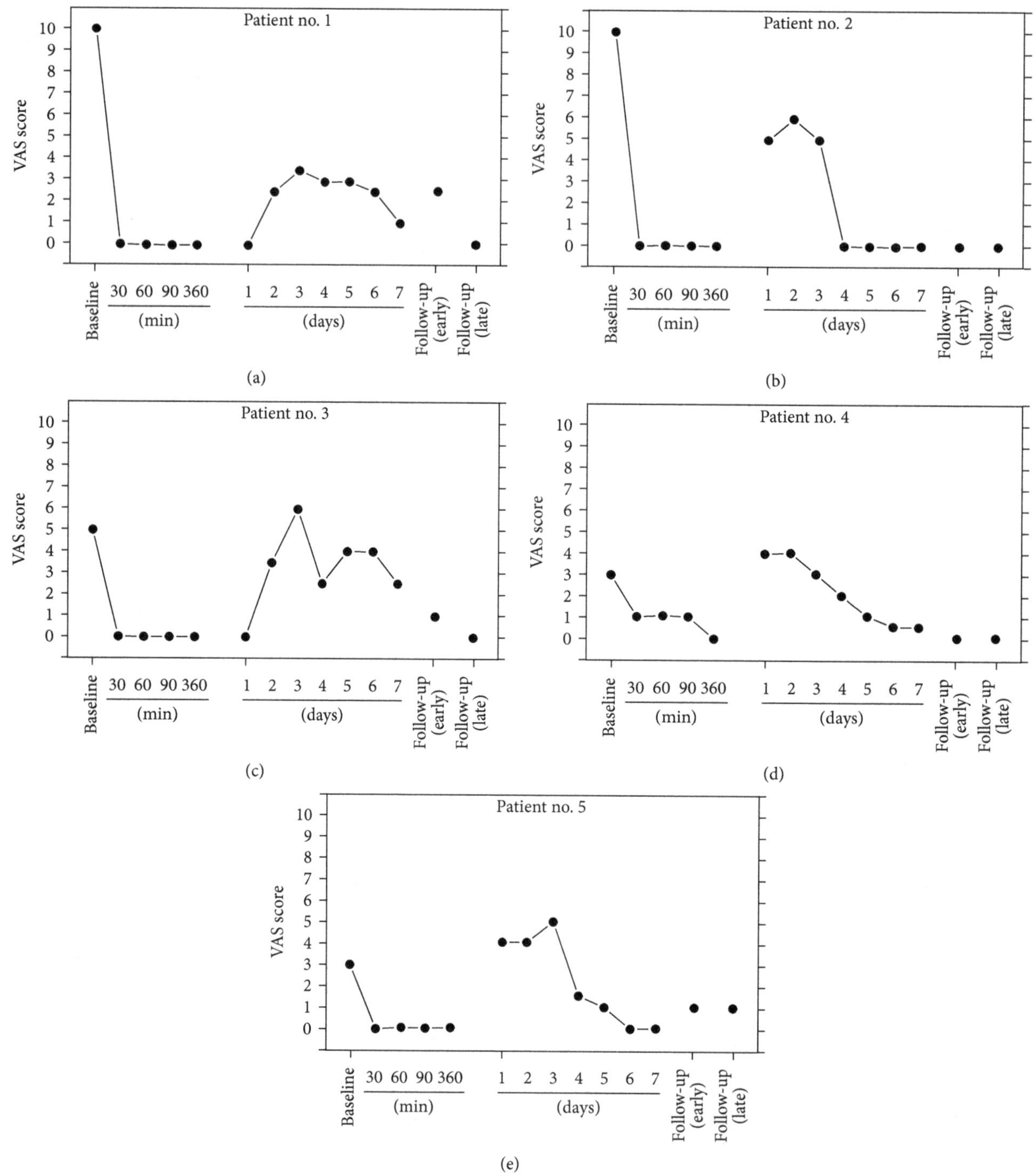


FIGURE 1: Baseline and postprocedure VAS scores for patients treated by intravenous regional blockade with phenoxybenzamine. Early follow-up evaluation times were at 6, 8, 11, 27, and 11 days after the procedure for patients 1, 2, 3, 4, and 5, respectively. The latest follow-up evaluations were at 17, 7, 5, 9, and 7 months for patients 1, 2, 3, 4, and 5, respectively. Reproduced with permission from *Anesthesiology*, 1998 [17].

exert an "immunomodulatory/anti-inflammatory" effect that may be part of its longer term contribution to the resolution of the neuropathic syndrome [19]. These effects may involve noncompetitive blockade of $\alpha_2$-adrenergic receptors on the surface membrane of immune elements, specifically, macrophages. The agonist activity of norepinephrine (and epinephrine) on $\alpha_2$-receptors of macrophages is reported to enhance the release of the inflammatory cytokine, tumor necrosis factor alpha (TNF-$\alpha$) [26, 27]. TNF-$\alpha$, substance P, and interleukin 1$\beta$ are all inflammatory cytokines that sensitize afferent sensory neurons [2, 23, 28, 29]. In this connection, phenoxybenzamine has been shown to decrease the

TABLE 1: Summary of clinical trials of phenoxybenzamine for treatment of CRPS.

| Predominant syndrome | Total number of patients | Target daily dose range (mg) | Number with favorable clinical outcome | Reference |
|---|---|---|---|---|
| CRPS II; causalgia | 15 | 40–160 | 11 | Moser et al., 1953 [13] |
| CRPS II; causalgia | 40 | 40–120 | 40 | Ghostine et al., 1984 [14] |
| CRPS I | 1 | 20 | 1 | Lefkoe and Cardenas, 1996 [16] |
| CRPS I and II | 33 | 120 | 17 | Muizelaar et al., 1997 [15] |
| CRPS I | 5 | 5 | 5 | Malik et al., 1998 [17] |
| CRPS I | 4 | 3–10 | 3 | Inchiosa and Kizelshteyn, 2008 [19] |

release of TNF-$\alpha$ from macrophages in endotoxin-challenged mice [30, 31]. A still further possible role of phenoxybenzamine in suppression of macrophage involvement relates to the fact that the release of cytokines is mediated by calmodulin [32], and phenoxybenzamine has been shown to have high potency for the inhibition of calmodulin [30, 33, 34]. The possible sites of action of phenoxybenzamine discussed above are summarized in Figure 2.

A recent publication by Chang et al. [35] has added considerable support to the relatively small body of clinical observations that show a possible therapeutic value of phenoxybenzamine for the treatment of CRPS. Their studies identified patterns of genes that were differentially expressed in the Complete Freund's Adjuvant (CFA) animal model. This model results in tactile allodynia and thermal hyperalgesia. Gene map arrays were obtained from RNA extracts of the L4 and L5 dorsal root ganglia of rats that had received intraplantar CFA for 4 days and compared with untreated matched controls. More than 100 genes from the CFA-treated animals were significantly (>1.5-fold; $P < 0.05$) up- or downregulated.

The genes that showed significant changes included many that are involved in immune function, inflammatory response, and neuron growth and survival. The total pattern of gene changes was considered to be a gene "signature" of the CFA model [35]. A search of the Broad Build02 database (and associated matching tool) [36] for pharmacologically active compounds that had strong inverse gene signatures in relation to that of the CFA pathology yielded phenoxybenzamine as one of five compounds with the strongest inverse matches of gene expression.

These investigators next compared phenoxybenzamine with naproxen for its effects on mechanical allodynia in the CFA 4-day model [35]. The drugs and vehicle control were administered by oral gavage on day 4, and behavioral responses to stimuli were measured two hours later. Phenoxybenzamine was found to have approximately equal potency to naproxen in this pain model. With both drugs at a single dose of 10 mg/kg, naproxen reversed the pain sensitivity by 93%, and phenoxybenzamine caused an 82% reversal.

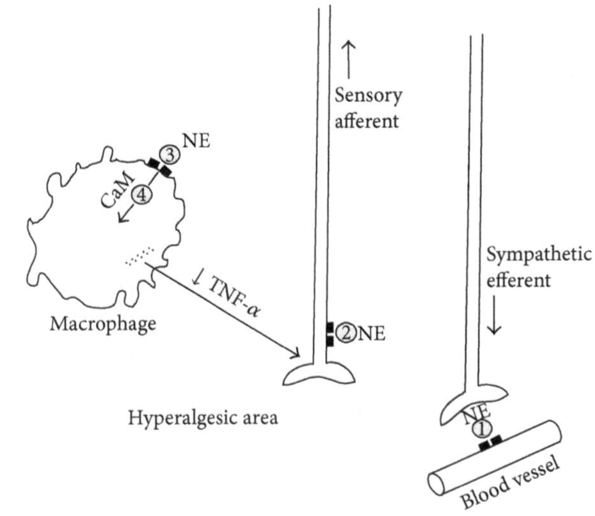


FIGURE 2: Depiction of possible sites of action of phenoxybenzamine in the suppression of neuropathic pain. Site 1) Blockade of norepinephrine (NE) effects on $\alpha_1$-adrenergic receptors on blood vessels, thereby promoting vasodilation; Site 2) blockade of adrenergic receptors that populate afferent sensory fibers; Site 3) blockade of $\alpha_2$-adrenergic receptors on the surface of macrophages, which appear to mediate release of proinflammatory cytokines, including tumor necrosis factor-$\alpha$ (TNF-$\alpha$); Site 4) inhibition of calmodulin (CaM), which is involved in the cytokine-release process. (Schematically based on Figure 4 of Jänig and Baron, 2003; [23] reproduced with permission from *Pain Practice*, 2008 [19]).

## 5. Side Effects

We have commented previously [19] on the fact that the most common side effects of phenoxybenzamine are related to its $\alpha$-adrenergic antagonist effects. These include postural hypotension, associated reflex tachycardia, and nasal congestion. These effects are relatively minor and are all dose related, and tolerance to these effects, when they appeared, took place after several doses in our own studies [19]. Inhibition of ejaculation has been reported in males, but it would seem that this occurs at higher doses of the drug than the doses used in our experience.

## 6. Controversies in Relation to Carcinogenic Risks

The labeling for the proprietary oral dosage form of phenoxybenzamine, Dibenzyline, carries a warning regarding possible carcinogenic and mutagenic risks, as observed in *in vitro* and small animal testing (WellSpring Pharmaceutical Corporation, Sarasota, FL). These findings are always of concern and warrant consideration of a risk to benefit evaluation. However, there is little or no evidence that the drug is carcinogenic in humans. Te [37] and Inchiosa and Kizelshteyn [19] have commented on the precedents of widely used drugs (e.g., spironolactone and several of the statin class drugs) that have evidence in animals of carcinogenicity at multiples of human doses. Te [37] has discussed the fact that these concerns have probably limited the valuable application of phenoxybenzamine for the treatment of urinary tract disorders and other pathologies. In his 2002 paper, he estimated that more than 20,000 patients would have been exposed to phenoxybenzamine since it was introduced in 1953. In a review of surveillance data up to 1961, and continuing with adverse event reporting, there were no reports of human cancer that would have appeared to have been related to treatment with phenoxybenzamine [37].

Early in 2013, through the United States Freedom of Information policies, I requested the Adverse Events Reporting data from the FDA for phenoxybenzamine for the past 10-year period. This would largely cover the period since Dr. Te's researches. There were 3 cases in which a malignant disease was recorded in a patient that had received phenoxybenzamine. One case of breast cancer can probably be discounted in regard to an association with phenoxybenzamine since cancer was already suspected at the time that the drug was started. The two other cases involved the use of the drug for urinary obstructive indications. The therapy seemed to have been beneficial for those conditions. Although the adverse event reports from the FDA do not list identifying information, it would appear that they are the same two cases cited in the package insert for Dibenzyline [38, 39]. Both patients had complicated medical histories; it may not be possible to assign cause and effect. It can be noted again that the drug has been in continuous clinical use for 60 years, and there is a paucity of documented evidence of an association with human cancer.

Of particular value in evaluating the question of carcinogenic concerns with phenoxybenzamine is a recent study from the Kaiser Permanente Medical Care Program [40]. This organization is a large chronic care institution with automated records of drugs dispensed and a cancer registry. They analyzed their databases for evidence of carcinogenicity in association with treatment with 9 drugs that are classified by the International Agency for Research on Cancer as probable or possible human carcinogens based on animal or limited human data. Phenoxybenzamine was one of the drugs investigated. It was used in the treatment of a total of 592 patients; there was no statistically significant association with any human cancer.

## 7. Conclusions

Phenoxybenzamine may be a reasonable drug for consideration in the treatment of CRPS, particularly, when a patient has not shown a satisfactory therapeutic response to more conventional therapies. It might also be considered before more invasive therapies, such as intraspinal opioid infusion or spinal cord stimulation, are undertaken. Also, it might be expected that a trial of treatment with phenoxybenzamine for a period of several days may be adequate to detect some improvement in symptoms if the drug is going to have a value for a particular patient [19]. Depending on a patient's current therapies, it may be possible to simply add the drug to the regimen, thereby eliciting some potential additive or synergistic effect. The hypotheses presented here that include potential immunomodulatory/anti-inflammatory effects of phenoxybenzamine appear to be consistent with evidence of an autoimmune contribution to the syndrome [41].

## Conflict of Interests

The author has no conflict of interests in relation to this review.

## Acknowledgments

The preparation of this review was supported by the Departments of Pharmacology and Anesthesiology of New York Medical College. The author is identified with a United States patent titled "Formulations of haloalkylamines and local anesthetics and methods for the treatment of reflex sympathetic dystrophy (RSD)." New York Medical College has sole ownership of this patent. There is currently no FDA-approved intravenous preparation of phenoxybenzamine available in the United States. The author appreciates the assistance of Venu M. Pothula, Department of Pharmacology, New York Medical College, in accessing and analyzing the FDA Adverse Events Reporting data bases.

## References

[1] M. Stanton-Hicks, W. Janig, S. Hassenbusch, J. D. Haddox, R. Boas, and P. Wilson, "Reflex sympathetic dystrophy: changing concepts and taxonomy," *Pain*, vol. 63, no. 1, pp. 127–133, 1995.

[2] R. J. Schwartzman, G. M. Alexander, and J. Grothusen, "Pathophysiology of complex regional pain syndrome," *Expert Review of Neurotherapeutics*, vol. 6, no. 5, pp. 669–681, 2006.

[3] H. Merskey and N. Bogduk, "Descriptions of chronic pain syndromes and definitions of pain terms," in *Classification of Chronic Pain*, pp. 40–43, IASP Press, Seattle, Wash, USA, 1994.

[4] P. J. Albrecht, S. Hines, E. Eisenberg et al., "Pathologic alterations of cutaneous innervation and vasculature in affected limbs from patients with complex regional pain syndrome," *Pain*, vol. 120, no. 3, pp. 244–266, 2006.

[5] A. L. Oaklander, J. G. Rissmiller, L. B. Gelman, L. Zheng, Y. Chang, and R. Gott, "Evidence of focal small-fiber axonal degeneration in complex regional pain syndrome-I (reflex sympathetic dystrophy)," *Pain*, vol. 120, no. 3, pp. 235–243, 2006.

[6] T. C. Westfall and D. P. Westfall, "Adrenergic agonists and antagonists," in *Goodman and Gilman's, the Pharmacological Basis of Therapeutics*, L. L. Brunton, Ed., pp. 267–268, McGraw-Hill, New York, NY, USA, 2006.

[7] C. Hamilton, H. Dalrymple, and J. Reid, "Recovery in vivo and in vitro of $\alpha$-adrenoceptor responses and radioligand binding after phenoxybenzamine," *Journal of Cardiovascular Pharmacology*, vol. 4, no. 1, supplement, pp. S125–S128, 1982.

[8] T. N. Weingarten, J. P. Cata, J. F. O'Hara et al., "Comparison of two preoperative medical management strategies for laparoscopic resection of pheochromocytoma," *Urology*, vol. 76, no. 2, pp. 508–511, 2010.

[9] R. S. Perez, P. E. Zollinger, P. U. Dijkstra et al., "Evidence based guidelines for complex regional pain syndrome type 1," *BMC Neurology*, vol. 10, article 20, 2010.

[10] L. Cossins, R. W. Okell, H. Cameron, B. Simpson, H. M. Poole, and A. Goebel, "Treatment of complex regional pain syndrome in adults: a systematic review of randomized controlled trials published from June 2000 to February 2012," *European Journal of Pain*, vol. 17, pp. 158–173, 2013.

[11] American Hospital Formulary Service, American Society of Health-System Pharmacists, Bethesda, Md, USA, 2013.

[12] D. S. Bennett and D. Brookoff, "Complex regional pain syndromes (reflex sympathetic dystrophy and causalgia) and spinal cord stimulation," *Pain Medicine*, vol. 7, no. 1, pp. S64–S96, 2006.

[13] M. MOSER, A. G. PRANDONI, J. A. ORBISON, and T. W. MATTINGLY, "Clinical experience with sympathetic blocking agents in peripheral vascular disease," *Annals of Internal Medicine*, vol. 38, no. 6, pp. 1245–1264, 1953.

[14] S. Y. Ghostine, Y. G. Comair, and D. M. Turner, "Phenoxybenzamine in the treatment of causalgia. Report of 40 cases," *Journal of Neurosurgery*, vol. 60, no. 6, pp. 1263–1268, 1984.

[15] J. P. Muizelaar, M. Kleyer, I. A. M. Hertogs, and D. C. DeLange, "Complex regional pain syndrome (reflex sympathetic dystrophy and causalgia): management with the calcium channel blocker nifedipine and/or the α-sympathetic blocker phenoxybenzamine in 59 patients," *Clinical Neurology and Neurosurgery*, vol. 99, no. 1, pp. 26–30, 1997.

[16] T. P. Lefkoe and D. D. Cardenas, "Reflex sympathetic dystrophy of the lower extremity in tetraplegia: case report," *Spinal Cord*, vol. 34, no. 4, pp. 239–242, 1996.

[17] V. K. Malik, M. A. Inchiosa Jr., K. Mustafa, M. Sanapati, M. C. Pimentel Jr., and E. A. M. Frost, "Intravenous regional phenoxybenzamine in the treatment of reflex sympathetic dystrophy," *Anesthesiology*, vol. 88, no. 3, pp. 823–827, 1998.

[18] M. De Mos, M. C. J. M. Sturkenboom, and F. J. P. M. Huygen, "Current understandings on complex regional pain syndrome," *Pain Practice*, vol. 9, no. 2, pp. 86–99, 2009.

[19] M. A. Inchiosa Jr. and G. Kizelshteyn, "Treatment of complex regional pain syndrome type I with oral phenoxybenzamine: rationale and case reports," *Pain Practice*, vol. 8, no. 2, pp. 125–132, 2008.

[20] R. N. Harden, S. Bruehl, M. Stanton-Hicks, and P. R. Wilson, "Proposed new diagnostic criteria for complex regional pain syndrome," *Pain Medicine*, vol. 8, no. 4, pp. 326–331, 2007.

[21] R. Baron and C. Maier, "Reflex sympathetic dystrophy: skin blood flow, sympathetic vasoconstrictor reflexes and pain before and after surgical sympathectomy," *Pain*, vol. 67, no. 2-3, pp. 317–326, 1996.

[22] P. D. Drummond, S. Skipworth, and P. M. Finch, "α1-Adrenoceptors in normal and hyperalgesic human skin," *Clinical Science*, vol. 91, no. 1, pp. 73–77, 1996.

[23] W. Jänig and R. Baron, "Complex regional pain syndrome: mystery explained?" *The Lancet Neurology*, vol. 2, no. 11, pp. 687–697, 2003.

[24] G. Wasner, J. Schattschneider, K. Heckmann, C. Maier, and R. Baron, "Vascular abnormalities in reflex sympathetic dystrophy (CRPS I): mechanisms and diagnostic value," *Brain*, vol. 124, no. 3, pp. 587–599, 2001.

[25] P. D. Drummond, P. M. Finch, S. Skipworth, and P. Blockey, "Pain increases during sympathetic arousal in patients with complex regional pain syndrome," *Neurology*, vol. 57, no. 7, pp. 1296–1303, 2001.

[26] R. N. Spengler, R. M. Allen, D. G. Remick, R. M. Strieter, and S. L. Kunkel, "Stimulation of α-adrenergic receptor augments the production of macrophage-derived tumor necrosis factor," *Journal of Immunology*, vol. 145, no. 5, pp. 1430–1434, 1990.

[27] I. J. Elenkov, R. L. Wilder, G. P. Chrousos, and E. S. Vizi, "The sympathetic nerve—an integrative interface between two supersystems: the brain and the immune system," *Pharmacological Reviews*, vol. 52, no. 4, pp. 595–638, 2000.

[28] M. Weber, F. Birklein, B. Neundörfer, and M. Schmelz, "Facilitated neurogenic inflammation in complex regional pain syndrome," *Pain*, vol. 91, no. 3, pp. 251–257, 2001.

[29] P. E. Molina, "Neurobiology of the stress response: contribution of the sympathetic nervous system to the neuroimmune axis in traumatic injury," *Shock*, vol. 24, no. 1, pp. 3–10, 2005.

[30] R. Bertini, S. Garattini, R. Delgado, and P. Ghezzi, "Pharmacological activities of chlorpromazine involved in the inhibition of tumour necrosis factor production in vivo in mice," *Immunology*, vol. 79, no. 2, pp. 217–219, 1993.

[31] N. Bloksma, F. Hofhuis, B. Benaissa-Trouw, and J. Willers, "Endotoxin-induced release of tumour necrosis factor and interferon in vivo is inhibited by prior adrenoceptor blockade," *Cancer Immunology, Immunotherapy*, vol. 14, no. 1, pp. 41–45, 1982.

[32] C.-J. Lo, I. Garcia, H. G. Cryer, and R. V. Maier, "Calcium and calmodulin regulate lipopolysaccharide-induced alveolar macrophage production of tumor necrosis factor and procoagulant activity," *Archives of Surgery*, vol. 131, no. 1, pp. 44–50, 1996.

[33] C. Q. Earl, W. C. Prozialeck, and B. Weiss, "Interaction of alpha adrenergic antagonists with calmodulin," *Life Sciences*, vol. 35, no. 5, pp. 525–534, 1984.

[34] T. J. Lukas, D. R. Marshak, and D. M. Watterson, "Drug-protein interactions: isolation and characterization of covalent adducts of phenoxybenzamine and calmodulin," *Biochemistry*, vol. 24, no. 1, pp. 151–157, 1985.

[35] M. Chang, S. Smith, A. Thorpe, M. J. Barratt, and F. Karim, "Evaluation of phenoxybenzamine in the CFA model of pain following gene expression studies and connectivity mapping," *Molecular Pain*, vol. 6, article 56, 2010.

[36] J. Lamb, E. D. Crawford, D. Peck et al., "The connectivity map: using gene-expression signatures to connect small molecules, genes, and disease," *Science*, vol. 313, no. 5795, pp. 1929–1935, 2006.

[37] A. E. Te, "A modern rationale for the use of phenoxybenzamine in urinary tract disorders and other conditions," *Clinical Therapeutics*, vol. 24, no. 6, pp. 851–861, 2002.

[38] O. Nettesheim, G. Höffken, M. Gahr, and M. Breidert, "Haematemesis and dysphagia in a 20-year-old woman with congenital spine malformation and situs inversus partialis," *Zeitschrift fur Gastroenterologie*, vol. 41, no. 4, pp. 319–324, 2003.

[39] S. Vaidyanathan, P. Mansour, B. M. Soni, P. L. Hughes, and G. Singh, "Chronic lymphocytic leukaemia, synchronous small cell carcinoma and squamous neoplasia of the urinary bladder in a paraplegic man following long-term phenoxybenzamine therapy," *Spinal Cord*, vol. 44, no. 3, pp. 188–191, 2006.

[40] G. D. Friedman, S.-F. Jiang, N. Udaltsova, C. P. Quesenberry Jr., J. Chan, and L. A. Habel, "Epidemiologic evaluation of pharmaceuticals with limited evidence of carcinogenicity," *International Journal of Cancer*, vol. 125, no. 9, pp. 2173–2178, 2009.

[41] A. Goebel and F. Blaes, "Complex regional pain syndrome, prototype of a novel kind of autoimmune disease," *Autoimmunity Reviews*, vol. 12, pp. 682–686, 2013.

# 11

# Achieving the Recommended Endotracheal Tube Cuff Pressure: A Randomized Control Study Comparing Loss of Resistance Syringe to Pilot Balloon Palpation

**Fred Bulamba,[1] Andrew Kintu,[2] Nodreen Ayupo,[2] Charles Kojjo,[2] Lameck Ssemogerere,[2] Agnes Wabule,[2] and Arthur Kwizera[2]**

[1]*Department of Anaesthesia and Critical Care, Faculty of Health Sciences, Busitema University, Mbale, Uganda*
[2]*Department of Anaesthesia and Critical Care, College of Health Sciences, Makerere University, Kampala, Uganda*

Correspondence should be addressed to Fred Bulamba; fredflybulamba@gmail.com

Academic Editor: Ferenc Petak

*Background.* Both under- and overinflation of endotracheal tube cuffs can result in significant harm to the patient. The optimal technique for establishing and maintaining safe cuff pressures (20–30 cm$H_2O$) is the cuff pressure manometer, but this is not widely available, especially in resource-limited settings where its use is limited by cost of acquisition and maintenance. Therefore, anesthesia providers commonly rely on subjective methods to estimate safe endotracheal cuff pressure. This study set out to determine the efficacy of the loss of resistance syringe method at estimating endotracheal cuff pressures. *Methods.* This was a randomized clinical trial. We enrolled adult patients scheduled to undergo general anesthesia for elective surgery at Mulago Hospital, Uganda. Study participants were randomized to have their endotracheal cuff pressures estimated by either loss of resistance syringe or pilot balloon palpation. The pressures measured were recorded. *Results.* One hundred seventy-eight patients were analyzed. 66.3% (59/89) of patients in the loss of resistance group had cuff pressures in the recommended range compared with 22.5% (20/89) from the pilot balloon palpation method. This was statistically significant. *Conclusion.* The loss of resistance syringe method was superior to pilot balloon palpation at administering pressures in the recommended range. This method provides a viable option to cuff inflation.

## 1. Background

High-volume low-pressure cuffed endotracheal tubes (ETT) are the standard of airway protection. However, they have potential complications [1–3]. Underinflation increases the risk of air leakage and aspiration of gastric and oral pharyngeal secretions [4, 5]. Cuff pressures less than 20 cm$H_2O$ have been shown to predispose to aspiration which is still a major cause of morbidity, mortality, length of stay, and cost of hospital care as revealed by the NAP4 UK study. In this cohort, aspiration had the second highest incidence of primary airway-related serious events [6].

On the other hand, overinflation may cause catastrophic complications. It has been demonstrated that, beyond 50 cm$H_2O$, there is total obstruction to blood flow to the tracheal tissues. This has been shown to cause severe tracheal lesions and morbidity [7, 8]. However, less serious complications like dysphagia, hoarseness, and sore throat are more prevalent [9–11]. There are a number of strategies that have been developed to decrease the risk of aspiration, but the most important of all is continuous control of cuff pressures.

To achieve the optimal ETT cuff pressure of 20–30 cm$H_2O$ [3, 8, 12–14], ETT cuffs should be inflated with a cuff manometer [15, 16]. However, these are prohibitively expensive to acquire and maintain in many operating theaters, and as such, many anesthesia providers resort to subjective methods like pilot balloon palpation (PBP) which is ineffective [1, 2, 16–20]. Alternative, cheaper methods like the minimum leak test that require no special equipment have produced inconsistent results.

A newer method, the passive release technique, although with limitations, has been shown to estimate cuff pressures better [21–24]. This method has been achieved with a modified epidural pulsator syringe [13, 18], a 20 ml disposable syringe, and more recently, a loss of resistance (LOR) syringe [21, 23, 24]. Compared with the cuff manometer, it would be cheaper to acquire and maintain a loss of resistance syringe especially in low-resource settings.

Our study set out to investigate the efficacy of the loss of resistance syringe in a surgical population under general anesthesia. ETT cuff pressures would be measured with a cuff manometer following estimation by either the PBP method or the LOR method. Our secondary objective was to determine the incidence of postextubation airway complaints in patients who had cuff pressures adjusted to 20–30 $cmH_2O$ range or 31–40 $cmH_2O$ range.

## 2. Materials and Methods

*2.1. Study Design and Setting.* This single-blinded, parallel-group, randomized control study was performed at Mulago National Referral Hospital, Uganda. The hospital has a bed capacity of 1500 inpatient beds, 16 operating rooms, and a mean daily output of 90 surgical operations. Anesthesia services are provided by different levels of providers including physician anesthetists (anesthesiologists), residents, and nonphysician anesthetists (anesthetic officers and anesthetic officer students). In the early years of training, all trainees provide anesthesia under direct supervision. In the later years, however, they can administer anesthesia either independently or under remote supervision.

*2.2. Study Population.* We included ASA class I to III adult patients scheduled to receive general anesthesia with endotracheal intubation for elective surgical operation. All patients with any of the following conditions were excluded: known or anticipated laryngeal tracheal abnormalities or airway trauma, preexisting airway symptoms, laparoscopic and maxillofacial surgery patients, and those expected to remain intubated beyond the operative room period.

*2.3. Randomization, Blinding, and Enrollment.* After screening, participants were allocated to either the PBP or the LOR group using block randomization, achieving a 1 : 1 allocation ratio. The allocation sequence was generated by an Internet-based application with the following input: nine sets of unsorted sequences, each containing twenty unique allocation numbers (1–20). Numbers 1–10 were labeled LOR, and numbers 11–20 were labeled PBP. The allocation sequence was concealed from the investigator by inserting it into opaque envelopes (according to the clocks) until the time of the intervention.

At the time of the intervention, the study investigator retrieved the next available envelope, which indicated the intervention group, from the next available block envelope and handed it to the research assistant. The patient was the only person blinded to the intervention group.

The anesthesia providers were either physician anesthetists (anesthesiologists or residents) or nonphysicians (anesthetic officer or anesthetic officer student). Students were under the supervision of a senior anesthetic officer or an anesthesiologist.

*2.4. Sample Size.* To detect a 15% difference between PBP and LOR groups, it was calculated that at least 172 patients would be required to be 80% certain that the limits of a 95%, two-sided interval included the difference.

*2.5. Intervention and Anesthetic Technique.* Every patient was wheeled into the operating theater and transferred to the operating table. Basic routine monitors were attached as per hospital standards. A wide-bore intravenous cannula (16- or 18-G) was placed for administration of drugs and fluids.

The patient was then preoxygenated with 100% oxygen and general anesthesia induced with a combination of drugs selected by the anesthesia care provider. These included an intravenous induction agent, an opioid, and a muscle relaxant. All patients received either suxamethonium (2 mg/kg, max 100 mg to aid laryngoscopy) or cisatracurium (0.15 mg/kg at for prolonged muscle relaxation) and were given optimal time before intubation. Using a laryngoscope, tracheal intubation was performed, ETT position confirmed, and secured with tape within 2 min. The size of ETT (POLYMED Medicure, India) was selected by the anesthesia care provider. With the patient's head in a neutral position, the anesthesia care provider inflated the ETT cuff with air using a 10 ml syringe (BD Discardit II). A research assistant (different from the anesthesia care provider) read out the patient's group, and one of the following procedures was followed.

PBP group (active comparator): in this group, the anesthesia care provider was asked to reduce or increase the pressure in the ETT cuff by inflating with air or deflating the pilot balloon using a 10 ml syringe (BD Discardit II) while simultaneously palpating the pilot balloon until a point he or she felt was appropriate for the patient. When this point was reached, the 10 ml syringe was then detached from the pilot balloon, and a cuff manometer (VBM, Medicintechnik Germany. Accuracy −2 $cmH_2O$) was attached. The pressure reading of the VBM was recorded by the research assistant.

LOR group (experimental): in this group, the research assistant attached a 7 ml plastic, luer slip loss of resistance syringe (BD Epilor, USA) containing air onto the pilot balloon. The cuff was then briefly overinflated through the pilot balloon, and the loss of resistance syringe plunger was allowed to passively draw back until it ceased. This point was observed by the research assistant and witnessed by the anesthesia care provider. The loss of resistance syringe was then detached, the VBM manometer was attached, and the pressure reading was recorded.

Cuff pressure adjustment: in both arms, very high and very low pressures were adjusted as per the recommendation by the ethics committee. In case of a very low pressure reading (below 20 $cmH_2O$), the ETT cuff pressure would be adjusted to 24 $cmH_2O$ using the manometer. On the other hand, high cuff pressures beyond 50 $cmH_2O$ were reduced to 40 $cmH_2O$.

Also, at the end of the pressure measurement in both groups, the manometer was detached, breathing circuit was

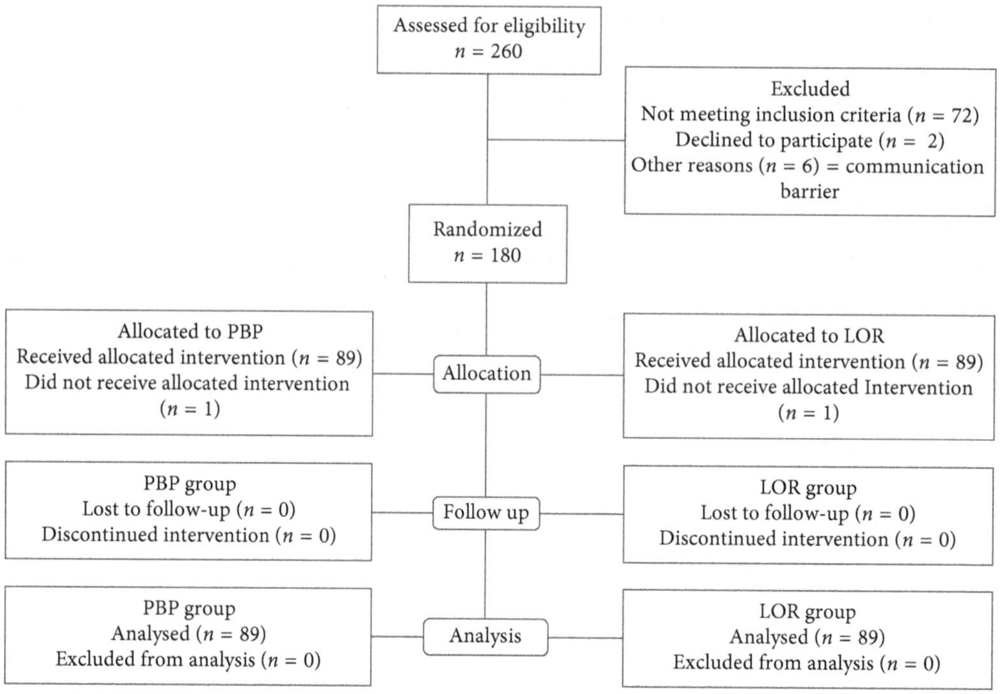


FIGURE 1: A CONSORT flow diagram of study patients. LOR = loss of resistance syringe method; PBP = pilot balloon palpation method.

attached to the ETT, and ventilation was started. The patient was maintained on isoflurane (1–1.8%) mixed with 100% oxygen flowing at 2 L/min. Anesthesia continued without further adjustment of ETT cuff pressure until the end of the case. Nitrous oxide and medical air were not used as these agents are unavailable at this hospital. All patients who received non-depolarizing muscle relaxants were reversed with neostigmine 0.03 mg/kg and atropine 0.01 mg/kg at the end of surgery.

*2.6. Primary Outcome.* Cuff pressure reading of the VBM manometer was recorded by the research assistant. The individual anesthesia care providers participated more than once during the study period of seven months.

*2.7. Secondary Outcome.* The patients were followed up and interviewed only once at 24 hours after intubation for presence of cough, sore throat, dysphagia, and/or dysphonia. Only two of the four research assistants reviewed the patients postoperatively, and these were blinded to the intervention arm. This outcome was compared between patients with cuff pressures from 20 to 30 $cmH_2O$ range and those from 31 to 40 $cmH_2O$ following the initial correction of cuff pressures.

*2.8. Data Management.* All data were double entered into EpiData version 3.1 software (The EpiData Association, Odense, Denmark), with range, consistency, and validation checks embedded to aid data cleaning. The data were exported to and analyzed using STATA software version 12 (StataCorp Inc., Texas, USA).

Categorical data are presented in tabular, graphical, and text forms and categorized into PBP and LOR groups. The chi-square test was used for categorical data. Continuous data are presented as the mean with standard deviation and were compared between the groups using the $t$-test to detect any significant statistical differences.

The magnitude of effect on the primary outcome was computed for 95% CI using the $t$-test for difference in group means. An intention-to-treat analysis method was used, and the main outcome of interest was the proportion of cuff pressures in the range 20–30 $cmH_2O$ in each group.

For the secondary outcome, incidence of complaints was calculated for those with cuff pressures from 20 to 30 $cmH_2O$ range and those from 31 to 40 $cmH_2O$.

*2.9. Data Safety Management Board.* The Data Safety Management Board (DSMB) comprised an anesthesiologist, a statistician, and a member of the SOMREC IRB who would be informed of any adverse event. The study would be discontinued if 5% of study subjects in one study group experienced an adverse event associated with the study interventions as determined by the DSMB, or if a $p$ value of $<0.001$ was obtained on an interim analysis performed halfway through patient accrual. None of these was met at interim analysis.

*2.10. Ethical Considerations.* The study was approved by the School of Medicine Research and Ethics Committee, Makerere University, and registered with http://www.clinicaltrials.gov (NCT02294422). All patients provided informed, written consent before the start of surgery.

## 3. Results

*3.1. Baseline Characteristics.* A total of 178 patients were enrolled from August 2014 to February 2015 with an equal

TABLE 1: Baseline characteristics of patients.

| Variable | Pilot balloon palpation ($n = 89$) | Loss of resistance ($n = 89$) | Total $N = 178$ | $p$ value |
|---|---|---|---|---|
| *Age group (years)* | | | | |
| Mean (sd, min-max) | 42.3 (15.6, 19–89) | 42.6 (15.2, 18–78) | — | 0.19 |
| *Sex, n (%)* | | | | |
| Female | 62 (69.7) | 74 (83.1) | 136 (76.4) | 0.034 |
| Male | 27 (30.3) | 15 (16.9) | 42 (23.6) | — |
| *ETT size in mm, n (%)* | | | | |
| 6.5 | 7 (7.9) | 9 (10.1) | 16 (8.99) | — |
| 7.0 | 38 (42.7) | 34 (38.2) | 72 (40.45) | — |
| 7.5 | 33 (37) | 45 (50.6) | 78 (43.82) | 0.028 |
| 8.0 | 6 (6.7) | 1 (1.1) | 7 (3.93) | — |
| 8.5 | 5 (5.7) | 0 (0) | 5 (2.81) | — |
| *Duration of intubation in hrs, n (%)* | | | | |
| ≤1 | 28 (31.2) | 17 (19.1) | 45 (25.3) | — |
| 1-2 | 42 (47.2) | 46 (51.7) | 88 (49.4) | — |
| >2 | 19 (21.6) | 26 (29.2) | 45 (25.3) | 0.14 |
| *Provider level, n (%)* | | | | |
| *Resident | 28 (31.5) | 72 (80.9) | 100 (56.2) | — |
| **AO | 51 (57.3) | 10 (11.2) | 61 (34.3) | — |
| AO students | 2 (2.2) | 3 (3.4) | 5 (2.8) | — |
| Anesthesiologist | 8 (9.0) | 4 (4.5) | 12 (6.7) | — |

*Anesthesiology resident, **anesthetic officer.

TABLE 2: ETT cuff pressure estimation by the PBP and LOR methods.

| Method | Cuff pressure ranges, $N$ (%) <20 | 20–30 | 31–40 | >40 | Mean (sd) | Proportion adjusted |
|---|---|---|---|---|---|---|
| PBP | 8 | 20 | 18 | 43 | 51 (28.9) | 51 (57.3) |
| LOR | 11 | 59 | 18 | 1 | 27 (5.8) | 12 (13.5) |

All those <20 and >40 were adjusted by the manometer.

distribution between arms as shown in the CONSORT diagram in Figure 1.

The study comprised more female patients (76.4%). In addition, most patients were below 50 years (76.4%). The study groups were similar in relation to sex, age, and ETT size (Table 1).

*3.2. ETT Cuff Pressures.* Generally, the proportion of ETT cuffs inflated to the recommended pressure was less in the PBP group at 22.5% (20/89) compared with the LOR group at 66.3% (59/89) with a statistically significant positive mean difference of 0.47 with $p$ value < 0.01 (0.343–0.602). Also to note, most cuffs in the PBP group were inflated to a pressure that exceeded the recommended range in the PBP group, and 51% of the cuff pressures attained had to be adjusted compared with only 12% in the LOR group (Table 2).

The distribution of cuff pressures (unadjusted) achieved by the different care providers is shown in Figure 2. The difference in the number of intubations performed by the different level of providers is huge with anesthesia residents and anesthetic officers performing almost all intubation and initial cuff pressure estimations.

*3.3. Postextubation Airway Symptoms.* The total number of patients who experienced at least one postextubation airway symptom was 113, accounting for 63.5% of all patients. The incidence of postextubation airway complaints after 24 hours was lower in patients with a cuff pressure adjusted to the 20–30 $cmH_2O$ range, 57.1% (56/98), compared with those whose cuff pressure was adjusted to the 30–40 $cmH_2O$ range, 71.3% (57/80). This however was not statistically significant ($p$ value 0.053) (Table 3).

## 4. Discussion

*4.1. Study Population.* We conducted a single-blinded randomized control study to evaluate the LOR syringe method in accordance with the CONSORT guideline (CONSORT checklist provided as Supplementary Materials available here).

At the study hospital, there are more females undergoing elective surgery under general anesthesia compared with males. In addition, over 90% of anesthesia care at this hospital was provided by anesthetic officers and anesthesia residents during the study period. Anesthetic officers provide over 80% of anesthetics in Uganda.

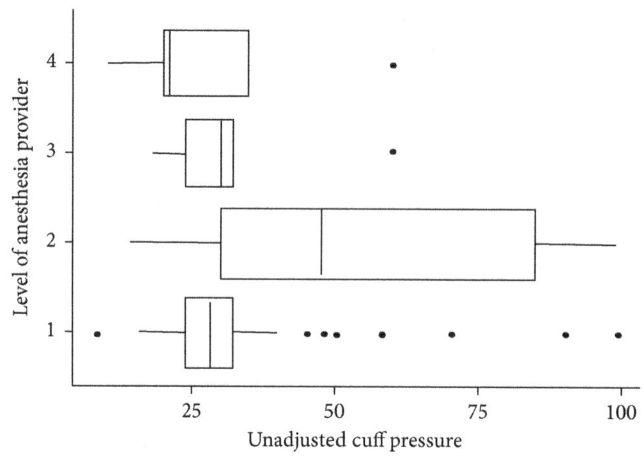


FIGURE 2: The distribution of cuff pressures achieved by the different levels of providers. 1: anesthesia resident; 2: anesthesia officer; 3: anesthesia officer student; 4: anesthesiologist.

TABLE 3: Incidence of postextubation airway complaints in the study population.

| Complaint, $n$ (%) | All participants, $N = 178$ | 20–30 $cmH_2O$, $N = 98$ | 31–40 $cmH_2O$, $N = 80$ | $p$ value |
|---|---|---|---|---|
| At least one | 113 (63.5) | 56 (57.1) | 57 (71.2) | 0.052 |
| None | 65 (36.5) | 42 (42.9) | 23 (28.8) | — |
| *With cough* | | | | |
| Yes | 45 (25.3) | 17 (17.3) | 28 (35.0) | 0.07 |
| No | 133 (74.7) | 81 (82.7) | 52 (65.0) | — |
| *With dysphagia* | | | | |
| Yes | 14 (8.0) | 8 (8.2) | 6 (7.5) | 0.87 |
| No | 164 (92.0) | 90 (91.8) | 74 (92.5) | — |
| *With dysphonia* | | | | |
| Yes | 16 (9.0) | 14 (14.3) | 2 (2.5) | 0.029 |
| No | 162 (91.0) | 84 (85.7) | 78 (97.5) | — |
| *With sore throat* | | | | |
| Yes | 89 (50.0) | 42 (42.9) | 47 (58.7) | 0.035 |
| No | 89 (50.0) | 56 (57.1) | 33 (41.3) | — |

*4.2. ETT Cuff Pressure.* The primary outcome of the study was to determine the proportion of cuff pressures in the optimal range from either group. The initial, unadjusted cuff pressures from either method were used for this outcome. When considering this primary outcome, the LOR syringe method had a significantly higher proportion compared to the PBP method. This adds to the growing evidence to support the use of the LOR syringe for ETT cuff pressure estimation. There are data regarding the use of the LOR syringe method for administering ETT cuff pressures [21, 23, 24], but studies on a perioperative population are scanty. In our study, 66.3% of ETT cuff pressures estimated by the LOR syringe method were in the optimal range. Kim and coworkers, who evaluated this method in the emergency department, found an even higher percentage of cuff pressures in the "normal range" (22–32 $cmH_2O$) in their study. Another study, using nonhuman tracheal models and a wider range (15–30 $cmH_2O$) as the optimal, had all cuff pressures within the optimal range [21]. It is however difficult to extrapolate these results to the human population since the risk of aspiration of gastric contents is zero while working with models when compared with patients.

There is a relatively small risk of getting ETT cuff pressures less than 30 $cmH_2O$ with the use of the LOR syringe method [23, 24], 12.4% from the current study. Secondly, this method is still provider-dependent as they decide when plunger draw-back has ceased. Precaution was taken to avoid premature detachment of the loss of resistance syringe in this study.

The PBP method, although commonly employed in operating rooms, has been repetitively shown to administer cuff pressures out of the optimal range (20–30 $cmH_2O$) [2, 3, 25]. Findings from this study were in agreement, with 25.3% of cuff pressures in the optimal range after estimation by the PBP method. It should however be noted that some of these studies have been carried out in different environments (emergency rooms) and on different kinds of patients (emergency patients) by providers of varying experience [2].

Another viable argument is to employ a more pragmatic solution to prevent overly high cuff pressures by inflating the cuff until no air leak is detected by auscultation. This method is cheap and reproducible and is likely to estimate cuff pressures around the normal range. Perhaps the LOR syringe method needs to be evaluated against the "no air leak on auscultation" method.

This study shows that the LOR syringe method is better at estimating cuff pressures in the optimal range when compared with the PBP method but still falls short in comparison to the cuff manometer. In low- and middle-income countries, the cost of acquiring ($ 250–300) and maintaining a cuff manometer is still prohibitive.

*4.3. Postextubation Airway Complaints.* The secondary objective of the study evaluated airway complaints in those who had cuff pressure in the optimal range (20–30 $cmH_2O$) and those above the range (31–40 $cmH_2O$). The difference in the incidence of sore throat and dysphonia was statistically significant, while that for cough and dysphagia was not. The overall trend suggests an increase in the incidence of postextubation airway complaints in patients whose cuff pressures were corrected to 31–40 $cmH_2O$ compared with those corrected to 20–30 $cmH_2O$. This however was not statistically significant ($p$ value 0.052).

Considering that this was a secondary outcome, it is possible that the sample size was small, hence leading to underestimation of the incidence of postextubation airway complaints between the groups. It is however possible that these results have a clinical significance.

The complaints sought in this study included sore throat, dysphagia, dysphonia, and cough. These were adopted from a review on postoperative airway problems [26] and were defined as follows: sore throat, continuous throat pain (which could be mild, moderate, or severe), dysphagia, uncoordinated swallowing or inability to swallow or eat, dysphonia, hoarseness or voice changes, and cough (identified by a discomforting, dry irritation in the upper airway leading to a cough). All these symptoms were of a new onset following extubation.

There is consensus that keeping ETT cuff pressures low decreases the incidence of postextubation airway complaints [11].

Previous studies have shown that the incidence of postextubation airway symptoms varies from 15% to 94% in various study populations [7, 9, 11, 27] and could be affected by the method of interview employed, such as the one used in our study (yes/no questions). This study was not powered to evaluate associated factors, but there are suggestions that the levels of anesthesia providers with varying skill set and technique at direct laryngoscopy may be associated with a high incidence of complications. However, this could be a site-specific outcome.

## 5. Conclusion

Although this was a single-blinded, single-centre study, results suggest that the LOR syringe method was superior to PBP at administering pressures in the optimal range.

The high incidence of postextubation airway complaints in this study is most likely a site-specific problem but one that other resource-limited settings might identify with.

We recommend the use of the cuff manometer whenever available and the LOR method as a viable option. Alternatively, cheaper, reproducible methods, like the minimum leak test that limit overly high cuff pressures should be sought and evaluated.

## Abbreviations

ETT: Endotracheal tube
PBP: Pilot balloon palpation
LOR: Loss of resistance
ASA: American Society of Anesthesiologists.

## Conflicts of Interest

The authors declare that they have no conflicts of interest.

## Authors' Contributions

Fred Bulamba, Andrew Kintu, Arthur Kwizera, and Arthur Kwizera were responsible for concept and design, interpretation of the data, and drafting of the manuscript. Charles Kojjo, Agnes Wabule, and Nodreen Ayupo were responsible for patient recruitment and data collection and analysis. All authors have read and approved the manuscript.

## Acknowledgments

The authors wish to thank Ms. Martha Nakiranda, Bachelors of Arts in Education, Makerere University, Uganda, for her assistance in editing this manuscript.

## References

[1] R. Fernandez, L. Blanch, J. Mancebo, N. Bonsoms, and A. Artigas, "Endotracheal tube cuff pressure assessment: pitfalls of finger estimation and need for objective measurement," *Critical Care Medicine*, vol. 18, no. 12, pp. 1423–1426, 1990.

[2] H. B. Ghafoui, H. Saeeidi, M. Yasinzadeh, S. Famouri, and E. Modirian, "Excessive endotracheal tube cuff pressure: is there any difference between emergency physicians and anesthesiologists?," *Signa Vitae*, vol. 7, no. 2, pp. 17–20, 2012.

[3] P. Sengupta, D. I. Sessler, P. Maglinger et al., "Endotracheal tube cuff pressure in three hospitals, and the volume required to produce an appropriate cuff pressure," *BMC Anesthesiology*, vol. 4, no. 1, p. 8, 2004.

[4] J. Rello, R. Soñora, P. Jubert, A. Artigas, M. Rué, and J. Vallés, "Pneumonia in intubated patients: role of respiratory airway care," *American Journal of Respiratory and Critical Care Medicine*, vol. 154, no. 1, pp. 111–115, 1996.

[5] M. L. Sole, X. Su, S. Talbert et al., "Evaluation of an intervention to maintain endotracheal tube cuff pressure within therapeutic range," *American Journal of Critical Care*, vol. 20, no. 2, pp. 109–117, 2011.

[6] T. M. Cook, N. Woodall, and C. Frerk, "Major complications of airway management in the UK: results of the Fourth National Audit Project of the Royal College of Anaesthetists and the Difficult Airway Society. Part 1: anaesthesia," *British Journal of Anaesthesia*, vol. 106, no. 5, pp. 617–631, 2011.

[7] J. Liu, X. Zhang, W. Gong et al., "Correlations between controlled endotracheal tube cuff pressure and postprocedural complications: a multicenter study," *Anesthesia and Analgesia*, vol. 111, no. 5, pp. 1133–1137, 2010.

[8] R. D. Seegobin and G. L. van Hasselt, "Endotracheal cuff pressure and tracheal mucosal blood flow: endoscopic study of effects of four large volume cuffs," *British Medical Journal*, vol. 288, no. 6422, pp. 965–968, 1984.

[9] P. Biro, B. Seifert, and T. Pasch, "Complaints of sore throat after tracheal intubation: a prospective evaluation," *European Journal of Anaesthesiology*, vol. 22, no. 4, pp. 307–311, 1995.

[10] C. Stein, G. Berkowitz, and E. Kramer, "Assessment of safe endotracheal tube cuff pressures in emergency care - time for change?," *South African Medical Journal*, vol. 101, no. 3, p. 172, 2011.

[11] N. Suzuki, K. Kooguchi, T. Mizobe, M. Hirose, Y. Takano, and Y. Tanaka, "Postoperative hoarseness and sore throat after tracheal intubation: effect of a low intracuff pressure of endotracheal tube and the usefulness of cuff pressure indicator," *Masui*, vol. 48, no. 10, pp. 1091–1095, 1999.

[12] W. N. Bernhard, L. Yost, D. Joynes, S. Cothalis, and H. Turndorf, "Intracuff pressures in endotracheal and tracheostomy tubes. Related cuff physical characteristics," *Chest*, vol. 87, no. 6, pp. 720–725, 1985.

[13] N. Lomholt, "A device for measuring the lateral wall cuff pressure of endotracheal tubes," *Acta Anaesthesiologica Scandinavica*, vol. 36, no. 8, pp. 775–778, 1992.

[14] U. Nordin, "The trachea and cuff-induced tracheal injury: an experimental study on causative factors and prevention," *Acta Oto-Laryngologica*, vol. 345, pp. S1–S71, 1977.

[15] J. R. Bouvier, "Measuring tracheal tube cuff pressures–tool and technique," *Heart and Lung*, vol. 10, no. 4, pp. 686–690, 1981.

[16] R. J. Hoffman, V. Parwani, and I. H. Hahn, "Experienced emergency medicine physicians cannot safely inflate or estimate endotracheal tube cuff pressure using standard techniques," *American Journal of Emergency Medicine*, vol. 24, no. 2, pp. 139–143, 2006.

[17] V. Foroughi and R. Sripada, "Sensitivity of tactile examination of endotracheal tube intra-cuff pressure," *Anesthesiology*, vol. 87, no. 3, p. 965A, 1997.

[18] E. Resnikoff and A. J. Katz, "A modified epidural syringe as an endotracheal tube cuff pressure-controlling device," *Anaesthesia and Analgesia*, vol. 70, no. 2, pp. 208–211, 1990.

[19] S. Stewart, J. A. Secrest, B. R. Norwood, and R. Zachary, "A comparison of endotracheal tube cuff pressures using estimation techniques and direct intracuff measurement," *American Journal of Nurse Anesthestists*, vol. 71, no. 6, pp. 443–447, 2003.

[20] S. W. Wangaka, *Estimation of endotracheal tube cuff pressures at Kenyatta National Hospital*, University of Nairobi, Nairobi, Kenya, 2006.

[21] C. K. Cho, H. U. Kwon, M. J. Lee, S. S. Park, and W. J. Jeong, "Application of perifix(R) LOR (loss of resistance) syringe for obtaining adequate intracuff pressures of endotracheal tubes," *Journal of Korean Society of Emergency Medicine*, vol. 21, no. 2, pp. 175–183, 2010.

[22] H. Jin, G. Y. Tae, K. K. Won, J. Young, and K. K. Duk, "Usefulness of new technique using a disposable syringe for endotracheal tube cuff inflation," *Korean Journal of Anesthesiology*, vol. 56, no. 5, pp. 513–518, 2009.

[23] H. M. Kim, J. K. No, Y. S. Cho, and H. J. Kim, "Application of a loss of resistance syringe for obtaining the adequate cuff pressures of endotracheal intubated patients in an emergency department," *Journal of the Korean Society of Emergency Medicine*, vol. 23, no. 6, pp. 769–775, 2012.

[24] K. C. Park, Y. D. Sohn, and H. C. Ahn, "Effectiveness, preference and ease of passive release techniques using a syringe for endotracheal tube cuff inflation," *Journal of the Korean Society of Emergency Medicine*, vol. 21, no. 6, pp. 795–800, 2010.

[25] L. Gilliland, H. Perrie, and J. Scribante, "Endotracheal tube cuff pressures in adult patients undergoing general anaesthesia in two Johannesburg Academic Hospitals," *Southern African Journal of Anaesthesia and Analgesia*, vol. 21, no. 3, pp. 81–84, 2015.

[26] L. Zuccherelli, "Postoperative upper airway problems," *Southern African Journal of Anaesthesia and Analgesia*, vol. 9, no. 2, p. 5, 2003.

[27] M. H. Bennett, P. R. Isert, and R. G. Cumming, "Postoperative sore throat and hoarseness following tracheal intubation using air or saline to inflate the cuff–a randomized controlled trial," *Anesthesia and Analgesia*, vol. 28, no. 4, pp. 408–413, 2000.

12

# Drug Errors and Protocol for Prevention among Anaesthetists in Nigeria

**U. U. Johnson and L. N. Ebirim**

*Department of Anaesthesiology, University of Port Harcourt Teaching Hospital, PMB 6173, Port Harcourt, Rivers State, Nigeria*

Correspondence should be addressed to U. U. Johnson; ujohnson360@gmail.com

Academic Editor: Jean Jacques Lehot

*Background.* Drugs are often prescribed, dispensed, and administered by the same person during anaesthesia, and this may increase the risk of drug error. *Objectives.* To assess the frequency of drug administration errors by anaesthetists, the drugs commonly involved, and the effects of such errors. *Method.* A questionnaire-based study was carried out among participants at an annual conference of Nigerian anaesthetists. Sixty-six of the 80 participants returned the completed questionnaire. The respondents comprised 1 nurse anaesthetist, 34 resident doctors, 3 doctors with diploma in anaesthesia, and 28 consultant anaesthetists. The collated data on drug errors, the effect of such errors on patients, and formulated protocols to prevent future occurrence were subjected to descriptive analysis using Microsoft Excel. *Result.* Drug error was reported by 71.21% and witnessed by 22.72% of the respondents. Most of the drug errors occurred during general anaesthesia (90.3%) for emergency procedures (51.61%), and muscle relaxants were most commonly involved (58.06%). *Conclusion.* Drug errors are common among anaesthetists in Nigeria and their incidence is greater during general anaesthesia for emergency procedures, largely as a result of ampoule swaps due to similarities in ampoule design and packaging. Guidelines on their prevention should be developed by all health institutions.

## 1. Introduction

Anaesthesia is a unique specialty in which drugs are prescribed, dispensed, and often urgently administered by the same person, and this may increase the risk of some drugs being administered in error [1]. Morbidity and mortality which result from medication errors impact negatively on the confidence the populace has on the health care facility [2] and litigation can be instituted for claims and even imprisonment on grounds of negligence [3]. One of the solutions by World Health Organization for improving patients' safety involves reducing such errors. Unfortunately drug errors are often underreported [4], and plans to prevent their occurrence are not formulated. This study therefore sought to highlight the frequency, cause, and effect of drug administration errors among anaesthetists in Nigeria.

## 2. Method

A cross-sectional questionnaire-based study was carried out among participants at an annual scientific conference of anaesthetists in Nigeria. A copy of the questionnaire on drug errors in anaesthesia was given to each of 80 participants at the conference to complete. Only 66 completed copies of the questionnaire were returned. Data was collected on anaesthetic drugs administration errors, cause of the errors, effect on the patients, and formulated protocols to prevent future occurrence. The data was subjected to descriptive analysis using Microsoft Excel.

## 3. Result

Sixty-six (82.5%) of the 80 distributed copies of the questionnaire were completed and returned, and the respondents comprised 1 (1.51%) nurse anaesthetist, 34 (51.15%) resident doctors, 3 (4.54%) doctors with postgraduate diploma in anaesthesia, and 28 (42.42%) consultants with fellowship qualifications in anaesthesia. Forty-seven (71.21%) of the respondents had administered drug in error while 15 (22.72%) only witnessed and 4 (6.06%) neither administered nor witnessed drugs administered in error as shown in Figure 1.

TABLE 1: Drug administered, type of error, and frequency.

| Drugs administered in error | Type and frequency of error | | | | | |
|---|---|---|---|---|---|---|
| | Inappropriate dosing | Ampoules swaps | Syringe swaps | Not indicated | Total | Percentage |
| Premedicants | — | 7 | 1 | — | 8 | 12.90 |
| Induction agents | — | — | 2 | — | 2 | 3.22 |
| Muscle relaxants | — | 25 | 11 | — | 36 | 58.06 |
| Analgesics | 1 | — | — | — | 1 | 1.61 |
| Vasopressors | — | 9 | — | — | 9 | 14.51 |
| Calcium injection | 1 | — | — | — | 1 | 1.61 |
| Reversal drugs | — | — | 1 | — | 1 | 1.61 |
| Not Indicated | — | — | — | 4 | 4 | 6.45 |
| Total | 2 | 41 | 15 | 4 | 62 | 100 |

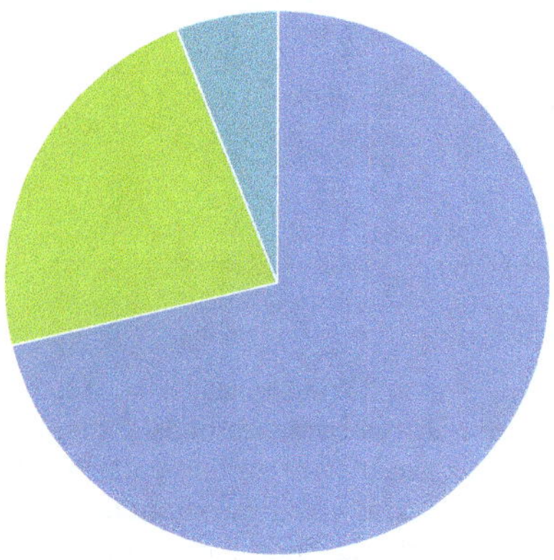


FIGURE 1: Incidence of drug errors.

Thirty-two (51.61%) of the errors occurred during emergency procedures, while 24 (38.70%) occurred during electives and 6 (9.67%) did not indicate the type of procedure. Fifty-six (90.32%) of the drug errors occurred during general anaesthesia, and 5 (8.06%) occurred during regional anaesthesia, while the type of anaesthesia was not indicated in 1 (1.61%). The drugs that were administered in error included premedicants, intravenous induction agents, muscle relaxants, analgesics, and vasopressors. Others included calcium injections and drugs for reversal of neuromuscular blockade as shown in Table 1.

Ampoules swaps accounted for 41 (66.12%) of the drug errors while syringe swaps were responsible for 15 (24.19%) and inappropriate dosing was recorded in 2 (3%) of the drug errors. An assistant was present in 45 (72.58%) of the cases, absent in 10 (16.12%), and not indicated in 7 (11.29%).

Effects of the drug errors were considered by the respondents to be mild in 16 (25.80%) cases, moderate in 22 (35.48%), severe in 9 (14.51%), and fatal in 2 (3.22%). In 13 (20.96%) of the cases there was no effect as shown in Table 2.

Guidelines for the prevention of drug error were not present in 8 (12.90%), but 54 (87.08%) used various methods either singly or combined as shown in Table 3.

TABLE 2: Effect of the drug errors.

| Effect | Number of patients | Percentage |
|---|---|---|
| None | 13 | 20.96 |
| Mild | 16 | 25.80 |
| Moderate | 22 | 35.48 |
| Severe | 9 | 14.51 |
| Fatal | 2 | 3.22 |
| Total | 62 | 100 |

## 4. Discussion

Drug errors are considered to be uncommon but this may be an underestimation as a result of underreporting of incidents in the health care system [4], However, the estimated frequency of drug errors has been reported to be 1 in every 133 anaesthetics [5]. Most anaesthetists admit making at least 1 drug error in the course of their practice [1].

The drug errors could be inappropriate dosing, wrong sequence of administration, administration of a drug different from what was intended, or administration of a drug which the patient is allergic to. Drug errors could occur as a result of syringe swaps or ampoule swaps. One study [6] observed more syringe swaps (44%) than ampoule swaps (14%), and this was attributed to similarity in syringe colour and size but in this study the incidence of ampoule swaps was 69% while that of syringe swaps was 27%. Several studies have attributed ampoule swaps to similarities in drug packaging and ampoule design [7–10].

Drug error has been reported to be commoner during general anaesthesia than during regional anaesthesia [6]. In this study, 90.32% of the drug errors occurred during general anaesthesia while only 8.06% took place during regional/local anaesthesia. This is probably due to the fact that fewer drugs are used for regional than for general anaesthesia. There is a correlation between the urgency in drug administration and the incidence of drug error [11]. This explains the higher incidence of drug error observed during emergency procedures (51.61%, electives 24%) in this study.

It is important for the practitioner to develop an awareness of the ubiquity of medication errors and the potential capacity of such errors to inflict serious harm or death on

TABLE 3: Preventive measures in respondents' health institutions.

| Guidelines for prevention | Number of respondents | Percentage |
|---|---|---|
| None | 8 | 12.90 |
| All drugs must be administered by anaesthetist | 1 | 1.61 |
| Legible drug labels + double check | 9 | 14.51 |
| Syringe coding + double check | 5 | 8.06 |
| Double check only | 29 | 46.77 |
| Syringe coding + double checks + prefilled syringes with label | 1 | 1.61 |
| Syringe coding only | 4 | 6.45 |
| Legible drug labels only | 1 | 1.61 |
| Magnifying glass + double check | 1 | 1.61 |
| Magnifying glass + syringe coding | 1 | 1.61 |
| Magnifying glass + legible drug labels + double check | 1 | 1.61 |
| All the options | 1 | 1.61 |
| Total | 62 | 100 |

patients [12]. The public perceives drug errors as negligence and suspension of the physician is considered an effective deterrent [2], and conviction for manslaughter could even be sought [13]. Education of staff is therefore crucial in the prevention of medication errors [14].

Understanding the causes and conditions that may lead to a medication error can help the practitioners to formulate a plan to prevent its occurrence. The causes of medication errors include lack of concentration by the attending physician, poor cart organization, ampoules looking alike, and unclear or unreadable drug labels [13]. Awareness should be created by the pharmacy department when drugs with similar label and packaging are procured to reduce the incidence of ampoule swaps. The legibility of some of the labels can be improved using magnifying glass and it was the practice by only 1.61% of the respondents. The use of magnifying glass can reduce the frequency of these errors and should therefore be encouraged.

Two-person confirmation or double check of drugs has been strongly advocated [15] and this was observed to be the practice in 46.77% of respondents in this study. However, double check can only be effective if the labels on the drugs are legible or readable and procurement of drugs with legible labels should be encouraged.

Another recommended method for confirming drugs before administration is the use of barcode technology [16]. Though very sensitive, the barcode technology is very expensive and cannot be afforded in the resource poor settings.

Medication errors can also be reduced by using syringe coding. Although it has been found [6] that syringe swaps occurred most often between syringes of equal size and the frequency was not reduced by introduction of colour coding of labels, standardized syringe sizes, with or without needles for particular drugs, can reduce the frequency of syringe swaps. Whereas the use of class-specific colour coding for syringe and ampoule might not reduce substitution of drugs in the same pharmacological class, it would have considerable potential for reducing interclass drug administration errors [17, 18]. About 6.45% of respondents in this study used only syringe coding. Various combinations of methods were used to prevent drug administration errors as indicated in Table 3.

Drug error has the potential for serious morbidity and even mortality. Whereas 20.96% were not affected by the drug errors reported, mild, moderate, and severe symptoms were observed in 25.80%, 35.48%, and 14.51%, respectively. Mortality was also reported in 3.22%. The death of any patient as a result of medication errors could be viewed as negligence by the public, and legal measures may be instituted against such personnel.

Despite many recommendations which have been made to minimize drug errors, their uptake in clinical practice is low. One barrier which has been consistently raised is that there remains a lack of class 1 evidence in favour of any of the recommended measures to reduce medication errors. Waiting for the evidence to emerge before implementing of change would inevitably run the risk of continuing significant patient harm [1]. However, a systematic review of the literature on the reduction of intravenous drug administration errors in anaesthesia has provided a strong support for the use of systematic countermeasures to decrease the incidence of intravenous drug administration errors in anaesthesia. Measures for the prevention of drug errors is therefore necessary and should be encouraged in our health institutions.

## 5. Conclusion

Drug administration errors are common among anaesthetists in Nigeria, and their incidence is greater during general anaesthesia for emergency procedures, largely as a result of ampoule swaps due to similarities in ampoule design and packaging. Legibility of the drug labels also contributed a significant percentage of drug errors. The pharmaceutical companies should therefore be encouraged to improve the ampoule design and legibility of labeling. Guidelines on the prevention of drug errors should be developed in all health institutions, and the use of magnifying lens for identification of drugs which was observed to be an uncommon practice in this environment should be encouraged.

## Conflicts of Interest

The researchers declare that there are no conflicts of interest in this work.

## References

[1] R. P. Mahajan, "Medication errors: can we prevent them?" *British Journal of Anaesthesia*, vol. 107, no. 1, pp. 3–5, 2011.

[2] R. J. Blendon, C. M. DesRoches, M. Brodie et al., "Views of practicing physicians and the public on medical errors," *The New England Journal of Medicine*, vol. 347, no. 24, pp. 1933–1940, 2002.

[3] J. Cranshaw, K. J. Gupta, and T. M. Cook, "Litigation related to drug errors in anaesthesia: an analysis of claims against the NHS in England 1995-2007," *Anaesthesia*, vol. 64, no. 12, pp. 1317–1323, 2009.

[4] R. P. Mahajan, "Critical incident reporting and learning," *British Journal of Anaesthesia*, vol. 105, no. 1, pp. 69–75, 2010.

[5] C. S. Webster, A. F. Merry, L. Larsson, K. A. McGrath, and J. Weller, "The frequency and nature of drug administration error during anaesthesia," *Anaesthesia and Intensive Care*, vol. 29, no. 5, pp. 494–500, 2001.

[6] S. Fasting and S. E. Gisvold, "Adverse drug errors in anesthesia, and the impact of coloured syringe labels," *Canadian Journal of Anesthesia*, vol. 47, no. 11, pp. 1060–1067, 2000.

[7] M. Currie, P. Mackay, C. Morgan et al., "The 'wrong drug' problem in Anaesthesia: an analysis of 2000 incident reports, Anaesth," *Intensive Care*, vol. 21, pp. 596–601, 1993.

[8] L. L. Leape, D. W. Bates, D. J. Cullen et al., "Systems analysis of adverse drug events," *The Journal of the American Medical Association*, vol. 274, no. 1, pp. 35–43, 1995.

[9] C. N. Mato and S. Fyneface-Ogan, "Drug errors in anaesthetic practice: case reports," *Nigerian journal of medicine : journal of the National Association of Resident Doctors of Nigeria*, vol. 12, no. 3, pp. 157–159, 2003.

[10] E. O. Nwasor, S. T. Sule, and D. B. Mshelia, "Audit of medication errors by anesthetists in North Western Nigeria," *Nigerian Journal of Clinical Practice*, vol. 17, no. 2, pp. 226–231, 2014.

[11] J. B. Cooper, R. S. Newbower, and R. J. Kitz, "An analysis of major errors and equipment failures in anesthesia management: Considerations for prevention and detection," *Anesthesiology*, vol. 60, no. 1, pp. 34–42, 1984.

[12] R. J. Glavin, "Drug errors: consequences, mechanisms, and avoidance," *British Journal of Anaesthesia*, vol. 105, no. 1, pp. 76–82, 2010.

[13] S. J. Wheeler and D. W. Wheeler, "Medication errors in anaesthesia and critical care," *Anaesthesia*, vol. 60, no. 3, pp. 257–273, 2005.

[14] R. Flin, R. Patey, R. Glavin, and N. Maran, "Anaesthetists' non-technical skills," *British Journal of Anaesthesia*, vol. 105, no. 1, pp. 38–44, 2010.

[15] R. Evley, J. Russell, D. Mathew, R. Hall, L. Gemmell, and R. P. Mahajan, "Confirming the drugs administered during anaesthesia: a feasibility study in the pilot National Health Service sites, UK," *British Journal of Anaesthesia*, vol. 105, no. 3, pp. 289–296, 2010.

[16] E. G. Poon, C. A. Keohane, C. S. Yoon et al., "Effect of bar-code technology on the safety of medication administration," *The New England Journal of Medicine*, vol. 362, no. 18, pp. 1698–1707, 2010.

[17] M. Harmer, C. S. Webster, and A. F. Merry, "British syringe label 'standards' are an accident waiting to happen," *Anaesthesia*, vol. 55, no. 6, p. 618, 2000.

[18] Webster C. S., Merry A. F., L. Larsson, and McGrath K. A., "A complex system-approach to safer drug administration in anaesthesia," *Journal of Clinical Monitoring and Computing*, vol. 16, pp. 150-151, 2000.

# 13

# Perioperative Elevation in Cell-Free DNA Levels in Patients Undergoing Cardiac Surgery: Possible Contribution of Neutrophil Extracellular Traps to Perioperative Renal Dysfunction

**Yu Qi,[1] Tokujiro Uchida,[1] Mamoru Yamamoto,[1] Yudai Yamamoto,[1] Koji Kido,[1] Hiroyuki Ito,[1] Nagara Ohno,[2] Miho Asahara,[2] Yoshitsugu Yamada,[2] Osamu Yamaguchi,[3] Chieko Mitaka,[1] Makoto Tomita,[4] and Koshi Makita[1]**

[1]*Department of Anesthesiology, Tokyo Medical and Dental University, Graduate School of Medical and Dental Sciences, 1-5-45 Yushima, Bunkyo-ku, Tokyo 113-8519, Japan*
[2]*Department of Anesthesiology, The University of Tokyo, Graduate School of Medicine, Tokyo, Japan*
[3]*Department of Critical Care Medicine, Yokohama City University Medical Center, Kanagawa, Japan*
[4]*Clinical Research Center, Tokyo Medical and Dental University Hospital of Medicine, Tokyo, Japan*

Correspondence should be addressed to Tokujiro Uchida; uchida.mane@tmd.ac.jp

Academic Editor: Ronald G. Pearl

*Background.* This study aimed to determine the perioperative change in serum double-strand DNA (dsDNA) as a marker potentially reflecting neutrophil extracellular trap concentration in samples from patients undergoing cardiac surgery and to analyze a relationship between serum dsDNA concentrations and perioperative renal dysfunction. *Methods.* Serum dsDNA concentrations in samples that were collected during a previously conducted, prospective, multicenter, observational study were measured. Eighty patients undergoing elective cardiac surgery were studied. Serum samples were collected at baseline, immediately after surgery, and the day after surgery (POD-1). *Results.* Serum dsDNA concentration was significantly increased from baseline (median, 398 ng/mL [interquartile range, 372–475 ng/mL]) to immediately after surgery (median, 540 ng/mL [437–682 ng/mL], $p < 0.001$), and they were reduced by POD-1 (median, 323 ng/mL [256–436 ng/mL]). The difference in serum creatinine concentration between baseline and POD-1 was correlated with dsDNA concentration on POD-1 ($r_s = 0.61$, $p < 0.001$). *Conclusions.* In patients undergoing cardiac surgery, serum dsDNA concentration is elevated postoperatively. Prolonged elevation in dsDNA concentration is correlated with perioperative renal dysfunction. Further large-scale studies are needed to determine the relationship between serum concentration of circulating dsDNA and perioperative renal dysfunction.

## 1. Introduction

Cell-free double-strand DNA (dsDNA) is thought to be one of danger associated molecular patterns, and its plasma concentration can be elevated in patients with sepsis [1, 2] and multiple trauma [3]. Among multiple sources of cell-free dsDNA including necrotic cells and apoptotic cells, neutrophil might be an important source, because activated neutrophils release dsDNA-based structures, called neutrophil extracellular traps (NETs), which forms fibrous structures to trap circulating microorganisms and kills them by antimicrobial proteins that are derived from neutrophil granules and the cytoplasm [4–6]. However, excessive release of NETs into plasma results in endothelial injury, which may result in tissue injury in major organs [6, 7]. Previous studies have shown that circulating cell-free dsDNA concentration reflects the amount of NET formation in the blood [1, 3, 8], and in patients with multiple trauma, circulating cell-free dsDNA concentration reflects the severity of injury [3]. Major surgery has some common characteristics with trauma, including tissue damage, inflammation, and activation of the endothelium and immune cells. However, the perioperative change in dsDNA concentration and its contribution to perioperative organ dysfunction have not been determined yet.

The objective of this study was to analyze perioperative changes in serum dsDNA concentration, as a marker reflecting NET formation, in patients undergoing cardiac surgery. To understand the kinetics of dsDNA, activity and antigen concentration of deoxyribonuclease-1 (DNase-I) were also studied. To determine the contribution of neutrophil activation to increased serum dsDNA concentration, we measured the concentration of S100A12 as a marker of neutrophil activation [9] and examined the correlation between S100A12 and dsDNA concentration. Finally, we investigated whether renal dysfunction is related to an elevation in dsDNA concentration. For these purposes, we studied clinical data and serum samples from a previously conducted multicenter, observational study for biomarkers of respiratory failure after cardiovascular surgery [10, 11].

## 2. Methods

*2.1. Study Design.* We studied clinical data and biological samples which were collected in a previously conducted study for biomarkers for respiratory failure after cardiac surgery [10, 11]. The original study is registered in the University Hospital Medical Information Network (UMIN) Clinical Trials Registry (ID: UMIN000010674; http://www.umin.ac.jp/ctr/index/htm/), and the details and results have been previously published in full [10, 11]. Briefly, a total of 87 patients undergoing cardiac surgery were enrolled in the original study. Serum concentrations of sRAGE and angiopoietin-2 were found to be elevated postoperatively, and the range in elevation was associated with respiratory failure morbidity after cardiac surgery. Three university hospitals participated in this study, and approval for the protocol was obtained from each institutional review board for clinical studies (Institutional Review Board, Clinical Research Center, Tokyo Medical and Dental University Hospital; Graduate School of Medicine and Faculty of Medicine, The University of Tokyo Research Ethics Committee; General Administration Division General Affairs Section, Yokohama City University Medical Center). Preoperative exclusion criteria were as follows: (i) age < 20 years; (ii) history of myocardial infarction within 30 days before the day of surgery; (iii) preoperative diagnosis of pneumothorax; (iv) diagnosis of chronic obstructive pulmonary disease; (v) neuromuscular disease; (vi) morbid obesity (body mass index > 40 $kg/m^2$); and (vii) systemic connective tissue disease. Postoperative exclusion criteria were as follows: (i) severe neurological complications requiring mechanical ventilation; (ii) the need for an extracorporeal circuit because of cardiac failure; and (iii) patients whose pulmonary artery occlusion pressure was >18 mmHg in the first postoperative week. As an additional exclusion criterion, patients who were treated with hemodialysis before surgery were excluded to study the relationship between serum dsDNA concentration and perioperative renal dysfunction. Each patient provided written informed consent. Details of clinical management (anesthesia, steroid use, and postoperative mechanical ventilation) are described in the report of the original study [10, 11]. Criteria for diagnosis of acute kidney injury (AKI) were based on the Acute Kidney Injury Network classification system [12].

*2.2. Measurements of Serum dsDNA Concentration.* Three patients who were treated with hemodialysis and four patients with limited availability of serum were excluded. Therefore, 80 patients were included in the current study. Serum samples were collected (i) immediately after induction of general anesthesia (baseline), (ii) immediately after surgery (PostOp), and (iii) the day after surgery (POD-1) [10, 11]. Serum dsDNA concentration was quantified by the method used in previous studies [3, 13], using Quant-iT PicoGreen dsDNA Reagent (#P7581, Molecular Probes, Eugene, OR, USA). Fluorescence was measured by the GloMax Fluorometer (Promega Japan) with filter setting of 485 nm (excitation) and 538 nm (emission).

*2.3. Enzyme-Linked Immunosorbent Assay (ELISA) for Biomarkers and DNase-I Antigen.* Commercially available ELISA kits were used to measure serum concentrations of S100A12 (S100A12/EN-RAGE ELISA Kit; Circulex, Nagano, Japan), serum neutrophil gelatinase-associated lipocalin (NGAL) concentration (DLCN20, R&D Systems, Minneapolis, MN, USA), the antigen of DNase-I (Human Deoxyribonuclease I ELISA Kit; Cusabio, Hubei, China), anti-nucleosome antibody concentration (Anti-Nucleosome, ELISA Kit; Orgentec Diagnostika, Mainz, Germany), and perinuclear anti-neutrophil cytoplasmic antibody (pANCA) concentration (ANCA-P ELISA Kit; Abnova, Taipei City, Taiwan). Data for PostOp serum interleukin- (IL-) 8, N-terminal pro-B-type natriuretic peptide (NT-proBNP), and troponin-T concentrations were obtained from the same samples of 80 patients from the results of the original study [10].

*2.4. DNase Activity Assay.* We used the ORG590 DNase Activity ELISA (Orgentec Diagnostika) with some modifications for the measurement of DNase activity. Serum samples (100 $\mu$L) without dilution were used for measurements. The results were calculated as % activity reduction/mL (%AR) from the calibration curve and this was plotted with the results of six calibrators of defined concentration. Finally, DNase activity in mKuU/mL was calculated from %AR values using the regression formula based on the data that were shown in the product insert. We could not measure one sample from a patient undergoing valve surgery because of a shortage of sample. Therefore, we measured samples from 79 patients.

*2.5. Statistical Analyses.* All statistical analyses were performed using STATA/IC software (version 14, StataCorp, College Station, TX, USA). We used the Mann–Whitney *U* test for two-group comparisons. For intergroup comparisons, we used the chi-square test for categorical data and the Kruskal–Wallis test for numerical data which are not following a normal distribution. In the latter case, post hoc multiple

TABLE 1: Patients' characteristics.

| | Total | On-pump surgery | Off-pump surgery | $p$ value |
|---|---|---|---|---|
| Number of patients | 80 | 51 | 29 | |
| | | | | Chi-square test |
| Male/female (male%) | 57/23 (71%) | 34/17 (67%) | 23/6 (79%) | 0.92 |
| | | | | Kruskal-Wallis test |
| Age (year) | 68 (58–74) | 67 (53–74) | 70 (60–74) | 0.08 |
| Body weight (kg) | 60 (53–68) | 59 (53–68) | 61 (57–68) | 0.54 |
| White blood cell count (cells/mm$^3$) | 5840 (4850–7100) | 5600 (4815–7100) | 5950 (4900–6900) | 0.70 |
| Hemoglobin (g/dL) | 12.7 (11.5–13.5) | 12.4 (11.4–13.3) | 13.1 (11.8–13.7) | 0.13 |
| Platelet count (10$^4$/mm$^3$) | 19.1 (15.5–23.8) | 18.5 (14.8–23.1) | 20.7 (16.5–25.6) | 0.21 |
| Total protein (g/dL) | 7.2 (6.6–7.4) | 7.2 (6.7–7.3) | 7.2 (6.6–7.6) | 0.13 |
| Albumin (g/dL) | 4.1 (3.8–4.4) | 4.2 (4.0–4.4) | 4.0 (3.8–4.3) | 0.21 |
| BUN (mg/dL) | 18.0 (14–22) | 17.5 (14.0–21.9) | 18.4 (15.4–22.0) | 0.59 |
| Creatinine (mg/dL) | 0.95 (0.75–1.2) | 0.92 (0.76–1.1) | 0.97 (0.75–1.2) | 0.83 |
| Mean blood pressure (mmHg) | 90 (82–98) | 85 (78–96) | 94 (87–103) | 0.006 |
| Heart rate (beats/min) | 70 (62–78) | 69 (62–77) | 70 (61–79) | 0.96 |
| $PaO_2/F_iO_2$ ratio | 427 (331-500) | 417 (342–500) | 428 (327–490) | 0.97 |
| Duration of surgery (min) | 385 (315–450) | 405 (346–486) | 320 (254–391) | 0.0004 |
| Duration of cardiopulmonary bypass (min) | | 197 (160–254) | | |
| Transfusion | | | | |
| Red cell (units[a]) | 0 (0–4) | 2 (0–4) | 0 (0–2) | 0.09 |
| Fresh frozen plasma (units[a]) | 0 (0–6) | 0 (0–8) | 0 (0–0) | 0.001 |
| Platelet (units[b]) | 0 (0–0) | 0 (0–20) | 0 (0–0) | 0.001 |

Values are median (interquartile range).
[a]One unit of packed red cells or fresh frozen plasma was derived from 200 mL of donated blood.
[b]One unit of packed platelet concentrate contained $2 \times 10^{10}$ platelets.
BUN: blood urea nitrogen.

comparisons were analyzed with Steel–Dwass's test. We used Spearman's test for correlation analyses and the correlation was graded depending on the $r_s$ value as follows: $r_s \geq 0.4$ and $<0.7$ as a moderate correlation and $r_s \geq 0.2$ and $<0.4$ as a weak correlation. We analyzed contributing factors to the morbidity of AKI by multiple logistic regression analysis, using variables selected by univariate analyses as possible confounding factors. These factors consisted of baseline creatinine concentration, type of surgery (on-pump or off-pump), dose of red cell transfusion, PostOp IL-8, troponin-T, NT-proBNP concentrations, and duration of surgery. In these multivariable tests, backward elimination was performed at $p > 0.15$. To assess discrimination ability of logistic regression models, area under the curve of receiver operating characteristic curve (AUROC) was calculated for each model. Statistical significance was defined as $p < 0.05$.

## 3. Results

Baseline demographic data and clinical variables are shown in Table 1. Fifty-one patients underwent on-pump surgery (19 patients underwent aortic surgery; 32 patients underwent valve surgery) and 29 patients underwent off-pump surgery (29 patients underwent coronary artery bypass grafting). The duration of surgery was significantly longer in the on-pump surgery group compared with the off-pump group ($p < 0.001$). Significantly more transfusions were required in the on-pump surgery group compared with the off-pump surgery group ($p = 0.001$ for fresh frozen plasma; and $p = 0.001$ for platelet transfusion, Table 1). One patient died on POD-24 and another patient died on POD-57.

*3.1. Perioperative Changes in dsDNA Concentration.* The perioperative changes in serum dsDNA concentration in patients who underwent cardiac surgery are shown in Figure 1(a). In the total cohort, PostOp serum dsDNA concentration was significantly higher than that at baseline (baseline median 398 ng/mL, interquartile range [IQR] 372–475 ng/mL versus PostOp median 540 ng/mL, IQR 437–682 ng/mL, $p < 0.001$) and had fallen significantly by POD-1 (median 323 ng/mL, IQR 256–436 ng/mL, Figure 1(a)). The off-pump surgery group had significantly lower serum dsDNA concentration than the on-pump surgery group at all three time points ($p = 0.014$ at baseline, $p = 0.014$ immediately after surgery, and $p < 0.001$ on POD-1, Figure 1(b)). There were eight patients mechanically ventilated more than 3 days, and these patients showed significantly higher concentration of serum dsDNA on POD-1 (median 477 ng/mL, IQR 367–608 ng/mL) than those extubated by POD-3 (median 315 ng/mL, IQR 215–419 ng/mL, $p = 0.017$).

Serum DNase activity was reduced in the entire cohort immediately after surgery. On POD-1, DNase activity varied

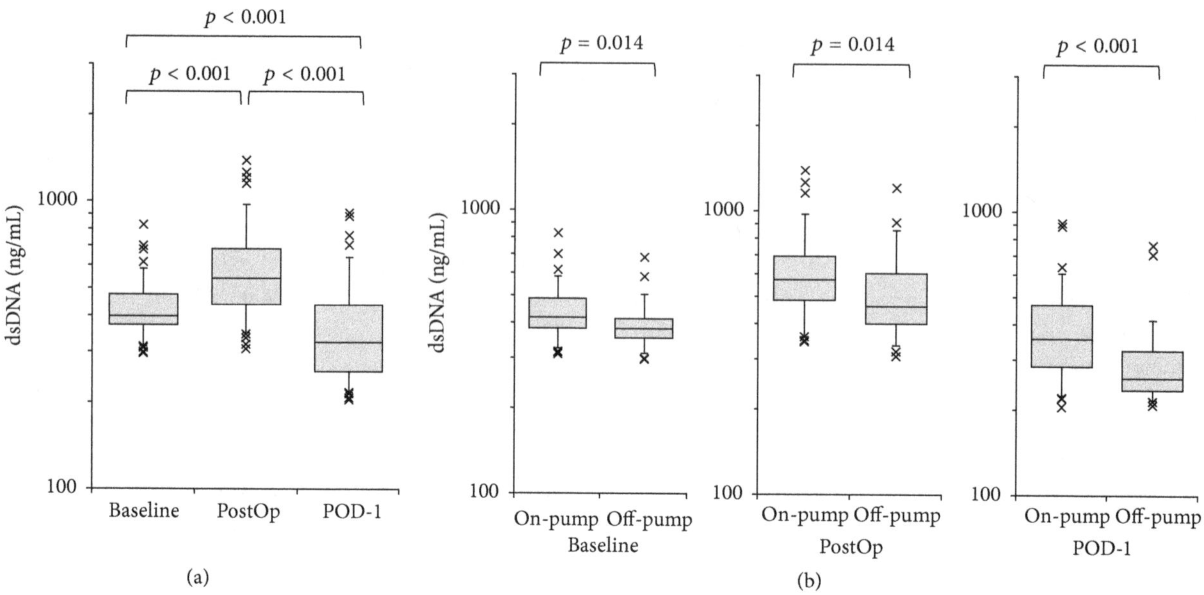


FIGURE 1: Perioperative changes in serum circulating double-strand DNA (dsDNA) concentration. (a) Perioperative changes in dsDNA concentration in the total cohort ($n = 80$). Measurements were performed at baseline, immediately after surgery (PostOp), and the day after surgery (POD-1). (b) Comparison of serum dsDNA concentration between on-pump ($n = 51$) and off-pump surgery ($n = 29$).

widely, which suggested that postoperative recovery of DNase activity was affected by perioperative factors (Figure 2(a)). We also measured the antigen concentration of DNase-I but found no significant difference at each of the three time points (Figure 2(b)). Patients in the off-pump surgery group tended to show more rapid recovery of DNase activity than those in the on-pump surgery group ($p = 0.016$, Figure 2(c)). Figure 3 shows the correlation between serum DNase activity and serum dsDNA concentration. When data from all three time points were combined (baseline, PostOp, and POD-1), a moderate negative correlation between these two variables was observed ($r_s = -0.45$, $p < 0.001$, Figure 3(d)). Samples with low DNase activity (<1 mKuU/mL) had significantly higher dsDNA concentration (median 472 ng/mL, IQR 380–585 ng/mL, and $n = 163$) compared with those with high DNase activity (≥1 mKuU/mL) (median 358 ng/mL, IQR 277–398 ng/mL, $n = 74$, and $p < 0.001$).

*3.2. Correlation between Neutrophil Activation and dsDNA Concentration.* To study the relationship between the dsDNA concentration and function of neutrophils, we measured S100A12 concentration, and the correlation between S100A12 and dsDNA concentration was examined. Concentrations of dsDNA were significantly correlated with S100A12 concentration at all three time points ($r_s = 0.54$, $p < 0.001$ at baseline, Figure 4(a); $r_s = 0.47$, $p < 0.001$ at PostOp, Figure 4(b); and $r_s = 0.50$, $p < 0.001$ on POD-1, Figure 4(c)). When the three measurements were combined, there was a significant correlation between S100A12 and dsDNA concentration ($r_s = 0.48$, $p < 0.001$, Figure 4(d)). S100A12 concentration showed a significant negative correlation with DNase activity at baseline ($r_s = -0.41$, $p < 0.001$, Figure 5(a)). PostOp concentration of S100A12 was elevated, DNase activity was reduced (Figure 5(b)), and S100A12 concentration on POD-1 varied widely, maintaining the negative correlation with DNase activity ($r_s = -0.52$, $p < 0.001$, Figure 5(c)). When the measurements from the three time points were combined, there was a significant negative correlation between S100A12 and DNase activity ($r_s = -0.61$, $p < 0.001$, Figure 5(d)), which suggested that activation of neutrophils resulted in an inhibitory effect on the activity of serum DNase.

*3.3. Relationship between Serum dsDNA Concentration and Renal Function.* Twenty-two patients were diagnosed with AKI (27.5%, three patients underwent off-pump surgery, and 19 patients underwent on-pump surgery). In one patient, renal replacement therapy was performed from POD-1 because of metabolic acidosis (stage 3 AKI), but all other patients with AKI had stage 1 impairment. Patients with postoperative AKI had higher baseline creatinine concentration than patients who did not develop AKI ($n = 58$). The duration of surgery was significantly longer ($p < 0.001$), and significantly more red cell transfusions were administered ($p = 0.002$) in those who developed AKI. Patients with AKI were found to have significantly higher serum IL-8 ($p < 0.001$), troponin-T ($p = 0.02$), and NT-proBNP ($p = 0.04$) concentrations immediately after surgery (Table 2). In the entire cohort, PostOp serum NGAL and creatinine concentrations on POD-1 were significantly correlated ($r_s = 0.56$, $p < 0.001$). Patients diagnosed with AKI exhibited significantly higher serum NGAL concentration immediately after surgery (median 136 ng/mL, IQR 81–218 ng/mL in patients with AKI compared with median 81 ng/mL, IQR 58–116 ng/mL in those without, $p = 0.005$). Figure 6(a) shows the relationship between serum creatinine concentration and dsDNA concentration. By the end of surgery,

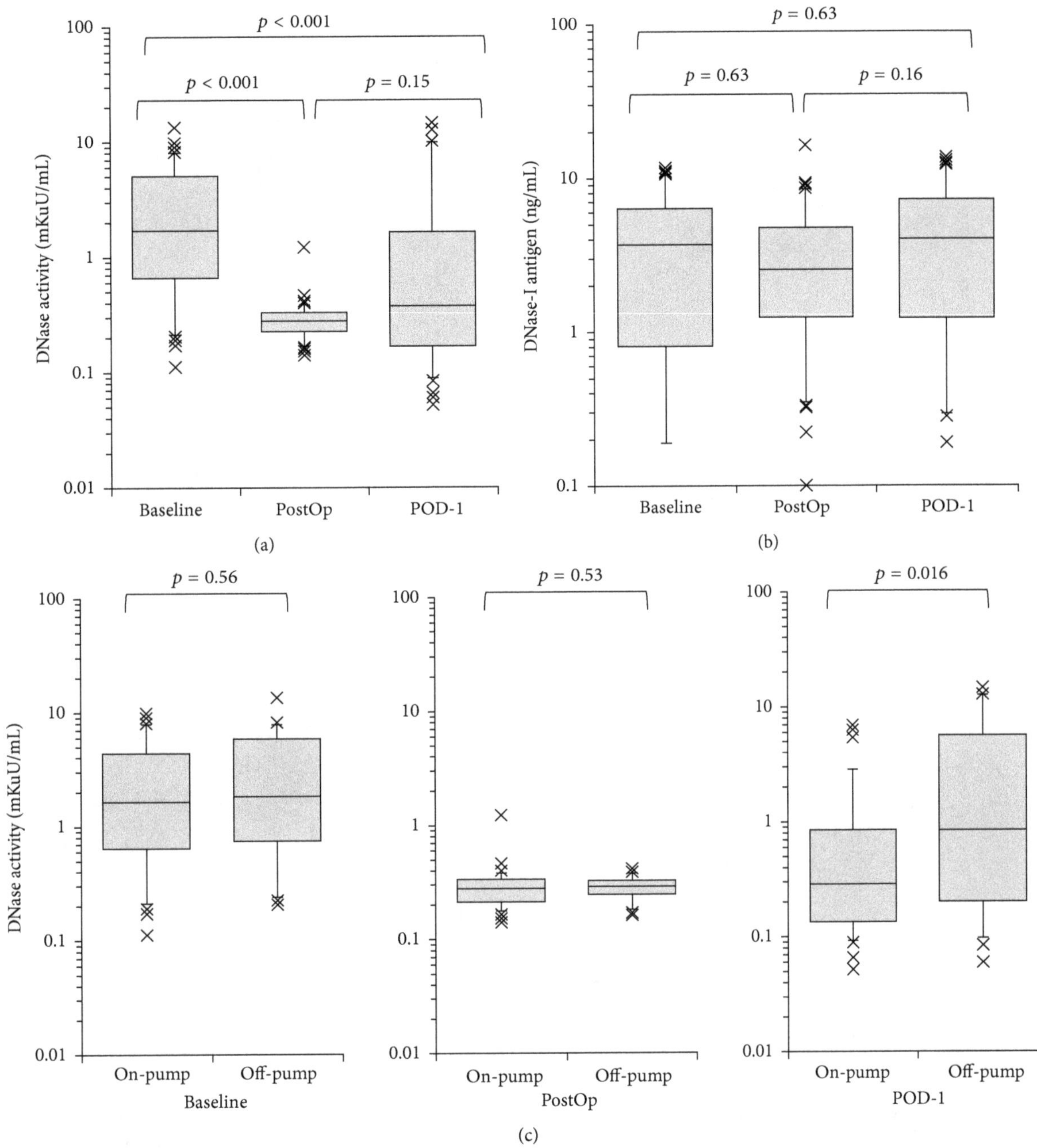


FIGURE 2: Perioperative changes in serum deoxyribonuclease (DNase) concentration. (a) Perioperative change in the activity of DNase in the total cohort. (b) Perioperative change in antigen concentration of DNase-I in the total cohort ($n$ = 80). (c) Comparison of the activity of DNase between on-pump ($n$ = 51) and off-pump surgery ($n$ = 29).

serum creatinine concentration was not significantly elevated, despite elevation in dsDNA concentration. However, on POD-1, patients with high dsDNA concentration showed elevated creatinine concentration, and there was a significant association between these two variables ($r_s = 0.43$, $p < 0.001$, Figure 6(a)). There was also a significant correlation between the perioperative change in serum creatinine concentration between baseline and POD-1 (Δcreatinine) and dsDNA concentration ($r_s = 0.61$, $p < 0.001$, Figure 6(b)). Patients with AKI (median 455 ng/mL, IQR 351–503 ng/mL) had significantly higher dsDNA concentration than those without (median 287 ng/mL, IQR 238–356 ng/mL, and $p < 0.001$, Figure 6(c)). We analyzed correlation between Δcreatinine and possible confounding factors for the morbidity AKI, including baseline creatinine concentration, type of surgery (on-pump or off-pump), amount of red cell transfusion, PostOp concentrations of IL-8, troponin-T, and NT-proBNP, and duration of surgery. Surgical duration ($p$ = 0.002) and dsDNA on POD-1 ($p$ = 0.003) were significantly contributing factors to AKI (Table 3), and the AUROC of this logistic

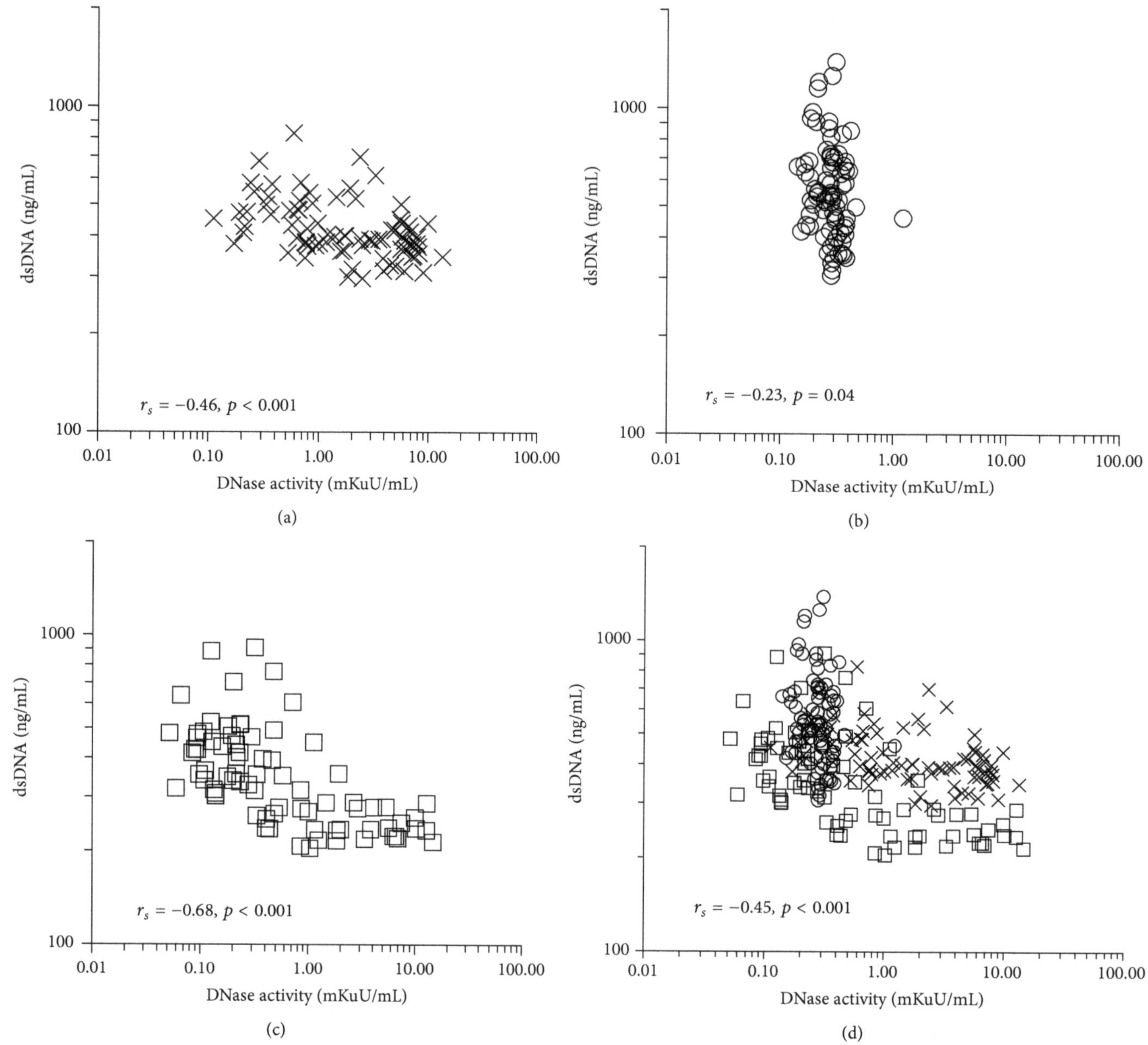


FIGURE 3: Relationship between serum double-strand DNA (dsDNA) concentration and the activity of deoxyribonuclease (DNase). Spearman's tests were performed at (a) baseline ($n = 79$), (b) immediately after surgery (PostOp, $n = 79$), and (c) the day after surgery (POD-1, $n = 79$). (d) When the data from all three time points (baseline, PostOp, and POD-1) were combined (merge), a moderate correlation between these two variables was observed ($r_s = -0.45$, $p < 0.001$). X marks, baseline; open circles, PostOp; open squares, POD-1. $r_s$: correlation coefficient calculated from Spearman's tests.

regression model was 0.86 for the discrimination of AKI. To determine the contribution of autoimmune antibodies to renal dysfunction, we measured anti-nucleosome antibody and pANCA concentration on POD-1. None of the patients showed positivity of these autoimmune antibodies.

## 4. Discussion

*4.1. Perioperative Kinetics of Circulating dsDNA in Patients Undergoing Cardiac Surgery.* We found that circulating dsDNA concentration was elevated postoperatively, and it fell by POD-1. These kinetics are similar to previously reported results from patients with multiple trauma [3]. Tissue damage, systemic inflammation, bleeding, and activation of hemostatic reactions are common characteristics of major surgery and trauma. Furthermore, recently published data showed that plasma histone levels were elevated both after severe trauma [14] and after pediatric cardiac surgery using cardiopulmonary bypass [15], which suggested that nucleosome components could be released immediately after cardiac surgery or trauma. Although dsDNA and histone could be released from multiple sources including damaged

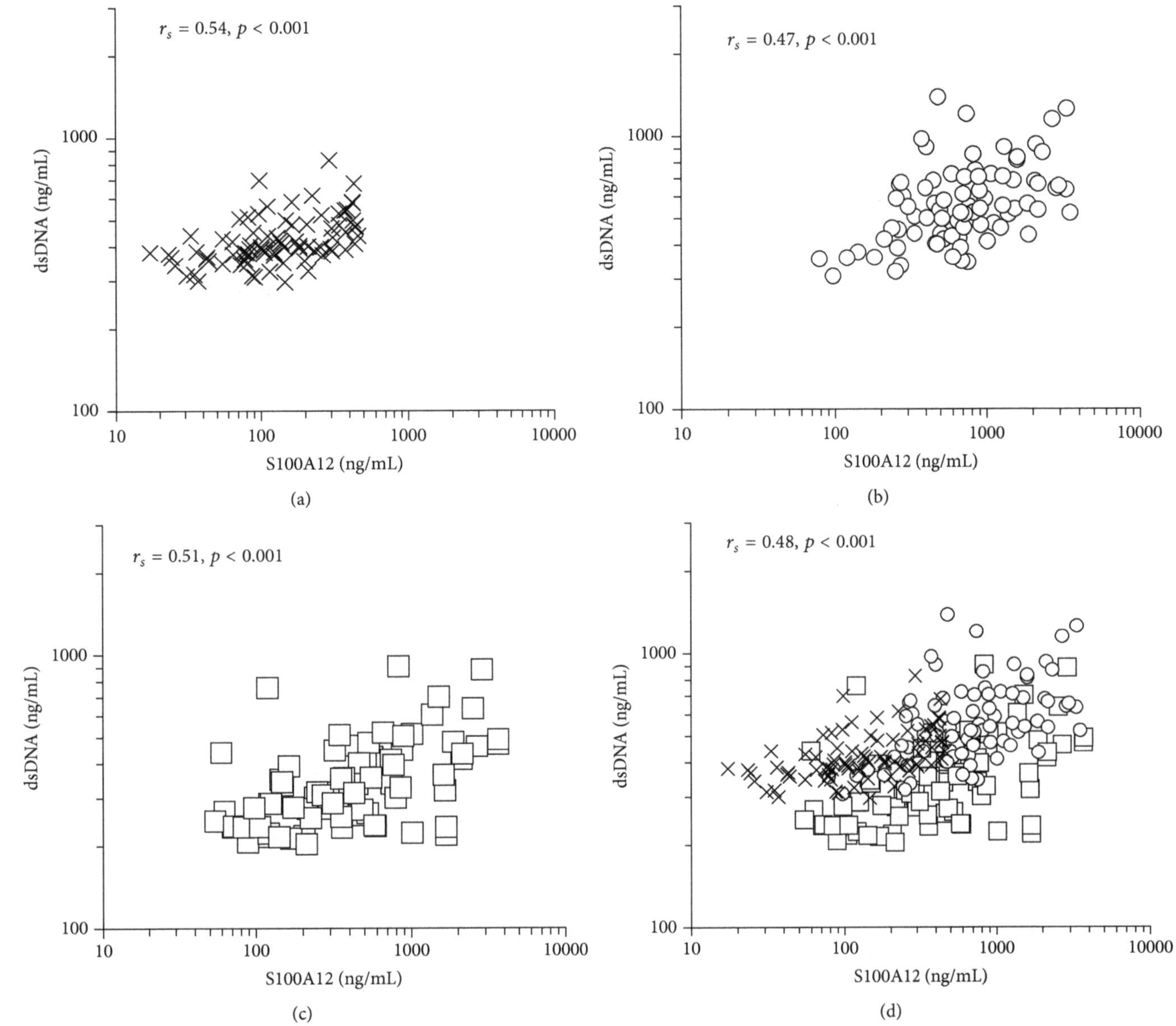


FIGURE 4: Association between the neutrophil activation marker S100A12 and serum double-strand DNA (dsDNA) concentration. (a) Baseline ($n$ = 80), (b) immediately after surgery (PostOp, $n$ = 80), and (c) the day after surgery (POD-1, $n$ = 80). (d) When the data from all three time points (baseline, PostOp, and POD-1) were combined (merge), a moderate correlation between these two variables was observed ($r_s$ = 0.48, $p$ < 0.001). X marks, baseline; open circles, PostOp; open squares, POD-1. $r_s$: correlation coefficient calculated from Spearman's tests.

tissue and apoptotic cells, neutrophils could be an important source, because use of cardiopulmonary bypass circuit and reuse of suctioned blood could activate neutrophils and could promote NET formation after cardiac surgery. Nevertheless the mechanisms underpinning these kinetics consist of production and release of free dsDNA into the serum and degradation by DNase-I.

We found that serum free dsDNA concentration was significantly correlated with the neutrophil activation marker S100A12. This finding suggests a major contribution of neutrophil-derived dsDNA to elevation in serum dsDNA concentration, supporting our use of dsDNA concentration as a marker of NET release. Immediately after surgery, a wide range of dsDNA concentrations was observed in the context of low DNase activity (Figure 3(b)), possibly reflecting a large variation in NET formation (as dsDNA concentration showed a significant correlation with S100A12 concentration at that time point, Figure 4(b)).

With regard to degradation of dsDNA, we found that serum DNase activity was reduced immediately after surgery, but there was no change in the antigen concentration of DNase-I. There was a negative correlation between dsDNA concentration and DNase activity (Figure 3). These findings suggest that postoperative elevation in circulating dsDNA concentration could be partially explained by the reduction in DNase activity. Furthermore, patients undergoing off-pump surgery tended to recover DNase activity more quickly than patients undergoing cardiopulmonary bypass

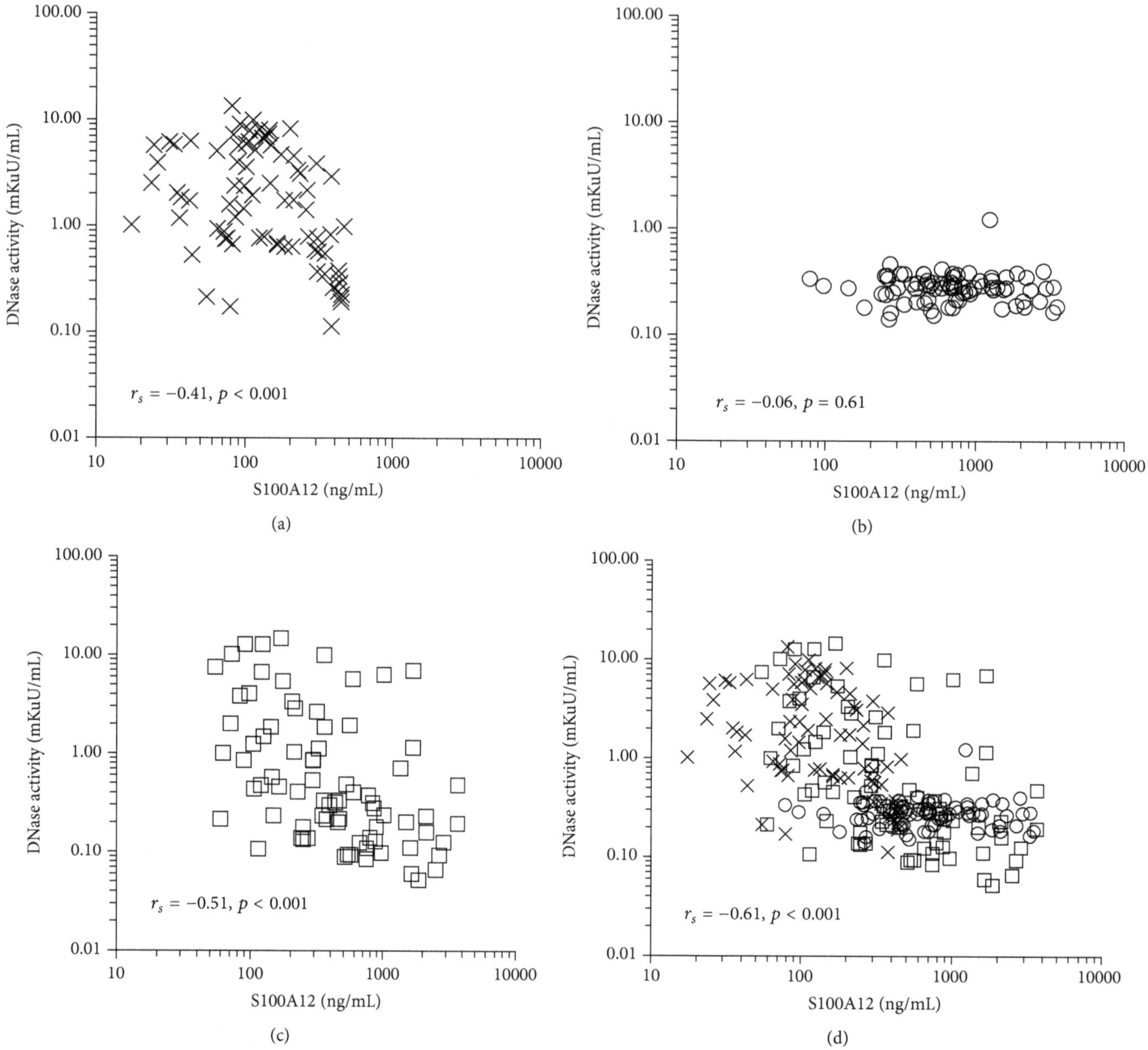


FIGURE 5: Relationship between the activity of deoxyribonuclease (DNase) and the neutrophil activation marker S100A12. (a) Baseline ($n$ = 79), (b) immediately after surgery (PostOp, $n$ = 79), and (c) the day after surgery (POD-1, $n$ = 79). (d) When the data from all three time points (baseline, PostOp, and POD-1) were combined (merge), a moderate correlation between these two variables was observed ($r_s = -0.61$, $p < 0.001$). X marks, baseline; open circles, PostOp; open squares, POD-1. $r_s$: correlation coefficient calculated from Spearman's tests.

(Figure 3(c)). This recovery might be the cause of lower circulating dsDNA concentration. A reduction in serum DNase activity has been reported in systemic lupus erythematosus [16] and chronic inflammatory bowel disease [17]. Therefore, inflammation might reduce DNase activity, and recovery from inflammation might be an important factor for reducing circulating dsDNA concentration. Interestingly, DNase-I antigen concentration did not change during the study period, suggesting the existence of an inhibitory factor for DNase-I. Furthermore, serum S100A12 concentration was negatively correlated with DNase activity. These findings may indicate that DNase activity and dsDNA concentration are regulated by mechanisms associated with activation of neutrophils.

*4.2. Potential Contribution of NETs to Perioperative Renal Dysfunction.* The perioperative incidence of AKI was 27.5% in our cohort; all patients with AKI exhibited an elevation in serum creatinine concentration of >0.3 mg/dL from baseline to POD-1. These patients showed a significant elevation in PostOp serum NGAL concentration compared with patients without AKI. The perioperative change in serum creatinine concentration showed a moderate association with serum dsDNA concentration on POD-1. Additionally, serum

TABLE 2: Characteristics of patients with or without acute kidney injury.

| | AKI | Non-AKI | $p$ value |
|---|---|---|---|
| Number of patients | 22 | 58 | |
| | | | Chi-square test |
| Male sex | 17 (77%) | 40 (69%) | 0.54 |
| Diabetes mellitus | 5 (22.7%) | 20 (34.5%) | 0.4 |
| Type of surgery (on-pump/off-pump) | 19/3 | 33/25 | 0.002 |
| | | | Mann–Whitney $U$ test |
| Age (year) | 68 (61–74) | 67 (56–74) | 0.66 |
| Body weight (kg) | 62 (58–68) | 60 (53–68) | 0.31 |
| Creatinine at baseline (mg/dL) | 1.06 (0.88–1.20) | 0.90 (0.74–1.11) | 0.047 |
| Data immediately after surgery | | | |
| White blood cell count (cells/mm$^3$) | 10300 (8658–12800) | 9980 (7875–13153) | 0.95 |
| Platelet count (10$^4$/mm$^3$) | 9.2 (8.2–10.5) | 10.6 (7.8–14.6) | 0.28 |
| Albumin (g/dL) | 3.5 (2.9–3.6) | 3.2 (2.7–3.6) | 0.22 |
| $PaO_2/F_IO_2$ ratio | 245 (168–319) | 279 (205–348) | 0.17 |
| Red cell transfusion (units[a]) | 4 (2–4) | 0 (0–4) | 0.002 |
| Serum interleukin-8 (pg/mL) | 97 (41–173) | 37 (2–62) | <0.001 |
| Serum troponin-T (ng/mL) | 0.70 (0.46–1.14) | 0.39 (0.19–0.71) | 0.02 |
| Serum NT-proBNP (pg/mL) | 329 (166–618) | 137 (69–567) | 0.04 |
| Duration of surgery (min) | 489 (400–580) | 353 (295–410) | <0.001 |
| Serum dsDNA concentration on POD-1 (ng/mL) | 455 (351–503) | 287 (238–356) | <0.001 |

[a]One unit of packed red cells or fresh frozen plasma was derived from 200 mL of donated blood.
AKI: patients diagnosed with acute kidney injury.
Non-AKI: patients without acute kidney injury.
POD-1: postoperative day-1 (the day after surgery).
OPCAB: off-pump coronary arterial bypass grafting.
NT-proBNP: N-terminal pro-B-type natriuretic peptide.

TABLE 3: Results of multiple logistic regression analyses for contributing factors to perioperative morbidity of acute kidney injury in the total study cohort.

| | Odds ratio | $p$ value |
|---|---|---|
| Duration of surgery (h) | 1.60 (1.19–2.13) | 0.003 |
| Serum dsDNA on POD-1 (per 100 ng/mL) | 2.09 (1.28–3.40) | 0.002 |

dsDNA: double-strand DNA.
POD-1: postoperative day-1 (the day after surgery).

dsDNA concentration on POD-1 was a significantly contributing factor to perioperative AKI in our cohort.

Although the exact mechanism could not be determined by the current study design, several mechanisms could be associated with this result. First, histone is one of the components of NETs, as well as dsDNA, and it could damage kidney tissue via toll-like receptor-2 and toll-like receptor-4 [18]. Second, granular antimicrobial proteins from neutrophils, including neutrophil elastase and myeloperoxidase, are also components of NETs, and they can damage endothelial tissue. Surgically induced elevation in NETs concentration could trigger endothelial dysfunction, and it might affect the microcirculation in renal tissue. Third, impairment of NET degradation is associated with renal dysfunction in some diseases, including systemic lupus erythematosus [16] and anti-neutrophil cytoplasmic antibody-associated vasculitis [19]. In these pathological conditions, inadequate degradation of NETs induces an autoimmune response to the residual NET components, including dsDNA and cytoplasmic proteins of neutrophils. Based on these facts, anti-nucleosomal antibody and pANCA were measured in this study, but neither of these autoimmune antibodies were positive, which suggested that none of these autoimmune responses contribute to the early phase of renal dysfunction. Nevertheless, based on the results of current study, further research will be necessary to study whether cell-free DNA or NETs induce kidney injury in more simplified experimental models and to illuminate the underlying pathophysiologic mechanisms.

*4.3. Study Limitations.* There are some limitations to this study. First, this study was designed as a reevaluation of a study for lung dysfunction after cardiac surgery, and patients with postoperative cardiac failure were excluded to eliminate cardiogenic pulmonary edema [10]. Therefore, the current results cannot be extrapolated to patients with postoperative cardiac failure. Second, in this study, we could not eliminate the sources of cell-free dsDNA other than neutrophils. The results of S100A12 suggested significant correlation between neutrophil activation and elevation in serum dsDNA

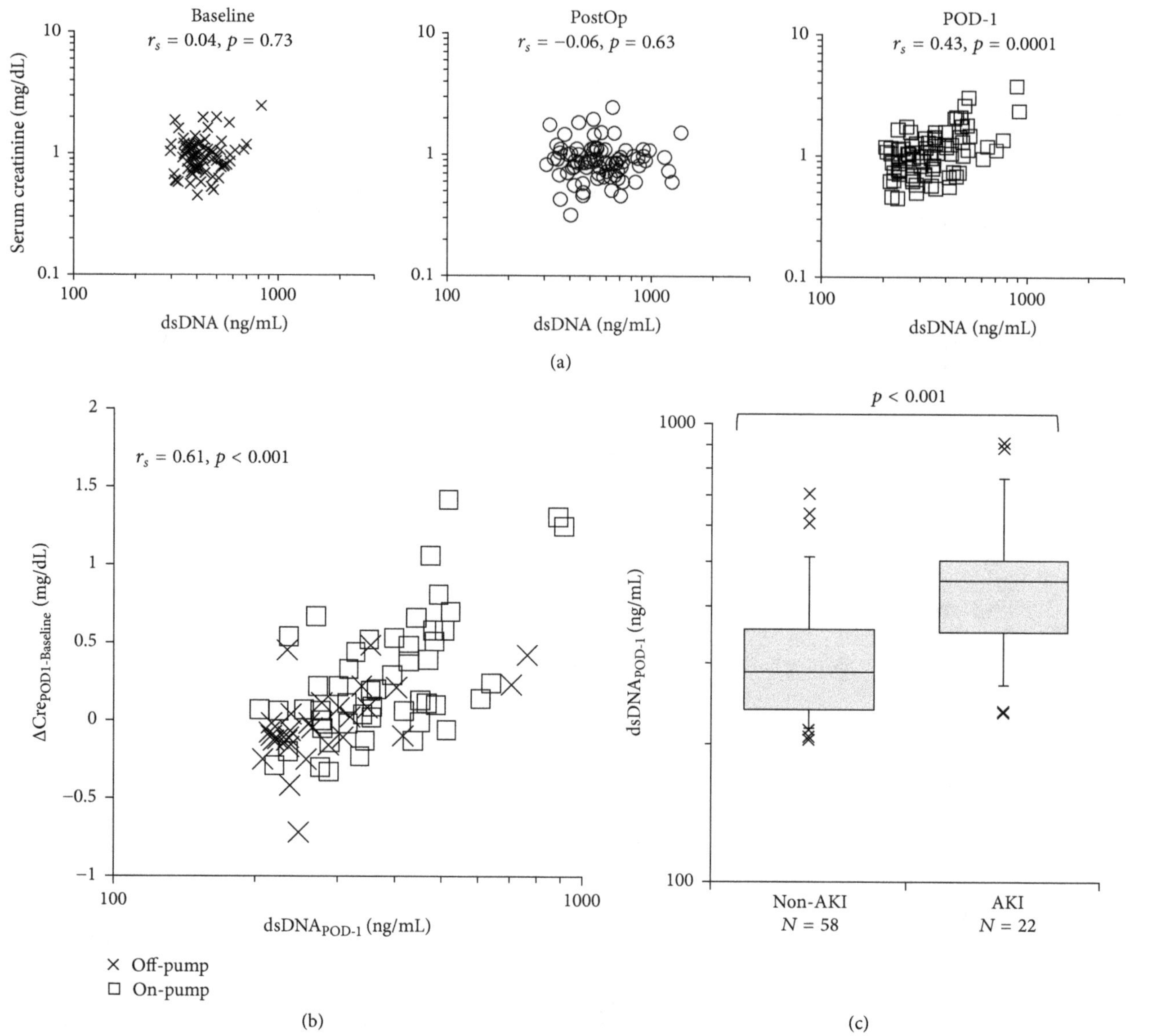


FIGURE 6: Association between serum double-strand DNA (dsDNA) concentration and serum creatinine concentration. (a) Relationship between serum dsDNA concentration and serum creatinine concentration. Spearman's tests were performed at baseline, immediately after surgery (PostOp), and the day after surgery (POD-1). X marks, baseline; open circles, PostOp; open squares, POD-1. (b) Relationship between the change in serum creatinine concentration from baseline to POD-1 ($\Delta Cre_{POD1\text{-}Baseline}$) and dsDNA concentration on POD-1. X marks, off-pump surgery; open squares, on-pump surgery. (c) Serum dsDNA concentration in patients with or without acute kidney injury (AKI). Patients with AKI showed a significantly higher value of dsDNA on POD-1 than those without AKI (non-AKI). $r_s$: correlation coefficient calculated from Spearman's tests.

concentration; however, we could not demonstrate whether the dsDNA bound neutrophil specific markers, such as myeloperoxidase and neutrophil elastase, because of sample shortage. Apoptosis and surgical destruction of tissues might be sources of dsDNA. At present, differentiation of the sources of dsDNA is difficult. Therefore, dsDNA from other sources might participate in the pathophysiology of perioperative organ dysfunction. Third, we could not eliminate the contribution of ischemia-reperfusion in the kidney because we could not detect intraoperative renal ischemia with high sensitivity. Although ischemia could cause neutrophil activation, we could not evaluate the relationship between ischemia and neutrophil activation. Multiple factors other than an elevation in serum dsDNA concentration could contribute to renal tissue damage, which could affect the relationship between the concentration of dsDNA and kidney function. Finally, the types of surgery were limited in the study cohort. Therefore, large-scale studies are required to determine the relationship between serum concentration of circulating dsDNA and perioperative renal dysfunction.

Subgroup analyses for different types of surgery might also be helpful for determining the contribution of confounding factors.

## 5. Conclusions

Serum dsDNA concentration is elevated after cardiac surgery, which might be explained by activation of neutrophils. Prolonged elevation in circulating dsDNA concentration was associated with perioperative renal dysfunction. These results could help in identifying dsDNA as a new biomarker for postoperative risk assessment of patients with cardiac surgery. Further large-scale prospective studies will be needed to illuminate the relationship between circulating dsDNA concentration and perioperative renal dysfunction and the potential pathophysiologic mechanisms that might be responsible.

## Competing Interests

The authors declare that they have no competing interests.

## Acknowledgments

This study was funded by Grants-in-Aid 15H05004 and 25462427 from JSPS, Japan.

## References

[1] T. Lögters, A. Paunel-Görgülü, C. Zilkens et al., "Diagnostic accuracy of neutrophil-derived circulating free DNA (cf-DNA/NETs) for septic arthritis," *Journal of Orthopaedic Research*, vol. 27, no. 11, pp. 1401–1407, 2009.

[2] D. J. Dwivedi, L. J. Toltl, L. L. Swystun et al., "Prognostic utility and characterization of cell-free DNA in patients with severe sepsis," *Critical Care*, vol. 16, article R151, 2012.

[3] S. Margraf, T. Lögters, J. Reipen, J. Altrichter, M. Scholz, and J. Windolf, "Neutrophil-derived circulating free DNA (CF-DNA/NETs): a potential prognostic marker for posttraumatic development of inflammatory second hit and sepsis," *Shock*, vol. 30, no. 4, pp. 352–358, 2008.

[4] V. Brinkmann, U. Reichard, C. Goosmann et al., "Neutrophil extracellular traps kill bacteria," *Science*, vol. 303, no. 5663, pp. 1532–1535, 2004.

[5] V. Papayannopoulos and A. Zychlinsky, "NETs: a new strategy for using old weapons," *Trends in Immunology*, vol. 30, no. 11, pp. 513–521, 2009.

[6] F.-C. Liu, Y.-H. Chuang, Y.-F. Tsai, and H.-P. Yu, "Role of neutrophil extracellular traps following injury," *Shock*, vol. 41, no. 6, pp. 491–498, 2014.

[7] M. Zawrotniak and M. Rapala-Kozik, "Neutrophil extracellular traps (NETs)—formation and implications," *Acta Biochimica Polonica*, vol. 60, no. 3, pp. 277–284, 2013.

[8] W. Meng, A. Paunel-Görgülü, S. Flohé et al., "Deoxyribonuclease is a potential counter regulator of aberrant neutrophil extracellular traps formation after major trauma," *Mediators of Inflammation*, vol. 2012, Article ID 149560, 8 pages, 2012.

[9] B. Meijer, R. B. Gearry, and A. S. Day, "The role of s100a12 as a systemic marker of inflammation," *International Journal of Inflammation*, vol. 2012, Article ID 907078, 6 pages, 2012.

[10] T. Uchida, N. Ohno, M. Asahara et al., "Soluble isoform of the receptor for advanced glycation end products as a biomarker for postoperative respiratory failure after cardiac surgery," *PLoS ONE*, vol. 8, no. 7, Article ID e70200, 2013.

[11] T. Uchida, H. Ito, H. Yamamoto et al., "Elevated levels of angiopoietin-2 as a biomarker for respiratory failure after cardiac surgery," *Journal of Cardiothoracic and Vascular Anesthesia*, vol. 28, no. 5, pp. 1293–1301, 2014.

[12] A. J. Bastin, M. Ostermann, A. J. Slack, G.-P. Diller, S. J. Finney, and T. W. Evans, "Acute kidney injury after cardiac surgery according to risk/injury/failure/loss/end-stage, acute kidney injury network, and kidney disease: improving global outcomes classifications," *Journal of Critical Care*, vol. 28, no. 4, pp. 389–396, 2013.

[13] Y. Arai, K. Yamashita, K. Mizugishi et al., "Serum neutrophil extracellular trap levels predict thrombotic microangiopathy after allogeneic stem cell transplantation," *Biology of Blood and Marrow Transplantation*, vol. 19, no. 12, pp. 1683–1689, 2013.

[14] S. T. Abrams, N. Zhang, J. Manson et al., "Circulating histones are mediators of trauma-associated lung injury," *American Journal of Respiratory and Critical Care Medicine*, vol. 187, no. 2, pp. 160–169, 2013.

[15] H. Gao, N. Zhang, F. Lu et al., "Circulating histones for predicting prognosis after cardiac surgery: a prospective study," *Interactive CardioVascular and Thoracic Surgery*, 2016.

[16] A. Hakkim, B. G. Fürnrohr, K. Amann et al., "Impairment of neutrophil extracellular trap degradation is associated with lupus nephritis," *Proceedings of the National Academy of Sciences of the United States of America*, vol. 107, no. 21, pp. 9813–9818, 2010.

[17] K. Malíčková, D. Ďuricová, M. Bortlík et al., "Impaired deoxyribonuclease I activity in patients with inflammatory bowel diseases," *Autoimmune Diseases*, vol. 2011, Article ID 945861, 5 pages, 2011.

[18] R. Allam, C. R. Scherbaum, M. N. Darisipudi et al., "Histones from dying renal cells aggravate kidney injury via TLR2 and TLR4," *Journal of the American Society of Nephrology*, vol. 23, no. 8, pp. 1375–1388, 2012.

[19] D. Nakazawa, U. Tomaru, and A. Ishizu, "Possible implication of disordered neutrophil extracellular traps in the pathogenesis of MPO-ANCA-associated vasculitis," *Clinical and Experimental Nephrology*, vol. 17, no. 5, pp. 631–633, 2013.

14

# Anesthesiologists' Preferences regarding Visitor Presence during Placement of Neuraxial Labor Analgesia

**Sangeeta Kumaraswami**,[1] **Suryanarayana Pothula,**[1] **Mario Anthony Inchiosa Jr.,**[2] **Keshar Paul Kubal,**[1] **and Micah Alexander Burns**[1]

[1]*Department of Anesthesiology, New York Medical College at Westchester Medical Center, 100 Woods Road, Macy Pavilion 2391, Valhalla, NY 10595, USA*
[2]*Department of Pharmacology and Anesthesiology, New York Medical College at Westchester Medical Center, 100 Woods Road, Macy Pavilion 2391, Valhalla, NY 10595, USA*

Correspondence should be addressed to Sangeeta Kumaraswami; sangeeta.kumaraswami@wmchealth.org

Academic Editor: Yukio Hayashi

*Introduction.* Neuraxial labor analgesia has become an integral part of modern obstetric anesthetic practice. Presence of a familiar person during its placement may be beneficial to the patient. A survey was sent to anesthesiologists practicing obstetric anesthesia in the USA to determine their views. *Methods.* The survey queried the following: existence of a written policy; would they allow a visitor; visitor's view, sitting or standing; reasons to allow or not allow a visitor; and influence by other staff on the decision. The responses were analyzed using multiple chi-square analyses. *Results.* Most practitioners supported allowing a visitor during placement. Reduction of patient anxiety and fulfillment of patient request were the major reasons for allowing a visitor. Sitting position and no view of the workspace were preferred. Visitor interference and safety were cited as the major reasons for precluding a visitor. Nonanesthesia providers rarely influenced the decision. Epidural analgesia was the preferred technique. Essentially no bias was found in the responses; there was statistical uniformity regardless of procedures done per week, years in practice, professional certification, geographic region (rural, urban, or suburban), or academic, private, or government responders. *Conclusion.* The practice of visitor presence during the placement of neuraxial labor analgesia is gaining acceptance.

## 1. Introduction

Over the last few decades, there have been increased in-hospital deliveries, and they account for 99% of all deliveries [1]. The need for psychological support of women in labor was recognized, and men were encouraged to provide support in the care of their partners during labor [2]. Though there was some initial opposition, this practice has become common now [3]. A pleasant birthing experience facilitates the creation of a strong bond between parents and the infant [4]. Continuous epidural anesthesia for pain management during childbirth has become a common practice in the United States of America and the rest of the world, with a significant number of women receiving neuraxial labor analgesia [5, 6].

With the involvement of anesthesiologists in vaginal deliveries in the form of labor pain management, responsibility for any visitor who is present during the procedure may belong to the anesthesiologist. No specific guidelines exist for the presence of a visitor in the room during placement of neuraxial labor analgesia. In an era where parental presence during pediatric anesthesia induction is encouraged [7], anesthesiologists may perhaps be divided in their opinions, regarding placement of neuraxial labor analgesia and presence of a visitor during the procedure.

The presence of a visitor during the placement of the neuraxial block may be desired and may benefit the parturient. It may increase patient satisfaction. There may be some disadvantages from the presence of a visitor during the procedure which may include interference and visitor safety. Anesthesiologists may have varying opinions regarding visitor presence during the placement of neuraxial labor analgesia. A survey among anesthesiologists may be useful in clarifying the concepts on this topic.

## 2. Methods

An obstetric anesthesia survey approved by the New York Medical College Institutional Review Board was designed on the SurveyMonkey® website and sent to anesthesiologists practicing obstetric anesthesia in the United States of America; no patients were involved in this study, which was strictly limited to a collection of personal responses from practicing physicians. The survey was distributed through the Society of Obstetric Anesthesia and Perinatology (SOAP), all anesthesiology residency programs, and several state anesthesia societies nonselectively. Resident physicians were not included in the study since they are unlikely to be practicing independently without supervision. To avoid duplication of responses, anesthesiologists were advised to refrain from answering the survey if they had taken it once. Participation in the survey was voluntary, and responses were completely anonymous.

SOAP is an organization of physicians who share an interest in the care of the pregnant patient and the newborn. The society sent the survey to all their members nationwide. Chairmen of the residency programs were contacted through e-mail with a request to forward the survey to physicians who practiced obstetric anesthesia in their department. State societies of all fifty states were contacted and thirty-three societies responded favorably. Those societies sent the survey to their members. The survey e-mail contained an Internet link in it, and responses were collected over a period of four months. Eighteen hundred completed responses were received. The survey first queried practitioners in relation to demographic categories. This was followed by questions related to actual clinical practice. The survey took about three to five minutes to complete.

*2.1. Statistical analyses.* We used multiple chi-square analyses (IBM-SPSS v.22 Statistical Software) to draw conclusions about the distribution of responses to the nine clinical practice-related questions of the survey. Bonferroni adjustments were applied to the critical thresholds for statistical significance (equivalent to $p \leq 0.05$). In some instances, the two leading responses that were not statistically different from each other were combined for the statistical comparisons with the other responses (Scheffe's method).

## 3. Results

The distribution of the responses to the six questions related to the demographic categories of responding physicians are presented in Table 1.

The detailed analysis of the responses to eight practice-related questions is presented in Figure 1.

TABLE 1: Survey demographics (categories of physicians).

| Questions | Physician category | Number (%) |
|---|---|---|
| Neuraxial procedures/week | <2 | 405 (22.50) |
| | 2–5 | 632 (35.11) |
| | 6–10 | 400 (22.22) |
| | >10 | 363 (20.16) |
| Years in practice | <2 | 175 (9.72) |
| | 2–5 | 323 (17.94) |
| | 6–15 | 472 (26.22) |
| | >15 | 830 (46.11) |
| Qualification | Board eligible | 130 (7.22) |
| | Board certified | 1463 (81.27) |
| | BE&F | 25 (1.38) |
| | BC&F | 182 (10.11) |
| Region of practice | Northeast | 666 (37.0) |
| | Midwest | 384 (21.33) |
| | South | 369 (20.50) |
| | West | 381 (21.16) |
| Practice setting | Rural | 134 (7.44) |
| | Suburban | 679 (37.72) |
| | Urban | 987 (54.83) |
| Nature of practice | Academic | 658 (36.55) |
| | Private | 1100 (61.11) |
| | Government | 42 (2.33) |

BE&F, board eligible and obstetric anesthesia fellowship trained; BC&F, board certified and obstetric anesthesia fellowship trained.

A summary of the responses to the nine practice-related questions is as follows:

**1: Does your practice or hospital have a written policy regarding allowing a patient's visitor in the room during placement of neuraxial labor analgesia? Yes, a written policy exists—Allows visitors; Yes, a written policy exists—Does not allow visitors; No written policy exists; I do not know.**

*Physicians most knowledgeable of the policy by category were ">5 procedures/week," ">15 years practice," "Board certified and obstetric anesthesia fellowship trained (BC&F)," and "Rural practice." These groups of physicians had, statistically, the smallest percentages who chose, "I do not know."*

**2: If no policy existed, would you be open to allowing a patient's visitor in the room during placement of neuraxial labor analgesia? Yes; No.**

*All physician categories favored allowing a visitor by at least 2 : 1.*

**3: If you allowed a visitor in the room during placement of neuraxial labor analgesia, you would want the** visitor always standing; visitor always sitting; does not matter.

*For all categories, combined "sitting" and "does not matter" responses were >85%.*

**4: If you allowed a visitor in the room during placement of neuraxial labor analgesia, you would want the visitor to be positioned such that,** the visitor has no view of the procedure (the patient is between the anesthesiologist and visitor); visitor has partial view of work space (but cannot see the patient's back); does not matter.

*For all categories, "no view" was favored over either "partial view" or "does not matter" by 1.5 : 1 or greater.*

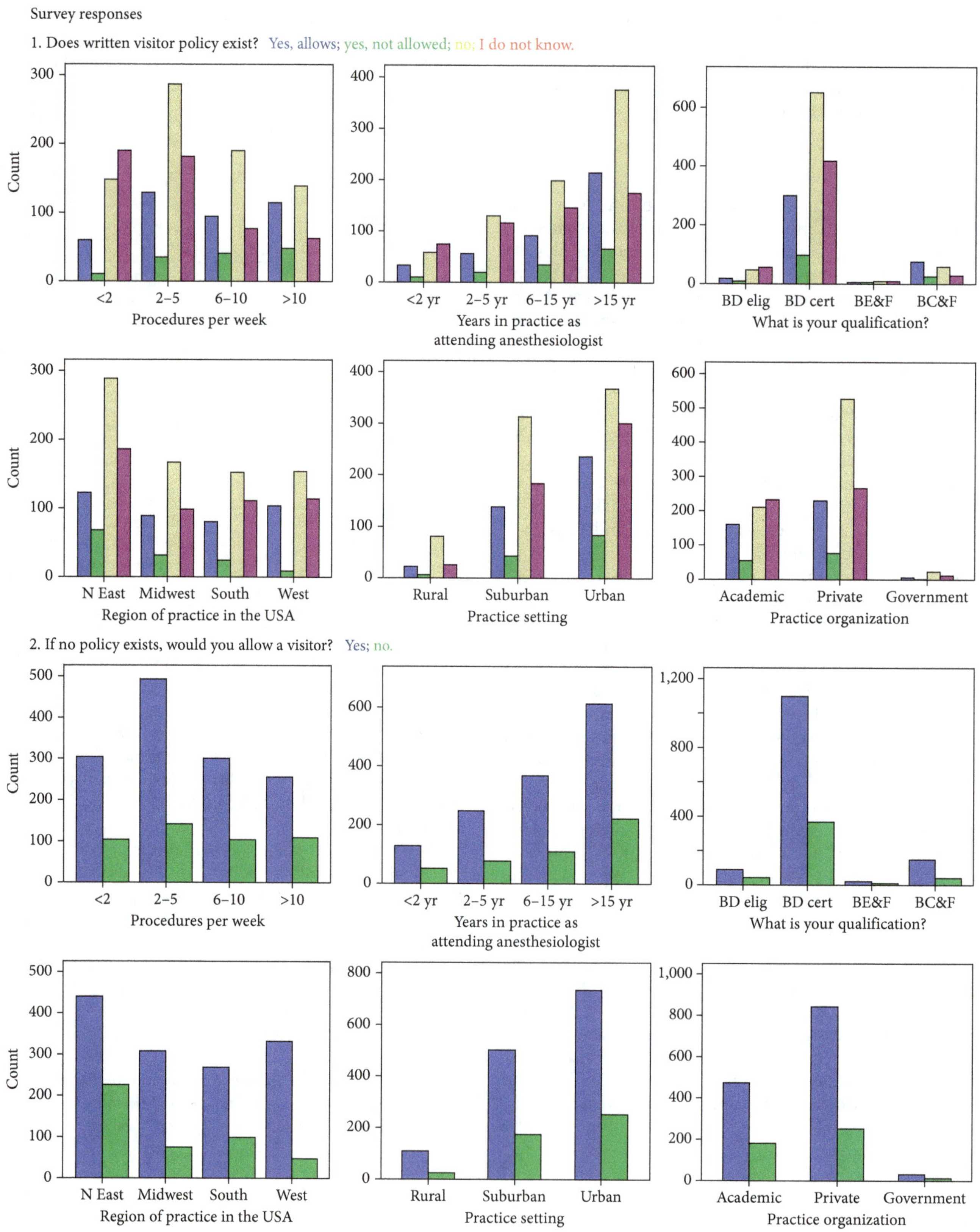


Figure 1: Continued.

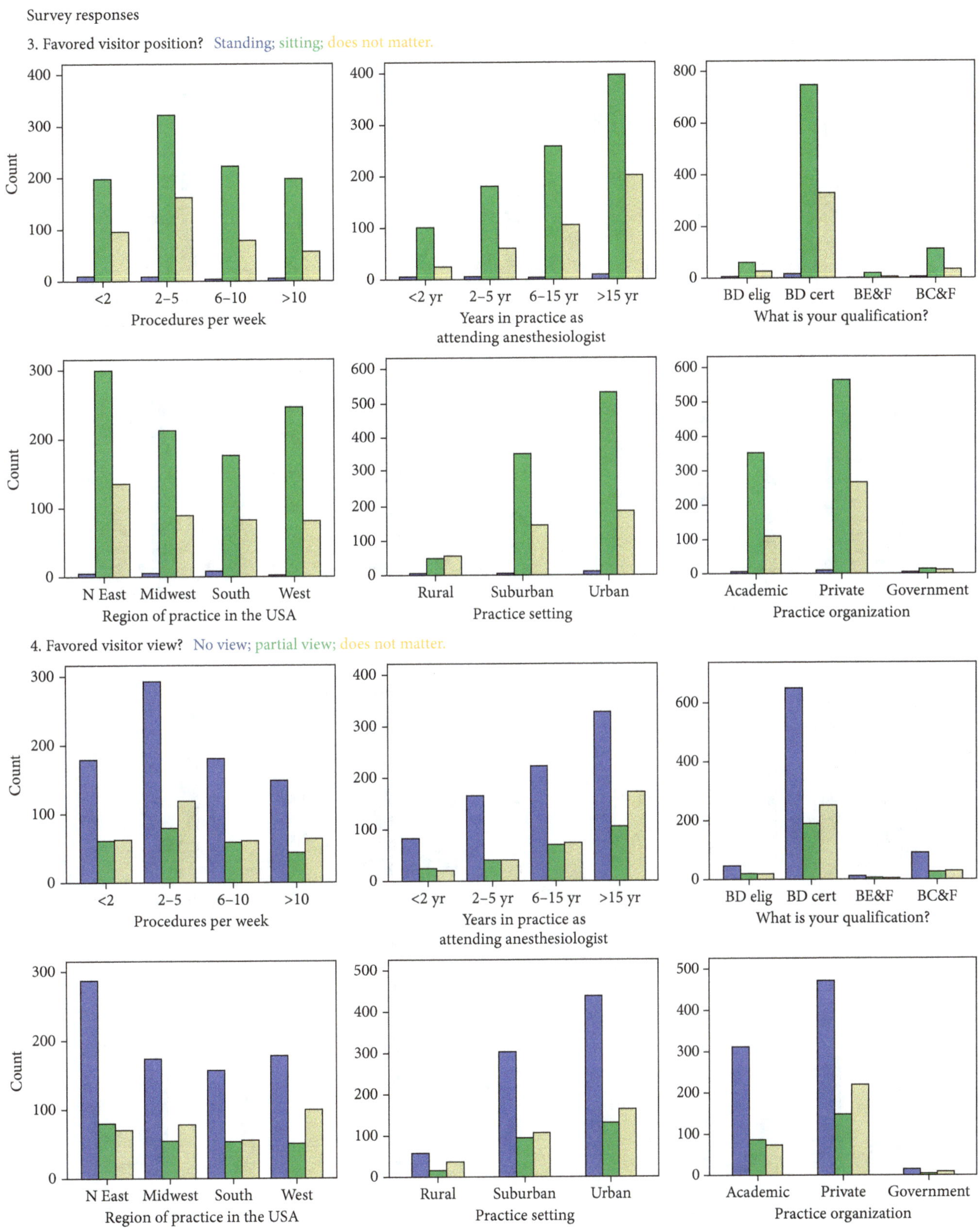


Figure 1: Continued.

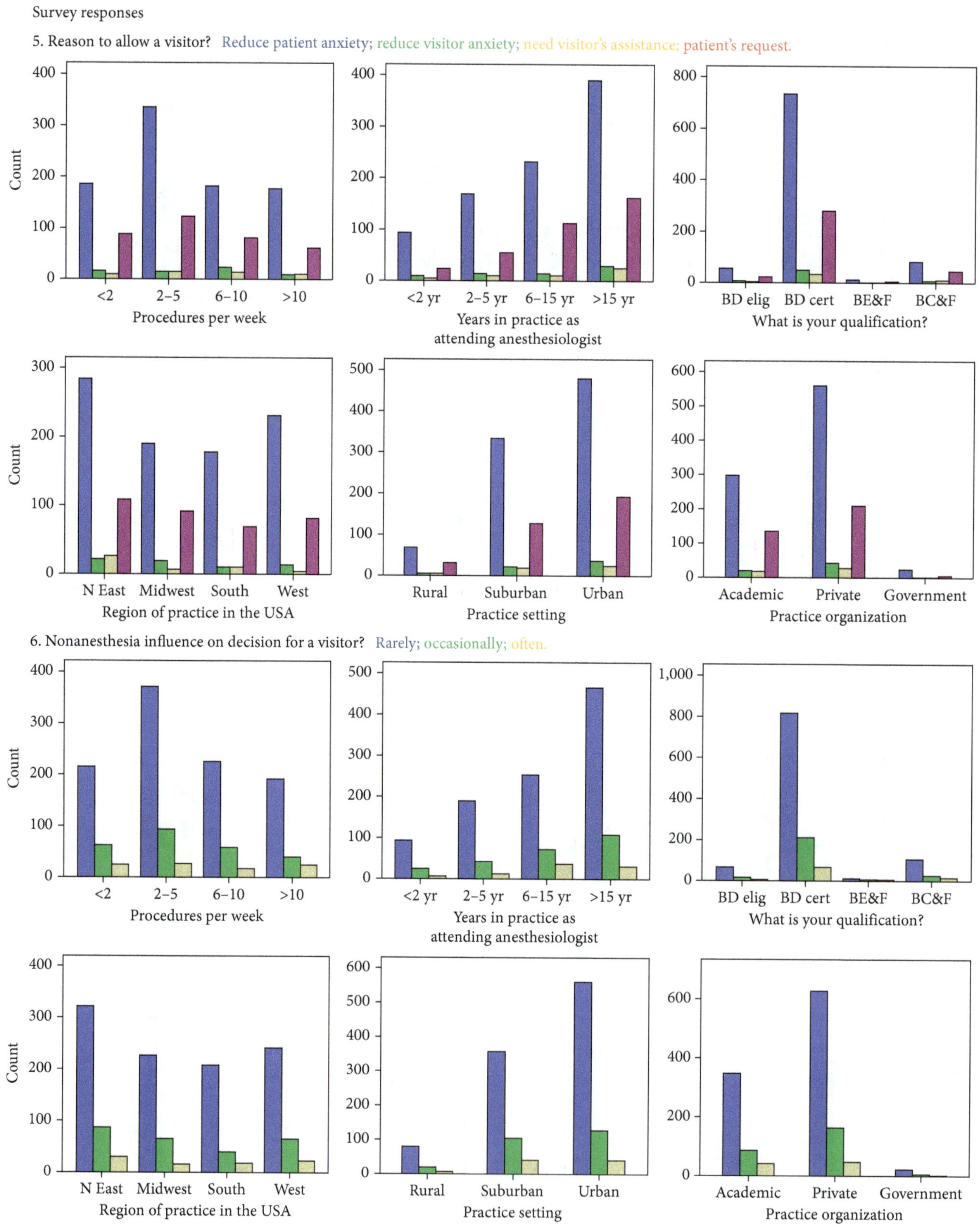


FIGURE 1: Continued.

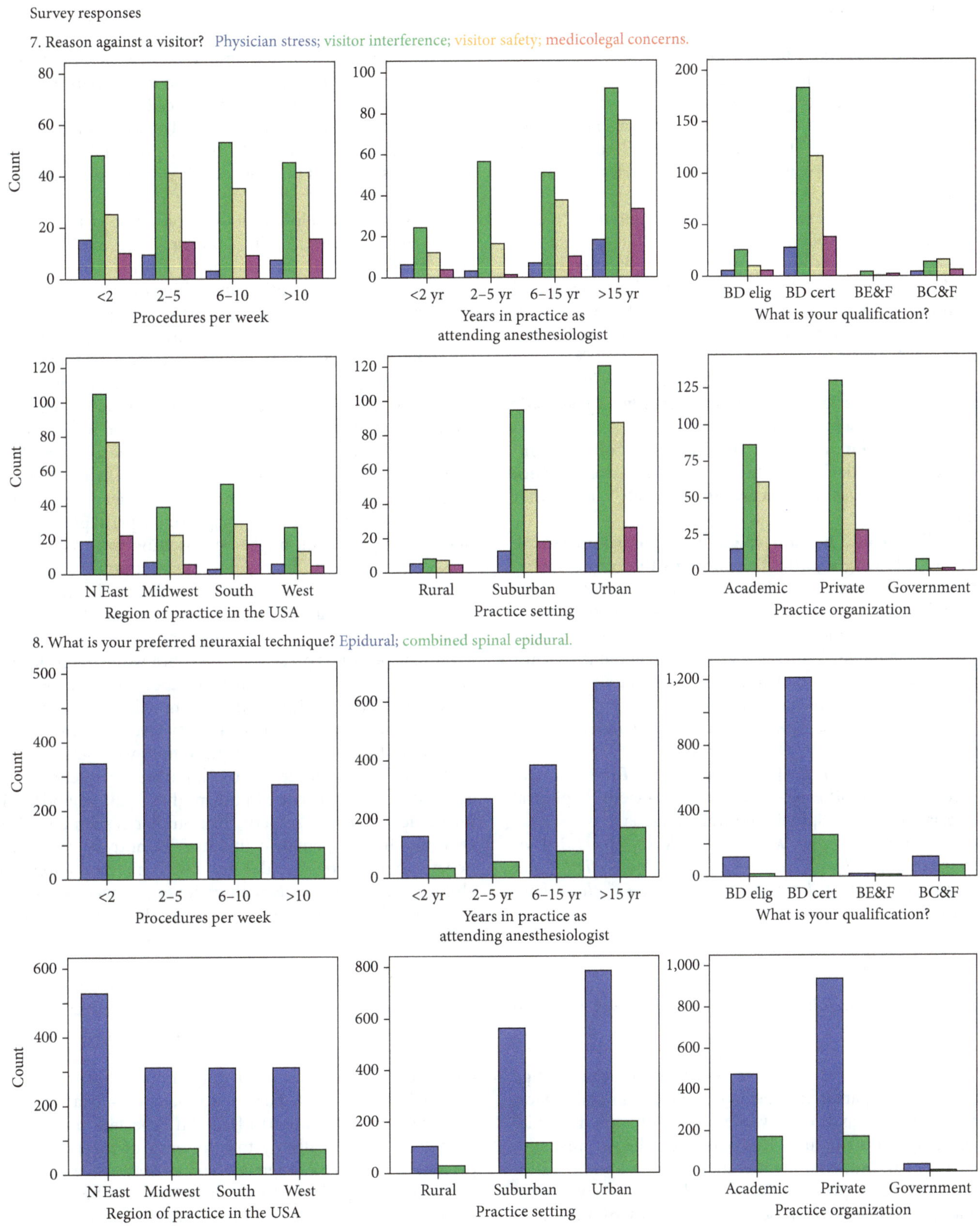


Figure 1: Detailed analysis of the distribution of responses to eight survey questions by the six categories of physician responders.

**5: What would be your single most important reason for allowing a patient's visitor in the room during placement of neuraxial labor analgesia?**

It would likely reduce patient anxiety; it would likely reduce visitor anxiety (e.g., if the visitor were very involved in patient care or if the patient were a teenager); visitor's assistance needed (e.g., if the visitor were a doula hired by the patient or if there was a language barrier); to fulfill patient request.

*For all categories, combined "reduce patient anxiety" and "to fulfill patient's request" responses were 85% or greater.*

**6: How often has another nonanesthesia member of the labor and delivery team (e.g., obstetrician or nurse) attempted to influence your decision to have a visitor present during placement of neuraxial labor analgesia?** Rarely (<5%); occasionally (5%–40%); often (>40%).

*All categories recorded "rarely" by 3:1 over other choices except for "Board eligible and obstetric anesthesia fellowship trained (BE&F)" which was 2:1.*

**7: (A similar question of frequency of a "nonanesthesia provider" to influence your decision to "not have a visitor" was also recorded as "rarely" over other choices.)**

**8: What would be your single most important reason for NOT allowing a patient's visitor in the room during placement of neuraxial labor analgesia?** Increase in anesthesiologist's stress; possible interference by the visitor (e.g., comments made if there is difficult epidural placement or if there is a medical emergency); concern about the visitor (e.g., passing out or not being able to maintain a sterile environment); medicolegal concerns.

*For all categories, combined visitor "interference" and "concern" responses were 80% or greater.*

**9: What is your preferred technique for neuraxial analgesia in an otherwise healthy parturient?** Epidural analgesia; combined spinal-epidural analgesia.

*All categories chose "Epidural analgesia" by 1.8:1 or greater except for "Qualification," and the "Board eligible and obstetric anesthesia fellowship trained (BE&F)" chose both options equally.*

## 4. Discussion

Most of the anesthesiologists in our survey were agreeable to the presence of a visitor in the room while doing the neuraxial labor analgesia procedure. The preferences of patients and their expectations of physicians can change with times. The parturient may like to have a familiar person in the room to reassure her while undergoing the neuraxial labor analgesia procedure. This person can be the husband, a partner, a friend, a family member, or even a nonmedical semiprofessional person like a doula. This may reflect a changing social environment. The specialty of anesthesiology may be adapting positively to those changes.

Of our respondents, 29.3% reported that their institutions had written policies regarding either specifically allowing or not allowing a visitor during the procedure. Any policy regarding the presence of a visitor should be written in detail with input from the department of risk management. It should preferably include a statement to remind staff members that they must use their judgement and individualize each decision. The presence of the spouse or a family member during placement of the neuraxial block should be discussed as part of the anesthetic plan. While the institution can have a policy, the final decision should be that of the anesthesiologist [8]. It may be preferable to mention visitor presence and possible disadvantages in the informed consent.

If a visitor was allowed in the room, then visitor "sitting" or "does not matter" with "no view" of workspace was preferred by most anesthesiologists. Sitting on a chair would minimize the risk of fainting and falling on the floor. Visitors involved with the care of a parturient might be sleep-deprived or hypoglycemic. Vasovagal syncope might be an added factor. Standing would only increase their risk of falling. Having no view of the workspace while the procedure was being done was preferred by many practitioners. This would mean that the visitor's position offered no view of the procedural field. Looking at an epidural needle may likely scare a layperson. Moreover, a potentially difficult or bloody placement of the epidural needle may lead to a messy procedural tray. A view of this, though perhaps commonplace for a physician, might be upsetting to a visitor.

According to the survey findings, important reasons for having a visitor in the room appeared to be to "reduce patient's anxiety" and "fulfill patient's request." Reduction in patient's anxiety may be thought of as being obvious if a familiar person is present in the room while the procedure is being performed. Contrary to expectations, a partner's presence during epidural catheter insertion for labor analgesia did not always decrease anxiety levels, instead anxiety and pain of epidural catheter placement were greater if the partner remained in the room [9]. Partner's presence can be associated with a decrease in the mother's pain memory with no reduction in her anxiety [10]. Similar results have been reported in the pediatric literature. Contrary to popular belief, parental presence did not always alleviate parents' or children's anxiety [11]. Not all patients may want a visitor in the room during epidural placement. There can be cultural influences and variations involved in deciding whether the partner is present in the delivery room during childbirth [12–14]. The partner's presence in the operating room during neuraxial anesthesia for cesarean delivery was associated with no significant difference in patient anxiety but was associated with decreased partner anxiety [15]. Epidural analgesia reduced paternal anxiety and stress and increased paternal involvement, participation, and satisfaction with the experience of childbirth [16]. An expectant mother may be helped emotionally by the presence of the partner, especially if there is a language barrier between the delivery team and the patient. This can be one of the prominent reasons for allowing a visitor during the placement of the epidural block. In view of these variations, it is scientifically prudent to conduct a new prospective study to clarify confusing observations regarding patient anxiety.

The influence by the nonanesthesiology members of the labor and delivery team in our decision making was found to be predominantly "rarely." This would be consistent with the statement endorsed by the American Congress of Obstetricians and Gynecologists and the Association of Women's Health, Obstetric and Neonatal Nurses, which states that optimal maternal and fetal outcomes can best be achieved in an atmosphere of multidisciplinary collaboration [17]. This indicates confidence in the decision-making capabilities of the anesthesiologists among the labor and delivery team.

"Interference by the visitor" and "concern about the visitor" were the leading causes for not wanting to have a visitor in the room. It is possible that one may encounter a disruptive visitor, which would be counterproductive to the care of the patient, especially if the placement of the block is difficult. Visitors in an operating room during a cesarean section made it more difficult to care for the patient with risks outweighing benefits [18]. Concerns about visitors include potential for fainting and compromise of sterility [19, 20]. Injuries to the visitor can occur, and the visitor may need to go to the emergency room for further medical care. Such injuries may lead to medicolegal complications [21]. A safety concern has been raised about nurses leaving the room during placement when there is an increase in patient census in the labor and delivery suite, which may result in the visitor helping with patient positioning [22]. Contamination of a sterile field is a concern. Respiratory droplets are known to travel three to four feet. It is recommended that visitors within four feet of the patient or procedural tray wear a mask during a neuraxial procedure. Wearing surgical masks would decrease sterile field contamination with nasal and oropharyngeal commensal bacteria [23, 24]. Allowing a visitor in the room while placing an epidural block may encourage the visitor to photograph or videotape the procedure. This may interfere with the medical procedure. The hospital policies regarding photography and videography should be ascertained and followed. This may involve medicolegal and privacy concerns.

Most anesthesiologists chose epidural over combined spinal-epidural analgesia as a preferred technique for labor analgesia. There are varied opinions about the practice of combined spinal-epidural versus epidural analgesia in labor [25]. Combined spinal-epidural analgesia (CSE) is considered superior and faster than epidural in the first but not in the second stage of labor [26]. It was of interest that most anesthesiologists preferred epidural rather than the combined technique. However, the "board eligible and obstetric anesthesia fellowship trained" anesthesiologists chose both techniques equally. It may be that the older generation of obstetric anesthesiologists were following the technique they were trained in during their residency, and younger recently trained members of the community are willing to explore both newer and traditional methods. If this assumption is true, this choice may change in the future.

One limitation of our survey is that we do not know the response rate among those who were invited to participate. We sacrificed the ability to determine the exact number of individuals who were successfully contacted by SOAP, departmental chairmen, or professional anesthesia state societies in favor of obtaining as large a response as possible.

The results of the survey strongly suggest that there is essentially no bias in the responses to the questions among the several categories of physicians; there is a marked statistical uniformity of responses from physicians regardless of procedures done per week, years in practice, professional certification, geographic region, practice setting (rural, urban, or suburban), or organization (academic, private, or government) (Figure 1).

## 5. Conclusion

The ASA task force on obstetric anesthesia guidelines supports a multidisciplinary approach to create favorable maternal and fetal outcomes [27]. Our research study was done to determine attitudes and opinions of obstetric anesthesiologists towards visitor presence. The practice of visitor presence during placement of neuraxial labor analgesia appears to be gaining acceptance with anesthesiologists. Patient's rights, visitor concerns, benefits, and risks should be weighed before a decision is made. Limited literature exists on this subject in obstetric anesthesia. Further studies need to be done to ascertain the advantages and disadvantages of this practice.

## Conflicts of Interest

The authors declare that they have no conflicts of interest.

## Acknowledgments

Sangeeta Kumaraswami appreciates helpful discussion with Samuel M. Barst, M.D., Department of Anesthesiology, New York Medical College at Westchester Medical Center, New York, during the early planning of the survey.

## References

[1] M. F. MacDorman, T. J. Mathews, and E. Declerq, *Home Births in the United States*, 1990–2009, NCHS data brief, no. 84, National Center for Health Statistics, Hyatsville, MD, USA, 2012.

[2] M. W. Enkin, M. J. N. C. Keirse, M. J. Renfrew, and J. P. Neilson, *A Guide to Effective Care in Pregnancy and Childbirth*, Oxford University Press, Oxford, UK, 2nd edition, 1995.

[3] J. Draper, "Whose welfare in the labour room? A discussion of the increasing trend of fathers' birth attendance," *Midwifery*, vol. 13, no. 3, pp. 132–138, 1997.

[4] E. D. Hodnett, S. Gates, G. J. Hofmeyr, and C. Sakala, "Continuous support for women during childbirth," *Cochrane Database of Systematic Reviews*, vol. 7, p. CD003766, 2013.

[5] B. A. Bucklin, J. L. Hawkins, J. R. Anderson, and F. A. Ullrich, "Obstetric anesthesia workforce survey: twenty-year update," *Anesthesiology*, vol. 103, no. 3, pp. 645–653, 2005.

[6] M. J. K. Osterman and J. A. Martin, "Epidural and spinal anesthesia use during labor: 27-state reporting area, 2008," *National Vital Statistics Reports*, vol. 59, no. 5, pp. 1–13, 2011.

[7] Z. N. Kain, A. A. Caldwell–Andrews, D. Krivutza, M. Weinberg, S. Wang, and D. Gaal, "Trends in the practice of parental presence during induction of anesthesia and the use of preoperative sedative premedication in the United States, 1995–2002: Results of a follow up national survey," *Anesthesia & Analgesia*, vol. 98, no. 5, pp. 1252–1259, 2004.

[8] N. Nathan and C. A. Wong, "Spinal, epidural, and caudal Anesthesia: anatomy, physiology, and technique," in *Chestnut's Obstetric Anesthesia: Principles and Practice*, D. H. Chestnut, C. A. Wong, L. C. Tsen et al., Eds., pp. 229–261, Elsevier Saunders, Philadelphia, PA, USA, 5th edition, 2014..

[9] S. Orbach-Zinger, Y. Ginosar, J. Sverdlik et al., "Partner's presence during initiation of epidural analgesia does not decrease maternal stress: a prospective randomized controlled trial," *Anesthesia & Analgesia*, vol. 114, no. 3, pp. 654–660, 2012.

[10] A. De Jong, L. Benayoun, B. Al Taweel Jr., and A. Wernet, "Spontaneous presence of partners reduces pain during epidural catheter placement," *International Journal of Obstetric Anesthesia*, vol. 22, no. 3, pp. 259-260, 2013.

[11] J. Chundamala, J. G. Wright, and S. M. Kemp, "An evidence-based review of parental presence during anesthesia induction and parent/child anxiety," *Canadian Journal of Anesthesia*, vol. 56, no. 1, pp. 57–70, 2009.

[12] Y. Bakhta and R. H. Lee, "A survey of Russian women regarding the presence of a companion during labor," *International Journal of Gynecology & Obstetrics*, vol. 109, no. 3, pp. 201–203, 2010.

[13] W. Y. Ip, "Relationships between partner's support during labour and maternal outcomes," *Journal of Clinical Nursing*, vol. 9, no. 2, pp. 265–272, 2000.

[14] I. W. Yim, "The effect of the husband's presence during labour in Hongkong," *Journal of Clinical Nursing*, vol. 6, no. 2, pp. 169-170, 1997.

[15] M. Prabhu, L. F. Wang, A. R. Tait, and A. S. Bullough, "A randomized controlled study of whether the partner's presence in the operating room during neuraxial anesthesia for cesarean delivery reduces patient anxiety," *International Journal of Obstetric Anesthesia*, vol. 18, no. 4, pp. 362–367, 2009.

[16] G. Capogna, M. Camorcia, and S. Stirparo, "Expectant fathers' experience during labor with or without epidural analgesia," *International Journal of Obstetric Anesthesia*, vol. 16, no. 2, pp. 110–115, 2007.

[17] K. Peddicord, "Quality patient care in labor and delivery: a call to action," *Journal of Obstetric, Gynecologic & Neonatal Nursing*, vol. 41, no. 1, p. 4, 2012.

[18] G. J. Reubins, A. Geller, R. L. Braid, S. J. Alvrez, D. S. Karayozyan, and M. I. Zakowski, *Survey of Soap Members on Practices and Policies of Operating Room Visitors for Cesarean Section*, ASA, Schaumbur, IL, USA, 2015.

[19] E. T. Crosby and S. H. Halpern, "Epidurals for labour, and fainting fathers," *Canadian Journal of Anaesthesia*, vol. 36, no. 4, p. 482, 1989.

[20] N. I. Gbingie, M. L. Alderson, and P. M. Barclay, "Informed consent, and fainting fathers," *Anaesthesia*, vol. 56, no. 6, pp. 603-604, 2001.

[21] J. S. Devore and R. Asrani, "Paternal fractured skull as a complication of obstetric anesthesia," *Anesthesiology*, vol. 48, no. 5, p. 386, 1978.

[22] M. C. Vallejo and S. Chaudhry, "Nursing and family-member assistance during labor epidural placement: a matter of safety," *International Journal of Obstetric Anesthesia*, vol. 17, no. 2, pp. 190-191, 2008.

[23] J. D. Siegel, E. Rhinehart, M. Jackson, L. Chiarello, and The Healthcare Infection Control Practices Advisory Committee, *Guideline for Isolation Precautions: Preventing Transmission of Infectious Agents in Healthcare Settings*Public Health Service, U.S. Department of Health and Human Services, Washington, DC, USA, 2007, https://www.cdc.gov/infectioncontrol/guidelines/isolation/.

[24] B. J. Philips, P. Armstrong, S. Fergusson, F. M. Anderson, and J. A. Wildsmith, "Surgical face masks are effective in reducing bacterial contamination caused by dispersal from the upper airway," *British Journal of Anaesthesia*, vol. 69, no. 4, pp. 407-408, 1992.

[25] S. W. Simmons, N. Taghizadeh, A. T. Dennis, D. Hughes, and A. M. Cyna, "Combined spinal-epidural versus epidural analgesia in labour," *Cochrane Database Syst Rev*, vol. 10, p. CD003401, 2012.

[26] D. Gambling, J. Berkowitz, T. R. Farrell, A. Pue, and D. Shay, "A randomized controlled comparison of epidural analgesia and combined spinal-epidural analgesia in a private practice setting: pain scores during first and second stages of labor and at delivery," *Anesthesia & Analgesia*, vol. 116, no. 3, pp. 636–643, 2013.

[27] Practice Guidelines for Obstetric Anesthesia, "An updated report by the American society of anesthesiologists task force on obstetric anesthesia and the society for obstetric anesthesia and perinatology," *Anesthesiology*, vol. 124, no. 2, pp. 270–300, 2016.

# 15

# Factors Associated with Postoperative Prolonged Mechanical Ventilation in Pediatric Liver Transplant Recipients

**Olubukola O. Nafiu,[1,2] Katari Carello,[1,2] Anjana Lal,[1,2] John Magee,[3] and Paul Picton[1]**

[1]*Department of Anesthesiology, University of Michigan, Ann Arbor, MI, USA*
[2]*Section of Pediatric Anesthesiology, University of Michigan, Ann Arbor, MI, USA*
[3]*Department of Surgery, University of Michigan, Ann Arbor, MI, USA*

Correspondence should be addressed to Olubukola O. Nafiu; onafiu@med.umich.edu

Academic Editor: Michael Frass

*Introduction.* Almost all pediatric orthotopic liver transplant (OLT) recipients require mechanical ventilation in the early postoperative period. Prolonged postoperative mechanical ventilation (PPMV) may be a marker of severe disease and may be associated with morbidity and mortality. We determined the incidence and risk factors for PPMV in children who underwent OLT. *Methods.* This was a retrospective analysis of data collected on 128 pediatric OLT recipients. PPMV was defined as postoperative ventilation ≥ 4 days. Perioperative characteristics were compared between cases and control groups. Multivariable logistic regression analysis was used to calculate odds ratios for PPMV after controlling for relevant cofactors. *Results.* An estimated 25% (95% CI, 17.4%–32.6%) required PPMV. The overall incidence of PPMV varied significantly by age group with the highest incidence among infants. PPMV was associated with higher postoperative mortality ($p = 0.004$) and longer intensive care unit ($p < 0.001$) and hospital length of stay ($p < 0.001$). Multivariable analysis identified young patient age, preoperative hypocalcemia, and increasing duration of surgery as independent predictors of PPMV following OLT. *Conclusion.* The incidence of PPMV is high and it was associated with prolonged ICU and hospital LOS and higher posttransplant mortality. Surgery duration appears to be the only modifiable predictor of PPMV.

## 1. Introduction

The vast majority of children undergoing orthotopic liver transplantation (OLT) are maintained on mechanical ventilation (MV) in the immediate postoperative period [1, 2]. Reasons for this practice include concerns about graft function, postoperative respiratory depression from opioids, preexisting malnutrition, and organ-recipient size mismatch as well as poor cooperation of young children with postoperative instructions [3]. With current improvements in the perioperative care of liver transplant recipients, there is increasing drive towards early extubation in both adults [4, 5] and children [3, 6].

Although many children require only a few days of MV following OLT, for some a more prolonged course is necessary. In general, prolonged postoperative mechanical ventilation (PPMV) in intensive care unit (ICU) patients is a marker of severe adverse events and is associated with higher morbidity and mortality as well as extraordinary resource utilization [3, 7]. Patients requiring PPMV have survived the acute phase of surgery but spend an increased amount of time in the ICU, consume about 50% of all intensive care unit (ICU) resources, and are more likely to die [7]. Consequently, investigating the incidence and factors predisposing to PPMV following liver transplant is an important area of research with the potential to reduce cost of care and improve long-term outcome for these patients.

To our knowledge, factors associated with PPMV following pediatric liver transplantation have not been comprehensively characterized. Here, we investigate the incidence and risk factors for PPMV in children who underwent liver transplant at a US tertiary hospital. We also explored the relationship between PPMV and a number of clinically important outcomes such as duration of intensive care unit (ICU) and total hospital length of stay (LOS) as well as 1-year posttransplant mortality rates.

## 2. Methods

This was a retrospective cohort study. Following Institutional Review Board approval *(IRB number HUM00068847)*, we queried our perioperative, clinical information system (Centricity® General Electric Healthcare, Waukesha, Wisconsin) and the Organ Transplantation Information System (OTIS) database. The records of all children with age $\leq$ 17 yr who underwent OLT at our institution were examined. We extracted the following clinical and anthropometric information from the database: age, gender, weight, American Society of Anesthesiology (ASA) physical status, and etiology of liver failure. All preoperative laboratory results were obtained from the blood drawn for preoperative evaluation on the day of operation.

*2.1. Case Definition and Variable Transformations.* Definition of PPMV following pediatric liver transplant is unavailable. Adult publications often utilize a 48 hr cut-point [8, 9]. This may not necessarily be a practical cut-point in children. Therefore, to estimate the incidence of PPMV, we used previously described cut-point which indicates that $\geq$96 hr mechanical ventilation was a marker of disease severity in pediatric intensive care unit (PICU) patients [10] to transform days of postoperative mechanical ventilation to a categorical variable (PPMV yes/no). Thus, the primary outcome (dependent) variable for this report, PPMV, was defined as requirement of mechanical ventilation for $\geq$4 consecutive postoperative days. This value also matched the 75th percentile number of days of postoperative ventilation in our study cohort.

Anesthesia duration was measured as the interval between documented "patient in room" and "anesthesia end." Similarly, duration of surgery was measured from the beginning of "surgical incision" to "surgery end." Surgery and anesthesia durations were considered prolonged if the times were $\geq$453 min and 592 min, respectively (each value corresponding to the 75th percentile times for the study cohort). Finally, length of stay (LOS) was calculated from the day of transplantation to ICU or hospital discharge. Mortality data were assessed as death occurring within one year from the day of liver transplantation.

*2.2. Exclusion Criteria.* Patients who required mechanical ventilation during the 48 hr preceding surgery (ventilator-dependent) were excluded. We also excluded patients who were older than 17 yr at the time of transplantation. Similarly, patients who died either in the operating room or within 96 hr of surgery were excluded. Including these patients in the analysis would result in a misclassification bias because they would have been included in the non-PMV group. Present analysis also excluded patients who were reintubated within 48 hr of successful extubation because reintubation is a known risk factor for prolonged intubation [10].

*2.3. Statistical Analysis.* Data analyses were carried out with Statistical Package for the Social Sciences (SPSS) for Windows, version 22.0, (SPSS Inc., Chicago, IL). Basic descriptive statistics including means, standard deviations, and percentages were calculated for demographic and anthropometric data. Distribution of skewed continuous variables such as age and hospital and ICU LOS was displayed with box and whisker plots after stratifying patients according to postoperative ventilation status. When necessary, continuous variables were transformed to categorical variables to emphasize clinical applicability. Pearson's Chi-square test for categorical variables and Student's $t$-test and one-way ANOVA for continuous variables were used to examine baseline clinical and perioperative factors associated with PMV. Prevalence of preoperative anemia, malnutrition, hyponatremia, and hypoalbuminemia were described as simple proportions. Furthermore, intraoperative uses of blood products (packed red blood cells, fresh frozen plasma, platelets, and cryoprecipitate) were described as simple proportions and compared across postoperative ventilation groups. We also explored the association between preoperative anemia and use of intraoperative blood transfusion.

*2.3.1. Multivariable Logistic Regression Analysis.* Multivariable analysis was performed using logistic regression (backward stepwise method) to calculate the adjusted odds ratios for the occurrence of PPMV.

To fit the logistic regression model, we estimated $\Pr(Y = 1 \mid X)$, where $Y$ is the binary dependent variable and $X$ is the vector of the covariates. Derivation of the response variable $Y$ (PPMV yes/no) is as detailed above. Model covariates were selected based on statistical significance or clinical relevance. Predictor variables were treated as continuous or categorical as needed. For example, to align with clinical utility, preoperative serum calcium and albumin were transformed into categorical variables (hypocalcemia or hypoalbuminemia, resp.). Similarly, intraoperative blood product utilization was coded as yes/no categorical variables for the regression model. Prior to performing multiple logistic regression analyses, variables were examined for multicollinearity by first creating a correlation matrix and scanning for highly correlated variables ($\geq$0.7). After collinearity diagnostics, all variables were entered into a nonparsimonious logistic regression model to determine independent predictors of PMV. All variables with a $p$ value $\leq 0.05$ were deemed independent predictors of PMV. Goodness of fit of the model was assessed using the Hosmer-Lemeshow test [11]. Furthermore, the model's predictive value was assessed using receiver operating characteristic (ROC) analyses and area under the curve (AUC). All reported $p$ values were 2-sided and a $p$ value of $<0.05$ was considered as statistically significant.

## 3. Results

One hundred and twenty-eight patients aged 4 mth to 17 yr who underwent liver transplant were included in this analysis. There were 22 (17.2%) infants, 37 (28.9%) preschool children, and 69 (53.9%) older children. The median duration of postoperative ventilation days for the total sample was 2

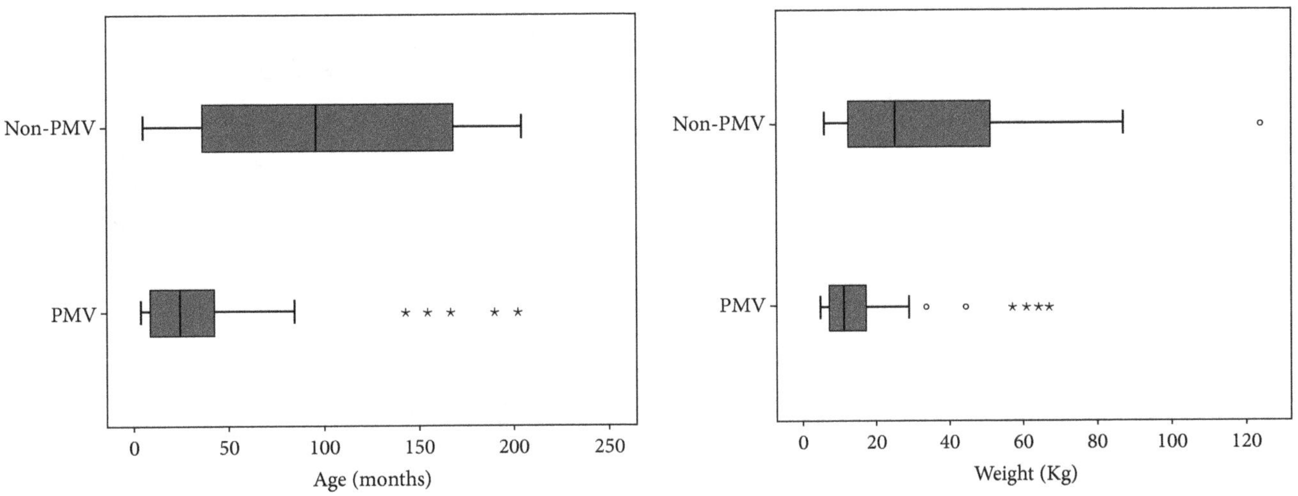


FIGURE 1: Box plots showing the distribution of age (months) and weight (Kg) stratified by postoperative ventilation status among 128 pediatric liver transplant recipients. Expectedly age and weight data were skewed. Children requiring prolonged postoperative ventilation were significantly younger ($p = 0.001$) and weighed less ($p = 0.005$) than those who were extubated early. PMV: prolonged mechanical ventilation. Circles and stars refer to outliers or extreme values.

(1,5) days. Overall, 32 (25%) patients required PPMV. Age and weight distribution in the study cohort displayed a slight right skew (Figure 1) with children who required PPMV being significantly younger ($p < 0.001$) and weighing less ($p = 0.005$) than those in the non-PPMV group (Figure 1).

Table 1 summarizes the baseline preoperative clinical and laboratory variables between the groups. In bivariable analyses, we identified a number of differences in the two study groups. Patients in the PPMV group were more likely to be infants and weigh below 10 kg. They were also more likely to have a preoperative liver diagnosis of biliary atresia. Furthermore, mean preoperative sodium, total protein, albumin, and calcium were significantly lower among children who required PMV. Similarly, preoperative WBC count, liver enzymes, and PT values were significantly higher in the PMV than in the non-PPMV group. Although baseline anemia was common in the study cohort, it was not significantly associated with PPMV.

Intraoperative and postoperative variables stratified by group allocation are detailed in Table 2. Mean duration of anesthesia and surgery was significantly longer in the PPMV compared to the non-PPMV group (Table 2). Intraoperative blood product utilization was very common in this group of patients, although only the use of fresh frozen plasma (FFP) and cryoprecipitate was significantly associated with PPMV (Table 2). Expectedly, intraoperative PRBC transfusion rates were significantly higher in patients with preoperative anemia compared to the nonanemic group (95.1% versus 78.4%; $p = 0.022$). Transfusion rates for FFP, platelets, and cryoprecipitate were similarly higher in the anemic group.

Total intensive care unit (ICU) and hospital LOS displayed a leptokurtic right skew (Figure 2). Mean ICU LOS was ten days longer in the PPMV group compared with that in those who were extubated early (16.4 days versus 6.6 days; $p < 0.001$). Similarly, mean posttransplant hospital LOS was 12 days longer among children requiring PPMV compared to

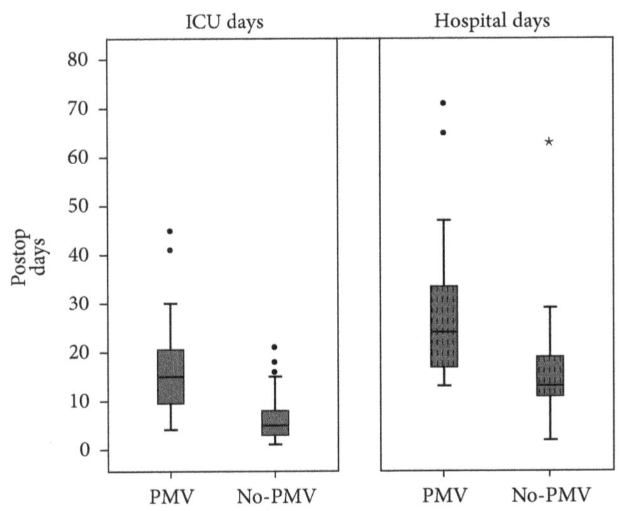


FIGURE 2: Box plot showing the distribution of postoperative ICU and hospital length of stay stratified according to duration of postoperative ventilation status. Patients in the PMV group had significantly longer ICU and hospital LOS compared with the non-PMV group. ICU: intensive care unit; LOS: length of stay; PMV: prolonged mechanical ventilation. Circles and stars refer to outliers or extreme values.

those who did not (27.7 days versus 15.2 days; $p < 0.001$). Overall posttransplant 1-year mortality was 5.5%. Children in the PPMV group had 8 times higher unadjusted odds of mortality compared with the control group (15.6% versus 2.1%, OR = 8.5; 95% CI = 11.6–47.3; $p = 0.011$).

*3.1. Multivariable Analyses.* In order to determine predictors of PMV, we performed multiple logistic regression analysis (backward stepwise method) with PMV as the dichotomous

Table 1: Baseline clinical and laboratory characteristics of the study cohort by PPMV status.

| Variables | All ($N$ = 128) | No ($N$ = 96) | Yes ($N$ = 32) | $p$ value |
|---|---|---|---|---|
| Male sex (%) | 53.9 | 51.0 | 62.1 | 0.260 |
| Infants (%) | 17.2 | 11.4 | 37.5 | 0.001 |
| Under five (%) | 51.1 | 37.7 | 77.4 | <0.001 |
| Weight (Kg) | 28.5 ± 24.4 | 33.9 ± 25.6 | 18.6 ± 18.4 | 0.003 |
| Height (cm) | 110.6 ± 38.6 | 119.2 ± 36.8 | 91.5 ± 36.0 | 0.002 |
| BMI | 19.9 ± 5.3 | 20.2 ± 5.6 | 19.5 ± 4.5 | 0.597 |
| Under 10 kg (%) | 26.0 | 16.7 | 50.0 | 0.001 |
| FTT (%) | 16.0 | 11.1 | 28.6 | 0.032 |
| Preoperative anemia (%) | 43.0 | 40.3 | 50.8 | 0.500 |
| Hepatopulmonary synd. | 8.5 | 4.9 | 15.2 | 0.09 |
| ASA > III (%) | 61 | 51.4 | 85.7 | 0.001 |
| PELD/MELD score | 20.10 ± 9.49 | 20.13 ± 10.1 | 20.04 ± 7.8 | 0.996 |
| *Liver disease etiology* (%) | | | | 0.014 |
| Biliary atresia | 33.0 | 23.0 | 51.5 | |
| Neonatal cholestasis | 13.8 | 14.8 | 12.1 | |
| Hepatitis | 17.0 | 16.4 | 18.2 | |
| Metabolic diseases | 12.8 | 12.8 | 0.0 | |
| Others* | 23.4 | 26.2 | 18.2 | |
| *Preoperative labs* | | | | |
| $\text{Sodium}_{(\text{mEq/L})}$ | 137.4 ± 4.0 | 138.2 ± 3.8 | 135.7 ± 3.7 | 0.004 |
| $\text{Potassium}_{(\text{mEq/L})}$ | 3.9 ± 0.5 | 3.9 ± 0.5 | 4.1 ± 0.48 | 0.315 |
| Serum $CO_{2\,(\text{mEq/L})}$ | 23.2 ± 3.3 | 24.0 ± 3.1 | 21.7 ± 3.1 | <0.001 |
| Calcium | 8.9 ± 0.85 | 9.1 ± 0.9 | 8.6 ± 0.6 | 0.007 |
| Magnesium | 2.0 ± 0.3 | 2.0 ± 0.3 | 1.9 ± 0.3 | 0.411 |
| $\text{Albumin}_{(\text{g/dL})}$ | 3.3 ± 0.7 | 3.5 ± 0.7 | 3.0 ± 0.5 | 0.007 |
| $\text{Protein}_{(\text{g/dL})}$ | 6.4 ± 1.1 | 6.6 ± 0.9 | 5.8 ± 1.2 | 0.004 |
| $\text{ALT}_{(\text{IU/L})}$ | 188.5 ± 323.3 | 177.4 ± 314.5 | 209.9 ± 343.8 | 0.652 |
| $\text{AST}_{(\text{IU/L})}$ | 308.3 ± 574.0 | 228.7 ± 337.3 | 510.0 ± 929.1 | 0.029 |
| Alk phos. | 592.4 ± 496.8 | 522.5 ± 436.4 | 769.7 ± 597.2 | 0.025 |
| PT | 16.3 ± 8.6 | 15.5 ± 7.9 | 18.5 ± 9.9 | 0.047 |
| PTT | 38.7 ± 16.5 | 36.6 ± 14.0 | 44.0 ± 21.2 | 0.047 |
| BUN | 11.8 ± 5.9 | 11.8 ± 5.8 | 11.4 ± 6.3 | 0.706 |
| $\text{Creatinine}_{(\text{mg/dL})}$ | 0.44 ± 0.2 | 0.49 ± 0.3 | 0.30 ± 0.2 | 0.001 |
| WBC | 7.8 ± 4.1 | 7.1 ± 3.4 | 9.5 ± 5.2 | 0.009 |

PPMV: prolonged postoperative mechanical ventilation; BMI: body mass index; FTT: failure to thrive; ASA: American Society of Anesthesiologists; MELD: Model for End-Stage Liver Disease; Alk Phos.: alkaline phosphate; BUN: blood urea nitrogen; WBC: white blood cells count. *Others: refers to other types of liver disease.

TABLE 2: Perioperative variables stratified according to PPMV status.

| Variables | All patients ($N$ = 128) | No ($N$ = 96) | No ($N$ = 32) | $p$ value |
|---|---|---|---|---|
| Operation time (min) | 397.0 ± 83.9 | 377.4 ± 86.1 | 435.6 ± 64.9 | <0.001 |
| Anesthesia time (min) | 538.1 ± 97.4 | 517.5 ± 99.4 | 578.7 ± 80.3 | 0.004 |
| PRBC (cc/kg) | 52.65 | 41.08 | 82.38 | 0.039 |
| FFP (cc/kg) | 53.57 | 38.41 | 92.55 | <0.001 |
| Platelets (cc/kg) | 5.96 | 4.61 | 9.47 | 0.092 |
| Crystalloid (cc/kg) | 69.12 | 58.78 | 95.71 | 0.157 |
| OR inotropes used | 8.5 | 8.2 | 9.1 | 0.882 |
| Split liver used (%) | 31.0 | 23.6 | 50.0 | 0.016 |
| ICU LOS (days) | 9.9 ± 8.0 | 6.6 ± 4.4 | 16.6 ± 9.5 | <0.001 |
| Hospital LOS (days) | 19.5 ± 12.4 | 15.3 ± 8.7 | 27.7 ± 14.2 | <0.001 |
| Reexploration | 37.0 | 25.0 | 67.9 | <0.001 |

PPMV: prolonged postoperative mechanical ventilation; PRBC: packed red blood cells; FFP: fresh frozen plasma; ICU LOS: intensive care unit length of stay; OR: operating room.

dependent variable and many of the baseline clinical and laboratory factors found to be significantly different in Tables 1 and 2 as independent (predictor) variables. Because duration of surgery and duration of anesthesia were highly correlated ($r$ = 0.91; $p$ < 0.001), only the former was included in the regression model. Furthermore, the number of variables included in our regression model was hampered by the overall sample size. Therefore, despite using the backward selection method, we had to utilize clinical judgement to select the most parsimonious model. Model performance was assessed with the Hosmer-Lemeshow (HL) goodness-of-fit test as well as receiver operating characteristic curve (ROC) analysis (reported as $c$-statistic) and the HL test revealed a good model fit to our data ($\chi^2$ = 10.22; df = 8; $p$ = 0.35). The $c$-statistic for the model was 0.82 (95% CI, 0.72–0.92), indicating good model discriminant ability. Furthermore, ROC curve analysis of the model's discriminant ability was good (Figure 3). The results of the multivariable logistic regression analysis are detailed in Table 3 and include the odds ratios for the initial and final models after backward exclusion. In the final model, under-five age group, increasing duration of surgery (per hour), high ASA status, and preoperative hypocalcemia were the most consistent factors associated with PMV. Specifically, for every additional hour of operation, the odds of PMV increased by 1.88. Similarly, under-five age group was associated with 9.5 times increased odds of PMV in this cohort of patients. Preoperative hypocalcemia was also a significant predictor of PMV in our patients.

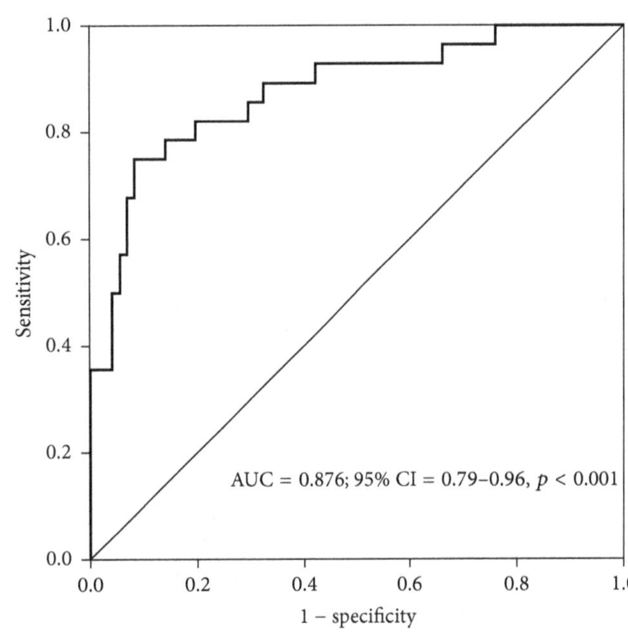


FIGURE 3: Receiver operator characteristic (ROC) curve evaluating the sensitivity and specificity of the model predicting PPMV. Area under the curve (AUC) for the predictors was 0.87 (95% CI = 0.79–0.96; $p$ < 0.001). AUC for the ROC indicates the usefulness of a test (our model) in predicting a binomial outcome (PMV yes/no). A value of 0.87 indicates "good" model predictive ability.

## 4. Discussion

We presented comprehensive data on the incidence and risk factors as well as clinically important outcomes associated with PMV following pediatric OLT. We have demonstrated that the incidence of PMV (≥4 days of postoperative mechanical ventilation) was high in this sample of children who underwent OLT. We also identified preoperative factors including young recipient age, prolonged duration of surgery, and preoperative hypocalcemia as being significantly associated with PMV. We further demonstrated that PMV was associated with considerably increased ICU and total hospital LOS and it is significantly associated with increased post-transplant mortality.

Pediatric liver transplantation has become an effective and widely accepted treatment for severe liver disease [12]. With improvement in anesthetic and surgical management in the last 25 yr, many pediatric OLT recipients are able to resume and maintain spontaneous ventilation soon after

Table 3: Multivariable logistic regression model and parameters for factors associated with PPMV ($N = 128$).

| Predictors | $\beta$ | SE | OR | 95% CI | $p$ value |
|---|---|---|---|---|---|
| *Beginning model* | | | | | |
| Constant | −5.5 | 1.8 | 0.004 | — | 0.005 |
| Under 5 yr | 2.96 | 1.07 | 19.44 | 2.37–158.97 | 0.003 |
| ASA ≥ 3 | 1.45 | 0.67 | 4.67 | 1.14–15.82 | 0.03 |
| Weight (Kg) | −0.032 | 0.02 | 1.03 | 0.97–1.09 | 0.24 |
| Sodium | −0.03 | 0.07 | 0.97 | 0.28–2.61 | 0.73 |
| WBC | 0.12 | 0.07 | 1.12 | 0.96–1.30 | 0.14 |
| Hypocalcemia (yes/no) | 1.42 | 0.72 | 4.14 | 1.22–15.51 | 0.024 |
| Surgery duration (hr.) | 0.71 | 0.23 | 2.03 | 1.27–3.26 | 0.003 |
| FFP transfusion (yes/no) | 0.88 | 0.98 | 2.43 | 0.35–16.68 | 0.36 |
| Cryoprecipitate (yes/no) | 0.50 | 0.71 | 1.65 | 0.41–6.68 | 0.48 |
| *Final model* | | | | | |
| Constant | −6.8 | 1.66 | 0.001 | — | <0.001 |
| Hypocalcemia (yes/no) | 1.46 | 0.62 | 4.32 | 1.27–13.90 | 0.019 |
| Surgery duration (hr.) | 0.63 | 0.20 | 1.88 | 1.25–2.81 | 0.013 |
| ASA status ≥ 3 | 1.24 | 0.65 | 4.42 | 1.29–16.69 | 0.019 |
| Under 5 yr | 2.29 | 0.62 | 9.51 | 2.75–32.55 | <0.001 |

PPMV: prolonged postoperative mechanical ventilation; FFP: fresh frozen plasma; ASA: American Society of Anesthesiologists; OR: odds ratio; SE: standard error.

surgery and typically only require a short period of postoperative mechanical ventilation. In children requiring PPMV, this may be due to the occurrence of a severe perioperative complication, which may be organ-specific or systemic. One of the primary objectives of the present investigation was to document the incidence of PPMV in pediatric OLT recipients and we found that, despite using a liberal definition of PPMV (≥4 days), the incidence was about 25%. Although this percentage appears to be quite high (and may reflect local practices), other investigators [13] have reported rates as high as 31.6% among adult OLT recipients who developed postoperative pneumonia. There is presently no comparable published data describing PPMV among pediatric OLT recipients. The present report therefore addresses key research needs on the subject of pediatric solid organ transplantation and it represents the necessary first steps towards delineating the scope of the problem. Large multicenter studies are necessary in order to compare practice across transplant units and determine median duration of postoperative mechanical ventilation in OLT recipients. This should help guide clinical practice and development of future pediatric OLT standards.

A second objective of the present analysis was to identify perioperative factors that are significantly associated with PPMV in pediatric OLT recipients. To this end, we found that patient's age was the strongest predictor of PPMV after adjusting for several clinical covariates. Although the confidence interval associated with the odds ratio for age group as a risk factor for PMV was very wide, under-five children had about 10 times increased odds of PPMV compared to their older peers in our regression model. This is an important point to consider when planning OLT in under-five children. They are a group that could be targeted for specific interventions to reduce the likelihood of PPMV.

In order to effectively prevent PPMV in children undergoing OLT, it is important to recognize factors that may predispose patients to this complication. Unfortunately, similar to the findings of previous investigators reporting on other types of surgical procedures [14, 15], many of the factors identified in our study are fairly intuitive but not necessarily modifiable. For example, factors such as under-five age group, preoperative hypocalcemia, prolonged duration of anesthesia, and surgery and intraoperative blood product transfusion are either part of the pathological process or indicative of severity of the underlying disease. However, despite these limitations, presence of these risk factors in a pediatric liver transplant patient may prove useful for alerting clinicians about the need for close follow-up and early intervention. Furthermore, identification of nonmodifiable factors may be helpful for risk stratification of patients and appropriate allocation of resources.

Most published data indicate that PPMV is associated with increased postoperative morbidity and mortality as well as significant medical expenditure. We found, as did previous investigators [16, 17], that one-year posttransplant death rate among patients requiring PPMV was higher than that in those who are not. It must be noted though that it is impossible to determine a causal relationship between PPMV and mortality from retrospective case-control data such as that we used in the present report. We also provided data for the first time in a pediatric OLT cohort, spotlighting the impact of PPMV on postoperative ICU and hospital LOS following liver transplant. Our results indicate that PPMV increased mean ICU and hospital LOS by 10 and 14 days, respectively. Although we do not have data on the charges associated with posttransplant complication in the present report, the total hospital cost associated with PPMV in the pediatric liver transplant is likely very high. Increased awareness among clinicians about the factors associated with PPMV among pediatric liver transplant patients is likely to lead to targeted interventions to reduce this complication.

Although it is impossible to determine the mechanisms underlying PPMV from a retrospective study such as ours, several putative mechanisms have been highlighted by previous reviews of the subject [18, 19]. Among these are increased respiratory demands due to pulmonary edema and pleura effusion and increased intrathoracic pressure from graft-size mismatch. Other possible causes include excessive sedation, preoperative malnutrition, and electrolyte abnormalities.

We also found that children undergoing primary liver transplant who have lower or deranged values of common metabolic variables were significantly more likely to require PPMV than those with normal values of these metabolic variables. This may simply reflect a more severe degree of preoperative hepatic dysfunction in children with lower values of these variables. Lower serum levels of biochemical parameters such as albumin and sodium may be associated with expanded total body water which may in turn lead to increased lung water [3]. This could make weaning from mechanical ventilation difficult in the postoperative period. These findings agree with those of previous investigators [20] demonstrating that electrolyte abnormalities such as hypocalcemia, hypomagnesaemia, and hypokalemia may be associated with respiratory muscle dysfunction, which could in turn predispose to longer requirement of ventilator support. Further studies to determine the mechanisms underlying these observations are warranted.

## 5. Study Limitations

This study has several strengths including single institution data, which ensures consistency of practice and robustness of the data collection process and the unambiguous, categorical outcome variable. However, there are some limitations to the study. The retrospective, cross-sectional nature of the study design did not dictate standardized care during the study period. Therefore, we cannot ascribe causality to any of the factors such as mortality and length of stay associated with PPMV in the present study. Also, we do not have data on several factors (including graft weight to recipient weight, history of obstructive sleep apnea, postoperative sedation status, postoperative pulmonary complications, and postoperative analgesia method) which could affect postoperative ventilation. However, whatever the final common pathway leading to PMV is, it is an important complication that is attended by significant morbidity and mortality in the pediatric OLT patient. To this end, PPMV may be a useful outcome measure for prognostication and quality improvement initiatives in pediatric liver transplant recipients.

In conclusion, we present the first pediatric data among recipients of OLT, which indicates a high incidence of PPMV among these patients. We also identified factors such as under-five age group, prolonged duration of surgery, and preoperative hypocalcemia as independent predictors of PPMV. Additionally, this article may be the first to describe increased postoperative ICU and hospital LOS following pediatric OLT. This important association has the potential for a multiplicative effect on the total cost associated with pediatric liver transplantation. Specific strategies to reduce the incidence of PPMV in the pediatric OLT patients are highly desirable. Furthermore, mechanisms underlying this important complication deserve further elucidation.

## Conflicts of Interest

The authors declare that there are no conflicts of interest regarding the publication of this paper.

## Acknowledgments

The National Institute of General Medical Sciences (NIGMS) (Grant no. K23 GM104354) supported Dr. Nafiu's work.

## References

[1] G. Neelakanta, M. Sopher, S. Chan et al., "Early tracheal extubation after liver transplantation," *Journal of Cardiothoracic and Vascular Anesthesia*, vol. 11, no. 2, pp. 165–167, 1997.

[2] M. S. Mandell, J. Lockrem, and S. D. Kelley, "Immediate tracheal extubation after liver transplantation: experience of two transplant centers," *Anesthesia and Analgesia*, vol. 84, no. 2, pp. 249–253, 1997.

[3] M. E. O'Meara, S. M. Whiteley, J. M. Sellors et al., "Immediate extubation of children following liver transplantation is safe and may be beneficial," *Transplantation*, vol. 80, no. 7, pp. 959–963, 2005.

[4] P. Zeyneloglu, A. Pirat, M. Guner, A. Torgay, H. Karakayali, and G. Arslan, "Predictors of Immediate Tracheal Extubation in the Operating Room After Liver Transplantation," *Transplantation Proceedings*, vol. 39, no. 4, pp. 1187–1189, 2007.

[5] M. S. Mandell, T. J. Stoner, R. Barnett et al., "A multicenter evaluation of safety of early extubation in liver transplant recipients," *Liver Transplantation*, vol. 13, no. 11, pp. 1557–1563, 2007.

[6] A. J. C. Mittnacht, M. Thanjan, S. Srivastava et al., "Extubation in the operating room after congenital heart surgery in children," *Journal of Thoracic and Cardiovascular Surgery*, vol. 136, no. 1, pp. 88–93, 2008.

[7] K. Stricker, H. U. Rothen, and J. Takala, "Resource use in the ICU: Short- vs. long-term patients," *Acta Anaesthesiologica Scandinavica*, vol. 47, no. 5, pp. 508–515, 2003.

[8] M. Glanemann, J. Langrehr, U. Kaisers et al., "Postoperative tracheal extubation after orthotopic liver transplantation," *Acta Anaesthesiologica Scandinavica*, vol. 45, no. 3, pp. 333–339, 2001.

[9] I. Garutti, J. Sanz, L. Olmedilla et al., "Extravascular Lung Water and Pulmonary Vascular Permeability Index Measured at the End of Surgery Are Independent Predictors of Prolonged Mechanical Ventilation in Patients Undergoing Liver Transplantation," *Anesthesia and Analgesia*, vol. 121, no. 3, pp. 736–745, 2015.

[10] V. Payen, P. Jouvet, J. Lacroix, T. Ducruet, and F. Gauvin, "Risk factors associated with increased length of mechanical ventilation in children," *Pediatric Critical Care Medicine*, vol. 13, no. 2, pp. 152–157, 2012.

[11] D. W. Hosmer, T. Hosmer, S. Le Cessie, and S. Lemeshow, "A comparison of goodness-of-fit tests for the logistic regression model," *Statistics in Medicine*, vol. 16, no. 9, pp. 965–980, 1997.

[12] U. Tannuri and A. C. A. Tannuri, "Postoperative care in pediatric liver transplantation," *Clinics*, vol. 69, no. 1, pp. 42–46, 2014.

[13] A. Echániz, S. Pita, A. Otero, F. Suárez, M. Gómez, and A. Guerrero, "Incidence, risk factors and influence on survival of infectious complications in liver transplantation," *Enfermedades Infecciosas y Microbiologia Clinica*, vol. 21, no. 5, pp. 224–231, 2003.

[14] F. Cislaghi, A. M. Condemi, and A. Corona, "Predictors of prolonged mechanical ventilation in a cohort of 3,269 CABG patients," *Minerva Anestesiologica*, vol. 73, no. 12, pp. 615–621, 2007.

[15] S. N. Prapas, I. A. Panagiotopoulos, A. Hamed Abdelsalam et al., "Predictors of prolonged mechanical ventilation following aorta no-touch off-pump coronary artery bypass surgery," *European Journal of Cardio-thoracic Surgery*, vol. 32, no. 3, pp. 488–492, 2007.

[16] C. Rajakaruna, C. A. Rogers, G. D. Angelini, and R. Ascione, "Risk factors for and economic implications of prolonged ventilation after cardiac surgery," *Journal of Thoracic and Cardiovascular Surgery*, vol. 130, no. 5, pp. 1270–1277, 2005.

[17] R. Ganschow, D. Nolkemper, K. Helmke et al., "Intensive care management after pediatric liver transplantation: a single-center experience," *Pediatric Transplantation*, vol. 4, no. 4, pp. 273–279, 2000.

[18] S. Faenza, M. S. Ravaglia, M. Cimatti, A. Dante, S. Spedicato, and A. M. M. Labate, "Analysis of the causal factors of prolonged mechanical ventilation after orthotopic liver transplant," *Transplantation Proceedings*, vol. 38, no. 4, pp. 1131–1134, 2006.

[19] M. Glanemann, U. Kaisers, J. M. Langrehr et al., "Incidence and indications for reintubation during postoperative care following orthotopic liver transplantation," *Journal of Clinical Anesthesia*, vol. 13, no. 5, pp. 377–382, 2001.

[20] C. Park, D. Kim, J. Choi, and E. Kim, "Intraoperative changes in hyponatremia as a risk factor for prolonged mechanical ventilation after living donor liver transplantation," *Transplantation Proceedings*, vol. 42, no. 9, pp. 3612–3616, 2010.

# 16

# Validation of Simple Methods to Select a Suitable Nostril for Nasotracheal Intubation

**Cattleya Thongrong,[1] Pattramon Thaisiam,[1] and Pornthep Kasemsiri[2]**

[1]*Department of Anesthesiology, Faculty of Medicine, Khon Kaen University, Khon Kaen, Thailand*
[2]*Division of Skull Base Surgery, Department of Otorhinolaryngology, Faculty of Medicine, Khon Kaen University, Khon Kaen, Thailand*

Correspondence should be addressed to Pornthep Kasemsiri; pkcolumbus99@gmail.com

Academic Editor: Davide Cattano

*Background.* Nasotracheal intubation is a blind procedure that may lead to complications; therefore, several tests were introduced to assess a suitable nostril for nasotracheal intubation. However, the value of simple tests in clinical practice was insufficient to evaluate. *Method.* A diagnostic prospective study was conducted in 42 patients, ASA classes I–III, undergoing surgery requiring nasotracheal intubation for general anesthesia. Two simple methods for assessing the patency of nostrils were investigated. Firstly, the occlusion test was evaluated by asking for the patient's own assessment of nasal airflow during occlusion of each contralateral nostril while in a sitting posture. Secondly, patients breathed onto a spatula held 1 cm below the nostrils while in a sitting posture. All patients were assessed using these two simple tests. Nasal endoscopic examination of each patient was used as a gold standard. *Results.* The diagnostic value of the occlusion test (sensitivity of 91.7%, specificity of 61.1%, PPV of 75.9%, NPV of 84.6%, LR+ of 2.36, and LR− of 0.14) seemed better than that of the spatula test (sensitivity of 95.8%, specificity of 25.0%, PPV of 63.0%, NPV of 81.8%, LR+ of 1.28, and LR− of 0.17). When both tests were combined in series, the diagnostic value increased (sensitivity of 87.9%, specificity of 70.8%, PPV of 80.1%, NPV of 81.4%, LR+ of 3.01, and LR− of 0.17). *Conclusion and Recommendations.* The simple occlusion test is more useful than the spatula test. However, combining the results from both tests in series helped to improve the diagnostic value for selecting a suitable nostril for nasotracheal intubation.

## 1. Introduction

Nasotracheal intubation is one of the most common methods for established airway management in patients undergoing surgeries, especially in the head and neck region. However, nasotracheal intubation is a blind procedure that may lead to complications such as epistaxis, avulsion of the middle and inferior turbinate [1–4], and tearing of the nasal septum. Numerous methods have been proposed to reduce these complications. Recommended methods include application of adrenaline [5], use of a smaller tracheal tube, use of a gastric tube or a suction tube for guidance [6, 7], softening the tracheal tube with warm water [8], and redesigning the nasotracheal tube tip [9–12].

Furthermore, the patency of the nostril is a very important factor in reducing injury to nasal passages. Recently, rhinomanometry has been introduced to evaluate the patency of nostrils [13–15]. However, this method is not commonly used in clinical practice because it is not simple and requires special equipment; thus, simpler techniques are preferred. Proposed simple methods include examining the pattern of condensation from expired breath on a spatula [16], inspecting the caudal end of the nasal septum [16], palpating the airflow from each nasal passage [17], and conducting a preanesthetic interview during which the patient is asked which one they perceive to be the clearer nostril [17, 18]. However, the diagnostic value of these simple techniques has not been studied adequately. This study was developed to compare the reliability of simple clinical assessment of the patency of nostrils with results from nasal endoscopic examination.

## 2. Materials and Methods

The Human Research Ethics Committee of Khon Kaen University approved this study protocol (HE601144), and written informed consent was obtained from each patient. All patients undergoing elective surgery and with the requirement of nasotracheal intubation in Srinagarind Hospital, Khon Kaen, Thailand, from July 1, 2017 to December 1, 2017, were enrolled. Patients of either gender aged less than 18 years or more than 75 years were excluded. Also excluded were patients conforming to physical status classification IV (American Society of Anesthesiologists), those with a history of nasal fracture or previous nasal surgery, those with a history of sinusitis or nasal tumor, and those with underlying blood dyscrasia.

We used two simple methods to assess the patency of nostrils. Firstly, the occlusion test, which was administered by asking for the patient's own assessment of nasal airflow during occlusion of the contralateral nostril while in a sitting posture. Nostrils were classified as left or right nostril clearer, or both equally clear. Secondly, patients breathed onto a spatula held 1 cm below the nostrils while in a sitting posture. The patterns of condensation on the spatula were used to determine whether or not one nostril was clearer than the other. If the area of condensation on one side had a diameter of 1 cm greater than that on the other, then that side was regarded as the clearer. These simple methods were assessed by one anesthesiologist. Subsequently, the nostrils were assessed with a 2.7 mm 0-degree nasal endoscope by one otorhinolaryngologist who did not know the previous anesthesiologist's results. The morphology of each nostril was graded in terms of nasal septum deviation (I = deviation 0–24%, II = deviation 25–49%, III = deviation 50–74%, and IV = deviation ≥75%) and inferior hypertrophy (I = nostril occluded by 0–24%, II = nostril occluded by 25–49%, III = nostril occluded by 50–74%, and IV nostril occluded by ≥75%). The standard left-facing bevel nasotracheal tube was prepared with thermo-softening and lubrication before it was inserted into the nostril that was regarded as more patent according to the nasal endoscopic finding. The number of attempts at intubation and severity of epistaxis were recorded.

Qualitative variables are presented as proportions, whereas quantitative variables are expressed as means and standard deviation. The nasal endoscopic examination was considered as the "gold standard" test for determining the patency of the nostril. The diagnostic value of each simple method was calculated using STATA version 10.0. Furthermore, we combined the results of the two simple tests in series and in parallel to see if this would yield improved diagnostic value. Sensitivity and specificity values are given, as well as predictive values and likelihood ratios, all with associated 95% confidence intervals.

## 3. Results

Patient characteristics are shown in Table 1. The majority of patients were undergoing maxillofacial surgery. Most patients had grade I deviation of the nasal septum, especially of the right side (Table 2). Only two patients had grade IV deviation of the nasal septum. Inferior turbinate hypertrophy is another troublesome factor for nasotracheal intubation. Almost half of patients had grade II enlargement of the inferior turbinate. The nasal endoscopic examination guided the choice of nostril for intubation. Nasotracheal intubation was successful on the first attempt for 33 of 42 patients. More than two attempts were required for one patient who presented with grade III hypertrophy of the inferior turbinate on both sides. Epistaxis was observed in 69.05% of cases, with mild bleeding. This epistaxis complication was not statistically significantly different between the right and left nostril ($p$ value > 0.05) (Table 3).

Table 1: Demographic data.

| Characteristics | Number | 95% CI |
|---|---|---|
| *Gender* | | |
| Male (%) | 14 (33.33) | 21.01–48.45 |
| Female (%) | 28 (66.77) | 51.55–78.99 |
| Age (yr, mean) | 47.98 (16.73) | 42.76–53.19 |
| Weight (kg, mean) | 54.81 (11.51) | 51.22–58.40 |
| Height (cm, mean) | 157.81 (7.95) | 155.33–160.29 |
| BMI | 21.90 (3.80) | 20.72–23.08 |
| *ASA class* | | |
| I (%) | 25 (59.52) | 44.49–72.96 |
| II (%) | 17 (40.78) | 27.04–55.51 |
| III (%) | 0 | 0 |
| *Underlying disease* | | |
| Diabetes mellitus | 5 (11.90) | 5.19–25.00 |
| Hypertension | 7 (16.67) | 8.32–30.60 |
| Dyslipidemia | 1 (2.38) | 0.42–12.32 |
| *Operation* | | |
| Endoscopic transoral thyroidectomy | 6 (14.29) | 6.72–27.84 |
| Wide excision with or without soft tissue reconstruction | 13 (30.95) | 19.07–46.03 |
| Maxillofacial surgery | 23 (54.76) | 39.95–68.78 |
| *Attempts at intubation* | | |
| Once | 33 (78.57) | 64.06–88.29 |
| Twice | 8 (19.05) | 9.98–33.30 |
| More than twice | 1 (2.38) | 0.42–12.32 |
| *Severity of epistaxis* | | |
| No bleeding | 13 (30.95) | 19.07–46.03 |
| Minimal bleeding | 29 (69.05) | 53.97–80.93 |

The diagnostic value of the simple tests was investigated (Table 4). The occlusion test seemed appropriate for assessing the suitable nostril for intubation due to its high sensitivity (91.7%) and fair specificity (61.1%). Combining the test results in series provided a better diagnostic value with good stratified sensitivity (87.9%) and higher specificity (70.8%).

## 4. Discussion

Assessment of nostrils before nasotracheal intubation is very important to reduce subsequent complications. Although rhinomanometry and endoscopy are more reliable than simple methods, they are not convenient for use in common practice. Simple methods are preferable to guide the choice of nostril to intubate. Smith and Reid [17] studied the accuracy of palpating the passage of air and asking for the patient's own assessment of nasal airflow. They used nasal endoscopic examination as the gold standard. They reported no significant difference between the overall diagnostic success rates of the two tests (44% and 47%, resp.).

Table 2: Nasal endoscopic finding.

| Nasal endoscopic finding: deviated nasal septum | Right nostril (%) | Left nostril (%) |
|---|---|---|
| Grade I: 0–24% | 29 (69.05) (95% CI: 53.97–80.93) | 19 (45.24) (95% CI: 31.22–60.05) |
| Grade II: 25–49% | 8 (19.05) (95% CI: 9.98–33.30) | 9 (21.43) (95% CI: 11.71–35.94) |
| Grade III: 50–74% | 4 (9.52) (95% CI: 3.77–22.07) | 13 (30.95) (95% CI: 19.07–46.03) |
| Grade IV: ≥75% | 1 (2.38) (95% CI: 0.42–12.32) | 1 (2.38) (95% CI: 0.42–12.32) |
| *Inferior turbinate hypertrophy* | | |
| Grade I: 0–24%; | 4 (9.52) (95% CI: 3.77–22.07) | 5 (11.90) (95% CI: 5.19–25.00) |
| Grade II: 25–49% | 20 (47.62) (95% CI: 33.36–62.28) | 28 (66.67) (95% CI: 51.55–78.99) |
| Grade III: 50–74% | 16 (38.10) (95% CI: 25.00–53.19) | 8 (19.05) (95% CI: 9.98–33.30) |
| Grade IV: ≥75% | 2 (4.76) (95% CI: 1.32–15.79) | 1 (2.38) (95% CI: 0.42–12.32) |

Table 3: Comparison of epistaxis complication between right and left nasotracheal intubation.

| Nasal endoscopic finding | Number | Side | Nasotracheal intubation: One attempt | | Two attempts | | More than two attempts | |
|---|---|---|---|---|---|---|---|---|
| | | | No bleeding | Minimal bleeding | No b leeding | Minimal bleeding | No bleeding | Minimal bleeding |
| More patent on the right side | 22 | Right | 5 (22.7)[†] (95% CI: 10.1–43.4) | 13 (59.1)[†] (95% CI: 38.7–76.7) | 0 | 4 (18.18)[††] (95% CI: 7.3–38.5) | 0 | 0 |
| Equal patent on both sides | 6 | Right | 3 (50.0)[†] (95% CI: 18.8–81.2) | 2 (33.3)[†] (95% CI: 9.7–70.0) | 0 | 0 | 0 | 0 |
| | | Left | 0 | 0 | 0 | 0 | 0 | 1 (16.7)[††] (95% CI: 0.3–56.4) |
| More patent on the left side | 14 | Left | 5 (35.7)[†] (95% CI: 16.3–61.2) | 5 (35.7)[†] (95% CI: 16.3–61.2) | 0 | 4 (28.6)[††] (95% CI: 11.7–54.7) | 0 | 0 |

[†]No statistically significant difference of no epistaxis event ($p = 0.84$) and minimal epistaxis ($p = 0.15$) between both nostrils at one attempt of intubation. [††]No statistically significant difference of minimal epistaxis between both nostrils at two attempts of intubation ($p = 0.34$) and more than two attempts of intubation ($p = 0.16$).

Table 4: Diagnostic value of the occlusion test, spatula test, and two tests combined (series test and parallel test).

| | Sensitivity | Specificity | Predictive value: Positive | Predictive value: Negative | Likelihood ratio: Positive | Likelihood ratio: Negative |
|---|---|---|---|---|---|---|
| Occlusion test | 91.7 (95% CI: 80.0–97.7) | 61.1 (95% CI: 43.5–76.9) | 75.9 (95% CI: 62.8–86.1) | 84.6 (95% CI: 65.1–95.6) | 2.36 (95% CI: 1.55–3.58) | 0.14 (95% CI: 0.05–0.36) |
| Spatula test | 95.8 (95% CI: 85.7–99.5) | 25.0 (95% CI: 12.1–42.2) | 63.0 (95% CI: 50.9–74.0) | 81.8 (95% CI: 48.2–97.7) | 1.28 (95% CI: 1.05–1.56) | 0.17 (95% CI: 0.04–0.73) |
| Series test | 87.9 (95% CI: 78.6–97.1) | 70.8 (95% CI: 56.0–85.7) | 80.1 (95% CI: 68.1–92) | 81.4 (95% CI: 69.5–93.3) | 3.01 (95% CI: 1.82–4.99) | 0.17 (95% CI: 0.08–0.38) |
| Parallel test | 99.7 (95% CI: 98.0–100) | 15.3 (95% CI: 3.5–27.0) | 61.1 (95% CI: 50.2–71.9) | 97.0 (95% CI: 83.5–100) | 1.18 (95% CI: 1.02–1.36) | NA |

Unfortunately, they found the tests had a diagnostic failure rate of approximately 45% when an abnormal nostril was present. Thus, they recommended that anesthesiologists should not rely on the two tests investigated. However, we reassessed the patient's own opinion of nasal airflow method. Its sensitivity was 91.7%, specificity was 61.1%, positive predictive value was 75.9, and positive likelihood ratio was 2.36.

For improved diagnostic value, the occlusion test was combined with the spatula test because it was a simple method with high sensitivity (95.8%). We investigated the diagnostic value of combining the results from the two tests in series and in parallel. When in series, both tests must be positive for an overall positive result to be accepted. Tests in series yielded a lower overall sensitivity than either alone, but the overall specificity was greater than for either alone. On the other hand, when in parallel, a positive result in either test should be taken as an overall positive result. Parallel interpretation of tests yielded greater overall sensitivity than either alone, but the overall specificity was less than for either alone. Therefore, the series approach was regarded as better than the parallel approach. In series, the tests provided a sensitivity of 87.9%, specificity of 70.8%, positive predictive value of 80.1, and positive likelihood ratio of 3.01. We therefore recommend use of results from both tests in series for guiding selection of the suitable nostril for nasotracheal intubation.

There have been several reports concerning selection of a nostril for nasotracheal intubation. In a randomized controlled trial, Boku et al. [18] found that nasal intubation via the right nostril produced less bleeding than did using the left nostril ($p = 0.0006$). These outcomes were similar to the study of Sanuki et al. [19], who reported that epistaxis during nasotracheal intubation was more frequent and severe when the left nostril was used. Nonetheless, Coe and Human [20] had demonstrated similar frequencies of epistaxis in both nostrils. This result was similar with our study. We found no statistically significant different epistaxis between both nostrils ($p > 0.05$) although we used the standard left-facing beveled nasotracheal tube. We gently inserted the well-lubricated nasotracheal tube with bevel of the tube against nasal septum or floor of nose for reduced injury to inferior turbinate. However, our small sample size was limited to indicate difference in this aspect. Furthermore, the dominant hand nature of the anesthesiologist is the other factor that may affect epistaxis complication from nasotracheal intubation. Usually, an anesthesiologist uses the dominant hand for the insertion tube; therefore, right-handed nature may prefer right nostril, whereas left-handed nature may prefer left nostril. We concern that the left-facing bevel of the tube may cause injury to inferior turbinate when introducing the tube through the left nostril due to the bevel of the tube against the turbinate. On the other hand, the bevel of the tube against the nasal septum when using the right nostril. It may help to reduce the chance of epistaxis on the right side. However, nasotracheal intubation on the left nostril is not a big deal. We recommend introducing the tube with some rotation to present the bevel against the floor of nose for avoiding injury to inferior turbinate. After the tip of the tube had been passed from the end of inferior turbinate to choana, the tube was rotated into the normal position for passing through the pharynx.

Accordingly, nasotracheal intubation is a blind procedure. The nasal examination will lead to a better understanding of the patency of each nostril and lead to reduction in complications. We urge anesthetists to assess the state of each nostril prior to intubation of their patients.

## 5. Conclusion

The simple occlusion test was better than the spatula test in guiding the choice of nostril for intubation. However, the combination of results from both tests in series provided the most reliable guidance.

## Conflicts of Interest

The authors declare that they have no conflicts of interest.


## Acknowledgments

The authors would like to acknowledge Professor David Blair for editing the manuscript via the Publication Clinic KKU, Thailand.


## References


[1] F. L. Scamman and R. W. Babin, "An unusual complication of nasotracheal intubation," *Anesthesiology*, vol. 59, no. 4, pp. 352-353, 1983.

[2] J. A. Wilkinson, R. D. Mathis, and D. J. Dire, "Turbinate destruction: a rare complication of nasotracheal intubation," *Journal of Emergency Medicine*, vol. 4, no. 3, pp. 209–212, 1986.

[3] R. Cooper, "Bloodless turbinectomy following blind nasal intubation," *Anesthesiology*, vol. 71, no. 3, p. 469, 1989.

[4] M. J. Kuo, A. P. Reid, and J. E. Smith, "Unilateral nasal obstruction: an unusual presentation of a complication of nasotracheal intubation," *Journal of Laryngology and Otology*, vol. 108, no. 11, pp. 991-992, 1994.

[5] K. Kameyama, S. Watanabe, T. Kano, and J. Kusukawa, "Effects of nasal application of an epinephrine and lidocaine mixture on the hemodynamics and nasal mucosa in oral and maxillofacial surgery," *Journal of Oral and Maxillofacial Surgery*, vol. 66, no. 11, pp. 2226–2232, 2008.

[6] Y. Morimoto, M. Sugimura, Y. Hirose, K. Taki, and H. Niwa, "Nasotracheal intubation under curve-tipped suction catheter guidance reduces epistaxis," *Canadian Journal of Anaesthesia*, vol. 53, no. 3, pp. 295–298, 2006.

[7] T. Elwood, D. M. Stillions, D. W. Woo, H. M. Bradford, and C. Ramamoorthy, "Nasotracheal intubation. A randomized trial of two methods," *Anesthesiology*, vol. 96, no. 1, pp. 51–53, 2002.

[8] Y. C. Kim, S. H. Lee, G. J. Noh et al., "Thermosoftening treatment of the nasotracheal tube before intubation can reduce epistaxis and nasal damage," *Anesthesia and Analgesia*, vol. 91, no. 3, pp. 698–701, 2000.

[9] S. Prior, J. Heaton, K. R. Jatana, and R. G. Rashid, "Parker flex-tip and standard-tip endotracheal tubes: a comparison during nasotracheal intubation," *Anesthesia Progress*, vol. 57, no. 1, pp. 18–24, 2010.
[10] J. H. Lee, C. H. Kim, J. H. Bahk, and K. S. Park, "The influence of endotracheal tube tip design on nasal trauma during nasotracheal intubation: magill-tip versus murphy-tip," *Anesthesia and Analgesia*, vol. 101, no. 4, pp. 1226–1229, 2005.
[11] K. Mizutani and N. Uno, "Another reason for easier right nasal intubation than for left nasal intubation," *Journal of Clinical Anesthesia*, vol. 27, no. 2, p. 181, 2015.
[12] M. J. Bucx, "A left bevelled tube is easier inserted from the right side," *Journal of Clinical Anesthesia*, vol. 27, no. 6, p. 531, 2015.
[13] K. Shohara, T. Goto, G. Kuwahara, Y. Isakari, T. Moriya, and T. Yamamuro, "Validity of rhinometry in measuring nasal patency for nasotracheal intubation," *Journal of Anesthesia*, vol. 31, no. 1, pp. 1–4, 2017.
[14] H. S. Lim, D. Kim, J. Lee, J. S. Son, J. R. Lee, and S. Ko, "Reliability of assessment of nasal flow rate for nostril selection during nasotracheal intubation," *Journal of Clinical Anesthesia*, vol. 24, no. 4, pp. 270–274, 2012.
[15] S. Sabour and E. V. Dastjerdi, "Reliability of assessment of nasal flow rate for nostril selection during nasotracheal intubation: common mistakes in reliability analysis," *Journal of Clinical Anesthesia*, vol. 25, no. 2, p. 162, 2013.
[16] R. Kayarkar, T. J. Woolford, and G. A. Francis, "Simple preoperative assessment to reduce the risk of traumatic epistaxis during nasotracheal intubation," *European Journal of Anaesthesiology*, vol. 19, no. 9, pp. 690-691, 2002.
[17] J. E. Smith and A. P. Reid, "Identifying the more patent nostril before nasotracheal intubation," *Anaesthesia*, vol. 56, no. 3, pp. 258–262, 2001.
[18] A. Boku, H. Hanamoto, Y. Hirose et al., "Which nostril should be used for nasotracheal intubation: the right or left? A randomized clinical trial," *Journal of Clinical Anesthesia*, vol. 26, no. 5, pp. 390–394, 2014.
[19] T. Sanuki, M. Hirokane, and J. Katoni, "Epistaxis during nasotracheal intubation: a comparison of nostril sides," *Journal of Oral and Maxillofacial Surgery*, vol. 68, no. 3, pp. 618–621, 2010.
[20] T. R. Coe and M. Human, "The peri-operative complications of nasal intubation: a comparison of nostril side," *Anesthesia*, vol. 56, no. 5, pp. 447–450, 2001.

# Analgesic Effects of Preincision Ketamine on Postspinal Caesarean Delivery in Uganda's Tertiary Hospital

**Richard Mwase,[1] Tonny Stone Luggya,[2] John Mark Kasumba,[3] Humphrey Wanzira,[4] Andrew Kintu,[2] Joesph V. B. Tindimwebwa,[2] and Daniel Obua[2]**

[1]*Uganda People's Defense Forces Directorate of Medical Services, Bombo Military Hospital, Bombo, Uganda*
[2]*Department of Anesthesia, College of Health Sciences, Makerere University, Kampala, Uganda*
[3]*Directorate of Surgical Services, Mulago Hospital, Kampala, Uganda*
[4]*Ministry of Health, Kampala, Uganda*

Correspondence should be addressed to Tonny Stone Luggya; tluggya@gmail.com

Academic Editor: Audun Stubhaug

*Background.* Good postoperative analgesic management improves maternal satisfaction and care of the neonate. Postoperative pain management is a challenge in Mulago Hospital, yet ketamine is accessible and has proven benefit. We determined ketamine's postoperative analgesic effects. *Materials and Methods.* We did an RCT among consenting parturients that were randomized to receive either intravenous ketamine (0.25 mg/kg) or placebo after spinal anesthetic. Pain was assessed every 30 mins up to 24 hours postoperatively using the numerical rating scale. The first complaint of pain requiring treatment was noted as "time to first breakthrough pain." *Results.* We screened 100 patients and recruited 88 that were randomized into two arms of 44 patients that received either ketamine or placebo. Ketamine group had 30-minute longer time to first breakthrough pain and lower 24-hour pain scores. Postoperative diclofenac consumption was lesser in the ketamine group compared to placebo and Kaplan-Meier graphs showed a higher probability of experiencing breakthrough pain earlier in the placebo group. *Conclusion.* Preincision intravenous ketamine (0.25 mg/kg) offered 30-minute prolongation to postoperative analgesia requirement with reduced 24-hour pain scores. We recommend larger studies to explore this benefit. This trial is registered with Pan African Clinical Trial Registry number PACTR201404000807178.

## 1. Introduction

Pain is a subjective and multidimensional experience often inadequately managed in medical practice [1], with a USA survey reporting a 50–70% likelihood of experiencing moderate to severe postoperative pain due to inadequate pain management [2]. Good postoperative pain control improves maternal satisfaction and baby care, decreases morbidity [3, 4], and is desired to increase mobility which reduces the incidence of deep vein thrombosis [5]. In a low resource setting like Uganda, the National Referral and Teaching Hospital, Mulago, (MNRTH) faces profound challenges, for example, overwhelming patient numbers and anecdotal clinical staff shortages with a nurse: patient ratio of 1:40 [6]. Only forty-five percent (45%) of anesthesia providers have full-time access to pethidine or morphine while twenty-one percent (21%) have no complete access to these drugs [7].

Ketamine is an N-methyl-D-aspartate (NMDA) receptor antagonist that produces analgesia by desensitization of sensitized NMDA receptors, thereby inhibiting pain transmission in the CNS [8, 9]. In subanesthetic doses, it has been shown to reduce first 24 hours analgesic requirements after surgery with decreased postoperative opioid requirements in elective Caesarean section patients [10, 11]. Also for chronic pain it is a "third line" treatment where conventional treatments have failed [12]. Ketamine is safe for use in late pregnancy and for neonates and studies done in Africa have shown that it reduced morphine requirement after delivery among parturients [13]. It was recently cleared for use in brain injury patients based on its stable hemodynamic profile and beneficial bronchodilating respiratory properties, which has led to increased clinical use especially in severe asthma treatment [14].

We hypothesized that nonsedating dose of 0.25 mg/kg of preincision ketamine would prolong the time to pain requiring treatment, based on ketamine's beneficial properties above and especially since studies showed its benefit as an adjuvant for postoperative analgesia in low-dose regimens ranges of 0.25–0.5 mg/kg [15]. We chose a randomized prospective controlled trial setting to study the twenty-four-hour (24-hour) postoperative analgesia effects when administered at preincision for elective Caesarean delivery performed under spinal anesthesia.

## 2. Materials and Methods

This study was approved by the Makerere University, School of Medicine Research and Ethics Committee (SOMREC), and was registered to the Pan African Clinical Trial Registry with identifier number PACTR201404000807178. This was a prospective, randomized, double-blind, placebo-controlled trial conducted from January to March 2014 at MNRTH, which is a 1500-bed capacity that receives on average 48,000 patients annually at its Accident and Emergency (A&E). The labor suit conducts 32,000 deliveries annually with Caesarean sections accounting for 15–20% [16].

Eligible patients due for elective Caesarean section under spinal anesthesia were taken through consent process and enrolled after getting written consent. Our inclusion criteria included parturients scheduled for elective Caesarean section with American Society of Anesthesiologists (ASA) physical statuses I and II. Exclusion criteria were patients with hypertension, hypersensitivity to ketamine or its preservatives, ASA class > II, psychiatric disease, those who received chronic opioid therapy, and also those who required conversion from spinal to general anesthesia.

Sample size was calculated based on a power of 80% and standard deviation of 25 from study by Menkiti et al. [17] who used a ketamine dose of 0.15 mg/kg and noticed lower postoperative pain scores in the ketamine group, with the minimum expected difference ($D$) between the two means ($\mu_1 - \mu_2$), at 120 minutes. This gave us a total patient estimate ($N$) of eighty-eight (88) patients with forty-four (44) in each arm of the study.

*2.1. Randomization and Concealment.* Block randomization with a block of 4 was used to randomly assign participants to receive either ketamine or placebo in equal numbers for the two groups. A computer program was used to generate the randomization sequence by an independent statistician.

The ketamine group received intravenous ketamine (0.25 mg/kg) and the placebo group received normal saline and blinding for both participants and study investigators was achieved by use of 10 mL syringes of similar appearance and consistency. The placebo was 10 mL of normal saline while ketamine was diluted to make 10 mL of 5 mg/mL solution. All syringes had 5 mg/mL colorless solution that catered for a lowest possible adult weight of 40 kg and a highest weight being 200 kg.

*Concealment.* Concealment was achieved by making sure that each syringe was labelled according to sequence-generated codes earlier presented as a list of sequential random treatment codes. The labelled syringes were brought in an opaque carrier envelope to the operating theatre and handed to the principle investigator every morning in the presence of a theatre nurse and study investigator. At the theatre receiving area a syringe was retrieved with its sticker code number, similar to computer generated number sequence, becoming the patients study number and then patient was weighed before transportation to the operating theatre (OR).

*2.2. Study Procedures.* Patient was weighed in the OR and received standard spinal anesthetic 2 mL of 0.5% heavy bupivacaine with 8% dextrose and 20 mcg of fentanyl and then placed supine with a left lateral tilt to achieve a sensory block height of T6 before surgery. Oxygen at 3 L/min was administered by nasal prongs to all patients. Immediately before surgical incision, the study drugs were administered as per randomized allocation of 0.05 mL/kg of study-drug or placebo as described above, followed by prophylactic intravenous antibiotics. Postoperative pain was assessed using the self-reporting numeric rating scale (NRS) with a rating of the lowest 0 = no pain, 10 = worst pain, 1–3 = mild pain, 4–6 = moderate pain, and 7–10 = severe pain. This was monitored every 30 mins for 24 hours or until first complaint of pain called the "time to first breakthrough pain" which was considered to be the pain requiring treatment (NRS ≥ 3). At this point rescue analgesic was administered firstly by intramuscular diclofenac (75 mg), then standard of care treatment, and then tramadol as secondary or meperidine/pethidine (100 mg) as tertiary for persistent pain.

*2.3. Data Management.* Interviewer-administered and pretested questionnaires were used for data collection. The data was cleaned, coded, and double-entered into Epidata version 3.1 and then exported and analyzed with STATA® Version 12 (Statacorp LP). The participants characteristics were presented as means and accompanying standard deviation for weight (kg), height (cm), and duration of surgery (in minutes) while median with range was estimated for age (in years) and parity as these were discreet variables. The differences in median (range) between those randomized to receive ketamine and those on placebo were assessed using a Wilcoxon rank sum test, while a $t$-test was used to test for the mean differences among the continuous variables. Survival analysis using the Kaplan-Meier survival curves was used to determine the probability of breakthrough pain between the two randomization arms with accompanying log-rank test to estimate the $p$ value. In analysis, a $p$ value of $\leq 0.05$ was considered statistically significant.

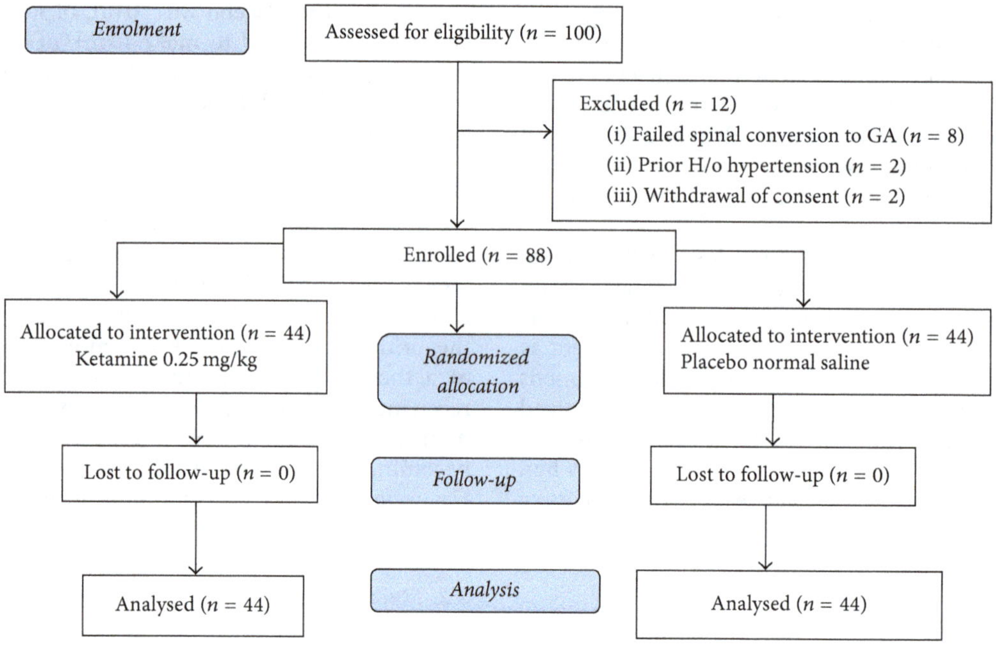


FIGURE 1: Flow chart and numerical scale.

TABLE 1: Patients' demographics.

| Variable | Overall | Randomization group | | $p$ value |
|---|---|---|---|---|
| | | Ketamine | Placebo | |
| Median age in years (range) | 29 (14–44) | 28 (14–44) | 29 (18–41) | 0.76 |
| Median parity (range) | 4 (1–9) | 4 (1–9) | 4 (1–7) | 0.55 |
| Mean weight in Kg (SD) | 67 (10.91) | 67 (10.96) | 67 (10.97) | 0.78 |
| Mean height in cm (SD) | 160 (5.85) | 160 (5.52) | 160 (6.22) | 0.94 |
| Mean duration of operation in minutes (SD) | 40 (12.73) | 40 (13.51) | 39 (12.03) | 0.72 |

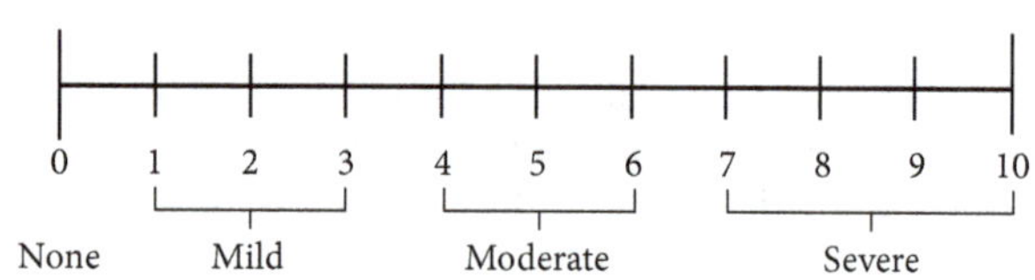


FIGURE 2: Numeric rating scale (NRS).

## 3. Results

*3.1. Baseline Characteristics.* We screened 100 participants for this study and 12 were excluded while 88 parturients were enrolled with 44 assigned to one of the two groups (Figure 1). Overall, the median (range) age was 29 (14–44) years, with a median (range) parity of 4 (1–9) as shown in Table 1. The average (standard deviation) weight and height of enrolled mothers were 67 kg (10.91) and 160 cm (5.85), respectively. On average each operation took 40 minutes (12.75) with baseline maternal demographics equally distributed in both arms. NRS scale (Figure 2) was used to assess patients pain.

*3.2. Breakthrough Pain.* The median (range) time (in minutes) to first "breakthrough pain" among both groups was significantly longer in the ketamine group [210 (90–270)] when compared to those that received placebo [180 (90–360)] with $p = 0.002$. The 24-hour median (range) NRS pain scores were higher and significant in the placebo group [5 (3–7)] compared to the ketamine group [7 (3–9)] ($p = 0.001$) (Table 2). Primary rescue analgesia dose of diclofenac was lower in the ketamine group [used up to 75 mg] in comparison to the placebo [used up to 150 mg] ($p$ value = 0.053). Secondary rescue analgesia with tramadol was equaled in both arms and therefore not statistically significant as shown in Figure 2 and Table 2. Eight patients (5-placebo and 3-ketamine) required a tertiary dose of pethidine (100 mg) due to persistent pain (Figure 3). At delivery all neonates scored APGAR 10 at 5 and 10 minutes while at study termination all mothers and newborns were in good general condition with stable vitals.

*3.2.1. Kaplan-Meier Survival Graph.* The probability of experiencing earlier breakthrough pain is significantly higher among those receiving placebo as compared to those who received ketamine with a log-rank test $p = 0.011$ (Figure 4). This showed ketamine significantly delayed the onset of breakthrough pain as compared to those who received placebo.

TABLE 2: Showing primary and secondary outcomes.

| Outcome | Randomization group<br>Ketamine<br>Median (range) | <br>Placebo<br>Median (range) | $p$ value |
|---|---|---|---|
| Time to breakthrough pain (minutes) | 210 (90–270) | 180 (90–360) | 0.002 |
| NRS at first breakthrough pain | 5 (3–7) | 7 (3–9) | 0.001 |
| Diclofenac used (mg) | 75 (75–150) | 150 (75–150) | 0.05 |
| Tramadol used (mg) | 100 (100–200) | 100 (100–200) | 0.75 |

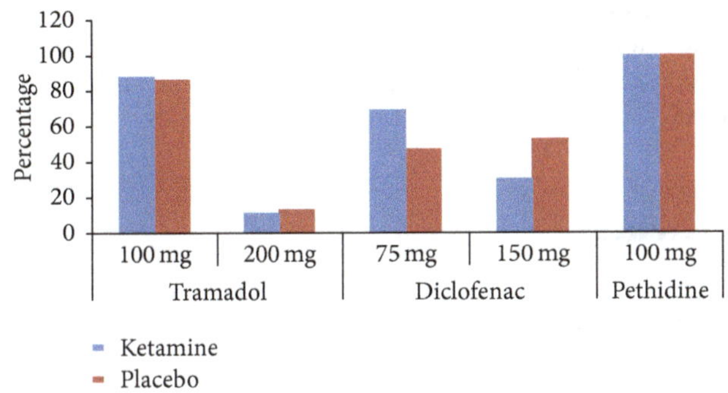


FIGURE 3: Graph showing postoperative analgesic drugs.

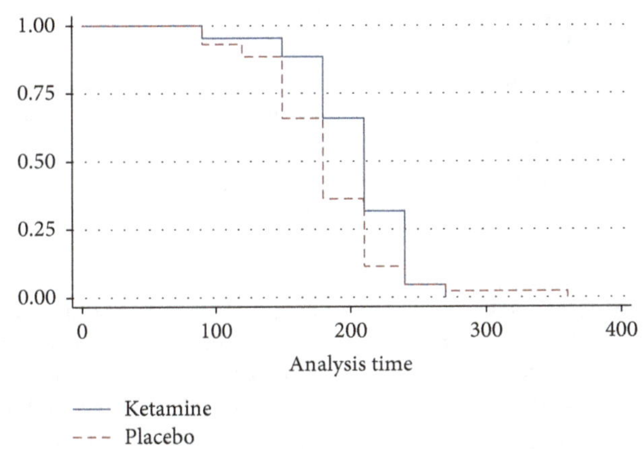


FIGURE 4: Kaplan-Meier survival curve. Ketamine versus placebo Kaplan-Meier survival estimates for breakthrough pain.

## 4. Discussion

We set out to determine the effects of low-dose ketamine on postoperative course when given intravenously at preincision after spinal anesthetic for Caesarean section delivery. Our study showed that preincision IV ketamine 0.25 mg/kg prolonged first requirement of pain treatment by 30 minutes with our ketamine group showing lower pain scores at 24 hours and also, albeit not statistically significant, had reduced cumulative analgesic administration. This showed promise for ketamine's postoperative clinical benefit especially in our resource limited setting. The first day after Caesarean delivery is crucial for maternal-child bonding and early initiation of breast feeding and a good long postoperative pain window allows clinicians to start other analgesic drugs before the anticipated onset of postoperative pain [17]. Our study findings are similar to clinical setting studies on ketamine that showed 10–30-minute prolongation breakthrough pain after outpatient knee arthroscopy [18].

Ketamine was chosen because it is a readily available drug in our setting and its multiple beneficial properties especially its NMDA blockade aid in postoperative analgesia based on the hypothesis that preemptive analgesia prevents induction of central sensitization by pain inputs [19]. Surgical tissue damage causes central pain pathway sensitization by glutamate release that is manifested clinically as heightened pain sensation, due to activation of postsynaptic NMDA receptors in the spinal cord [20]. Also NMDA receptors found both pre- and postsynaptically at pain fiber terminations in the dorsal horn contribute to "wind-up," central sensitization plus long-term potentiation (LTP), all of which may contribute to initiation of abnormal pain; hence NMDA antagonists may prevent induction of central sensitization and diminish hypersensitivity [19]. Studies from West Indies showed ketamine reduced postoperative opioid requirement with coupled improved patient satisfaction [21]; however our study did not capture this as our local postoperative standard of care at study time was diclofenac followed by tramadol secondarily and then pethidine/meperidine as tertiary options for "persistent" pain. Ketamine in subanesthetic doses offered persistent analgesia on awakening because of its two main active metabolites and its elimination half-life of 180 minutes with analgesia [22]; we therefore postulated that ketamine be used for analgesia since studies have shown, other than the intravenous route, its efficacy after intramuscular and oral administration [23, 24]. Also its formulation is stable at room temperature with no need of special storage conditions and produces general anaesthesia within 30–60 seconds that lasts 10 to 15 minutes with ability to use repeated 1–3 mg/min boluses for maintenance which has made it easy to use in emergency prehospital care [25].

This obstetrics study was a pioneer ketamine RCT in MNRTH to show ketamine's potential as a postoperative adjunct to analgesia and was undertaken because globally postoperative pain remains an issue even in first world systems despite wide knowledge, new analgesics, and delivery techniques [2].

Our findings of 30-minute extension to time to breakthrough pain could in part be because we considered the lower threshold cutoff for pain as 3 on numerical scale unlike similar studies that used a higher threshold at the moderate pain level (4 for NRS and <2 for VAS) as a point of intervention [18], or because we gave it at preincision rather than at end of surgery hence observing a "shortened" time to next analgesic. We thus recommend more ketamine studies addressing and incorporating our perceived shortcomings that affected this study's time variable. However clinically in this study, ketamine was tolerated well among women and neonates with insignificant adverse effects and had similar outcomes to other studies [21].

*4.1. Study Limitations.* Limitations of this study are the following: low powered study unable to give statistically significant finings, inability to draw a solid conclusion for maternal and neonatal safety without monitoring ketamine serum levels as liquid chromatography- (LC-) tandem mass spectrometry for its metabolites were not available and would have been a steep cost for self-funded research, and failure to capture ketamine's long-term effects, preferably in postnatal clinic at 6 weeks as per MNRTH protocol, because we premised it on the subanesthetic dose used and study terminated at 48 hours postoperatively.

## 5. Conclusion

For Caesarean delivery Mulago, preincision intravenous ketamine (0.25 mg/kg) given after spinal anesthetic had a good safety profile and gave 30-minute prolongation to postoperative analgesia requirement with reduced 24 hr pain scores and findings are generalizable as biological interventions are usually similar across populations. However we recommend larger studies to further explore ketamine benefits and get the right dose estimate for prolongation of postoperative pain.

## Abbreviations

MNRTH: Mulago National Referral and Teaching Hospital
NMDA: N-Methyl-D-aspartate
ASA: American Society of Anesthesiologists
NRS: Numeric rating scale.

## Competing Interests

The authors declare that they have no competing interests either financial or nonfinancial.

## Authors' Contributions

Dr. Mwase hand in hand with his supervisors developed this idea from conceptualization to final proposal and then primarily assisted in data collection and trained research assistants. Dr. Tonny Stone Luggya, Daniel Obua, and John Mark Kasumba supervised proposal development and oversaw study design, data analysis, and results review through to dissertation completion. Dr. Joesph V. B. Tindimwebwa and Andrew Kintu helped with final thesis and manuscript review to improve its quality, and Dr. Humphrey Wanzira helped with the statistical analysis through to finalization.

## Acknowledgments

The authors acknowledge all the colleagues at the Department of Anesthesia at Makerere University and the tireless and dedicated staff of Mulago National Referral Hospitals Labor Suite and Obstetrics Department. They, moreover, extend their sincere thanks to their partners in education, that is, Association of Anesthesiologists of Great Britain and Ireland (AAGBI) and Global Partners of Anesthesia and Surgery (GPAS).

## References

[1] H. Y. V. Ip, A. Abrishami, P. W. H. Peng, J. Wong, and F. Chung, "Predictors of postoperative pain and analgesic consumption: a qualitative systematic review," *Anesthesiology*, vol. 111, no. 3, pp. 657–677, 2009.

[2] J. L. Apfelbaum, C. Chen, S. S. Mehta, and T. J. Gan, "Postoperative pain experience: results from a national survey suggest postoperative pain continues to be undermanaged," *Anesthesia and Analgesia*, vol. 97, no. 2, pp. 534–540, 2003.

[3] C. Miaskowski, "Patient-controlled modalities for acute postoperative pain management," *Journal of Perianesthesia Nursing*, vol. 20, no. 4, pp. 255–267, 2005.

[4] L. Niemi-Murola, R. Pöyhiä, K. Onkinen, B. Rhen, A. Mäkelä, and T. T. Niemi, "Patient satisfaction with postoperative pain management—effect of preoperative factors," *Pain Management Nursing*, vol. 8, no. 3, pp. 122–129, 2007.

[5] N. P. Yost, S. L. Bloom, M. K. Sibley, J. Y. Lo, D. D. McIntire, and K. J. Leveno, "A hospital-sponsored quality improvement study of pain management after cesarean delivery," *American Journal of Obstetrics and Gynecology*, vol. 190, no. 5, pp. 1341–1346, 2004.

[6] D. Ozgediz, M. Galukande, J. Mabweijano et al., "The neglect of the global surgical workforce: experience and evidence from Uganda," *World Journal of Surgery*, vol. 32, no. 6, pp. 1208–1215, 2008.

[7] S. C. Hodges, C. Mijumbi, M. Okello, B. A. Mccormick, I. A. Walker, and I. H. Wilson, "Anaesthesia services in developing countries: defining the problems," *Anaesthesia*, vol. 62, no. 1, pp. 4–11, 2007.

[8] P. Paoletti and J. Neyton, "NMDA receptor subunits: function and pharmacology," *Current Opinion in Pharmacology*, vol. 7, no. 1, pp. 39–47, 2007.

[9] M. Niesters, A. Dahan, M. Swartjes et al., "Effect of ketamine on endogenous pain modulation in healthy volunteers," *Pain*, vol. 152, no. 3, pp. 656–663, 2011.

[10] R. F. Bell, J. B. Dahl, R. A. Moore, and E. Kalso, "Perioperative ketamine for acute postoperative pain," *Cochrane Database of Systematic Reviews*, 2006.

[11] M. Haliloglu, M. Ozdemir, N. Uzture, P. O. Cenksoy, and N. Bakan, "Perioperative low-dose ketamine improves postoperative analgesia following Cesarean delivery with general anesthesia," *Journal of Maternal-Fetal and Neonatal Medicine*, vol. 29, no. 6, pp. 962–966, 2016.

[12] G. Hocking and M. J. Cousins, "Ketamine in chronic pain management: an evidence-based review," *Anesthesia and Analgesia*, vol. 97, no. 6, pp. 1730–1739, 2003.

[13] P. Kashefi, "The benefits of intraoperative small-dose ketamine on postoperative pain after cesarean section," *Anesthesiology*, vol. 104, no. 27, 2006.

[14] F. Aroni, N. Iacovidou, I. Dontas, C. Pourzitaki, and T. Xanthos, "Pharmacological aspects and potential new clinical applications of ketamine: reevaluation of an old drug," *Journal of Clinical Pharmacology*, vol. 49, no. 8, pp. 957–964, 2009.

[15] M. Berti, M. Baciarello, R. Troglio, and G. Fanelli, "Clinical uses of low-dose ketamine in patients undergoing surgery," *Current Drug Targets*, vol. 10, no. 8, pp. 707–715, 2009.

[16] Africa Business Pages, "Health and beauty category: Mulago hospital," http://directory.africa-business.com/business/496bd3238f/Mulago-Hospital.

[17] I. D. Menkiti, I. Desalu, and O. T. Kushimo, "Low-dose intravenous ketamine improves postoperative analgesia after caesarean delivery with spinal bupivacaine in African parturients," *International Journal of Obstetric Anesthesia*, vol. 21, no. 3, pp. 217–221, 2012.

[18] C. Menigaux, B. Guignard, D. Fletcher, D. I. Sessler, X. Dupont, and M. Chauvin, "Intraoperative small-dose ketamine enhances analgesia after outpatient knee arthroscopy," *Anesthesia and Analgesia*, vol. 93, no. 3, pp. 606–612, 2001.

[19] H. Xie, X. Wang, G. Liu, and G. Wang, "Analgesic effects and pharmacokinetics of a low dose of ketamine preoperatively administered epidurally or intravenously," *Clinical Journal of Pain*, vol. 19, no. 5, pp. 317–322, 2003.

[20] B. A. Orser, P. S. Pennefather, and J. F. MacDonald, "Multiple mechanisms of ketamine blockade of N-methyl-D-aspartate receptors," *Anesthesiology*, vol. 86, no. 4, pp. 903–917, 1997.

[21] M. Thomas, I. Tennant, R. Augier, G. Gordon-Strachan, and H. Harding, "The role of pre-induction ketamine in the management of postoperative pain in patients undergoing elective gynaecological surgery at the University Hospital of the West Indies," *West Indian Medical Journal*, vol. 61, no. 3, pp. 224–229, 2012.

[22] F. Camu and C. Vanlersberghe, "Pharmacology of systemic analgesics," *Best Practice & Research Clinical Anaesthesiology*, vol. 16, no. 4, pp. 475–488, 2002.

[23] I. S. Grant, W. S. Nimmo, L. R. Mcnicol, and J. A. Clements, "Ketamine disposition in children and adults," *British Journal of Anaesthesia*, vol. 55, no. 11, pp. 1107–1111, 1983.

[24] I. S. Grant, W. S. Nimmo, and J. A. Clements, "Pharmacokinetics and analgesic effects of i.m. and oral ketamine," *British Journal of Anaesthesia*, vol. 53, no. 8, pp. 805–810, 1981.

[25] K. Porter, "Ketamine in prehospital care," *Emergency Medicine Journal*, vol. 21, no. 3, pp. 351–354, 2004.

[26] M. Richard, *Effect of 0.25mg/kg intravenous ketamine during spinal Anaesthesia on post caesarean analgesic requirement in elective caesarean sections in Mulago, a randomized clinical trial [M.S. thesis]*, Department of Anaesthesia of Makerere University, 2014.

18

# Effects of Intraoperative Dexamethasone and Ondansetron on Postoperative Nausea and Vomiting in Microvascular Decompression Surgery

**Cattleya Thongrong,[1] Patitha Chullabodhi,[1] Pornthep Kasemsiri,[2] Amnat Kitkhuandee,[3] Narin Plailaharn,[1] Lumyai Sabangban,[1] and Thirada Jimarsa[1]**

[1]*Department of Anesthesiology, Faculty of Medicine, Khon Kaen University, Khon Kaen, Thailand*
[2]*Division of Skull Base Surgery, Department of Otorhinolaryngology, Faculty of Medicine, Khon Kaen University, Khon Kaen, Thailand*
[3]*Division of Neurosurgery, Department of Surgery, Faculty of Medicine, Khon Kaen University, Khon Kaen, Thailand*

Correspondence should be addressed to Pornthep Kasemsiri; pkcolumbus99@gmail.com

Academic Editor: Michael Frass

*Background.* Postoperative nausea and vomiting (PONV) is a common problem and may lead to catastrophic complications, especially in neurosurgical cases. The aim of this study was to evaluate the effects of dexamethasone and ondansetron for preventing PONV in patients who underwent microvascular decompression (MVD) surgery. *Methods.* A prospective, double-blinded, randomized control trial was conducted with 54 patients who underwent MVD. Patients were allocated into two groups. The study group (Gr. D) received intraoperative dexamethasone 4 mg iv and ondansetron 4 mg iv, whereas the control group (Gr. N) received placebo (0.9% normal saline 1 ml iv and 0.9% normal saline 2 ml iv). The incidence and severity of PONV were observed at 1, 2, 4, and 24 hr postsurgery. *Results.* At 1, 2, 4, and 24 hr postsurgery, Gr. D had a lower incidence (7.4%, 11.1%, 29.6%, and 66.7%) and lower severity of PONV than Gr. N (18.5%, 29.6%, 37.0%, and 81.5% at 1, 2, 4, and 24 hr; $p > 0.05$). The requirement for antiemetic drugs was not significantly different between the groups ($p > 0.05$). *Conclusion.* Administration of dexamethasone and ondansetron 4 mg seemed to decrease the incidence of PONV in the first 24 hours but not significantly. Therefore, further studies are to be carried out by escalating either dexamethasone dose or the dose of ondansetron or both.

## 1. Introduction

Postoperative nausea and vomiting (PONV) is a common complication. The consequences of PONV are unfavorable and can prolong the length of a hospital stay because of complications, such as, discomfort, aspiration pneumonia, bleeding from the surgical wound, and wound dehiscence [1]. PONV can be influenced by multiple factors, including sex, age, type of anesthesia, type of surgery, and intraoperative analgesic drugs [1, 2].

Approximately 40–70% of patients who undergo neurosurgery suffer from PONV in the first 24 hours [2–5]. But the incidence of PONV following microvascular decompression (MVD) surgery hovers around 70% [5]. Such high incidence of PONV is due to the close proximity of the operating field to the chemoreceptor trigger zone or the area postrema (vomiting center). PONV in a neurosurgical operation may induce increased intracranial pressure or even cause life-threatening brain herniation and death [6–8].

Dexamethasone and ondansetron are commonly used for prophylaxis of PONV [9–13] due to their negligible adverse effects. They are prescribed in several surgical procedures, including laparoscopic cholecystectomy, obstetrical-gynecological surgery, and craniotomy. Literature search did not reveal any clinical trial on the intraoperative use of dexamethasone and ondansetron for prevention of PONV in patients following MVD. To address the above issue, a double-blinded, randomized controlled clinical study was carried out.

## 2. Methods

This prospective, randomized double-blinded controlled trial was conducted at Srinagarind Hospital, Khon Kaen, Thailand, from August 7, 2014, to February 16, 2016. Patients who were scheduled for MVD of the trigeminal nerve root were enrolled. The study group (Gr. D) received intra-operative dexamethasone 4 mg and ondansetron 4 mg, whereas the control group (Gr. N) received placebo (0.9% normal saline 1 ml and 0.9% normal saline 2 ml). Patients of either gender who were at least 18 years old, those who had a physical status classification of I to III according to the American Society of Anesthesiologists, and those who had a body mass index of 18–35 kg/m$^2$ were included. The exclusion criteria were patients on long-term administration of dexamethasone or ondansetron, those with a history of allergic reactions to dexamethasone or ondansetron, those who had undergone antiemetic therapy within 24 hr before surgery, those with underlying liver or renal failure, those who were pregnant, or those who had undergone emergency surgery. This research was approved by the Human Research Ethics Committee of Khon Kaen University (HE571218). In addition, this study was registered with the ClinicalTrial.gov (NCT03685032). The sample size was calculated on the basis of the incidence of PONV following MVD in our hospital database. An 80% different incidence of PONV was considered as a clinically relevant difference. Considering a significance level of 0.05 and power of 0.8, we needed 27 patients for each group.

Fifty-four patients were allocated into 2 groups (Gr. D 27 patients and Gr. N 27 patients) by computer-generated randomization (block of four). All patients received 100% oxygen for 3 minutes before induction with fentanyl 1–1.5 mcg/kg, 2% xylocaine 1–1.5 mg/kg, propofol 1.5–2 mg/kg, and cis-atracurium 0.15 mg/kg. Subsequently, endotracheal tubes were intubated and connected to the anesthetic circuit with controlled ventilation. The ventilation settings were a respiratory rate of 12 times per minute, a tidal volume of 6–8 ml/kg, and an end-tidal $CO_2$ of 30–35 mmHg. Ventilation was assisted with 2% sevoflurane in an adjusted oxygen airflow of 1:1 liter per minute. After patients received general anesthesia, a sequentially numbered opaque sealed envelope was opened. Gr. D was administered 4 mg of dexamethasone in 1 ml iv, and Gr. N received normal saline 1 ml iv. At the end of the operation when suturing the dura mater, Gr. D received ondansetron 4 mg in 2 ml iv while Gr. N received normal saline 2 ml iv. The study drugs based on a sequentially numbered list were prepared in the same way. These drugs had similar characteristics, including clear color and no observable particles, and were loaded into syringes labeled for each group. The attending anesthesiologists, anesthetic nurses, and ward nurses, as well as the patients were blinded to the computer-generated randomization lists.

After completing the operation, the patients were evaluated for the incidence and severity of PONV and a pain score at 1 and 2 hr in the postoperative period in the recovery room and at 4 and 24 hr in the ward by anesthetic nurses. The patients could request antiemetic and opioid analgesic medications, and the doses were recorded as well as the level of satisfactory reduction of PONV (0 = no symptoms; 1 = mild: few symptoms and not requiring treatment; 2 = moderate: presented symptoms and needed ondansetron 8 mg iv; 3 = severe: persisted symptoms after received ondansetron 8 mg iv and needed re-administration of ondansetron 8 mg iv). If symptoms still persist after re-administration of ondansetron, metoclopramide 10 mg iv will be administrated. The intensity of postoperative pain was measured with a numeric rating scale (NRS: 0 = no pain and 10 = severe pain). An independent *t*-test, chi-squared test, and Fisher's exact test were used as appropriate for data analysis. $P < 0.05$ was considered statistically significant.

## 3. Results

Fifty-four patients were allocated into two groups (Gr. N and Gr. D), and there were no differences in the demographic baseline data ($p > 0.05$) (Table 1). Important confounding factors included the consumption of opioids, which showed no statistically significant differences in the postoperative period ($p > 0.05$) (Table 2). At 1, 2, 4, and 24 hr in the postoperative period, Gr. D had a lower incidence of PONV than Gr. N ($p > 0.05$) (Table 3). The requirement for antiemetic drugs did not differ significantly between the groups ($p > 0.05$) (Table 4).

## 4. Discussion

PONV is a common serious problem, especially in neurosurgical patients, because of the morbidity and mortality complications resulting from elevated intracranial and arterial pressure [14]. The incidence of PONV following MVD is high. Meng and Quinlan [8] and Vengkatraghavan et al. [15] reported an incidence of 60% within the first 24 hr. Joo et al. [5] found that 69.7% of patients undergoing MVD developed PONV. Additionally, Ha et al. [16] found the high incidences despite the use of antiemetic prophylaxis. The ramosetron prophylaxis allowed the incidences of nausea of 87.1% and vomiting of 51.6%, whereas ondansetron prophylaxis allowed the incidence of nausea of 93.6% and vomiting of 61.3%.

In the present study, the incidence of PONV was similar to that in other studies. It was found that patients had a higher incidence of PONV following postoperative duration. In Gr. N, incidences of 18.5%, 29.6%, 37.0%, and 81.5% were observed at 1, 2, 4, and 24 hr, respectively. This trend of incidence was similar in the other group that was administered dexamethasone 4 mg and ondansetron 4 mg. For this group, the incidences were reported to be 7.4%, 11.1%, 29.6%, and 66.7% at 1, 2, 4, and 24 hr, respectively. Although the administration of dexamethasone and ondansetron was found to decrease the incidence of PONV, this decrease was not significantly different ($p > 0.05$).

Table 1: Demographic data.

| | Gr. N ($n$ = 27) | Gr. D ($n$ = 27) | $p$ value |
|---|---|---|---|
| *Gender* | | | |
| Male (%) | 8 (29.6) | 9 (33.3) | 0.77 |
| Female (%) | 19 (70.4) | 18 (66.7) | |
| Age (yr, mean) | 35–69 (56.07) | 29–74 (55.62) | 0.868 |
| Weight (kg, mean) | 44–97 (64.70) | 32–90 (61.11) | 0.357 |
| Height (cm, mean) | 140–175 (159.92) | 145–175 (159.48) | 0.824 |
| *ASA class* | | | |
| I (%) | 11 (40.7) | 14 (51.9) | |
| II (%) | 16 (59.3) | 13 (48.1) | 0.373 |
| III (%) | 0 | 0 | |
| *Age < 50 yr* | | | |
| Yes (%) | 6 (22.2) | 9 (33.3) | 0.362 |
| No (%) | 21 (77.8) | 18 (66.7) | |
| *Smoking* | | | |
| Yes (%) | 3 (11.1) | 4 (14.8) | 0.500 |
| No (%) | 24 (88.9) | 23 (85.2) | |
| *Motion sickness* | | | |
| Yes (%) | 4 (14.8) | 4 (14.8) | 0.648 |
| No (%) | 23 (85.2) | 23 (85.2) | |
| *History of PONV* | | | |
| Yes (%) | 2 (7.4) | 5 (18.5) | 0.21 |
| No (%) | 25 (92.6) | 22 (81.5) | |
| *Duration of surgery (min, mean)* | 55–150 (103.33) | 55–145 (98.89) | 0.452 |
| *Fentanyl used intraoperative (mcg, mean)* | 100–200 (143.51) | 100–225 (136.11) | 0.365 |

Table 2: Pain score and opioid analgesics consumed in the 24 hr postoperative period.

| | Gr. N ($n$ = 27) | Gr. D ($n$ = 27) | $p$ value |
|---|---|---|---|
| *Postoperative pain score (mean NRS)* | | | |
| At 1 hr | 4.6 (95% CI: 0–10) | 4.0 (95% CI: 0–8) | 0.725 |
| At 2 hr | 3.2 (95% CI: 0–8) | 2.9 (95% CI: 0–7) | 0.640 |
| At 4 hr | 2.7 (95% CI: 0–6) | 2.6 (95% CI: 0–6) | 0.562 |
| At 24 hr | 4.4 (95% CI: 0–10) | 4.0 (95% CI: 0–8) | 0.691 |
| *Mean opioid consumption* | | | |
| *Fentanyl (mcg, mean)* | | | |
| At 1 hr | 31.5 (95% CI: 0–75) | 28.7 (95% CI: 0–100) | 0.738 |
| At 2 hr | 5.6 (95% CI: 0–50) | 3.7 (95% CI: 0–25) | 0.539 |
| At 4 hr | 1.9 (95% CI: 0–25) | 0.9 (95% CI: 0–25) | 0.561 |
| At 24 hr | 0 | 0 | 0 |
| *Morphine (mg, mean)* | | | |
| At 24 hr | 3.11 (95% CI: 0–6) | 2.44 (95% CI: 0–6) | 0.245 |

Table 3: Incidence of postoperative nausea and vomiting and its severity in the 24 hr postoperative period.

| Postoperative time | | PONV and grading ($n$) | | | | $p$ value |
|---|---|---|---|---|---|---|
| | | Mild | Moderate | Severe | Total, $n$ (%) | |
| At 1 hr | Gr. N ($n$ = 27) | 1 (95% CI: 0.7–18.3) | 3 (95% CI: 3.9–28.1) | 1 (95% CI: 0.7–18.3) | 5 (18.5) (95% CI: 8.2–36.7) | 0.669 |
| | Gr. D ($n$ = 27) | 1 (95% CI: 0.7–18.3) | 1 (95% CI: 0.7–18.3) | 0 | 2 (7.4) (95% CI: 2.1–23.3) | |
| At 2 hr | Gr. N ($n$ = 27) | 7 (95% CI: 13.2–44.7) | 0 | 0 | (95% CI: 13.2–44.7) | 0.175 |
| | Gr. D ($n$ = 27) | 3 (95% CI: 3.9–28.1) | 0 | 0 | 3 (11.1) (95% CI: 3.9–28.1) | |
| At 4 hr | Gr. N ($n$ = 27) | 10 (95% CI: 21.5–55.8) | 0 | 0 | (95% CI: 21.5–55.8) | 0.372 |
| | Gr. D ($n$ = 27) | 6 (95% CI: 10.6–40.7) | 1 (95% CI: 0.7–18.3) | 1 (95% CI: 0.7–18.3) | 8 (29.6) (95% CI: 15.9–48.5) | |
| At 24 hr | Gr. N ($n$ = 27) | 16 (95% CI: 40.7–75.5) | 6 (95% CI: 10.6–40.7) | 0 | (95% CI: 63.3–91.8) | 0.202 |
| | Gr. D ($n$ = 27) | 10 (95% CI: 21.5–55.8) | 6 (95% CI: 10.6–40.7) | 2 (95% CI: 2.1–23.3) | 18 (66.7) (95% CI: 47.8–81.4) | |

Table 4: Antiemetics used in the 24-hr postoperative period.

| | | | Postoperative period (n) | | | |
|---|---|---|---|---|---|---|
| | | | 1 hr | 2 hr | 4 hr | 24 hr |
| N ($n = 27$) | Ondansetron | 8 mg | 4 (95% CI: 5.9–32.5) | 0 | 0 | 3 (95% CI: 3.9–28.1) |
| | Metoclopramide | 10 mg | 0 | 0 | 0 | 4 (95% CI: 5.9–32.5) |
| D ($n = 27$) | Ondansetron | 8 mg | 1 (95% CI: 0.6–18.3) | 0 | 2 (95% CI: 2.1–23.4) | 5 (95% CI: 8.2–36.7) |
| | Metoclopramide | 10 mg | 0 | 0 | 0 | 3 (95% CI: 3.9–28.1) |
| $p$ value | Ondansetron | | 0.167 | — | 0.161 | 0.453 |
| | Metoclopramide | | — | — | — | 0.731 |

However, these results were different from the findings of Kathirvel et al. [10], who compared dexamethasone 4 mg iv alone with dexamethasone 4 mg iv and ondansetron 4 mg iv in patients who underwent elective craniotomy for resection of various intracranial tumors and vascular lesions. They found that the incidence of postoperative emesis was significantly reduced in patients who received dexamethasone and ondansetron (11%) compared with those who received dexamethasone alone (39%) ($p < 0.001$). Regarding our results, administration of dexamethasone 4 mg and ondansetron 4 mg may not be statistically significant effective therapy in MVD because this operation is a high probability of PONV. Furthermore, the efficacy of another antiemetic prophylactic drug (i.e., ramosetron) in MVD was investigated. There was no difference in preventive efficacy between ramosetron and ondansetron [16]. Currently, antiemetic prophylaxis against PONV is a lack of sufficient emphasis in MVD. However, antiemetic prophylaxis in the infratentorial craniotomy reported that a larger dose of ondansetron 8 mg at the time of wound closure decreased the incidence of PONV [17]. Therefore, further studies should be conducted to investigate this hypothesis in MVD with a larger sample size and escalating either doses of dexamethasone or ondansetron or both.

Furthermore, the incidence of PONV was higher at 24 hr after surgery, whereas a lower incidence of PONV at 1 hr, 2 hr, and 4 hr was found. This result may have been affected by propofol. Several previous studies reported that propofol alone reduces PONV. Sneyd et al. [18], who analyzed prospective randomized comparator studies, suggested that there was a reduction in PONV following maintenance of anesthesia with propofol compared with inhalational agents. They found a significantly lower incidence of PONV in the propofol group. Regarding the severity of PONV, the present study found that most patients had mild PONV, and half of these patients needed antiemetic rescue, especially at 24 hr. Unfortunately, the differences between using antiemetic drugs between the two groups were not statistically significant ($p > 0.05$).

There are several possible limitations of this study. First, doses of dexamethasone and ondansetron were too small to provide the antiemetic prophylactic effect following MVD because this operation, relative to other neurosurgical procedures, has a potentially high risk for PONV. Second, it was overestimated that dexamethasone 4 mg and ondansetron 4 mg could reduce the incidence of PONV from a control group by 80%. This estimation led to a small sample size with a low power of preventive emesis effect.

## 5. Conclusion

Administration of dexamethasone 4 mg and ondansetron 4 mg as intraoperative medications for patients who underwent MVD seemed to decrease the incidence of PONV but did not reach statistical significance. Therefore, further studies should be developed by escalating either dexamethasone dose or ondansetron dose or both.

## Abbreviations

PONV: postoperative nausea and vomiting
MVD: microvascular decompression surgery
iv: intravenous.

## Conflicts of Interest

The authors declare that they have no conflicts of interest.

## Acknowledgments

This study was supported by the Invitation Research Grant from the Faculty of Medicine, Khon Kaen University (Grant No. I58126). Furthermore, we would like to acknowledge Emeritus Prof. James A. Will, University of Wisconsin, Madison, for editing the manuscript via Publication Clinic KKU, Thailand.

## References

[1] B. Latz, C. Mordhorst, T. Kerz et al., "Postoperative nausea and vomiting in patients after craniotomy: incidence and risk factors," *Journal of Neurosurgery*, vol. 114, no. 2, pp. 491–496, 2011.

[2] N. Kurita, M. Kawaguchi, K. Nakahashi et al., "Retrospective analysis of postoperative nausea and vomiting after craniotomy," *Masui*, vol. 53, no. 2, pp. 150–155, 2004.

[3] P. H. Manninen, S. K. Raman, K. Boyle, and H. El-Beheiry, "Early postoperative complications following neurosurgical procedures," *Canadian Journal of Anesthesia/Journal Canadien d'anesthésie*, vol. 46, no. 1, pp. 7–14, 1999.

[4] S. A. Irefin, A. Schubert, E. L. Bloomfield, G. E. DeBoer, E. J. Mascha, and Z. Y. Ebrahim, "The effect of craniotomy location on postoperative pain and nausea," *Journal of Anesthesia*, vol. 17, no. 4, pp. 227–231, 2003.

[5] J. D. Joo, J. H. Han, Y. H. Kim et al., "The incidence of postoperative nausea and vomiting after microvascular decompression," *Journal of Korean Skull Base Society*, vol. 7, no. 2, pp. 13–16, 2012.

[6] C. Tan, C. R. Ries, K. Mayson, A. Gharapetian, and D. E. G. Griesdale, "Indication for surgery and the risk of postoperative nausea and vomiting after craniotomy: a case-control study," *Journal of Neurosurgical Anesthesiology*, vol. 24, no. 4, pp. 325–330, 2012.

[7] K. Sato, S. Sai, and T. Adachi, "Is microvascular decompression surgery a high risk for postoperative nausea and vomiting in patients undergoing craniotomy?," *Journal of Anesthesia*, vol. 27, no. 5, pp. 725–730, 2013.

[8] L. Meng and J. J. Quinlan, "Assessing risk factors for postoperative nausea and vomiting: a retrospective study in patients undergoing retromastoid craniectomy with microvascular decompression of cranial nerves," *Journal of Neurosurgical Anesthesiology*, vol. 18, no. 4, pp. 235–239, 2006.

[9] L. López-Olaondo, F. Carrascosa, F. J. Pueyo, P. Monedero, N. Busto, and A. Sáez, "Combination of ondansetron and dexamethasone in the prophylaxis of postoperative nausea and vomiting," *British Journal of Anaesthesia*, vol. 76, no. 6, pp. 835–840, 1996.

[10] S. Kathirvel, H. H. Dash, A. Bhatia, B. Subramaniam, A. Prakash, and S. Shenoy, "Effect of prophylactic ondansetron on postoperative nausea and vomiting after elective craniotomy," *Journal of Neurosurgical Anesthesiology*, vol. 13, no. 3, pp. 207–212, 2001.

[11] M. Elhakim, M. Nafie, K. Mahmoud, and A. Atef, "Dexamethasone 8 mg in combination with ondansetron 4 mg appears to be the optimal dose for the prevention of nausea and vomiting after laparoscopic cholecystectomy," *Canadian Journal of Anesthesia/Journal Canadien d'anesthésie*, vol. 49, no. 9, pp. 922–926, 2002.

[12] B. Gautam, B. R. Shrestha, P. Lama, and S. Rai, "Antiemetic prophylaxis against postoperative nausea and vomiting with ondansetron-dexamethasone combination compared to ondansetron or dexamethasone alone for patients undergoing laparoscopic cholecystectomy," *Kathmandu University Medical Journal*, vol. 6, no. 3, pp. 319–328, 2008.

[13] F. Bano, S. Zafar, S. Aftab, and S. Haider, "Dexamethasone plus ondansetron for prevention of postoperative nausea and vomiting in patients undergoing laparoscopic cholecystectomy: a comparison with dexamethasone alone," *Journal of College of Physicians and Surgeons Pakistan*, vol. 18, no. 5, pp. 265–269, 2008.

[14] A. S. Habib, J. C. Keifer, C. O. Borel, W. D. White, and T. J. Gan, "A comparison of the combination of aprepitant and dexamethasone versus the combination of ondansetron and dexamethasone for the prevention of postoperative nausea and vomiting in patients undergoing craniotomy," *Anesthesia and Analgesia*, vol. 112, no. 4, pp. 813–818, 2011.

[15] L. Venkatraghavan, L. Lil, T. Bailey, P. H. Manninen, and M. Tymianski, "Sumatriptan improves postoperative quality of recovery and reduces postcraniotomy headache after cranial nerve decompression," *British Journal of Anaesthesia*, vol. 117, no. 1, pp. 73–79, 2016.

[16] S. H. Ha, H. Kim, H. M. Ju, D. J. Nam, and K. T. Min, "Comparison of the antiemetic effect of ramosetron with ondansetron in patients undergoing microvascular decompression with retromastoid craniotomy: a preliminary report," *Korean Journal of Anesthesiology*, vol. 68, no. 4, pp. 386–391, 2015.

[17] J. M. Fabling, T. J. Gan, H. E. EI-Moalem, D. S. Warner, and C. O. Borel, "A randomized, double-blind comparison of ondansetron versus placebo for prevention of nausea and vomiting after infratentorial craniotomy," *Journal of Neurosurgical Anesthesiology*, vol. 14, no. 2, pp. 102–107, 2002.

[18] J. R. Sneyd, A. Carr, W. D. Bytom, and A. J. T. Bilski, "A meta-analysis of nausea and vomiting following maintenance of anaesthesia with propofol or inhalational agents," *European Journal of Anaesthesiology*, vol. 15, no. 4, pp. 443–445, 1998.

# Regional Anaesthesia is Associated with Shorter Postanaesthetic Care and Less Pain than General Anaesthesia after Upper Extremity Surgery

**Sven Grauman,[1] Jakob Boethius,[1] and Joakim Johansson[1,2]**

[1]*Department of Anaesthesia and Intensive Care, Östersund Hospital, Östersund, Sweden*
[2]*Department of Surgical and Perioperative Sciences, Anesthesiology and Intensive Care, Unit of Research, Education and Development-Östersund, Umeå University, Umeå, Sweden*

Correspondence should be addressed to Joakim Johansson; joakim.johansson@regionjh.se

Academic Editor: Audun Stubhaug

*Introduction.* For surgery on the upper extremity, the anaesthetist often has a choice between regional anaesthesia (RA) and general anaesthesia (GA). We sought to investigate the possible differences between RA and GA after upper extremity surgery with regard to postoperative patient comfort. *Methods.* This is a retrospective observational study that was performed at an acute care secondary referral centre. One hundred and eighty-seven procedures involving orthopaedic surgery on the upper extremity were included. The different groups (RA and GA) were compared regarding the primary outcome variable, length of stay in Postanaesthesia Unit, and secondary outcome variables, opioid consumption and nausea treatment. *Results.* RA was associated with significantly shorter median length of stay (99 versus 171 minutes). In the GA group, 32% of the patients received opioid analgesics and 21% received antiemetics. In the RA group, none received opioid analgesics and 3% received antiemetics. *Conclusion.* In this observational study, RA was superior to GA for surgery of the upper extremity regarding Postanaesthesia Care Unit length of stay, number of doses of analgesic, and number of doses of antiemetic administered.

## 1. Introduction

Regional anaesthesia (RA) is used more commonly than general anaesthesia (GA) for surgery on the lower extremity [1]. RA is believed to be associated with less postoperative pain, less resource utilisation in the PACU (Postanaesthesia Care Unit), and fewer complications.

There is not a similar preference for RA in surgery of the upper limb [2, 3].

However, for surgery on the upper extremity, RA has gained popularity during recent years, probably depending on increase in ultrasound (US) availability [2–4].

The brachial plexus is the dominant type of RA used for surgery on the upper extremity. There are a number of different methods of brachial plexus block (interscalene, supraclavicular, infraclavicular, and axillary) and also different methods to ensure deposition of local anaesthetics in proximity to the nerves (anatomical landmarks, nerve stimulator, and/or US). It is possible that this heterogeneity of techniques has hampered the development of a general recommendation on anaesthetic preference for surgery of the upper extremity [1, 5].

RA is an attractive alternative to GA since it can be associated with less perioperative resource utilisation [1, 5]. The risk of perioperative complications is generally considered to be lower with RA as compared to GA [1, 5–7].

It has been shown that RA decreases postoperative pain and time spent in the PACU after hand and shoulder surgery [8–11]. There is less consensus regarding the rate of complications associated with different brachial plexus approaches [2–4, 7]. It is likely that such information, even if it is found, is outdated due to the fast development of the US-guided technique [2–4].

Most studies comparing RA with GA for upper limb surgery are conducted in specialised clinics. Thereby, it is uncertain if the results may be applied to larger, nonspecific units with a bulk of other cases, a mix of urgent and elective procedures, and with a proportion of the physicians in training.

Despite the recent advancements in techniques for RA, postoperative pain and nausea continue to be a major problem [12]. Resource utilisation (PACU LOS (length of stay) and opioid and antiemetic consumption) may reflect the wellbeing of patients.

We wanted to explore the impact of the choice of anaesthesia (RA versus GA) on resource utilisation in the PACU.

## 2. Methods

Ethical approval for this study (2014/396-31) was provided by the Regional Ethics Review Board (Etikprövningsnämnden Umeå, Samverkanshuset, 901 87 Umeå, Sweden). Due to the observational design of the study and no handling of sensitive data, this study did not require informed consent from participants.

This is a retrospective case control study. Our hospital has 10 theatres with mixed cases from all surgical specialties except neurosurgery and thoracic surgery. A total of 8000 procedures are performed annually. The anaesthetists perform all types of anaesthetics, in addition to intensive care. All the RAs and GAs in this study were done in a setting where all physicians, including residents, rotate between all the different positions. No personnel knew of the study at the time of the anaesthesia. Our PACU is open weekdays from 07.00 to 21.00 and takes care of the patients until they are ready to go home (outpatients) or to the ward (inpatients).

A power calculation based on 100 minutes in the PACU for the RA group and 150 minutes for the GA group, 80 minutes standard deviation, power 80%, and level of significance 0.05 revealed that a sample size of 41 in each group was sufficient.

We included all patients in our department that had orthopaedic surgery done on or distal to the elbow from January 1 to June 30, 2012, that were 21 years or older. We did not include cases operated on during on-call hours. Other exclusion criteria were concomitant surgical procedures not on the upper extremity during the same operation, patients not planned for PACU admission after the surgery, or those in which a combination of RA and GA was planned beforehand. If the same patient had more than one procedure on the upper extremity during the study, all such procedures were registered as separate cases. Patient characteristics and all other relevant information were collected from the medical records database.

Two groups were identified to categorise the patients.

(1) General anaesthesia (GA), defined as anaesthesia with the use of an endotracheal tube or a supraglottic laryngeal mask. Induction and maintenance of anaesthesia was performed with propofol or thiopental and sevoflurane. Perioperative pain control was achieved with fentanyl, alfentanil, and/or morphine.

(2) Regional anaesthesia (RA), defined as a brachial plexus block with local anaesthetics. Ropivacaine was the drug used in almost all cases. Sedation with midazolam or propofol was given in some of these cases.

Almost all patients in the GA group and none in the RA group received local anaesthetics in the surgical area in conjunction with the above-described strategy.

The outcome variables were

(i) PACU length of stay,

(ii) number of doses of opiates given in the PACU, defined as an occasion with intravenous administration of morphine, ketobemidone, alfentanil, or fentanyl, regardless of the choice of drug and dose,

(iii) Number of doses of antiemetics given in the PACU, defined as an occasion with intravenous administration of haloperidol, granisetron, ondansetron, betamethasone, or metoclopramide, regardless of the choice of drug and dose,

(iv) Regional anaesthesia performed in the PACU ("rescue RA"), defined as a brachial plexus or other conduction block during the time spent in the PACU,

(v) Unplanned overnight admission to the hospital postoperatively.

Other collected data were ASA-class, duration of the surgical procedure, age, planned out- or inpatient surgery and type of surgery (fracture or no fracture surgery).

*2.1. Statistical Analysis.* Median and interquartile range (ICR) or mean and confidence interval (CI) were used to describe the parameters. For comparison between groups, we used the Mann–Whitney or $t$-test as appropriate. For comparison of binary variables, Fischer's exact test was used. The eight patients with failed RA (that had a GA in addition) are included in the RA group in order to perform an intention to treat analysis (ITT).

A multiple linear regression was performed on the primary outcome (PACU length of stay), looking at the possibly independent variables RA/GA, age, sex, time of surgery, and fracture/no fracture.

## 3. Results

Figure 1 shows how the study groups were defined. 187 patients were included, 87 in the group RA and 100 in the group GA.

The RA group was significantly older ($p > 0.001$), of a significantly higher ASA-class ($p = 0.023$), and had a longer a duration of surgery ($p = 0.029$) than the GA group, but there was no difference in proportion of planned outpatient surgery or proportion of fracture surgery (Table 1).

The primary outcome variable, PACU length of stay, was significantly shorter after RA than GA (Table 2).

The secondary outcome, administration of opiates and antiemetics, differed significantly between the two groups (Table 2).

Thirteen patients (13%) in the GA group had rescue RA in the PACU and ten (10%) were converted from planned outpatient to inpatient surgery (Table 2).

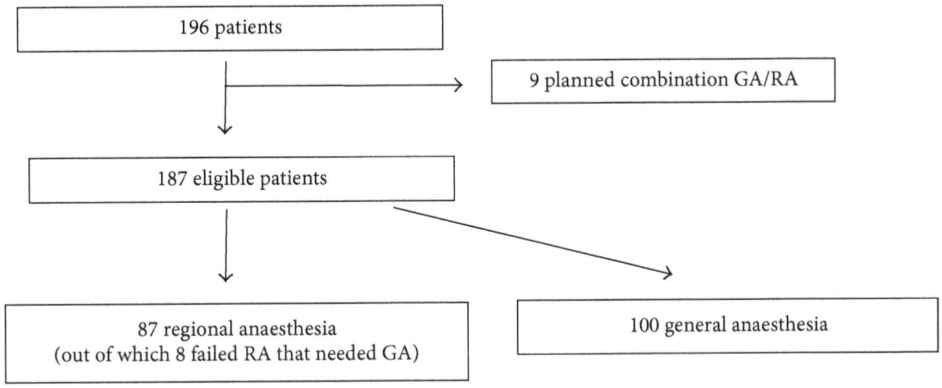


FIGURE 1: CONSORT-diagram illustrating the study. The 8 patients with failed RA that needed unplanned general anaesthesia was still included in the RA group for an intention to treat analysis.

TABLE 1: Demographics and study variables in the two groups.

| | RA | GA | $p$ |
|---|---|---|---|
| $n$ | 87 | 100 | — |
| Sex (male, %) | 47 | 45 | 0.883 |
| Age (years, median, IQR) | 60 (54–70) | 54 (33–63) | <0.001 |
| ASA (mean, CI) | 1.80 (1.66–1.95) | 1.59 (1.47–1.71) | 0.023 |
| Outpatient (%) | 80 | 77 | 0.381 |
| Duration of surgery (minutes, median, IQR) | 87 (59–117) | 74 (42–105) | 0.029 |
| Fracture surgery, yes/no | 44% | 39% | 0.309 |

ASA, American Society of Anesthesiologists.

TABLE 2: Outcome in the two groups.

| | RA | GA | $p$ |
|---|---|---|---|
| $n$ | 87 | 100 | — |
| PACU LOS (minutes, median, IQR) | 99 (70–136) | 171 (115–251) | <0.001 |
| Opiates in PACU, yes/no | 0 | 32% | <0.001 |
| Opiates, mean number of doses in PACU | 0 | 0.53 | na |
| Antiemetics in PACU, yes/no | 3% | 21% | <0.001 |
| Antiemetics, number of doses in PACU | 0.04 | 0.44 | <0.001 |
| Rescue block in PACU, yes/no | 0 | 13% | <0.001 |
| Unplanned stay overnight | 0 | 10% | 0.002 |

PACU, Postanaesthesia Care Unit. LOS, length of stay. Na, not applicable.

A multiple regression analysis revealed that independent factors significantly associated with PACU LOS were RA/GA, fracture surgery, and duration of surgery but not age or sex (Table 3).

This multiple regression also suggested looking closer at the group that had surgery in relation to a fracture, since this factor also was related to a longer time spent in the PACU.

A univariate subgroup analysis showed that, in cases with intended RA, the difference in PACU LOS between fracture and nonfracture cases was small (109 versus 94 minutes). The GA group on the other hand doubled their PACU LOS (248 versus 124) (Table 4) if their surgery was in relation to a fracture.

Table 5 demonstrates that in the case of an intended RA other procedures related parameters do not matter that much. On the other hand, for cases where GA was intended, duration of surgery and fracture/nonfracture surgery were both markedly related to PACU LOS.

TABLE 3: Multiple regression on PACU-time.

| | Coefficient of regression | $p$ |
|---|---|---|
| Age | −0.06 | 0.32 |
| Sex | 0.01 | 0.82 |
| Fracture surgery (yes/no) | 0.33 | <0.001 |
| Duration of surgery | 0.15 | 0.025 |
| RA/GA (yes/no) | 0.46 | <0.001 |

RA, regional anaesthesia. GA, general anaesthesia. PACU, Postanaesthesia Care Unit.

TABLE 4: Univariate analyses within the subgroups RA/GA concerning fracture surgery or not.

| | RA ($n$ = 87) | | | GA ($n$ = 100) | | |
|---|---|---|---|---|---|---|
| | Fracture ($n$ = 38) | No fracture ($n$ = 49) | $p$ | Fracture ($n$ = 39) | No fracture ($n$ = 61) | $p$ |
| PACU LOS (min) | 109 (80–149) | 94 (61–121) | 0.057 | 248 (186–300) | 124 (102–180) | < 0.001 |

Median (IQR). PACU, Postanaesthesia Care Unit. LOS, length of stay.

TABLE 5: Multiple regressions on PACU length of stay for subgroups RA and GA.

| | RA ($n$ = 87) | | GA ($n$ = 100) | |
|---|---|---|---|---|
| | Coefficient of regression | $p$ | Coefficient of regression | $p$ |
| Age | 0.09 | 0.45 | −0.09 | 0.28 |
| Sex | 0.13 | 0.25 | −0.07 | 0.41 |
| Duration of surgery | −0.04 | 0.73 | 0.25 | 0.01 |
| Fracture surgery (yes/no) | 0.25 | 0.03 | 0.42 | <0.001 |

PACU, Postanaesthesia Care Unit. RA, regional anaesthesia. GA, general anaesthesia.

## 4. Discussion

Our results show that patients that had RA, as compared to those that had only GA, spent a shorter time in the PACU and consumed less analgesic and antiemetic drugs, suggesting less experienced pain and less experienced postoperative nausea and vomiting.

The results corroborate earlier studies to some degree, confirming superiority of an RA approach in upper extremity surgery [1, 5–7]. Despite this knowledge, RA remains underused for different reasons [12]. We theorize that there may be some apprehension to use RA outside of specialised units. What is new is that our study was performed in a secondary referral unit (regional acute care hospital), where surgery on the upper extremity constitutes a small part of the total number of procedures. The procedures involved are both urgent and elective and we have no subspecialised anaesthetists that handle these cases. In addition, approximately 25% of our staff of physicians were residents, representative for a typical acute care general facility. This makes the results applicable to the great majority of care facilities, not only to specialised units.

In the RA group, there was no need for postoperative analgesic intervention and virtually no antiemetic drugs.

From Tables 4 and 5 it is reasonable to conclude that RA intention is most important for fracture surgery, supposedly because of more postoperative pain compared to nonfracture surgery.

There are reasons to believe that the increasing use of US for regional blocks has had an impact on procedure related parameters, such as the learning curve and success rate. All our blocks were done with the support of US and our standard block for arm surgery is the supraclavicular brachial plexus block. The success rate was 92% during this study period, defined as surgery without GA when RA alone was planned on beforehand.

The study has some strengths. It is consecutive and cases included were anaesthetised under real working conditions by nonspecialist regional anaesthetists, including physicians under education. Further, it was not known to participants, anaesthetists, or personnel in the PACU that the case was to be included in a study.

The primary outcome variable, PACU LOS, is somewhat complicated to assess. It is affected by many factors not related to the surgery itself; for example, the surgeon often wants to speak to the patient before he/she leaves the PACU or a postsurgical X-ray often is warranted. In addition to these factors, the outpatients will have to wait for home transportation at the PACU. It is reasonable to suppose that these factors affect both the RA- and the GA group to the same degree and hence that this factor did not have any major effect on the results.

The study also has several weaknesses. Since it is a retrospective study, there was no randomisation; hence the choice between RA and GA was done at the presurgical visit by the anaesthetist. This may introduce confounding variables and the results may not have been the same with randomisation. As can be seen from Table 1, the RA group was significantly older and had longer duration of surgery, so groups were not matched perfect.

As it is a retrospective study, there was no uniform protocol for induction and maintenance of GA and no strict protocol for the blocks.

Furthermore, the study only included patients operated at daytime since our PACU is closed at night. The same personnel join the operation theatre and supply Postanaesthesia Care during on-call hours. It is reasonable to believe that the results would have been the same if on-call hours would have been studied as well.

The outcome variable used for postoperative pain was number of doses of opioids administered. If a patient has severe pain in the PACU, this may call for a single larger dose. Thereby the results may have differed in that patients in severe pain had relatively fewer doses administered. If this was so, it would have counteracted the results found and hence it is not a major limitation.

In light of the exceptional development of RA in recent years, a prospective randomised trial, testing the hypothesis that we have tried to explore here, is indeed warranted and could probably add substantial evidence to the establishment of a gold standard regarding the choice between RA and GA for different types of surgery on the upper extremity.

The results of this study are applicable to a nonspecialised unit where this specific type of surgery constitutes a small part of all procedures and where anaesthetists are not subspecialised, are on a rotating schedule, and include physicians under training.

On this behalf, we conclude that this observational study supports the use of regional anaesthesia as opposed to general anaesthesia for orthopaedic surgery on or below the elbow of the arm. Regional anaesthesia was associated with shorter time spent in the Postanaesthesia care unit and less administered doses of opioids and antiemetics.

## Competing Interests

None of the authors have any conflict of interests in relation to this manuscript.

## Acknowledgments

Thanks are due to Lars Söderström for statistical advice.

## References

[1] P. Gulur, M. Nishimori, and J. C. Ballantyne, "Regional anaesthesia versus general anaesthesia, morbidity and mortality," *Best Practice & Research: Clinical Anaesthesiology*, vol. 20, no. 2, pp. 249–263, 2006.

[2] B. G. Bruce, A. Green, T. A. Blaine, and L. V. Wesner, "Brachial plexus blocks for upper extremity orthopaedic surgery," *Journal of the American Academy of Orthopaedic Surgeons*, vol. 20, no. 1, pp. 38–47, 2012.

[3] K. Russon, T. Pickworth, and W. Harrop-Griffiths, "Upper limb blocks," *Anaesthesia*, vol. 65, supplement 1, pp. 48–56, 2010.

[4] J. M. Maga, L. Cooper, and R. E. Gebhard, "Outpatient regional anesthesia for upper extremity surgery update (2005 to present) distal to shoulder," *International Anesthesiology Clinics*, vol. 50, no. 1, pp. 47–55, 2012.

[5] E. Tziavrangos and S. A. Schug, "Regional anaesthesia and perioperative outcome," *Current Opinion in Anaesthesiology*, vol. 19, no. 5, pp. 521–525, 2006.

[6] S. E. Mason, A. Noel-Storr, and C. W. Ritchie, "The impact of general and regional anesthesia on the incidence of post-operative cognitive dysfunction and post-operative delirium: a systematic review with meta-analysis," *Journal of Alzheimer's Disease*, vol. 22, no. 3, pp. S67–S79, 2010.

[7] R. Sripada and C. Bowens Jr., "Regional anesthesia procedures for shoulder and upper arm surgery upper extremity update—2005 to present," *International Anesthesiology Clinics*, vol. 50, no. 1, pp. 26–46, 2012.

[8] C. J. L. McCartney, R. Brull, V. W. S. Chan et al., "Early but no long-term benefit of regional compared with general anesthesia for ambulatory hand surgery," *Anesthesiology*, vol. 101, no. 2, pp. 461–467, 2004.

[9] C. L. Wu, L. M. Rouse, J. M. Chen, and R. J. Miller, "Comparison of postoperative pain in patients receiving interscalene block or general anesthesia for shoulder surgery," *Orthopedics*, vol. 25, no. 1, pp. 45–48, 2002.

[10] A. Hadzic, B. A. Williams, P. E. Karaca et al., "For outpatient rotator cuff surgery, nerve block anesthesia provides superior same-day recovery over general anesthesia," *Anesthesiology*, vol. 102, no. 5, pp. 1001–1007, 2005.

[11] A. R. Brown, R. Weiss, C. Greenberg, E. L. Flatow, and L. U. Bigliani, "Interscalene block for shoulder arthroscopy: comparison with general anesthesia," *Arthroscopy*, vol. 9, no. 3, pp. 295–300, 1993.

[12] N. Rawal, "Current issues in postoperative pain management," *European Journal of Anaesthesiology*, vol. 33, no. 3, pp. 160–171, 2016.

# Job Satisfaction and Associated Factors among Anesthetists Working in Amhara National Regional State, Northwest Ethiopia, May 2017

**Demeke Yilkal Fentie, Henos Enyew Ashagrie, and Habtamu Getinet Kasahun**

*Department of Anesthesia, School of Medicine, Gondar College of Medicine and Health Sciences, University of Gondar, Gondar, Ethiopia*

Correspondence should be addressed to Demeke Yilkal Fentie; dyilkal97@gmail.com

Academic Editor: Ronald G. Pearl

*Background.* Job satisfaction is an important determinant of health staff's motivation, retention, and performance. Difficulties in critical decision-making and problems with lack of respect and recognition lead to lower job satisfaction level among anesthetists. It leads to high turnover intention, dropout from the profession, burnout, impaired health status of anesthetists, and lower work performance. *Objective.* The aim of this multicenter cross-sectional study was to assess the level of job satisfaction and associated factors among anesthetists working in Amhara National Regional State. *Methods.* A multicenter cross-sectional study was conducted from April 1 to June 30, 2017. Ninety-eight anesthetists that were working in Amhara National Regional State Hospitals were involved in this study. The structured questionnaire was scored on five-point Likert scales. Data were analyzed using Statistical Package for Social Sciences version 20. Binary logistic regression was used to measure statistical significance between dependent and each independent variable. Variables with $P$ value of ≤0.2 on crude analysis were taken into multivariate analysis, and $P$ value 0.05 and 95% CI was used as cut off point. *Result.* 98 out of 104 participants were involved in this study with a response rate of 94.3%. The overall level of job satisfaction was 46.9%. Anesthetists in academic working position were satisfied with the odds of about 2.3 (AOR = 2.269; CI = 1.137–6.740) compared to those in clinical working position. Anesthetists were least satisfied with coworker relationships (37.8%), work schedule (43.9%), professional opportunity (46.9%), and recognition (49%) while they were most satisfied from their control of responsibility (59.2%), social interaction (55%), and salary and benefits (51%). *Conclusion and Recommendation.* Job satisfaction of anesthetists was low, and we suggest that facilitation of professional development, creation of smooth relationship in working environment, increasing the number of anesthetists, and recognition of the anesthesia professional are of paramount importance to increase job satisfaction of anesthetists.

## 1. Introduction

Anesthetists are experts in intensive care, perioperative patient care, acute and chronic pain management, as well as research, and teaching, both at undergraduate and postgraduate levels [1]. Involving in stressful and overloaded working areas results in higher turnover intention, burnout, and job dissatisfaction [2, 3]. Demand-supply imbalance of anesthetists has greatly increased, and they are overworking [4]. Workload and stress due to difficulties in critical decision-making have been shown as problems with the specialty of anesthesia [5]. Anesthetists lack recognition and feedback from patients and even colleagues despite working within a team [5, 6]. All these produce lower job satisfaction that might impair the health of anesthetists their job performance [7].

The WHO in 2013 reported that health-care worker shortages are common globally and the world will be debt of 12.9 million health workers by 2035. Shortage and misdistribution of anesthetists is a social problem in many countries leading to workload, job dissatisfaction, and finally burnout [8]. Lack of recognition from management and lack of public and client awareness towards the role of anesthetists and feedback towards anesthesia have been indicated as causes of low job satisfaction [1, 5, 9].

A study conducted in Switzerland suggests that employees' satisfaction needs to be evaluated, to improve their working condition and to ensure strategies and coping mechanisms to reduce professional stress [5]. Little is known about anesthetists' levels of job satisfaction or workload stress despite their key role in the operating room, ICU, emergency department, and involvement in research and teaching [4]. Lack of job support, long working hours, and challenges in managing life threatening scenarios has been shown to be associated with increased stress and low level of job satisfaction [10].

A study of Netherlands found that job satisfaction as one of the most important and well-investigated work attitudes in organizational behavior, and turnover intention is related to dissatisfaction with job [11]. Another study identified autonomy, collegial relationship, patient-care giver interaction, payment, and availability of resources and educational status as factors that determine job satisfaction of physicians. [12]. One investigation found no difference in satisfaction among men and women anesthetists [13]. A study performed in Kenya showed that inhospitable working condition, limited promotion opportunities, and weak health-care systems result in dissatisfaction and demotivation with work and leaving the country [14]. According to a study in Ethiopia, reasons for dissatisfaction of health-care workers were lack of motivation, inadequate salary, insufficient training opportunities, and inadequate number of human resources, and satisfiers were getting satisfaction from helping others and professional gratification [15]. Control over decision-making and allowing anesthetists to have more influence on their own work pace and flexible work schedule improves working conditions which leads to better job satisfaction and motivation among Switzerland anesthetists [2]. A study conducted in Australia found that high standard of practice and practical aspects of the job were satisfying, whereas poor recognition and long hours were the dissatisfying aspects of the job [6]. Lack of achievement and lack of recognition are identified as dissatisfiers than working conditions and interactions with the seniors [16].

One review commented that improving overall health and improving work satisfaction may decrease burnout among operation theatre team members [17]. Company policies, opportunities for advancement, and the relation between pay and the amount of work are also suggested to be job dissatisfiers among health workers [18]. A meta-analysis conducted in the United Kingdom found that job satisfaction level is an important factor influencing the health of workers [19]. Anesthesia specialty has been identified as a specialty at risk of professional burnout which is associated with poor health including marital difficulties, anxiety, and depression might contribute to alcoholism and drug addiction [7].

Particularly, stress, arising from handling severe illness and death, operating complex equipments, and experiencing a lack of recognition with members of other occupational groups or managers lead to burnout and job dissatisfaction [2, 6, 20]. A study done in Austria showed that one-quarter of anesthetists working in teaching hospitals were at risk for burnout syndrome (characterized by mental and physical exhaustion), and 50% of anesthetists had greater job dissatisfaction (P 0.002) with their job and plan to future dropout from their profession [21].

Table 1: Sociodemographic characteristics of anesthetists working in Amhara National Regional State April to May, 2017 ($N = 98$). Data are expressed in frequency and percentage.

| Variables | Frequency | Percent |
|---|---|---|
| *Gender* | | |
| Male | 77 | 78.6 |
| Female | 21 | 21.4 |
| *Age* | | |
| <25 | 17 | 17.3 |
| 25–30 | 61 | 61.2 |
| 31–35 | 11 | 11.9 |
| >35 | 9 | 9.2 |
| *Marital status* | | |
| Single | 57 | 58.2 |
| Married | 41 | 41.8 |
| *Educational status* | | |
| BSc | 62 | 63.3 |
| Diploma | 19 | 19.4 |
| MSc | 17 | 17.3 |
| *Religion* | | |
| Orthodox | 70 | 71.4 |
| Muslim | 16 | 16.3 |
| Protestant | 12 | 12.3 |
| *Salary in ETB* | | |
| <5000 | 17 | 17.3 |
| 5000–7000 | 38 | 38.8 |
| 7000–9000 | 27 | 27.6 |
| >9000 | 16 | 16.3 |

Job satisfaction of anesthetists is an important key issue for their well being and for improved quality of patient care. The specialty of anesthesia has been classified as high risk for the development of job dissatisfaction. Dropout from the profession due to stress, fatigue, and long working hours is the problem of anesthetists throughout the world. According to the report by Ethiopian Association of Anesthetists, there are a total of 1200 anesthetists serving a population of 100 million in the country showing that there is shortage of anesthesia professionals which may lead to increased workload and job dissatisfaction.

In Ethiopia, the number of anesthetists in intention of turnover, dropout from the profession, and leaving the working area is increasing which is a challenge for the health-care system. One study also showed that job satisfaction is determinant factor for motivation and increased work effectiveness, efficiency, and quality [16]. A cross-sectional study performed in Ethiopia showed that less than half (45.8%) of anesthetists were satisfied with their job [9]. There are limited published data on job satisfaction of anesthetists.

The present study was designed to assess the overall job satisfaction and determine factors affecting the level of job satisfaction among anesthetists which may help health policy makers to implement health policies that focus on incentives, conducive working conditions, fair workloads, and employee retention.

TABLE 2: Satisfaction level among participants by job satisfaction subscales in Amhara National Regional State April to May, 2017 ($N$ = 98). Data are expressed in percentage.

| Job satisfaction subscales | Level of satisfaction | |
|---|---|---|
| | Satisfied $n$ (%) | Dissatisfied $n$ (%) |
| Control and responsibility | 58 (59.2) | 40 (40.8) |
| Scheduling | 43 (43.9) | 55 (56.1) |
| Social interaction | 54 (55.1) | 44 (44.9) |
| Professional opportunities | 46 (46.9) | 53 (54.1) |
| Salary and benefits | 50 (51) | 48 (49) |
| Praise and recognition | 48 (49) | 50 (51) |
| Coworker | 37 (37.8) | 61 (62.2) |
| Overall | 46 (46.9) | 53 (53.1) |

## 2. Methods

Multicenter cross-sectional study was conducted from April to May 2017 in Amhara National Regional State, Northwest Ethiopia.

*2.1. Study Area.* There are five referral and 12 general hospitals in Amhara National Regional State. According to the information from the Amhara Regional Health Bureau, there are about 104 anesthetists working in the region.

*2.2. Source Population.* All anesthetists working in Amhara National Regional State were included in this study.

*2.3. Study Population.* Anesthetists working in Amhara National Regional State who were available during data collection period were included in this study.

*2.4. Dependent Variable.* Level of job satisfaction which was recorded on a five-point Likert scale was the dependent variable.

*2.5. Independent Variables.* Sociodemographic variables including, age, gender, religion, educational status, marital status, years of practice, work-related characteristics, working position, salary, and working hours per week were independent variables.

Job satisfaction subscales such as control responsibility, schedule, coworker interaction, praise and recognition, and social interaction were also incorporated as independent variables.

*2.6. Operational Definitions. Job satisfaction*: one's positive perceived emotion on the appraisal of his/her job which is measured by taking the mean (average) score of different 24 items by using five-point Likert scale (from 1 = very dissatisfied to 5 = very satisfied). The overall job satisfaction score was calculated by taking the average (mean) score of all the subscales.

To measure level of job satisfaction of each individual, the mean (average) value of all subscales was calculated. Mean value of subscales was taken as a cut point value to determine whether an anesthetist was satisfied with his/her job or not. As a result, anesthetists for whom score was below mean were considered as dissatisfied and those with mean and above were regarded as satisfied.

*Likert scale*: the sum of response to several Likert items.

*Likert items*: the statement that the respondents are asked to evaluate in the survey.

*2.7. Data Collection Procedures.* Having approval from Institutional Ethical Review Board of University of Gondar, a self-administered questionnaire consisting of sociodemographic variables and 24-item of job satisfaction tool was sent through hand-delivered questionnaire for all anesthetists working in Amhara regional state, and the data were collected by five data collectors within a month after administration of the questionnaires, and it was supervised by the principal investigator.

*2.8. Data Quality Management.* Study participants were oriented on how to fill the questionnaire, and data collection was supervised by the supervisor. The data were cleaned and checked for completeness using Epi info.

*2.9. Data Processing and Analysis Procedures.* Data was coded, entered, and analyzed using SPSS version 20 statistical software. Each item of the job satisfaction was measured by a 5 point Likert scale having a total of 24 items as validated by Tourangeau et al. The reliability coefficient (Cronbach's alpha) of this instrument for our total respondents was 0.88. The 24 items were further divided into seven subscales. Predictor items were also summated accordingly to determine agreement status of the respondent by using computed mean for each sub scale and the higher means score indicating higher satisfaction from the subscales. Descriptive statistics was presented as frequency and percentage.

Using binary logistics regressions model, bivariate and multivariate analyses were employed to determine the association between dependent and independent variables. Variables with $P$ value of $<0.2$ from bivariate analysis were taken to multivariate analysis. $P$ values $<0.05$ were considered statistically significant.

TABLE 3: Multivariate analysis for predictors of job satisfaction of anesthetists, Amhara National Regional State April to May, 2017 ($N = 98$). Data are expressed in COR and AOR.

| Independent predictors | Job satisfaction | | COR (95% CI) | AOR (95% CI) |
|---|---|---|---|---|
| | Satisfied | Dissatisfied | | |
| *Gender* | | | | |
| Male | 39 | 38 | 2.05 (0.74–5.64)* | |
| Female | 7 | 14 | 1 | *** |
| *Age* | | | | |
| <25 | 9 | 8 | 1 | *** |
| 25–30 | 23 | 38 | 0.53 (0.18–1.59) | |
| 31–35 | 6 | 5 | 1.06 (0.23–4.88) | |
| >35 | 8 | 1 | 7.11 (0.72–6.85)* | |
| *Marital status* | | | | |
| Single | 24 | 33 | 1.23 (0.55–2.76) | |
| Married | 16 | 25 | 1 | *** |
| *Working position* | | | | |
| Academic | 25 | 17 | 2.45 (1.08–5.56)* | 2.91 (1.20–7.05)** |
| Clinical | 21 | 35 | 1 | 1 |
| *Working hour/week* | | | | |
| ≤50 | 14 | 13 | 2.38 (0.83–6.83) | |
| 51–70 | 11 | 8 | 2.62 (0.81–08.43) | |
| 71–90 | 7 | 13 | 1.56 (0.49–4.90) | |
| >90 | 8 | 24 | 1 | *** |
| *Educational status* | | | | |
| MSc | 5 | 12 | 2.66 (0.67–10.58) | |
| BSc | 25 | 37 | 2.4 (0.75–7.62) | |
| Diploma | 10 | 9 | 1 | *** |
| *Salary* | | | | |
| <5000 | 9 | 8 | 1 | *** |
| 5000–7000 | 12 | 26 | 0.64 (0.20–2.04) | |
| 7000–9000 | 11 | 16 | 0.71 (0.25–2.40) | |
| >9000 | 8 | 8 | 1.14 (0.29–4.50) | |
| *Work experience* | | | | |
| 1–3 | 23 | 33 | 1 | *** |
| 4–6 | 11 | 21 | 1.17 (0.49–2.81) | |
| 7–9 | 1 | 1 | 1.33 (0.07–22.41) | |
| ≥10 | 5 | 3 | 4.00 (0.74–21.58) | |
| *Resource and supply* | | | | |
| Inadequate | 22 | 33 | 1 | *** |
| Adequate | 24 | 19 | 1.89 (0.84–4.25)* | |

*$P$ value $< 0.2$; **$P < 0.05$ and ***did not appear.

*2.10. Ethical Consideration.* Ethical clearance was obtained from the School of Medicine Ethics Committee of University of Gondar. Written informed consent was obtained from each study participant after clear explanation on what the study entails. Anyone not willing to participate in the study was informed that they have full right not to participate or stop at any time. Confidentiality was ensured by keeping the secrecy of personal identification, completed questionnaires, and results in well secured area.

## 3. Results

*3.1. Sociodemographic Characteristics.* Out of 104 eligible anesthetists working in Amhara National Regional State, 98 responded the self-administered questionnaire, giving a response rate of 94%. Of study participants, 77 (78.6%) were male while 21 (21.4) were females and most of the respondents were unmarried 57 (58.2%). Of study subjects, 61 (62.2%) were in the age group of 25–30 years followed by 9 (9.2%) above 30 years. Of the total respondents, 62 (63.3%) were BSc, 17 (17.3%) MSc, and 19 (19.4%) were diploma anesthetists (Table 1).

*3.2. Work Related Characteristics.* Regarding work experience of anesthetists more than half of them were served about 1–5 years and 6 (6.1%) of them served above 9 years. Of the study participants, 56 (57.1%) were clinical staffs, and 42 (42.9%) were academic staffs.

*3.3. Job Satisfaction of Anesthetists.* Overall, forty six (46.9%) of respondents were satisfied (Table 2). Regarding each subscales, more than half of study participants 58 (59.5%) were satisfied with their control and responsibility at the work place and 54 (55.1%) of anesthetists were satisfied with interaction with patients. Coworker relationship (37; 37.8%), work scheduling (43; 43.9%), professional opportunities, and recognition (48; 49%) were among factors for which less than half of respondents were satisfied.

*3.4. Factors Associated with Job Satisfaction.* Univariate analysis indicated that age of respondents, gender, working position, and medical resource and supply were significantly associated with job satisfaction. The cut point for statistical significance was $P < 0.20$ in crude analysis. All this significant variables in crude analysis were taken into multivariate analysis, and multivariate analysis showed that anesthetists in academic position were about three times more satisfied (AOR = 2.91; CI = 1.20–7.056.740) (Table 3) compared to those in clinical position. Others (age, gender, medical resource, and supply) were not associated significantly with job satisfaction.

## 4. Discussion

Job satisfactions of health-care workers play a vital role in improving the quality of client care. The finding of the present study indicated that less than half (46.9%) of anesthetists were satisfied with their job which is in line with a study conducted in Jimma (Ethiopia) where 45.8% of anesthetists and 41.4% of health workers were satisfied with their job [9, 15].

The result of the present study is inconsistent with the survey conducted in Canada and Nigeria which indicated that 75% and 58.7% of anesthesiologists, respectively, reported overall satisfaction with their job [1, 3]. This might be due to high surgical regard and public image, working in a standard set up, and fair salary and incentives in case of the Canadian and Nigerian studies.

The result of our study showed that anesthetists in academic position were more satisfied compared to those of clinical staffs (AOR = 2.91; CI = 1.20–7.056.740). This might be due to advancing opportunities and difference in salary and incentives. Additionally, professional development might build up the confidence of anesthetists and increase their satisfaction.

In contrast to earlier findings [22, 23] which showed 59.3% and 51.6% of health workers were satisfied, only 37.8% of anesthetists were satisfied to coworker interaction of their respective hospitals. Lack of trained OR assistance and misunderstanding with surgeons might result in lower job satisfaction in the study area. Although our results differ considerably from previous studies, it could be argued that managing critical events, communication problems, [4] and stress might lead to bad reactions to coworkers.

In our study, satisfaction with working schedule was low (43.9%) in accordance with [9, 22, 24] in which heavy work load and less flexible scheduling impaired job satisfaction. This might also be explained by shortage of anesthesia professionals in the study area. This study showed low (46.9%) satisfaction from professional development. This is consistent with a study conducted in Dutch [25] which showed providing sufficient opportunities for learning and growing would produce high job satisfaction level. Scholars reported that acquiring advanced skills and promotion motivate employees and achieve high job satisfaction [26].

The result of the present study showed respondents were less (51%) satisfied with recognition. It could be argued by the reasons that the anesthesia professional is a new specialty in our country and public awareness about the role of anesthetists might be low. Scholars promote that acknowledging employees for their good work is motivator for job satisfaction.

This study revealed that strong control over work and responsibility produces higher job satisfaction (59.5%) in good agreement with [2]. A study conducted in Nigeria suggests that giving enough job freedom and power might help employee to feel own of the results and greater job satisfaction [26]. Supported by the result of a study in Ethiopia, our study indicated that satisfaction with social interaction like helping others and patient outcome was relatively high [9]. This might be due to the fact that anesthetists work to relief pain and suffering diseases of their clients.

## 5. Limitation of the Study

The possible weakness may come from the small sample size, and there is not a special standardized job satisfaction measurement tool for anesthetists, and we modified the job satisfaction scale developed for nurses.

## 6. Conclusion

Job satisfaction of anesthetists working in Amhara National Regional State is low. The only factor associated with job satisfaction was working position. Anesthetists were most satisfied with their control and responsibility and least satisfied with coworker interaction.

## Abbreviations

ETB: Ethiopian birr
ICU: Intensive care unit
JS: Job satisfaction
WHO: World Health Organization
UOG: University of Gondar.

## Conflicts of Interest

The authors declare that there are no conflicts of interest regarding the publication of this paper.

## References


[1] K. Jenkins and D. Wong, "A survey of professional satisfaction among Canadian anesthesiologists," *Canadian Journal of Anesthesia*, vol. 48, no. 7, pp. 637–645, 2001.

[2] J. F. Kinzl, H. Knotzer, C. Traweger, W. Lederer, T. Heidegger, and A. Benzer, "Influence of working conditions on job satisfaction in anaesthetists," *British Journal of Anaesthesia*, vol. 94, no. 2, pp. 211–215, 2005.

[3] A. Rukewe, "Job satisfaction among anesthesiologists at a tertiary hospital in Nigeria," *Saudi Journal of Anaesthesia*, vol. 6, no. 4, pp. 341–344, 2012.

[4] B. Report, "Evaluation of stressors and coping strategies for stress in Indian anaesthesiologists," *Indian Journal of Anaesthesia*, vol. 55, no. 2, p. 193, 2011.

[5] P. Rama-maceiras, S. Parente, and P. Kranke, "Job satisfaction, stress and burnout in anaesthesia: relevant topics for anaesthesiologists and healthcare managers," *European Journal of Anaesthesiology*, vol. 29, no. 7, pp. 311–319, 2012.

[6] M. T. Kluger, K. Townend, and T. Laidlaw, "Job satisfaction, stress and burnout in Australian specialist anaesthetists," *Anaesthesia*, vol. 58, no. 4, pp. 339–345, 2003.

[7] E. Michinov, M. Laffon, and E. Rusch, "Job satisfaction, life satisfaction and burnout in French anaesthetists," *Journal of Health Psychology*, vol. 15, no. 6, pp. 948–958, 2010.

[8] K. Kawasaki, M. Sekimoto, T. Ishizaki, and Y. Imanaka, "Work stress and workload of full-time anesthesiologists in acute care hospitals in Japan," *Journal of Anesthesia*, vol. 23, no. 2, pp. 235–241, 2009.

[9] N. Desalegn, L. Akalu, and M. Haile, "Ethiopian anesthetists job satisfaction level and factors affecting their level of job satisfaction," *Journal of Anesthesiology*, vol. 3, no. 5, pp. 17–24, 2015.

[10] T. Shams and R. El-Masry, "Job stress and burnout among academic career anaesthesiologists at an Egyptian University Hospital," *Sultan Qaboos University Medical Journal*, vol. 13, no. 2, pp. 287–295, 2013.

[11] C. B. Mahoney, C. Brown-mahoney, and A. A. J. Van Zundert, "Understanding nurse anesthetists' intention to leave their job: how burnout and job satisfaction mediate the impact of personality and workplace characteristics," *Health Care Management Review*, vol. 36, no. 2, pp. 155–163, 2015.

[12] T. R. Konrad, E. S. Williams, M. Linzer et al., "Brief report measuring physician job satisfaction in a changing workplace and a challenging environment," *Medical Care*, vol. 37, no. 11, pp. 1174–1182, 2010.

[13] J. P. Leigh, R. L. Kravitz, M. Schembri, S. J. Samuels, and S. Mobley, "Physician career satisfaction across specialties," *Archives of Internal Medicine*, vol. 162, no. 14, pp. 1577–1584, 2017.

[14] K. Goetz, M. Marx, I. Marx et al., "Working atmosphere and job satisfaction of health care staff in Kenya: an exploratory study," *BioMed Research International*, vol. 2015, Article ID 256205, 7 pages, 2015.

[15] A. Yami, L. Hamza, A. Hassen, C. Jira, and M. Sudhakar, "Original article job satisfaction and its determinants among health workers in specialized hospital, Southwest Ethiopia," *American Journal of Agriculture and Forestry*, vol. 4, no. 5, p. 112, 2016.

[16] R. J. House and L. A. Wigdor, "Herzberg's dual-factor theory of job satisfaction and motivation: a review of the evidence and a criticism," *Personnel Psychology*, vol. 20, no. 4, pp. 369–390, 1959.

[17] J. S. Schildcrout, N. D. Mercaldo, and M. B. Weinger, "Risk of burnout in perioperative clinicians a survey study and literature review," *Anesthesiology*, vol. 114, no. 1, pp. 194–204, 2017.

[18] S. Rothmann, "Job satisfaction, occupational stress, burnout and work engagement as components of work-related well-being," *SA Journal of Industrial Psychology*, vol. 34, no. 3, pp. 11–16, 2002.

[19] B. Street, "The relationship between job satisfaction and health: a meta-analysis," *Occupational and Environmental Medicine*, vol. 62, no. 2, pp. 105–112, 2005.

[20] B. X. Tran, H. V. Minh, and N. D. Hinh, "Factors associated with job satisfaction among commune health workers: implications for human resource policies," *Global Health Action*, vol. 6, no. 1, pp. 1–6, 2013.

[21] W. Lederer and C. Traweger, "Significance of working conditions on burnout in anesthetists," *Acta Anaesthesiologica Scandinavica*, vol. 50, no. 1, pp. 58–63, 2014.

[22] E. T. Bekru, A. Cherie, and A. A. Anjulo, "Job satisfaction and determinant factors among midwives working at health facilities in Addis Ababa city, Ethiopia," *PLoS One*, vol. 12, no. 2, article e0172397, 2017.

[23] A. Geleto, N. Baraki, G. E. Atomsa, and Y. Dessie, "Job satisfaction and associated factors among health care providers at public health institutions in Harari region, eastern Ethiopia: a cross-sectional study," *BMC Research Notes*, vol. 8, no. 1, pp. 1–7, 2015.

[24] V. M. Ma, K. Van Dam, and A. Van Zundert, "Job satisfaction amongst Dutch nurse anaesthetists: the influence of emotions on events," *International Nursing Review*, vol. 57, no. 1, pp. 85–91, 2010.

[25] K. Van Dam, C. Brown-mahoney, and H. T. A. Knape, "Work climate related to job satisfaction. Among Dutch nurse anesthetists," *AANA Journal*, vol. 79, no. 1, pp. 63–70, 2011.

[26] S. I. Dugguh, "Job satisfaction theories: traceability to employee performance in organizations," *IOSR Journal of Business and Management*, vol. 16, no. 5, pp. 11–18, 2014.

# 21

# Efficacy of Continuous S(+)-Ketamine Infusion for Postoperative Pain Control

**Luiz Eduardo de Paula Gomes Miziara,[1] Ricardo Francisco Simoni,[1,2] Luís Otávio Esteves,[1] Luis Henrique Cangiani,[1] Gil Fernando Ribeiro Grillo-Filho,[1] and Anderson Garcia Lima e Paula[1]**

[1]*Department of Anesthesiology, Centro Médico Campinas, Rua Edilberto Luis Pereira da Silva 150, Campinas, SP, Brazil*
[2]*Department of Pharmacology, Universidade de Campinas (UNICAMP), Centro Médico Campinas, Rua Edilberto Luis Pereira da Silva 150, 13083-190 Campinas, SP, Brazil*

Correspondence should be addressed to Luiz Eduardo de Paula Gomes Miziara; miziara.luiz@cmcnet.com.br

Academic Editor: Jean Jacques Lehot

*Aim.* A double-blind, randomized, placebo-controlled trial was designed to evaluate the efficacy of continuous intraoperative infusion of S(+)-ketamine under intravenous anesthesia with target-controlled infusion of remifentanil and propofol for postoperative pain control. *Methods.* Forty-eight patients undergoing laparoscopic cholecystectomy were assigned to receive continuous S(+)-ketamine infusion at a rate of 0.3 $mg{\cdot}kg^{-1}{\cdot}h^{-1}$ ($n$ = 24, intervention group) or an equivalent volume of saline at the same rate ($n$ = 24, placebo group). The same target-controlled intravenous anesthesia was induced in both groups. Pain was assessed using a 0 to 10 verbal numeric rating scale during the first 12 postoperative hours. Pain scores and morphine consumption were recorded in the postanesthesia care unit (PACU) and at 4 and 12 hours after surgery. *Results.* Pain scores were lower in the intervention group at all time points. Morphine consumption did not differ significantly between groups during PACU stay, but it was significantly lower in the intervention group at each time point after PACU discharge ($P$ = 0.0061). At 12 hours after surgery, cumulative morphine consumption was also lower in the intervention group (5.200 ± 2.707) than in the placebo group (7.525 ± 1.872). *Conclusions.* Continuous S(+)-ketamine infusion during laparoscopic cholecystectomy under target-controlled intravenous anesthesia provided better postoperative pain control than placebo, reducing morphine requirement.

## 1. Introduction

Postoperative pain control with multimodal analgesia is important not only to relieve pain but also to reduce postoperative side effects, such as nausea, vomiting, need for sedation, and length of hospital stay. Therefore, adjuvant drugs with proven efficacy in this type of analgesia are very useful for anesthesiologists.

Several experimental and clinical studies suggest that the administration of potent short-acting opioids, such as remifentanil, is associated with central sensitization to pain, a phenomenon known as opioid-induced hyperalgesia [1–4]. The activation of N-methyl-D-aspartate (NMDA) receptors has been suggested to be the main mechanism facilitating the response to sensory stimuli and leading to opioid-induced hyperalgesia, along with a state of excitability in the spinal cord dorsal horn.

One of the two subunits of the NMDA, namely, subunit 2B (NR2B), has an important role in the genesis of remifentanil-induced hyperalgesia and inflammatory hyperalgesia caused by the induction of long-term potentiation. A previous study found that increased tyrosine phosphorylation in this subunit may be prevented with the use of ketamine [5].

Although ketamine acts on several receptors, its analgesic effects result mainly from the fact that it is a NMDA receptor antagonist that prevents central sensitization [2, 6] and inhibits this receptor by reducing mean time and frequency of NMDA receptor channel opening, the latter through an allosteric mechanism. Therefore, ketamine has been widely used to investigate the role of the NMDA receptor in several animal and human models.

S(+)-ketamine is a ketamine isomer that acts by changing channel opening time through noncompetitive blockade [7]. Furthermore, compared with the racemic mixture, it has a twofold higher analgesic potency [7, 8] and a three- to fourfold greater affinity for the intrachannel phencyclidine receptor site, which is the site of action of S(+)-ketamine.

The present study was designed to evaluate the efficacy of continuous intraoperative infusion of S(+)-ketamine for pain control after laparoscopic cholecystectomy under target-controlled total intravenous anesthesia, testing the hypothesis that S(+)-ketamine is more effective than placebo in the control of postoperative pain.

## 2. Methods

This double-blind, randomized, placebo-controlled trial was conducted at Centro Médico Campinas, Brazil, from June 2012 to February 2014, and participants were recruited among patients scheduled for laparoscopic cholecystectomy during this period. After approval of the study by the Research Ethics Committee, all participants signed the informed consent form. The trial is registered at ClinicalTrials.gov, number NCT02421913. Eligible participants were all patients aged 18–65 years with American Society of Anesthesiologists Physical Status (ASA PS) classes 1-2. Exclusion criteria were use of alcohol or illicit drugs, H2 inhibitors, opioids, or calcium channel blockers in the last 10 days, chronic pain, myocardial ischemia, or psychiatric disorders.

Sample size was calculated based on the results of a previous pilot study. To detect a difference of at least 38% in pain scores in the postanesthesia care unit (PACU) between the intervention and placebo groups, with an alpha error of 5% and a beta error of 20%, a sample size of at least 21 patients per group was required to achieve 80% power and a 95% confidence interval. Three more patients were added to each group to account for possible losses to follow-up during the trial.

Participants were randomly assigned in a 1:1 ratio to receive either S(+)-ketamine or placebo during laparoscopic cholecystectomy. The randomization sequence was created by an anesthesiologist with no involvement in the care of participants using the Randomizer software (https://www.randomizer.org/). All participants and the anesthesiologist performing the laparoscopic cholecystectomy were kept blind to group assigment. The allocation sequence was concealed in sequentially numbered, sealed envelopes. In order to preserve the double-blind nature of the study, the envelopes were opened by a third person with no involvement in the anesthetic procedure, who prepared a 50 mL syringe containing either S(+)-ketamine (intervention group) or saline (placebo group). In case of emergency, the anesthesiologist responsible for the care of the patient was allowed to violate the protocol and be informed about the group to which the patient was assigned.

No preanesthetic medication was administered to patients. Mean noninvasive blood pressure (MBP), ECG, pulse oximetry ($SpO_2$), bispectral index (BIS), and capnography were monitored in all patients after tracheal intubation.

After venipuncture, patients received intravenous parecoxib sodium (40 mg). Anesthesia was induced with midazolam at a dose of $0.05\ mg{\cdot}kg^{-1}$ and target-controlled infusions of propofol (target dose of $3.0\ \mu{\cdot}mL^{-1}$) and remifentanil (target dose of $6.0\ ng{\cdot}mL^{-1}$) using the Marsh pharmacokinetic model with ke0 of $1.21\ min^{-1}$ and the Minto pharmacokinetic model, respectively. Unconsciousness was determined by loss of corneal and palpebral reflexes and confirmed by a BIS $< 50$. Rocuronium ($0.6\ mg{\cdot}kg^{-1}$) was then administered. Immediately after tracheal intubation, the target dose of propofol was adjusted to maintain BIS between 35 and 50 and the target dose of remifentanil was reduced to $3\ ng{\cdot}mL^{-1}$. Five minutes before surgery, patients assigned to the intervention group received continuous S(+)-ketamine infusion at a rate of $0.3\ mg{\cdot}kg^{-1}{\cdot}h^{-1}$, and patients assigned to the placebo group received an equivalent volume of saline at the same rate.

At the beginning of surgery, the target dose of remifentanil was increased to 5 ng·mL and adjusted intraoperatively to maintain MBP ± 15% of baseline levels, while the target dose of propofol was adjusted intraoperatively to maintain BIS between 35 and 50. At the end of the procedure, neuromuscular blockade was reversed with sugammadex. Additionally, propofol and remifentanil infusions were discontinued, as well as S(+)-ketamine and saline infusions in the intervention and placebo groups.

The duration of anesthesia, duration of surgery, time until awakening (spontaneous opening of the eyes and/or BIS $> 70$), and overall dose of S(+)-ketamine, remifentanil, and propofol infused per total body weight were recorded. Patients were extubated in the operating room and transferred to the PACU, where postoperative pain was assessed using a 0 to 10 verbal numeric scale (VNS). Patients were considered pain-free if they scored $\leq 2$ and in pain if they scored $\geq 3$ on the VNS. Morphine was administered at a dose of $0.05\ mg{\cdot}kg^{-1}$ when the patient reported pain for the first time and at a dose of $0.025\ mg{\cdot}kg^{-1}$ on subsequent occasions. Pain scores were recorded in the PACU and at 4 and 12 hours after the end of surgery, and patients were continuously monitored during their PACU stay by one of the anesthesiologists responsible for this clinical trial. Patients were assessed by the same anesthesiologist every 20 minutes after being discharged from PACU and within the first 4 hours after surgery and every 40 minutes from the fourth to the twelfth hour after surgery. All patients were instructed to call for the presence of the anesthesiologist responsible for the surgical procedure, either verbally or using an individual alarm device, at any time between these assessments in case of pain or any other unpleasant effect.

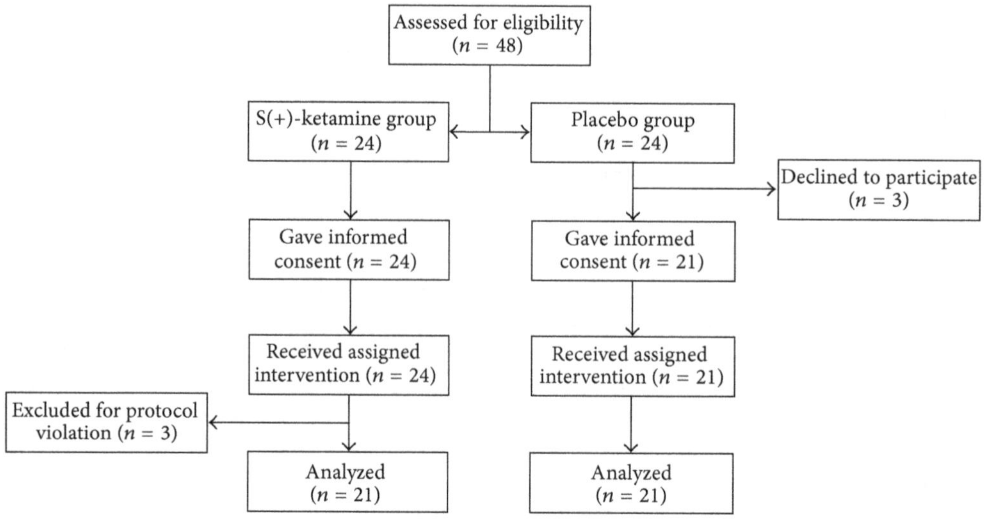


FIGURE 1: Patient flow chart.

Parametric variables were analyzed using Student's $t$-test, and nonparametric variables were analyzed using the Mann-Whitney $U$ test. Variables were expressed as mean and standard deviation (SD). Differences were considered significant when the $P$ value was less than 0.05.

## 3. Results

A total of 48 patients were enrolled in the trial: 24 were randomized to S(+)-ketamine and 24 to placebo. Three patients from the placebo group refused to participate in the study. Of 24 patients who received continuous S(+)-ketamine infusion, three were excluded for protocol violation. Therefore, the final analysis included 42 patients, 21 in the S(+)-ketamine group and 21 in the placebo group (Figure 1).

Patients' demographic data were similar in both groups. There was no difference between groups regarding duration of surgery, duration of anesthesia, and time until awakening. There was no significant statistical difference between the two groups with regard to length of stay, but all patients stayed at the unit for 120 minutes for a more accurate evaluation of the outcomes of interest.

Mean (SD) remifentanil consumption was 0.170 (0.054) $mcg{\cdot}kg^{-1}{\cdot}min^{-1}$ in the S(+)-ketamine group and 0.228 (0.042) $mcg{\cdot}kg^{-1}{\cdot}min^{-1}$ ($P = 0.0175$) in the placebo group, and mean (SD) propofol consumption was 72.194 (11.539) $mcg{\cdot}kg^{-1}{\cdot}min^{-1}$ in the S(+)-ketamine group and 84.895 (13.739) $mcg{\cdot}kg^{-1}{\cdot}min^{-1}$ in the placebo group, with a significant difference between groups ($P = 0.0286$).

Median pain scores on the VNS during PACU stay were 5.5 in the S(+)-ketamine group and 8.5 in the placebo group ($P < 0.0001$). Pain scores decreased to 0.0 in the S(+)-ketamine group and 7.0 in the placebo group ($P = 0.0004$) at 4 hours after surgery and to 0.0 and 5.0, respectively, at 12 hours after surgery ($P = 0.0309$) (Figure 2).

There was no difference in morphine consumption during PACU stay between patients who received S(+)-ketamine

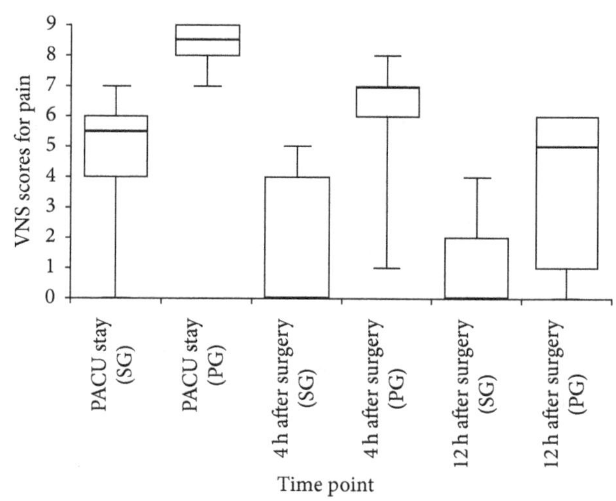


FIGURE 2: Pain scores during PACU stay and at 4 and 12 h after surgery. PACU: postanesthesia care unit; PG: placebo group; SG: S(+)-ketamine group.

(4.00 [SD, 2.29] mg) and placebo (4.30 [SD, 0.83] mg) ($P = 0.5770$). The mean (SD) dose of morphine used was 0.750 (1.198) mg in the S(+)-ketamine group and 1.825 (0.689) mg in the placebo group ($P = 0.0108$) from PACU discharge up to 4 hours after surgery and 0.450 (0.93) mg and 1.400 (0.99) mg, respectively, ($P = 0.0089$) between 4 and 12 hours after surgery, with statistically significant differences at these time points. Cumulative morphine consumption was significantly lower in the S(+)-ketamine group than in the placebo group (5.200 [SD, 2.707] mg versus 7.525 [SD, 1.872] mg; $P = 0.0061$) (Figure 3).

The following postoperative side effects were recorded: nausea (1 patient in the S(+)-ketamine and 2 patients in the placebo group), agitation (2 patients in the S(+)-ketamine group), and hallucination (1 patient in the S(+)-ketamine group), with no difference between groups.

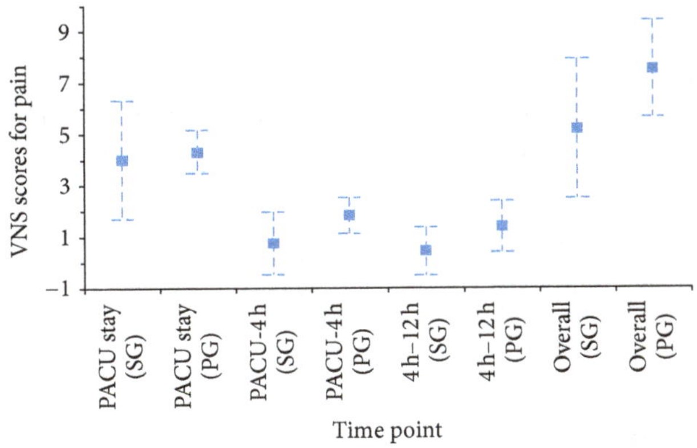


FIGURE 3: Morphine consumption during PACU stay and at 4 and 12 h after surgery. 4 h–12 h: from 4 to 12 h after surgery; PACU: postanesthesia care unit; PACU-4 h: from PACU discharge up to 4 h after surgery; PG: placebo group; SG: S(+)-ketamine group.

## 4. Discussion

In the current study, continuous intraoperative infusion of S(+)-ketamine (at a rate of 0.3 mg·kg$^{-1}$·h$^{-1}$) in patients under intravenous anesthesia with target-controlled infusion of remifentanil and propofol provided better postoperative pain control than placebo over the first 12 hours after laparoscopic cholecystectomy.

Continuous infusion of remifentanil has been associated with the development of opioid-induced hyperalgesia [9, 10]. Experimental studies have shown that patients become rapidly tolerant to infusion of potent short-acting opioids such as remifentanil. The mechanisms involved in this tolerance include activation of NMDA receptors in the spinal cord dorsal horn [2, 6, 11], inactivation of $\mu$-opioid receptors [12], spinal dynorphin release [13], and upregulation of cyclic adenosine monophosphate [14].

The time of recovery from anesthesia with remifentanil is relatively dose independent. Thus, this drug can be administered at high doses during surgery with low risk of delayed postoperative recovery or respiratory depression. However, high doses of remifentanil administered intraoperatively are more closely related to the induction of postoperative secondary hyperalgesia as compared to long-acting opioids [2, 4, 15], requiring higher doses of morphine in the postoperative period to provide appropriate analgesia [16]. In a study with healthy human volunteers, a skin area with preexisting mechanical hyperalgesia was significantly enlarged 60–90 minutes after remifentanil infusion [17].

NMDA receptors are complexes formed by at least two types of subunits: NR1A/B and NR1A/2B. Subunit 2B (NR2B) is particularly important, because of its role in the organization of sensory pathways and in the development of neuropathic pain [18, 19].

A previous study has shown that propofol acts as a NMDA receptor antagonist on the NR1 subunit. This phenomenon was mediated by a signaling mechanism involving the activation of protein phosphatase 2A and thus may have some effect on reducing opioid-induced hyperalgesia [20].

Tyrosine phosphorylation in the NR2B subunit has an important role in the induction of long-term potentiation, a phenomenon associated with central sensitization [21] and with the onset and development of inflammatory hyperalgesia [11]. Remifentanil-induced hyperalgesia has been shown to lead to a considerable increase in tyrosine phosphorylation in the NR2B subunit, and this increase may be prevented by ketamine [5]. Yuan et al. suggest that glycogen synthase kinase- (GSK-) 3 beta contributes to the development of remifentanil-induced hyperalgesia through the regulation of NMDA receptor subunits (NR1 and NR2B) in the spinal cord and that inhibition of GSK-3 beta may be effective in the treatment of hyperalgesia [22].

Kingston et al. [20] showed the antagonist effect of propofol on NMDA receptors. Cerebral mechanisms may be important for the results obtained by the interaction between remifentanil and S-ketamine, because several pain pathways are influenced differently by one of the two drugs. Remifentanil directly inhibits nociceptive information through opioid receptors located in the nervous system, whereas S(+)-ketamine acts on brain structures such as insula and anterior cortex, thus modulating the emotional aspect of pain [23]. Gupta et al. suggest an important synergism between ketamine and opioids [24]. In the S(+)-ketamine group, there was a decrease in propofol and remifentanil consumption, but future studies are needed to establish more accurate correlations and conclusions on the specific interactions between these drugs.

The blockade of NMDA receptor with the administration of ketamine suppressed the development of opioid-induced hyperalgesia and injury-induced central sensitization even when ketamine was given at subanesthetic doses [25]. Clinical studies have demonstrated the efficacy of ketamine in the control of acute postoperative pain in several surgical procedures. Results have shown reduced pain scores and analgesic consumption even after the end of the duration of action of ketamine.

A systematic review concluded that intravenous ketamine is an effective adjunct for postoperative analgesia, being particularly beneficial in abdominal, thoracic, and orthopedic surgeries [6]. However, an opposite result was found by a meta-analysis on the use of NMDA receptor antagonists to control pain and remifentanil-induced hyperalgesia [2].

The reduced remifentanil consumption in the S(+)-ketamine group may have contributed to reduction of postoperative hyperalgesia. Guignard et al. concluded that higher doses of remifentanil in the intraoperative period lead to an increase in pain and in the postoperative consumption of morphine [9].

Hang et al. concluded that the effective dose of ketamine in 50% and 95% of patients ($ED_{50}$ and $ED_{95}$) for prevention of postoperative hyperalgesia after remifentanil-based anesthesia was 0.24 mg/kg and 0.33 mg/kg, respectively [15]. In another study, Untergehrer et al. used S(+)-ketamine at continuous infusion rates from 0.25 to 0.50 mg·kg·h as subanesthetic doses [1].

The rate of continuous S(+)-ketamine infusion used in this study (0.3 mg·kg$^{-1}$·h$^{-1}$) is associated with effective analgesia [1, 15], whereas higher doses of S(+)-ketamine are associated with side effects leading to cognitive changes, such as hallucinations and unpleasant dreams, and with mood, perception, and consciousness changes. According to the pharmacokinetic model proposed by White et al. [26], a 0.3 mg/kg/h infusion for 16 minutes would lead to a concentration effect of 70 ng/mL. Since our surgical team started to perform surgery 11 minutes after anesthetic induction, on average, we decided to start the infusion 5 minutes before anesthetic induction. Koppert et al. used a similar dose of S ketamine in another study, also without an initial bolus [27].

The current study evaluated the effect of S(+)-ketamine using pain scores and overall consumption of morphine recorded over a 12-hour period after the end of surgery. The presence of any postoperative side effects was also noted. Despite the lower morphine requirement in the S(+)-ketamine group, the incidence of postoperative side effects did not differ significantly between groups.

The main limitation of this study is the lack of a longer follow-up throughout the postoperative period, which prevented us from drawing a more comprehensive conclusion on postoperative pain control. The decision to evaluate patients throughout a 12-hour period is based on the mean postoperative length of stay of patients undergoing laparoscopic cholecystectomy in our service. In addition, we believe that studying pain control in this surgery is of paramount importance, because this procedure is capable of releasing nociceptive mediators and requires a short hospital stay [28].

## 5. Conclusions

The present study tested the hypothesis that continuous infusion of low-dose S(+)-ketamine is more effective than placebo in the control of postoperative pain. Despite the lack of statistical difference in morphine consumption during PACU stay, this hypothesis is supported by our findings that continuous S(+)-ketamine infusion at a rate of $0.3\,mg{\cdot}kg^{-1}{\cdot}h^{-1}$ during laparoscopic cholecystectomy under target-controlled intravenous anesthesia reduced the overall need for postoperative morphine and VNS pain scores at all time points assessed. However, we recognize that further studies with longer postoperative follow-up are required to better understand the correlations found in this study.

## Abbreviations

ASA PS: American Society of Anesthesiologists Physical Status
GSK: Glycogen synthase kinase
NMDA: N-Methyl-D-aspartate
PACU: Postanesthesia care unit
VNS: Verbal numeric scale.

## Conflict of Interests

The authors declare that they have no competing interests.

## Authors' Contribution

Luiz Eduardo de Paula Gomes Miziara conceived the study, participated in its development and coordination, and helped to draft the paper. Ricardo Francisco Simoni participated in the design of the study, performed the statistical analysis, and helped to draft the paper. Luís Otávio Esteves, Luis Henrique Cangiani, Gil Fernando Ribeiro Grillo-Filho, and Anderson Garcia Lima e Paula participated in the development and design of the study. All authors read and approved the final paper.

## References

[1] G. Untergehrer, D. Jordan, S. Eyl, and G. Schneider, "Effects of propofol, sevoflurane, remifentanil, and (S)-ketamine in subanesthetic concentrations on visceral and somatosensory pain-evoked potentials," *Anesthesiology*, vol. 118, no. 2, pp. 308–317, 2013.

[2] Y. Liu, Y. Zheng, X. Gu, and Z. Ma, "The efficacy of NMDA receptor antagonists for preventing remifentanil-induced increase in postoperative pain and analgesic requirement: a meta-analysis," *Minerva Anestesiologica*, vol. 78, no. 6, pp. 653–667, 2012.

[3] X. Li, M. S. Angst, and J. D. Clark, "Opioid-induced hyperalgesia and incisional pain," *Anesthesia and Analgesia*, vol. 93, no. 1, pp. 204–209, 2001.

[4] N. Derrode, F. Lebrun, J.-C. Levron, M. Chauvin, and B. Debaene, "Influence of peroperative opioid on postoperative pain after major abdominal surgery: sufentanil TCI versus remifentanil TCI. A randomized, controlled study," *British Journal of Anaesthesia*, vol. 91, no. 6, pp. 842–849, 2003.

[5] X. Gu, X. Wu, Y. Liu, S. Cui, and Z. Ma, "Tyrosine phosphorylation of the N-Methyl-D-Aspartate receptor 2B subunit in spinal cord contributes to remifentanil-induced postoperative hyperalgesia: The preventive effect of ketamine," *Molecular Pain*, vol. 5, article 76, 2009.

[6] K. Laskowski, A. Stirling, W. P. McKay, and H. J. Lim, "A systematic review of intravenous ketamine for postoperative analgesia," *Canadian Journal of Anesthesia*, vol. 58, no. 10, pp. 911–923, 2011.

[7] P. C. Leal, R. K. Sakata, R. Salomão, E. J. Sadatsune, and A. M. Issy, "Avaliação do efeito da cetamina associada à remifentanila na dor pós-operatória," *Revista Brasileira de Anestesiologia*, vol. 63, pp. 178–182, 2013.

[8] W. Jaksch, S. Lang, R. Reichhalter, G. Raab, K. Dann, and S. Fitzal, "Perioperative small-dose S(+)-ketamine has no incremental beneficial effects on postoperative pain when standard-practice opioid infusions are used," *Anesthesia and Analgesia*, vol. 94, no. 4, pp. 981–986, 2002.

[9] B. Guignard, A. E. Bossard, C. Coste et al., "Acute opioid tolerance: intraoperative remifentanil increases postoperative pain and morphine requirement," *Anesthesiology*, vol. 93, no. 2, pp. 409–417, 2000.

[10] H. R. Vinik and I. Kissin, "Rapid development of tolerance to analgesia during remifentanil infusion in humans," *Anesthesia and Analgesia*, vol. 86, no. 6, pp. 1307–1311, 1998.

[11] W. Guo, F. Wei, S. Zou et al., "Group I metabotropic glutamate receptor NMDA receptor coupling and signaling cascade mediate spinal dorsal horn NMDA receptor 2B tyrosine phosphorylation associated with inflammatory hyperalgesia," *Journal of Neuroscience*, vol. 24, no. 41, pp. 9161–9173, 2004.

[12] J. A. Trafton, C. Abbadie, K. Marek, and A. I. Basbaum, "Postsynaptic signaling via the $\mu$-opioid receptor: responses of dorsal horn neurons to exogenous opioids and noxious stimulation," *Journal of Neuroscience*, vol. 20, no. 23, pp. 8578–8584, 2000.

[13] L. R. Gardell, R. Wang, S. E. Burgess et al., "Sustained morphine exposure induces a spinal dynorphin-dependent enhancement of excitatory transmitter release from primary afferent fibers," *The Journal of Neuroscience*, vol. 22, no. 15, pp. 6747–6755, 2002.

[14] S. L. Borgland, "Acute opioid receptor desensitization and tolerance: is there a link?" *Clinical and Experimental Pharmacology and Physiology*, vol. 28, no. 3, pp. 147–154, 2001.

[15] L.-H. Hang, D.-H. Shao, Y.-P. Gu, L. A. Colvin, and M. T. Fallon, "The ED50and ED95of ketamine for prevention of postoperative hyperalgesia after remifentanil-based anaesthesia in patients undergoing laparoscopic cholecystectomy," *Swiss Medical Weekly*, vol. 141, Article ID w13195, 2011.

[16] V. Joly, P. Richebe, B. Guignard et al., "Remifentanil-induced postoperative hyperalgesia and its prevention with small-dose ketamine," *Anesthesiology*, vol. 103, no. 1, pp. 147–155, 2005.

[17] M. S. Angst, W. Koppert, I. Pahl, D. J. Clark, and M. Schmelz, "Short-term infusion of the mu-opioid agonist remifentanil in humans causes hyperalgesia during withdrawal," *Pain*, vol. 106, no. 1-2, pp. 49–57, 2003.

[18] W. Zhang, C.-X. Shi, X.-P. Gu, Z.-L. Ma, and W. Zhu, "Ifenprodil induced antinociception and decreased the expression of NR2B subunits in the dorsal horn after chronic dorsal root ganglia compression in rats," *Anesthesia and Analgesia*, vol. 108, no. 3, pp. 1015–1020, 2009.

[19] X. Gu, J. Zhang, Z. Ma et al., "The role of N-methyl-d-aspartate receptor subunit NR2B in spinal cord in cancer pain," *European Journal of Pain*, vol. 14, no. 5, pp. 496–502, 2010.

[20] S. Kingston, L. Mao, L. Yang, A. Arora, E. E. Fibuch, and J. Q. Wang, "Propofol inhibits phosphorylation of N-methyl-D-aspartate receptor NR1 subunits in neurons," *Anesthesiology*, vol. 104, no. 4, pp. 763–769, 2006.

[21] J. A. P. Rostas, V. A. Brent, K. Voss, M. L. Errington, T. V. P. Bliss, and J. W. Gurd, "Enhanced tyrosine phosphorylation of the 2B subunit of the N-methyl-D-aspartate receptor in long-term potentiation," *Proceedings of the National Academy of Sciences of the United States of America*, vol. 93, no. 19, pp. 10452–10456, 1996.

[22] Y. Yuan, J.-Y. Wang, F. Yuan, K.-L. Xie, Y.-H. Yu, and G.-L. Wang, "Glycogen synthase kinase-3beta contributes to remifentanil-induced postoperative hyperalgesia via regulating N-methyl-D-aspartate receptor trafficking," *Anesthesia and Analgesia*, vol. 116, no. 2, pp. 473–481, 2013.

[23] T. Sprenger, M. Valet, R. Woltmann et al., "Imaging pain modulation by subanesthetic S-(+)-ketamine," *Anesthesia & Analgesia*, vol. 103, no. 3, pp. 729–737, 2006.

[24] A. Gupta, L. A. Devi, and I. Gomes, "Potentiation of $\mu$-opioid receptor-mediated signaling by ketamine," *Journal of Neurochemistry*, vol. 119, no. 2, pp. 294–302, 2011.

[25] J.-P. Laulin, P. Maurette, J.-B. Corcuff, C. Rivat, M. Chauvin, and G. Simonnet, "The role of ketamine in preventing fentanyl-induced hyperalgesia and subsequent acute morphine tolerance," *Anesthesia and Analgesia*, vol. 94, no. 5, pp. 1263–1269, 2002.

[26] M. White, P. de Graaff, B. Renshof, E. van Kan, and M. Dzoljic, "Pharmacokinetics of S(+) ketamine derived from target controlled infusion," *British Journal of Anaesthesia*, vol. 96, no. 3, pp. 330–334, 2006.

[27] W. Koppert, R. Sittl, K. Scheuber, M. Alsheimer, M. Schmelz, and J. Schüttler, "Differential modulation of remifentanil-induced analgesia and postinfusion hyperalgesia by S-ketamine and clonidine in humans," *Anesthesiology*, vol. 99, no. 1, pp. 152–159, 2003.

[28] R. F. Simoni, L. M. Cangiani, A. M. S. A. Pereira, M. P. Abreu, L. H. Cangiani, and G. Zemi, "Efficacy of intraoperative methadone and clonidine in pain control in the immediate postoperative period after the use of remifentanil," *Revista Brasileira de Anestesiologia*, vol. 59, no. 4, pp. 421–430, 2009.

22

# Intubation Success through I-Gel® and Intubating Laryngeal Mask Airway® using Flexible Silicone Tubes

**Latha Naik,[1] Neerja Bhardwaj,[1] Indu Mohini Sen,[1] and Rakesh V. Sondekoppam[2]**

[1] *Department of Anaesthesia and Intensive Care Medicine, Postgraduate Institute of Medical Education and Research, Chandigarh 160012, India*
[2] *Department of Anesthesia and Perioperative Medicine, Schulich School of Medicine and Dentistry, Western University, London, ON, Canada N6A 5A5*

Correspondence should be addressed to Latha Naik; lathabmc@gmail.com

Academic Editor: Kouichiro Minami

*Introduction.* The study aims to test whether flexible silicone tubes (FST) improve performance and provide similar intubation success through I-Gel as compared to ILMA. Our trial is registered in CTRI and the registration number is "CTRI/2016/06/006997." *Methods.* One hundred and twenty ASA status I-II patients scheduled for elective surgical procedures needing tracheal intubation were randomised to endotracheal intubation using FST through either I-Gel or ILMA. In the ILMA group ($n$ = 60), intubation was attempted through ILMA using FST and, in the I-Gel group ($n$ = 60), FST was inserted through I-Gel airway. *Results.* Successful intubation was achieved in 36.67% (95% CI 24.48%–48.86%) on first attempt through I-Gel ($n$ = 22/60) compared to 68.33% (95% CI 56.56%–80.1%) in ILMA ($n$ = 41/60) ($p$ = 0.001). The overall intubation success rate was also lower with I-Gel group [58.3% (95% CI 45.82%–70.78%); $n$ = 35] compared to ILMA [90% (95% CI 82.41%–97.59%); $n$ = 54] ($p < 0.001$). The number of attempts, ease of intubation, and time to intubation were longer with I-Gel compared to ILMA. There were no differences in the other secondary outcomes. *Conclusion.* The first pass success rate and overall success of FST through an I-Gel airway were inferior to those of ILMA.

## 1. Introduction

Supraglottic airway (SGA) devices are commonly used adjuncts to secure the airway during anesthesia or resuscitation and are an integral part of difficult airway algorithm for either elective or rescue use [1, 2]. Commonly used SGAs such as classic or proseal LMA are not ideal intubation aids as the airway conduit is either too narrow to accommodate an adult diameter endotracheal tube (ETT) or too long for the tracheal tube to reach the trachea. Additionally, CLMA is not sufficiently rigid to align the LMA with the glottic inlet [3]. The Intubating Laryngeal Mask Airway (ILMA) was introduced in 1997 for clinical use and is currently the "gold standard" for tracheal intubation through SGA either blindly or by fiberscope guidance [4–7]. I-Gel is a SGA with a noninflatable cuff made of medical grade thermoplastic called Styrene Ethylene Butadiene Styrene (SEBS). The device is known to be easier to insert [8, 9], by segregating the laryngeal opening from the oropharyngeal orifice allowing better support of the perilaryngeal structures. It results in higher sealing pressures by matching the peripharyngeal anatomy despite the absence of an inflatable cuff [10]. In a cadaveric study full glottis view was obtained in 60% of the cases soon after I-Gel insertion while some glottic opening was visible in 95% of the cases [11]. The airway channel is situated deep inside the bowl of the cuff and along with the epiglottic rest is known to ensure fresh gas flow irrespective of the downfolding of epiglottis. I-Gel has also been used as a conduit for endotracheal intubation in both mannequin and humans [12, 13].

Intubation through an ILMA requires the use of a wire-reinforced flexible silicone tube (FST). The FST is proposed

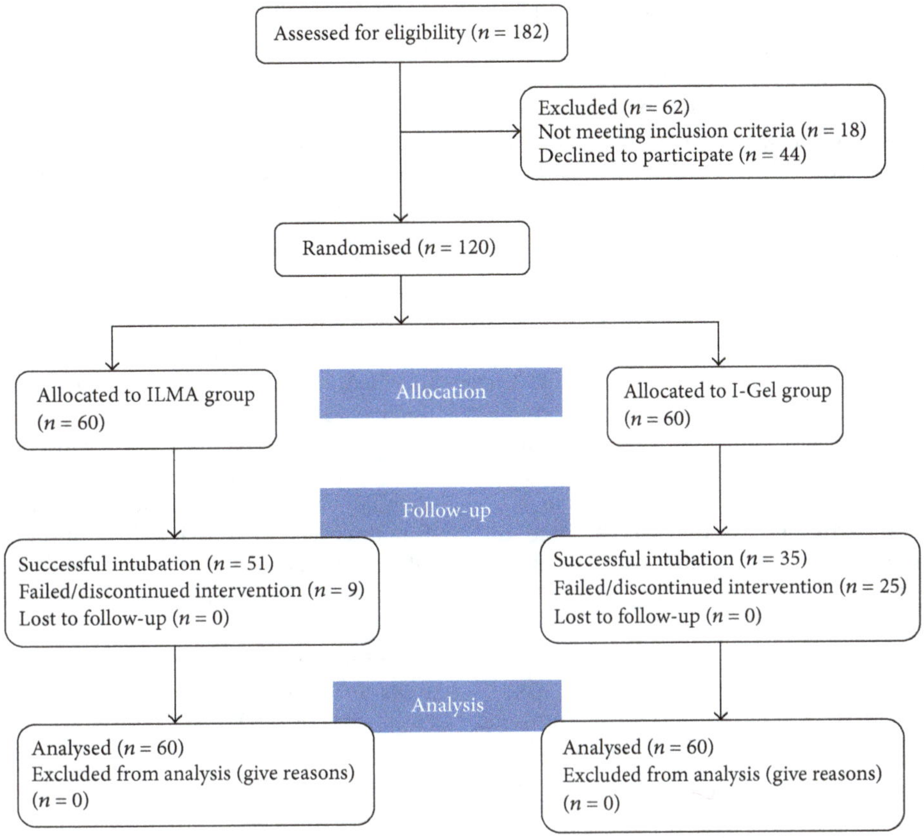


FIGURE 1: CONSORT diagram.

to have unique features best suited for its use through an SGA and include the soft moulded tip, the position of the inflation balloon within the tube wall, and the low volume cuff all of which make it easier to enter the laryngeal inlet compared to conventional PVC tubes. The wire-reinforced FST is also known to emerge at a lower angle than a normal PVC tube (47°) and hence does not abut anteriorly against the larynx, cricothyroid membrane, or trachea. The reported first pass success rate of intubation with an ILMA using the FST is in the range of 50–78.9% [14–17] whereas the same using a PVC tube ranges within 78.5%–86.7% [18, 19]. Although FST has been used for intubation through ILMA, success rate of intubation using FST through I-Gel has not been studied in normal airways. Since FST follows the curvature of the SGA, and I-Gel has been shown to conform well with the laryngeal inlet, we hypothesised that intubation success would be noninferior between the two devices utilizing FST for intubation. The primary outcome measure was the first pass success rate and the secondary outcome measures were the overall success rate, adverse events, and time to insertion and intubation of the two devices.

## 2. Materials and Methods

The study was conducted in a public tertiary care hospital in India between January 2012 and October 2012. Ethical approval for the study (8561/PG-2Trg/2010/9) was provided by the Postgraduate Institute of Medical Education and Research ethics committee, PGIMER, Chandigarh, India, on 11 December 2011. After taking informed consent, a total of 120 patients of either sex were included in the study on an intention to treat analysis basis (Figure 1: CONSORT diagram). The inclusion criteria for the study were age between 18 and 60 years, American Society of Anesthesiologists (ASA) physical status scores of I-II, 50–90 kg weight, and being scheduled to undergo elective surgical procedures requiring tracheal intubation. The patients were randomised into two groups: ILMA group (Group I, $n = 60$) and I-Gel group (Group G, $n = 60$) based on computer generated random number table (generated by NB). Patients with an ASA score III or IV, any contraindication to the use of muscle relaxants, presence of predictors of difficulty in intubation or ventilation, any increased risk of aspiration, or having a history of symptomatic gastroesophageal reflux were excluded from the study. Patients with high arched palate, restricted neck movement, or tonsillar hypertrophy were also excluded from the study.

All patients fasted overnight and received premedication with oral alprazolam 0.25 mg and ranitidine 150 mg the night before and on the morning of surgery. Preinduction monitoring included electrocardiography (ECG), noninvasive blood pressure (NIBP), and oxygen saturation ($SpO_2$). Neuromuscular monitoring using train of four (TOF) was instituted after induction of anesthesia. After securing intravenous access, patients were preoxygenated for 3 minutes. Anesthesia was induced with 2 μg/kg fentanyl and propofol 2 mg/kg. After confirming adequate bag-mask ventilation, atracurium 0.5 mg/kg was administered. Anesthesia was maintained with propofol infusion (100–150 μg/kg/min) and 100% oxygen. After complete neuromuscular blockade (TOF count 0) the supraglottic device size 4 was inserted according to the group allocation. SGA was inserted keeping the patient's head in neutral position in both the groups and in the ILMA group the cuff was inflated with 30 mL of air. Blind intubation was attempted using 7.0 mm ID FST. Appropriate placement of the device and intubation was confirmed by observation of adequate chest expansion and appearance of $ETCO_2$ waveform. Once the successful intubation was confirmed, SGA was removed using a stabilising rod. A maximum of three attempts were allowed per patient before considering the device as a failure. Intraoperatively, haemodynamic parameters were monitored every 1 minute for the first ten minutes and at 10-minute intervals thereafter till 30 minutes. Time (seconds) to successful insertion of the device (from picking the device to visible chest rise), number of attempts taken to insert the device, time to successful intubation (from the time of picking the tube from the table to visible chest rise), ease of intubation (easy/no resistance = 1, minimal resistance = 2, significant resistance = 3, or impossible = 4), airway reaction (laryngospasm, bronchospasm, coughing, and gagging), visible blood on the airway device, and any evidence of regurgitation were also noted.

On completion of the surgical procedure, propofol infusion was stopped. The duration of the surgical procedure and total propofol administered in the first hour were noted. When the TOF count was 3 or 4, neuromuscular blockade was reversed with neostigmine 0.05 mg/kg and glycopyrrolate 0.01 mg/kg. ETT was removed at TOF ratio of 90% and patient's responsiveness was assessed.

In the Post-Anaesthesia Care Unit (PACU), patients were queried for sore throat (visual analogue scale (VAS); VAS > 3 was considered significant), dysphagia (dysphagia scoring system; 0 = able to eat normal diet/no dysphagia, 1 = able to swallow some solid foods, 2 = able to swallow only semisolid foods, 3 = able to swallow liquids only, and 4 = unable to swallow anything/total dysphagia), ear/jaw/neck pain, and hoarseness of voice soon after the procedure (0 hour) and after 24 hours.

## 3. Statistical Analysis

The success rate of blind endotracheal intubation through the ILMA in first attempt using PVC has been found to be 66% [3, 4] (ranging from 50 to 80% [20]). Assuming similar success rates (74%) [18] with the use of silicone tubes in both SGA and a noninferiority limit of 30%, a total of 54 patients (27 patients per group) were required to be 80% sure that the upper limit of a one-sided 95% confidence interval (or equivalently a 90% two-sided confidence interval) will exclude a difference in favour of the standard group of more than 30% [21]. Hence we recruited a total of 120 patients (60 patients per group) to account for possible attrition of cases.

The statistical analysis was carried out using statistical package for social sciences (SPSS Inc., Chicago, IL, version 17 for windows). Normality of distribution was calculated using Shapiro-Wilk's test. Normally distributed data were compared using Student's "$t$" test and skewed data or scores were compared using Mann-Whitney $U$ test. Qualitative or categorical variables were described as frequencies or proportions and compared using Fishers exact test. Repeated measures ANOVA was used for the continuous variables, namely, heart rate and systolic and diastolic blood pressure. Each variable was first tested for the assumption of sphericity using Mauchly's test. All the variables had violation of sphericity and hence the differences in the observations of a variable over time were assessed using Greenhouse-Geisser and Huynh-Feldt corrections both within groups and between the groups. If there was a significant difference within a variable, pairwise comparison was used to find out at what time intervals the individual variations differed significantly with the baseline measurement. Bootstrapping for insertion parameters of the SGA and ETT was performed with 5000 bootstrap samples and the mean (95% CI) was obtained. The bootstrapped means were also compared between the two groups. All statistical tests were 2-sided and performed at a significance level of $\alpha = 0.05$.

## 4. Results

In this prospective, randomised clinical trial, a total of 182 patients were approached for the study (from November 2011 to October 2012) out of which 62 were found to be ineligible for the study (44 had some predictors of difficult airway; 18 did not consent for the study) and finally 120 patients were included. All recruited patients completed the study and hence were included for the final analysis (Figure 1). The two groups were comparable for age, weight, gender distribution, ASA physical status, and airway assessment (Table 1).

The number of attempts required for placement of I-Gel was comparable to that with ILMA ($p = 0.171$). The placement of I-Gel was easy in 42 patients, moderate in 16 patients, and difficult in 2 patients whereas the placement of ILMA was easy in 43 patients, moderate in 17 patients, and not difficult in any patient ($p = 0.755$). The time required for placement of I-Gel airway was comparable to that of ILMA ($p = 0.860$).

The overall intubation success rate was 58.3% (95% CI 45.82% to 70.78%) with I-Gel group ($n = 35/60$) compared to 90% (95% CI 82.41% to 97.59%) with ILMA ($n = 54$) ($p < 0.001$). The first pass success rate was 36.67% (95% CI 24.48% to 48.86%) with I-Gel ($n = 22/60$) compared to 68.33% (95% CI 56.56% to 80.1%) with ILMA ($n = 41/60$) ($p = 0.001$). The comparisons of 95% confidence intervals for the primary outcome of first pass success rate revealed the inferiority of intubating FST through the I-Gel in comparison to ILMA. The number of intubation attempts ($p = 0.027$) and time to intubation ($p = 0.007$) were significantly more with I-Gel compared to ILMA. Out of 35 successful attempts at insertion of device, intubation through I-Gel airway was easy in 17 cases, moderate in 13 cases, and difficult in 5 cases. Out of 54 successful attempts at device insertion

TABLE 1: Patient characteristics.

| Variable | Group G ($n = 60$) Median (95% CI) | Group I ($n = 60$) Median (95% CI) | $p$ value (sig < 0.05) |
|---|---|---|---|
| Age | 32.00 (28.52, 42.82) | 42.00 (35.68; 46.52) | 0.94 |
| Weight | 60.00 (58.88; 64.86) | 58.00 (56.52; 63.98) | 0.75 |
| Sex (M : F) | 13 : 47 | 17 : 43 | 0.39 |
| Duration of surgery | 75.00 (68.74; 115.26) | 77.50 (71.34; 95.16) | 0.86 |
| ASA status (1 : 2) | 50 : 10 | 43 : 17 | 0.12 |
| MMP (1 : 2) | 35 : 25 | 33 : 27 | 0.71 |
| TMD (cm) | 6.55 (6.55; 6.68) | 6.50 (6.53; 6.66) | 0.57 |

ASA: American Society of Anesthesiologists physical status; MMP: Mallampati score; TMD: thyromental distance.

TABLE 2: Device insertion and intubation parameters.

| Variable | Group G ($n = 60$) Median (95% CI) | Group I ($n = 60$) Median (95% CI) | $p$ value (sig < 0.05) |
|---|---|---|---|
| Number of SGA attempts | 1.00 (1.19; 2.01) | 1.00 (1.22; 1.98) | 0.171 |
| Ease of SGA insertion | 1.00 (1.05; 1.75) | 1.00 (1.01; 1.39) | 0.755 |
| Time to SGA placement | 9.28 (7.99; 13.25) | 8.50 (7.54; 10.86) | 0.860 |
| Ease of intubation | 2.00 (1.41; 1.91) | 1.00 (1.17; 1.46) | 0.017* |
| Intubation success | 58.3% ($n = 35$) | 90% ($n = 54$) | 0.000* |
| Time to intubation | 16.10 (13.49; 18.84) | 7.90 (7.81; 13.87) | 0.007* |
| Number of intubation attempts | 1.00 (0.94; 1.33) | 1.00 (0.95; 1.15) | 0.027* |
| Attempts at intubation; number (percentage) | | | |
| One | 22 (36.67) | 41 (68.3) | |
| Two | 8 (13.33) | 9 (15.0) | 0.001* |
| Three | 5 (8.3) | 4 (6.67) | |
| VAS 0 | 1.00 (0.36; 1.37) | 1.00 (1.04; 2.16) | 0.833 |
| Dysphagia 0 | 1.00 (0.92; 1.21) | 1.00 (1.04; 1.46) | 0.853 |
| VAS 24 | 0.00 (−0.03; 0.43) | 0.50 (0.28; 0.92) | 0.052 |
| Dysphagia 24 | 0.00 (−0.03; 0.15) | 0.00 (−0.02; 0.06) | 0.299 |

SGA: supraglottic airway device; VAS: visual analogue scale; * indicates $p < 0.05$.

through ILMA, intubation was easy for 39 cases, moderate for 13 cases, and difficult for 2 cases and this difference was statistically significant ($p = 0.017$) (Table 2). The bootstrapped confidence intervals for insertion parameters of SGA and ETT continued to show a statistically significant difference in time to intubation and the ease of intubation between the two groups while the rest of these parameters were comparable between the two groups (Table 3).

No airway reactions like gagging, laryngospasm, bronchospasm, or obstruction were noted during insertion of airway device in both groups. On removal of the airway device, laryngospasm was noted in one patient in each group. Blood on device was noted in 10 cases in I-Gel group and in 9 cases in ILMA group although this difference was not statistically significant. No patient had any evidence of gagging, bronchospasm, nausea/vomiting, or regurgitation on removal of devices in both the groups. There was no significant difference in the incidence of sore throat, dysphagia, and ear/jaw/neck pain between the two groups at 0 and 24 hours after surgery. The systolic blood pressure was lower from 1st min to 4th min after induction when compared to the baseline, but this was statistically significant only at 4th min ($p = 0.04$). At rest of the time intervals systolic blood pressure was comparable to the baseline (Figure 2). The heart rate and diastolic blood pressure did not show any significant difference compared to baseline in both I-Gel and ILMA groups. When the two groups were compared there were no significant differences in HR, SBP, and DBP. There was no significant difference in oxygen saturation both within group and in between groups. In no patient oxygen saturation ($SpO_2$) decreased below 95%. $EtCO_2$ levels were maintained in the normal range (35–45) in all the patients in both the groups.

## 5. Discussion

Our study shows the first pass success rate and the overall success of intubation using FST through an I-Gel airway to be inferior to that of ILMA. Intubation using FST through I-Gel had significantly higher insertion attempts and more failures and took longer intubation times in comparison to ILMA. The ease of intubation and the time to intubation

TABLE 3: Bootstrapped mean (95% CI) for device insertion and intubation parameters.

| Variable | Group G ($n = 60$) BS mean (95% CI) | Group I ($n = 60$) BS mean (95% CI) | $p$ value (sig < 0.05) |
|---|---|---|---|
| Number of SGA attempts | 1.20 (1.07; 1.36) | 1.04 (1.00; 1.08) | 0.088 |
| Ease of insertion | 1.40 (1.22; 1.60) | 1.24 (1.14; 1.35) | 0.180 |
| Ease of intubation | 1.66 (1.43; 1.89) | 1.31 (1.19; 1.46) | 0.023* |
| Time to SGA placement (min) | 10.27 (9.07; 11.65) | 9.60 (8.80; 10.44) | 0.418 |
| Time to intubation (min) | 13.39 (11.41; 15.39) | 10.11 (8.76; 11.53) | 0.012* |
| Number of intubation attempts | 1.51 (1.29; 1.76) | 1.31 (1.17; 1.48) | 0.191 |

SGA: supraglottic airway device; * indicates $p < 0.05$.

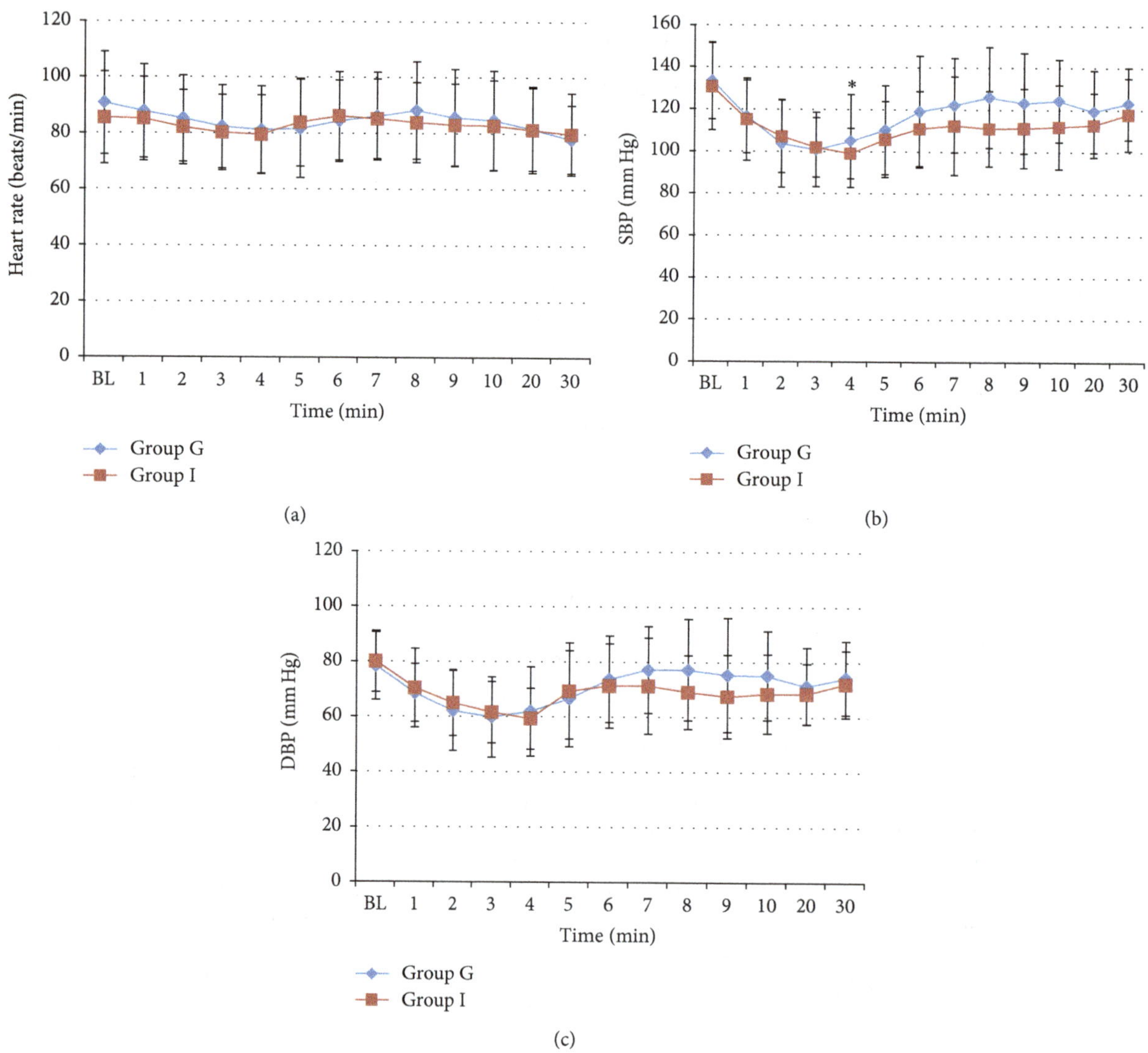


FIGURE 2: (a) Heart rate variation between two groups. (b) Systolic blood pressure variation between two groups. *$p = 0.04$, repeated measures ANOVA test. (c) Diastolic blood pressure variation between two groups.

were significantly longer with I-Gel even when corrected for skewed distribution using bootstrapping.

SGA is an integral part of difficult airway algorithm and resuscitation protocols [22]. It is also commonly used as a rescue device when a "cannot intubate, cannot ventilate" scenario arises [23]. In many scenarios the SGA could be used as a conduit for endotracheal intubation, either using a fiberscope or by blind passage. SGAs are also commonly used in out-of-hospital cardiopulmonary arrest (OHCA) and have been shown to reduce the time from collapse to

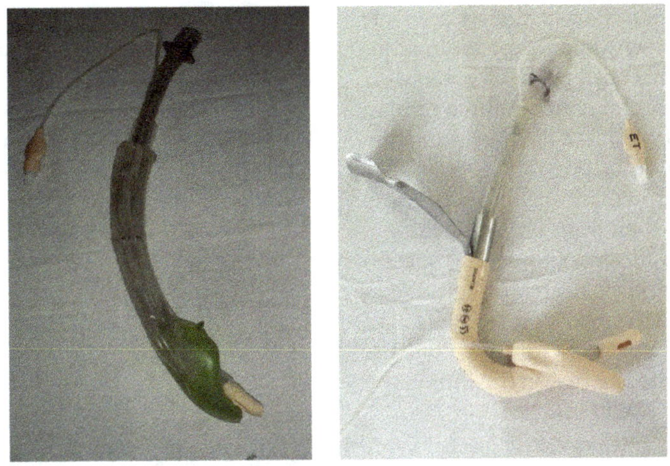

(a) (b)

FIGURE 3

securing the airway [24]. Recently the resuscitation outcomes such as survival to hospital discharge, return of spontaneous circulation, and 24-hour survival were shown to be better following endotracheal intubation in comparison to SGA when used for OHCA [25, 26]. Intubating through a SGA may thus potentially combine the best of both the devices for such scenarios. Among the studies comparing intubation success through ILMA versus I-Gel, most of the studies have utilized PVC endotracheal tubes through the I-Gel while using FST or PVC tubes through the ILMA [18, 19, 27]. Halwagi et al. [18] used PVC ETT through both devices and found that first pass success rate is 69% with the I-Gel and 74% with ILMA. The overall success rate was 73% with I-Gel and 91% with ILMA. A similar study by Kapoor et al. [19] showed that the first pass success rate of PVC ETT through the two devices was 66 and 74% while the overall success rate of intubation was 96 and 82% in I-Gel and ILMA, respectively. In a study comparing different endotracheal tubes (FST versus PVC tubes) through I-Gel and single use ILMA in patients with difficult airways, Theiler et al. [27] noted a blind intubation success rate of 15% with McGill PVC tubes and 21% with single use FST through I-Gel while the same was 69 and 60% with ILMA, respectively. The patients in the study by Theiler et al. [27] had some predictors of difficult airway which may explain the lower intubation success in their study in comparison to the present study.

The success rate of FST passage through ILMA in our study is in agreement with other studies. Whether FST is the ideal tube for blind endotracheal intubation through SGA or whether ordinary PVC tubes can be used instead has been studied by many investigators. Sharma et al. [28] found the first pass success rate through ILMA for FST to be similar to that of PVC tubes (95 versus 90 for FST and PVC, resp.). The overall success rate was 97 and 96% for FST and PVC tubes, respectively, but the time taken to perform the intubation and the number of manoeuvres were higher for PVC tubes. A recent study by Shah et al. [29] has also shown similar success rates between FST and PVC tubes through ILMA. While a study by Kundra et al. [30] showed a similar first pass (86%) and overall success rate of intubation (96%) for FST and PVC tubes, Kanazi et al. [31] showed an inferior performance of both Parker tube and PVC tubes through ILMA. The prewarming of PVC tubes [30] and use of repositioning manoeuvres did influence the success rates in both the studies [30, 31]. Although comparative studies of different endotracheal tubes through I-Gel are limited to a few studies, studies looking at the first pass and overall intubation success of PVC tubes through I-Gel report range within 65–69% and 73–87.7%, respectively [32, 33].

The overall success rate was significantly lower with I-Gel in our study (58.3%) and also intubation times were significantly longer in I-Gel group than in the ILMA group. The study by Halwagi et al. [18] contrastingly showed a longer intubation times with ILMA in comparison to I-Gel and could reflect the improvement in intubation success with ILMA on subsequent attempts in their study. The higher first pass and overall failure rate seen with I-Gel in comparison to ILMA could be explained based on the structural properties of the SGA and the FST. The flexible silicon tipped tube is a well-designed, straight, soft, wire-reinforced silicon tube which lacks wire reinforcement in the distal inch and terminates like a conical soft tip for use with ILMA. This combined with the enhanced curved shape of the ILMA leads these flexible tubes towards the plane of the glottis at an angle of 35°. The relatively straight shape of the I-Gel stem and the ending of the airway channel deep into the bowl of the cuff may direct the soft tip of FST posteriorly thereby increasing the risk of oesophageal intubation or snaring on the arytenoids (Figure 3). The more rigid PVC tubes have a fixed curvature directed anteriorly thereby better aligning the tube towards laryngeal inlet than FST when advanced through an I-Gel.

There are several limitations in our study. The patient population included in this study consists of patients with normal airways. Our current findings might not apply to patients with difficult airways. We did not perform any external laryngeal manipulation or use cricoid pressure in our study which could also have impacted the success rate of intubation in either group [33]. Although the intubations were performed by a single experienced performer, blinding to the device is not possible which may be a source of bias. Lack of visualisation of the position of the devices in relation to the laryngeal structures is another possible limitation of the present study. In addition a good mask larynx relationship was ascertained clinically rather than from fibreoptic view.

In conclusion, the first pass success and overall success rate of FST through I-Gel are inferior to those through ILMA. Further studies incorporating bronchoscopic visualisation for intubation attempts and manoeuvres to reposition the airway device may better illustrate the reason for intubation failure in I-Gel airway when FST are used.

## Competing Interests

The authors declare that there are no competing interests regarding the publication of this work.

## Acknowledgments

The study was submitted by Dr. Latha Naik for the dissertation thesis as a part of Anesthesia Residency Program (M.D. anesthesia) in Postgraduate Institute of Medical Education and Research, Chandigarh, India.

## References

[1] J. L. Benumof, "Laryngeal mask airway and the ASA difficult airway algorithm," *Anesthesiology*, vol. 84, no. 3, pp. 686–699, 1996.

[2] J. L. Benumof, "The laryngeal mask airway: indications and contraindications," *Anesthesiology*, vol. 77, no. 5, pp. 843–846, 1992.

[3] A. I. J. Brain, C. Verghese, E. V. Addy, A. Kapila, and J. Brimacombe, "The intubating laryngeal mask. II: a preliminary clinical report of a new means of intubating the trachea," *British Journal of Anaesthesia*, vol. 79, no. 6, pp. 704–709, 1997.

[4] G. Caponas, "Intubating laryngeal mask airway," *Anaesth Intensive Care*, vol. 30, no. 5, pp. 551–569, 2002.

[5] D. Z. Ferson, W. H. Rosenblatt, M. J. Johansen, I. Osborn, and A. Ovassapian, "Use of the intubating LMA-fastrach in 254 patients with difficult-to-manage airways," *Anesthesiology*, vol. 95, no. 5, pp. 1175–1181, 2001.

[6] H. G. Wakeling and A. Bagwell, "The intubating laryngeal mask airway in emergency failed intubation," *Anaesthesia*, vol. 54, pp. 305–306, 1999.

[7] X. Combes, B. Leroux, and S. Saubat, "Use of intubating laryngeal mask airway in obese patients," *Anesthesiology*, vol. 99, p. 1491, 2003.

[8] N. M. Wharton, B. Gibbison, D. A. Gabbott, G. M. Haslam, N. Muchatuta, and T. M. Cook, "I-gel insertion by novices in manikins and patients," *Anaesthesia*, vol. 63, no. 9, pp. 991–995, 2008.

[9] C. Leventis, A. Chalkias, M. A. Sampanis, X. Foulidou, and T. Xanthos, "Emergency airway management by paramedics: comparison between standard endotracheal intubation, laryngeal mask airway, and I-gel," *European Journal of Emergency Medicine*, vol. 21, no. 5, pp. 371–373, 2014.

[10] C. Janakiraman, D. B. Chethan, A. R. Wilkes, M. R. Stacey, and N. Goodwin, "A randomised crossover trial comparing the i-gel supraglottic airway and classic laryngeal mask airway," *Anaesthesia*, vol. 64, no. 6, pp. 674–678, 2009.

[11] R. M. Levitan and W. C. Kinkle, "Initial anatomic investigations of the I-gel airway: a novel supraglottic airway without inflatable cuff," *Anaesthesia*, vol. 60, no. 10, pp. 1022–1026, 2005.

[12] P. Michalek, P. Hodgkinson, and W. Donaldson, "Fiberoptic intubation through an I-gel supraglottic airway in two patients with predicted difficult airway and intellectual disability," *Anesthesia & Analgesia*, vol. 106, no. 5, pp. 1501–1504, 2008.

[13] P. Michalek, W. Donaldson, C. Graham, and J. D. Hinds, "A comparison of the I-gel supraglottic airway as a conduit for tracheal intubation with the intubating laryngeal mask airway: a manikin study," *Resuscitation*, vol. 81, no. 1, pp. 74–77, 2010.

[14] H. S. Joo and D. K. Rose, "The intubating laryngeal mask airway with and without fiberoptic guidance," *Anesthesia and Analgesia*, vol. 88, no. 3, pp. 662–666, 1999.

[15] P.-P. Lu, C.-H. Yang, A. C. Y. Ho, and M.-H. Shyr, "The intubating LMA: a comparison of insertion techniques with conventional tracheal tubes," *Canadian Journal of Anesthesia*, vol. 47, no. 9, pp. 849–853, 2000.

[16] K. Murashima, T. Fukutome, and J. Brimacombe, "A comparison of two silicone-reinforced tracheal tubes with different bevels for use with the intubating laryngeal mask," *Anaesthesia*, vol. 54, no. 12, pp. 1198–1200, 1999.

[17] E. H. Liu, R. W. Goy, Y. Lim, and F.-G. Chen, "Success of tracheal intubation with intubating laryngeal mask airways: a randomized trial of the LMA fastrach™ and LMA CTrach™," *Anesthesiology*, vol. 108, no. 4, pp. 621–626, 2008.

[18] A. E. Halwagi, N. Massicotte, A. Lallo et al., "Tracheal intubation through the I-gelTM supraglottic airway versus the LMA FastrachTM: a randomized controlled trial," *Anesthesia and Analgesia*, vol. 114, no. 1, pp. 152–156, 2012.

[19] S. Kapoor, D. D. Jethava, P. Gupta, D. Jethava, and A. Kumar, "Comparison of supraglottic devices i-gel® and LMA Fastrach® as conduit for endotracheal intubation," *Indian Journal of Anaesthesia*, vol. 58, no. 4, pp. 397–402, 2014.

[20] P. J. F. Baskett, M. J. A. Parr, J. P. Nolan et al., "The intubating laryngeal mask. Results of a multicentre trial with experience of 500 cases," *Anaesthesia*, vol. 53, no. 12, pp. 1174–1179, 1998.

[21] W. C. Blackwelder, "'Proving the null hypothesis' in clinical trials," *Controlled Clinical Trials*, vol. 3, no. 4, pp. 345–353, 1982.

[22] J. L. Apfelbaum, C. A. Hagberg, R. A. Caplan et al., "Practice guidelines for management of the difficult airway: an updated report by the American Society of Anesthesiologists Task Force on Management of the Difficult Airway," *Anesthesiology*, vol. 118, no. 2, pp. 251–270, 2013.

[23] Difficult airway society guidleines for "can't ventilate, can't intubate" situation, https://www.das.uk.com/files/cvci-Jul04-A4.pdf.

[24] K. Kajino, T. Iwami, T. Kitamura et al., "Comparison of supraglottic airway versus endotracheal intubation for the prehospital treatment of out-of-hospital cardiac arrest," *Critical Care*, vol. 15, no. 5, article R236, 2011.

[25] H. E. Wang, D. Szydlo, J. A. Stouffer et al., "Endotracheal intubation versus supraglottic airway insertion in out-of-hospital cardiac arrest," *Resuscitation*, vol. 83, no. 9, pp. 1061–1066, 2012.

[26] J. McMullan, R. Gerecht, J. Bonomo et al., "Airway management and out-of-hospital cardiac arrest outcome in the CARES registry," *Resuscitation*, vol. 85, no. 5, pp. 617–622, 2014.

[27] L. Theiler, M. Kleine-Brueggeney, N. Urwyler, T. Graf, C. Luyet, and R. Greif, "Randomized clinical trial of the i-gel™ and Magill tracheal tube or single-use ILMA™ and ILMA™ tracheal tube for blind intubation in anaesthetized patients with a predicted difficult airway," *British Journal of Anaesthesia*, vol. 107, no. 2, pp. 243–250, 2011.

[28] M. U. Sharma, S. Gombar, K. K. Gombar, B. Singh, and N. Bhatia, "Endotracheal intubation through the intubating laryngeal mask airway (LMA-Fastrach™): a randomized study of LMA- Fastrach™ wire-reinforced silicone endotracheal tube versus conventional polyvinyl chloride tracheal tube," *Indian Journal of Anaesthesia*, vol. 57, no. 1, pp. 19–24, 2013.

[29] V. R. Shah, G. P. Bhosale, T. Mehta, and G. P. Parikh, "A comparison of conventional endotracheal tube with silicone wire-reinforced tracheal tube for intubation through intubating laryngeal mask airway," *Saudi Journal of Anaesthesia*, vol. 8, no. 2, pp. 183–187, 2014.

[30] P. Kundra, N. Sujata, and M. Ravishankar, "Conventional tracheal tubes for intubation through the intubating laryngeal mask airway," *Anesthesia and Analgesia*, vol. 100, no. 1, pp. 284–288, 2005.

[31] G. E. Kanazi, M. El-Khatib, V. G. Nasr et al., "A comparison of a silicone wire-reinforced tube with the parker and polyvinyl chloride tubes for tracheal intubation through an intubating laryngeal mask airway in patients with normal airways undergoing general anesthesia," *Anesthesia and Analgesia*, vol. 107, no. 3, pp. 994–997, 2008.

[32] A. Pournajafian, M. Alimian, F. Rokhtabnak, M. Ghodraty, and M. Mojri, "Success rate of airway devices insertion: laryngeal mask airway versus supraglottic gel device," *Anesthesiology and Pain Medicine*, vol. 5, no. 2, Article ID e22068, 2015.

[33] G. Bhandari, K. Shahi S, and R. Bhakuni, "A comparative study of tracheal intubation through i-gel and intubating laryngeal mask airway," *People's Journal of Scientific Research*, vol. 6, pp. 24–29, 2013.

# 23

# Effect of Fluid Flow Rate on Efficacy of Fluid Warmer: An In Vitro Experimental Study

**Vorasruang Thongsukh, Chanida Kositratana, and Aree Jandonpai**

*Department of Anesthesiology, Faculty of Medicine Ramathibodi Hospital, Mahidol University, Bangkok 10400, Thailand*

Correspondence should be addressed to Vorasruang Thongsukh; ravts@yahoo.com

Academic Editor: Yukio Hayashi

*Introduction.* In patients who require a massive intraoperative transfusion, cold fluid or blood transfusion can cause hypothermia and potential adverse effects. One method by which to prevent hypothermia in these patients is to warm the intravenous fluid before infusion. The aim of this study was to determine the effect of the fluid flow rate on the efficacy of a fluid warmer. *Methods.* The room air temperature was controlled at 24°C. Normal saline at room temperature was used for the experiment. The fluid was connected to an infusion pump and covered with a heater line, which constantly maintained the temperature at 42°C. The fluid temperature after warming was measured by an insulated thermistor at different fluid flow rates (100, 300, 600, 900, and 1200 mL/h) and compared with the fluid temperature before warming. Effective warming was defined as an outlet fluid temperature of >32°C. *Results.* The room temperature was 23.6°C ± 0.9°C. The fluid temperature before warming was 24.95°C ± 0.5°C. The outlet temperature was significantly higher after warming at all flow rates ($p < 0.001$). The increases in temperature were 10.9°C ± 0.1°C, 11.5°C ± 0.1°C, 10.2°C ± 0.1°C, 10.1°C ± 0.7°C, and 8.4°C ± 0.2°C at flow rates of 100, 300, 600, 900, and 1200 mL/h, respectively. The changes in temperature among all different flow rates were statistically significant ($p < 0.001$). The outlet temperature was >32°C at all flow rates. *Conclusions.* The efficacy of fluid warming was inversely associated with the increase in flow rate. The outlet temperature was <42°C at fluid flow rates of 100 to 1200 mL/h. However, all outlet temperatures reached >32°C, indicating effective maintenance of the core body temperature by infusion of warm fluid.

## 1. Introduction

The normal core body temperature in humans is maintained by the hypothalamus and typically ranges from 36.5°C to 37.5°C. The interthreshold range is usually only 0.2°C to 0.4°C. Both general and regional anesthesia inhibit central thermoregulation and increase the interthreshold range to 2°C to 4°C, leading to hypothermia [1, 2]. Hypothermia is defined as a decrease in the core body temperature to <36°C [1]. The combination of hypothermia, acidosis, and coagulopathy has been identified as the "lethal triad" in trauma patients because it increases the risk of morbidity [3]. Intraoperative hypothermia is associated with postoperative myocardial ischemia, impaired coagulation, an increased risk of wound infection, and atrioventricular arrhythmia [3, 4]. Massive cold fluid or blood infusion is one cause of hypothermia. One liter of fluid at room temperature will reduce the mean body temperature by approximately 0.25°C [5]. Induction of mild hypothermia without extracorporeal circulation, a 30-min infusion of 2 L of normal saline at 4°C, decreases the core body temperature by 2.5°C [6]. The theoretical impact of fluid infusion on the body temperature can be calculated as follows:

$$\text{change in mean body temperature} = \frac{\text{thermal stress of infused fluids}}{(\text{weight} \times \text{sp heat})}, \quad (1)$$

where thermal stress = difference between core body temperature and temperature of infused fluid (°C) × specific heat of infused fluid × volume of infused fluid (L/h), weight = weight of patient (kg), and sp heat = specific heat of patient (0.83 kcal/L/°C). Sp heat of infused fluid: blood, 0.87 kcal/L/°C; saline, 1 kcal/L/°C [7, 8].

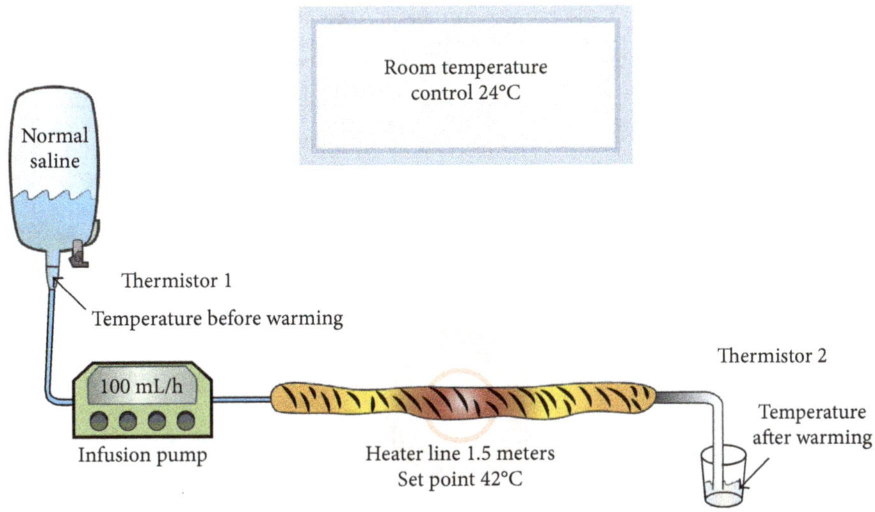


FIGURE 1: Schematic diagram of the experimental set-up.

According to this equation, the temperature of the infused fluid should not be <36°C in a normothermic patient to prevent a decrease in the mean body temperature during anesthesia. Jung et al. [9] developed a fluid warming device and suggested that effective warming was indicated by a warmed fluid temperature of >32°C. According to the above equation, when infusing fluid at 32°C at a flow rate of 2 L/h to a normothermic patient whose core body temperature is 36°C and body weight is 50 kg, the mean body temperature will decrease by only 0.2°C.

Warm intravenous infusion is a direct, active method of warming the core body temperature and is suitable for patients who require massive transfusion [10]. The temperature of the warmed intravenous fluid should not exceed 40°C to 42°C to avoid denaturation of plasma proteins [11]. The aim of this experimental study was to determine the effect of the infusion rate on the temperature of warmed fluid. Very high flow rate may cause ineffective fluid warming due to short transit time. The hypothesis was that increasing the infusion rate may decrease the efficacy of warming by the heat line. The fluid temperature before warming was the control variable, the different infusion rates were independent variables, and the difference in the fluid temperature after warming was the dependent variable.

## 2. Methods

This experimental study was performed in the general operating room at Ramathibodi Hospital. The ambient temperature was controlled at 24°C via a room air conditioning system which was close to the operating condition in our institution. Normal saline was used in this study because it is commonly used as an isotonic solution for fluid replacement in operating rooms. The fluid was maintained at the temperature of the operating room, then connected to the infusion pump (Terofusion; Terumo Europe, Leuven, Belgium), which was adjusted to flow rates of 100, 300, 600, 900, and 1200 mL/h, and these ranges of fluid flow rate were commonly infused in major abdominal operation in local setting. A 1.5 m heater line (Barkey autocontrol 3XPT; Barkey, Leopoldshöhe, Germany) covered the infusion line. The heater line was set at 42°C. After rinsing the warmed fluid for 5 min at each flow rate to maintain a constant temperature after warming, we recorded the room temperature by the electronic thermometer and the temperature of the fluid before and after passing through the heater line. Each flow rate was studied five times. The outlet temperature was measured at the immediate end of the heater line with an insulated digital thermistor (Life Scope i; Nihon Kohden, Tokyo, Japan) sealed in a 4 mL test tube. Before the study, the reliability and accuracy of thermistor were checked by repeatedly measuring the neonatal incubator temperature. Effective warming was defined as an outlet temperature of >32°C [9]. The experiment and data collection were completely done in one day. The schematic diagram is depicted in Figure 1.

Statistical analyses were performed using SPSS v.20.0 for Windows (IBM SPSS Inc., Armonk, NY), and a data chart was produced using Microsoft Excel 2007. All fluid temperatures are reported as mean ± standard deviation. The normality assumption for continuous variables was assessed by the Shapiro–Wilk test. A paired $t$-test or Wilcoxon's test was used to assess the statistical significance of the changes in temperature before and after warming, and an independent $t$-test or the Mann–Whitney $U$ test was used to assess the changes in temperature between each flow rate and the next higher one. All statistical analyses were two-sided with a significance level at $p$ value < 0.05.

## 3. Results

The room temperature during the experiment was 23.6°C ± 0.9°C. The temperature of the fluid before warming was 24.9°C ± 0.5°C. The outlet temperature significantly increased after warming at all infusion rates ($p < 0.001$). The maximum outlet temperature was 36.9°C at a flow rate of

TABLE 1: Fluid temperature before and after warming.

| Infusion rate (mL/h) | Fluid temperature before warming (°C) | Fluid temperature after warming (°C) | Difference in fluid temperature (°C) | $p$ value |
|---|---|---|---|---|
| 100 | 25.0 ± 0.1 | 35.9 ± 0.1 | 10.9 ± 0.1 | <0.001* |
| 300 | 24.8 ± 0.1 | 36.3 ± 0.2 | 11.5 ± 0.1 | <0.001* |
| 600 | 25.0 ± 0.2 | 35.2 ± 0.1 | 10.2 ± 0.1 | <0.001* |
| 900 | 24.1 ± 0.7 | 34.2 ± 0.0 | 10.1 ± 0.7 | <0.001* |
| 1,200 | 24.5 ± 0.2 | 33.0 ± 0.2 | 8.4 ± 0.2 | <0.001* |

Data are presented as mean ± standard deviation. *Statistically significant at $p < 0.001$.

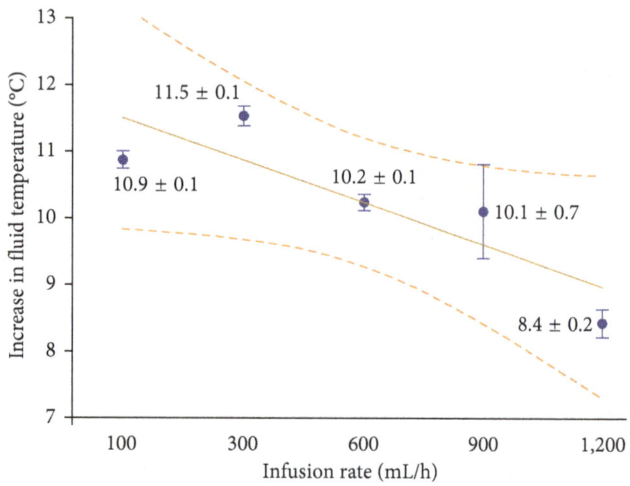


FIGURE 2: Increasing temperatures after warming at different infusion rates.

300 mL/h. The fluid temperature increased by 10.9°C ± 0.1°C, 11.5°C ± 0.1°C, 10.2°C ± 0.1°C, 10.1°C ± 0.7°C, and 8.4°C ± 0.2°C at flow rates of 100, 300, 600, 900, and 1200 mL/h, respectively (Table 1 and Figure 2). For all flow rates except 300 mL/h, the outlet temperature did not reach the ideal temperature of 36°C; however, all of the outlet temperatures were >32°C. The change in temperature was significantly different among all flow rates ($p < 0.001$) except the change between 600 and 900 mL/h. A linear trend was found for the entire set of flow rates (as shown in Figure 2), suggesting that the effectiveness of warming tended to be inversely correlated with the increase in flow rate.

## 4. Discussion

One of the main factors that affected the warming capacity in this experimental study was the ambient temperature. The operative room air conditioning system caused an ambient temperature fluctuation of 23.6°C ± 0.9°C, leading to variation in the fluid temperature before warming. However, the recommended operating room temperature that can prevent perioperative hypothermia ranges from 20°C to 24°C, which was within our range [12, 13]. The initial temperature of the fluid before warming is 24.9°C ± 0.5°C, higher than the room temperature may be from the different location of measurement and not well distributed of airflow. The heater line was constantly maintained at 42°C, but the outlet temperature at each flow rate was <42°C. Only the outlet temperature at a flow rate of 300 mL/h was >36°C. Nevertheless, the outlet temperature at all flow rates was >32°C, indicating effective warming. With respect to the warming efficacy of other devices, the Hotline (Smiths Medical, St. Paul, MN) can warm the fluid to 34.8°C at a flow rate of 80 mL/h, and the Astotherm (Armstrong Medical, Coleraine, Northern Ireland) can warm the fluid to 30°C at the same flow rate [7]. In clinical practice, infusion of warmed fluid more effectively maintains the patient's core body temperature than does infusion of room temperature fluid [14].

In the present study, the efficacy of fluid warming decreased as the flow rate increased. The change in temperature was dependent upon the duration of time that the venous line was in contact with the heater line for heat exchange. Therefore, the fluid can be completely heated at lower flow rates. However, we found that the efficacy of warming was lower at a flow rate of 100 than 300 mL/h; this may have been due to the higher rate of heat dispersal after warming to the atmosphere in the temperature measurement technique.

Based on our study, fluid warming with the heater line (Barkey autocontrol 3XPT®, Germany) can effectively increase infused fluid temperature for replacement therapy in uneventful abdominal operation. However, further research is required to see if more rapid flow rate can still generate optimal temperature or not. It is also worthwhile to compare the performance of some traditional fluid warming devices because some devices can effectively warm the fluid at higher flow rate than in our study.

## 5. Conclusion

Intravenous fluid warming is an alternative warming method by which to prevent hypothermia in patients who required a massive fluid transfusion. In the present study, the effectiveness of warming was inversely associated with the increase in the flow rate. Although the outlet temperature was <42°C as the set point of the heater line, all tested flow rates (100–1,200 mL/h) were able to increase the outlet temperature to >32°C, which was considered to be effective fluid warming fluid.

## Abbreviations

Sp heat: Specific heat.

## Additional Points

*Limitations.* The main limitation of the present study is that by its inherent nature, it cannot be extrapolated to the clinical setting. The effectiveness of the warming device and flow rate cannot represent the actual core body temperature after infusion of warmed fluid. However, the findings of this study will serve as a baseline for future clinical studies. Lee et al. [15] suggested that both the flow rate and length of the catheter from the warmer outlet to the patient influence the effectiveness of the warmer. A longer catheter may be associated with more heat loss to the ambient; thus, the outlet fluid should be located as close as possible to the patient.

## Conflicts of Interest

The authors declare that there are no conflicts of interest regarding the publication of this article.

## Authors' Contributions

Vorasruang Thongsukh conceived and designed the study and critically revised the final draft for important intellectual content. Chanida Kositratana and Aree Jandonpai performed the experiment. Vorasruang Thongsukh and Chanida Kositratana performed the statistical analysis and drafted the manuscript. All authors read and approved the final version of the manuscript.

## Acknowledgments

This study was supported by the general operating room staff of Ramathibodi Hospital. The authors thank Rojnarin Komonhirun for assisting with the statistical analysis and the preparation and submission of our manuscript.

## References

[1] D. I. Sessler, "Temperature monitoring and perioperative thermoregulation," *Anesthesiology*, vol. 109, no. 2, pp. 318–338, 2008.

[2] J. F. Butterworth, D. C. Mackey, and J. D. Wasnick, "Thermoregulation hypothermia, & malignant hyperthermia," in *Morgan and Mikhail's Clinical Anesthesiology*, J. Butterworth, D. C. Mackey, and J. Wasnick, Eds., pp. 1183–1191, McGraw-Hill Medical, New York, NY, USA, 5th edition, 2013.

[3] E. E. Moore, "Thomas G. Orr Memorial Lecture. Staged laparotomy for the hypothermia, acidosis, and coagulopathy syndrome," *American Journal of Surgery*, vol. 172, no. 5, pp. 405–410, 1996.

[4] B. J. Tsuei and P. A. Kearney, "Hypothermia in the trauma patient," *Injury*, vol. 35, no. 1, pp. 7–15, 2004.

[5] D. I. Sessler, "Temperature monitoring," in *Miller's Anesthesia*, R. D. Miller, Ed., pp. 1571–1597, Elsevier Churchill Livingstone, Philadelphia, PA, USA, 6th edition, 2005.

[6] A. Rajek, R. Greif, D. I. Sessler, J. Baumgardner, S. Laciny, and H. Bastanmehr, "Core cooling by central venous infusion of ice-cold (4 degrees C and 20 degrees C) fluid: isolation of core and peripheral thermal compartments," *Anesthesiology*, vol. 93, no. 3, pp. 629–637, 2000.

[7] C. E. Smith and W. Karl, "Principles of fluid and blood warming in trauma," *ITACCS*, vol. 8, no. 1, pp. 71–79, 2008.

[8] P. E. Horowitz, M. A. Delagarza, J. J. Pulaski, and R. A. Smith, "Flow rates and warming efficacy with Hotline and Ranger blood/fluid warmers," *Anesthesia and Analgesia*, vol. 99, no. 3, pp. 788–792, 2004.

[9] S. W. Jung, T. H. Han, J. Y. Lee et al., "Performance characteristics of high efficiency fluid and blood warmer using print circuit board heater at various flow rates," *Korean Journal of Anesthesiology*, vol. 51, no. 5, pp. 598–605, 2006.

[10] S. Kumar, P. F. Wong, A. C. Melling, and D. J. Leaper, "Effects of perioperative hypothermia and warming in surgical practice," *International Wound Journal*, vol. 2, no. 3, pp. 193–204, 2005.

[11] R. Vazquez and D. F. Larson, "Plasma protein denaturation with graded heat exposure," *Perfusion*, vol. 28, no. 6, pp. 557–559, 2013.

[12] AORN Recommended Practices Committee, "Recommended practices for the prevention of unplanned perioperative hypothermia," *AORN Journal*, vol. 85, no. 5, pp. 972–974, 2007.

[13] Pennsylvania Patient Safety Advisory Group, "Prevention of inadvertent perioperative hypothermia," *Patient Safety Authority*, vol. 5, no. 2, pp. 44–52, 2008.

[14] C. E. Smith, E. Geddes, S. Swede et al., "Warming intravenous fluids reduces perioperative hypothermia in women undergoing ambulatory gynecology surgery," *Anesthesia and Analgesia*, vol. 87, no. 1, pp. 37–41, 1998.

[15] S. H. Lee, H. K. Kim, S. C. Park, E. S. Kim, T. K. Kim, and C. S. Kim, "The effect of infusion rate and catheter length on the temperature of warming fluid," *Korean Journal of Anesthesiology*, vol. 58, no. 1, pp. 31–37, 2010.

# 24

# Percutaneous Nephrolithotomy: Current Clinical Opinions and Anesthesiologists Perspective

**Indira Malik and Rachna Wadhwa**

*Department of Anesthesiology and Critical Care, Dr. Baba Saheb Ambedkar Hospital, Rohini, Delhi 85, India*

Correspondence should be addressed to Rachna Wadhwa; drrachnawadhwa@gmail.com

Academic Editor: Yukio Hayashi

Percutaneous nephrolithotomy (PCNL), a minimally invasive method for removal of renal calculi, was initially started in the 1950s but gained popularity about two decades later and has now become standard practice for management. There has been an immense improvement in technique and various guidelines have been established for treatment of renal stones. However, it has its own share of complications which can be attributed to surgical technique as well as anesthesia related complications. PubMed and Google search yielded more than 30 articles describing the different complications seen in this procedure, out of which 15 major articles were selected for writing this review. The aim of this review article is to describe the implications of the complications associated with PCNL related to the anesthesiologist. The anesthesiologist is as much responsible for the management of the patient perioperatively as the surgeon. Therefore, it is mandatory to be familiar with the various complications, some of which may be life threatening and he should be able to manage them efficiently. The paper also analyses the advantages and drawbacks of the available options in anesthesia, that is, general and regional, both of which are employed for PCNL.

## 1. Introduction

Percutaneous nephrolithotomy (PCNL) is an established, minimally invasive procedure for removal of renal calculi more than 2 centimetres in size. In 1976, Fernstorm and Johansson reported the removal of renal calculus through a nephrostomy tract for the first time [1]; since then PCNL has become the most common procedure performed for the management of renal stones. It facilitates a direct approach to the calculus while the kidney and surrounding structures are subjected to lesser trauma as compared to the open approach, and hence a great deal of surgical expertise is required for percutaneous access to the kidney and stone removal. Many changes and modifications have been done to minimise morbidity, analgesic requirements, and duration of hospitalization, including use of regional blocks, single step dilatation, "Mini-Perc" technique, tubeless PCNL, and sandwich therapy [2–4].

Though the entire surgical team shoulders the responsibility for the outcome, the role of the anesthesiologist is not less. They not only help in providing optimal working conditions for the surgeon, but also recognise and deal with the complications related to anesthesia and the procedure as a whole.

## 2. Method for Data Collection and Synthesis

The keywords PCNL, complications, and anesthesia were searched in PubMed and Google and 30 articles were retrieved. Out of these, 15 articles were considered pertinent to our review. The data from these articles was retrieved and results of the related studies are compared and compiled to synthesize this review.

## 3. Background

The incidence and prevalence of renal calculi have increased globally across all ages, sex, and race, probably due to change in dietary habits and global warming [5]. The conventional and perhaps the oldest method of removing renal stones was open nephrolithotomy. Later, with the advent of uretero-scopes, ureteric stones were removed with the help of dormia

Table 1: Classification of surgical complications according to the modified Clavien grading system [6].

| Grade | Description of complication |
|---|---|
| I | Any deviation from the normal postoperative course without the need for pharmacological treatment or surgical, endoscopic and radiological interventions. Allowed therapeutic regimens are as follows: drugs as antiemetics, antipyretics, analgesics, diuretics, electrolytes, and physiotherapy. This grade also includes wound infections opened at the bedside. |
| II | Requiring pharmacological treatment with drugs other than such allowed for grade I complications. Blood transfusion and total parenteral nutrition are also included. |
| III | Requiring surgical, endoscopic, or radiological intervention. |
| IIIa | Intervention under regional anesthesia. |
| IIIb | Intervention under general anesthesia. |
| IV | Life threatening complication requiring ICU management. |
| IVa | Single organ dysfunction (including dialysis). |
| IVb | Multiorgan dysfunction. |
| V | Death. |

Modified and adapted from [6].

baskets. Percutaneous method of removing renal calculi was first described in the 1950s but it was actually performed almost two decades later in the 70s and 80s for routine removal of renal stones. Simultaneously, other procedures for removal of renal stones, such as extracorporeal shock wave lithotripsy (ESWL), also came into vogue and PCNL remained an underutilized procedure, until the last decade, which witnessed a surge in this specific procedure vis-à-vis improvement in technique, increased prevalence of renal stones, and delineation of clear cut indications for PCNL [7]. Currently, PCNL is the procedure of choice for managing kidney stones and continues to evolve and has largely replaced open stone surgery. Advances in technology and equipment have resulted in stone removal with less morbidity, shorter convalescence, and reduced cost compared with open surgery [8].

Currently, the indications for PCNL include large size renal calculi (>1.5–2 cm), staghorn calculi, upper tract calculi not responding to other modalities of treatment, lower pole stones, cystine nephrolithiasis, and stones in anatomically abnormal kidneys [7]. Generally two approaches are followed for PCNL.

*Standard PCNL.* The procedure is performed with the patient in prone position. A small incision 1.3 cm is given on the back overlying the affected kidney and a track is created from the skin to the kidney. It is then enlarged using a series of Teflon dilators or bougies with a sheath being placed over the last dilator to hold the track open. After this, nephroscope (fibre optic light source with two additional channels for renal visualisation and irrigation) is inserted; smaller stones may be removed with the help of a device with a basket at its end while larger stones may be fragmented by a Holmium laser lithotripter, ultrasonic or electrohydraulic probe. After removing the stones, a catheter is placed to drain the urinary system and a nephrostomy tube is placed to drain the fluid from the kidney to a drainage bag. They are usually removed before the patient is discharged.

*Mini PCNL.* It is performed with miniaturized nephroscope and has been found to have 99% efficacy in removal of stones 1–2.5 cm in size. Though not useful for larger calculi, it offers the advantages of shorter operating and recovery time and fewer complications.

Like all minimally invasive procedures, PCNL too has its share of complications, related to both the procedure and the underlying pathology. Early recognition and management of many of these complications reduce the morbidity and mortality considerably. A multicentre study of 5803 patients, conducted by the Clinical Research of the Endourological Society (CROES), reported an overall complication rate of 21.5%, using the modified Clavien system [9], which was developed in 1992 and later modified in 2004, for classification of complications [10, 11] and comparison of complication rates in radical prostatectomy and cystectomy. The modified Clavien system of classification of complications was first adopted by Tefekeli et al. in 2008 to stratify complications following PCNL [12] (Table 1).

## 4. Anesthetic Technique

There has been considerable debate regarding the ideal anesthetic technique for PCNL. The procedure is usually performed under general anesthesia (GA) and the published literature regarding the use of spinal anesthesia for PCNL is sparse [8]. Over the years, both these techniques have been used and they have their advantages and drawbacks. The advantages offered by GA include safety as the patient's airway is secured in prone position, feasibility to control tidal volume during percutaneous access puncture to minimise injury to the pleura and lungs, and prolonged anesthesia duration allowing the surgeon to make multiple and higher punctures with minimal patient discomfort, especially in cases with large stone load.

Regional anesthesia (RA) for PCNL was first described in 1988 [13]. Since then, a few studies have been done regarding use of regional anesthesia for PCNL [14–19]. It has its own merits in the form of less postoperative pain, less blood loss, and early recovery and discharge thereby reducing stay in the hospital.

A randomized, controlled trial including 200 patients compared the efficacy of GA versus RA in PCNL patients and concluded that both the groups had comparable intraoperative hemodynamics. However, postoperative Visual Analogue Score (VAS) scores were comparatively less after one hour postoperatively in the RA group while the GA group patients received analgesics within the first postoperative hour itself. Therefore, the consumption of systemic analgesics was greater in the patients who underwent GA. Incidence of postoperative nausea and vomiting was significantly higher in the GA group, but the overall patient satisfaction was also better. The patients who received RA had an increased incidence of shivering but the procedures were completed successfully without conversion to GA [20].

Mehrabi and Shirazi evaluated the intraoperative and postoperative anesthetic and surgical outcomes in patients who underwent PCNL under spinal anesthesia in prone position and concluded that spinal anesthesia is not only safe and effective for performing PCNL, but it is also a good alternative for GA in adult patients [16]. Borzouei et al. did a large study regarding the use of spinal anesthesia in PCNL and reported that spinal anesthesia is feasible, safe, and well tolerated especially in elderly patients with significant comorbidities such as pulmonary disease [15].

Other authors have previously compared the two techniques and found that while RA provided the advantage of better analgesia and shorter recovery times, GA was more comfortable for the patients in prone position and also safer, in case the procedure was prolonged [21, 22]. Kuzgunbay et al., 2009, found no significant difference between the GA and RA groups in terms of operative time, success rate, hemoglobin level, hospital stay, and complications. However, patients' satisfaction was higher in the RA group [17]. In a large retrospective study, involving 1004 patients, complications were graded according to Clavien classification and comparison of the two groups was done which revealed that the overall rate of complications was greater in the GA group [23].

The many specific anesthesia concerns in PCNL mandate a fine coordination between the surgical and anesthesia teams for optimal results. The choice of anesthesia depends, to a great extent, upon the patient's preference, the position for surgery favoured by the surgeon, surgical expertise, and estimated time of the procedure determined by the stone size, number, and location. The anesthesiologist should be fully aware of all the possible complications, irrespective of the choice of anesthetic technique, that occur intraoperatively as well as postoperatively.

*4.1. Preoperative Considerations.* Patients belonging to varying age groups may present for PCNL. Elderly patients may have many comorbidities like ischemic heart disease, respiratory dysfunction, and diabetes while young children may be highly uncomfortable and uncooperative. Hydronephrosis causing deranged renal functions and sepsis, in addition to the above, may add to the above. It is essential to communicate with the surgical team and confirm the adequacy of renal function by intravenous pyelogram (IVP), DMSA, or DTPA scan [24]. DMSA (dimercaptosuccinic acid) is a renal imaging tool to evaluate renal structure and morphology and DTPA (diethylene triamine pentaacetic acid) renal scan is performed to evaluate the blood supply and function and excretion of urine from the kidneys. This test can also find out what percentage each kidney contributes to the total kidney function. There is no indication for performing PCNL if the kidney is nonfunctional; such patients should be taken up for nephrectomy. Stabilization of the existing comorbidities in the preoperative period reduces intra- and postoperative complications, overall morbidity, and mortality. There should not be any active focus of infection preoperatively.

*4.2. Intraoperative Considerations.* Although GA has been considered to be the safest technique for PCNL worldwide, it has its own hazards like accidental extubation and kinking of endotracheal tube (ET) during positioning of the patient; hence, it is desirable to use a reinforced ET tube or an oral airway along with a regular ET tube and the tube should be firmly secured. Position of bolsters should be carefully checked to allow unhampered ventilation. Torsion of the neck veins may lead to facial edema, ocular edema, and ecchymosis.

Care should be taken to avoid pressure on the eyeballs in the prone position as this may lead to postoperative visual loss; if the external pressure on the globe exceeds the mean arterial pressure (MAP), perfusion to the optic nerve is hampered, leading to blindness. Pressure on the pinna should be avoided as it can cause pressure necrosis. In female patients, the breasts should be positioned medially to avoid pressure necrosis. The arms should be abducted and brought upwards with the elbows flexed equally to prevent overstretching of the brachial plexus on either side. All the pressure points like the elbows, wrists, knees, and ankles should be adequately padded to prevent peripheral nerve injuries.

When RA is used, many of the issues related to positioning are resolved as the patients are conscious and can position himself/herself in the prone position according to their comfort. However, there is a risk of sudden hypotension after making the patient prone. Patient discomfort increases with the duration of the procedure and the surgeon may not feel comfortable in making skin punctures, especially those close to the 11th rib, if the patient is unable to coordinate breath holding at that time.

## 5. Complications Related to Surgical Procedure and Their Anesthetic Implications

Various authors have studied complications related to PCNL per se (Table 2). Besides the definite risk of injury to the surrounding organs and major blood vessels, these patients

Table 2: Studies on complications of PCNL.

| Sl number | Author | Transfusion | Massive hemorrhage | Fever | Sepsis | Colonic injury | Pleural injury | Extravasation of urine | Mortality |
|---|---|---|---|---|---|---|---|---|---|
| 1 | El-Nahas et al. 2012 ($n = 241$) | 16% | 2% | 1.2% | 0.4% | NA | 2.4% | 8% | 0.4% |
| 2 | Mousavi-Bahar et al. 2011, ($n = 671$) | 0.6% | 1.5% | 1% | 0 | 0.3% | 0.7% | 5.2% | 0.3% |
| 3 | De la Rossette et al. 2011, ($n = 5803$) | 5.7% | NA | 10.5% | NA | NA | 1.8% | 3.4% | 0.3% |
| 4 | Shin et al. 2011, [6] ($n = 88$) | 6.9% | 1.4% | 11% | 0.6% | 0.7% | 1.1% | 0.4% | 0.4% |
| 5 | Rana et al. 2007, ($n = 667$) | 1.49% | 0.14% | NA | 1.79% | 0 | 0.14% | NA | 0 |
| 6 | Osman et al. 2005, ($n = 315$) | 0 | 0.3% | 32% | 0.3% | 0 | 0 | NA | 0.3% |
| 7 | Lee et al. 1987, ($n = 582$) | 11.2% | NA | 22.4% | 0.8% | 0.2% | 3.1% | 7.2% | 0.3% |

are also at considerable risk for sepsis. Each of these complications adds to the morbidity and sometimes mortality of patients. The majority of the complications occur in the intraoperative and immediate postoperative period; therefore, the anesthesiologist must be aware of the complications and be well equipped to deal with them effectively and minimise morbidity.

The overall rate of pleural injury ranges between 0.3 and 1% during percutaneous access puncture for PCNL. It may manifest as hydrothorax, pneumothorax, or hydropneumothorax and 64% of them may require chest tube drainage [25]. Since they are mostly diagnosed in the immediate postoperative period with shortness of breath, fever, and radiological evidence of pleural injury [26], it is desirable to fluoroscopically monitor the chest during the procedure and obtain a chest radiograph in the postoperative period.

Chances of pleural and lung injury are higher during upper pole access due to the close proximity of these structures. Preminger et al. (2005) reported 16% pleural injuries with supracostal approach as opposed to 4.5% with subcostal approach [27]. Ideally, the working sheath should be inserted under the 11th rib and above the 12th rib with ventilatory standstill; however, punctures above the 11th rib increase the risk of intrathoracic complications to 23.1% as compared to 1.5–12% for punctures above the 12th rib; the risk is 0.5% for subcostal approach [28]. Pulmonary injuries are likely to occur in 29% of cases on the right side and in 14% of cases on the left side [29]. A higher nephrostomy tract predisposes the patient to greater risk of incurring intrathoracic injury; therefore, when multiple or higher punctures are required to remove a greater stone load, GA would be safer and desirable and vigilance is required throughout the procedure, for raised airway pressures and end tidal $CO_2$, and falls in oxygen saturation indicating pleural or lung injury which should be managed promptly by maintaining ventilation with 100% oxygen and if pneumothorax is diagnosed intraoperatively, placement of chest tube.

Adjacent solid organs are also at risk for injury during percutaneous access approach. Hepatic or splenic injury may occur in case of coexisting hepatomegaly or splenomegaly. Currently there is no general consensus regarding management of splenic injuries; however, the majority of articles support conservative management. Similarly, liver injury is managed best with conservative approach. However, all gall bladder injuries necessitated cholecystectomy, the timing of diagnosis being the decisive factor between laparoscopic and open techniques [30].

Injuries to hollow organs like the small bowel and colon have been reported in 0.2–1% of cases [30, 31]. Bowel injury is more complicated to deal with due to intraperitoneal involvement and requires laparotomy. Gall bladder or small bowel perforation may lead to secondary peritonitis, sepsis, and septic shock with a mortality rate of 30%, if not managed early [32].

El-Nahas et al. retrospectively reviewed 5093 PCNL cases of which 15 patients (0.3%) suffered colonic perforation. Out of these 15 patients, 66.6% had left percutaneous access and 80% underwent lower calyceal puncture. Advanced age, thin built, female sex, and horse shoe kidney and cases with previous bowel or renal surgery were also independent risk factors for colonic injuries [33, 34].

In addition, the great vessels are also at risk for damage during percutaneous access puncture, in about 0.5% of cases [31]. Multiple attempts at initial percutaneous access, upper pole access, inexperienced surgeon, solitary kidney, and staghorn calculus may increase the risk of bleeding. The potential for massive bleeding during percutaneous access to the renal pelvis may occur due to the close proximity of the major hilar blood vessels and scanty parenchymal tissue to provide tamponade in case of injury [7]. Initial bleeding during the access may be from the renal capsule or parenchyma and is venous in nature and hence is controllable with balloon dilator and Kaye's tamponade catheter. Adequate hydration, large nephrostomy tube, and mannitol may also be helpful.

Improved techniques have significantly reduced transfusion rates and interventional control of delayed hemorrhage is now possible [6].

A series was conducted by El-Nahas et al., 2007, in 39 patients of PCNL complicated with severe bleeding who underwent arteriography and embolization. Pseudoaneurysms and arteriovenous fistulae were the most common causes of hemorrhage in them. Superselective angioembolization successfully controlled bleeding in 92% of cases, remaining cases required exploration, and one patient underwent nephrectomy [35]. A retrospective study by Srivastava et al., including 1854 patients for PCNL, reported major bleeding requiring angioembolization in 1.6% of cases. Pseudoaneurysm was found in 48.1% of bleeding patients on renal arteriography and 91.6% were successfully treated with angioembolization; the common factor between all the patients was increased stone size (>4.1 cm) [36]. Other factors responsible for increased risk of bleeding are diabetes mellitus, utilization of mature nephrostomy tract, concomitant surgical complications, access tracts passing through atrophic parenchyma, and the modality used for guiding access (fluoroscopy versus ultrasound) [37, 38].

Injury to the renal collecting system occurs in 8% of patients, causing extravasation and absorption of irrigation fluid leading to electrolyte disturbances, altered mental status, and intravascular volume overload. Decrease in the drainage of irrigation fluid, abnormal hemodynamic parameters, and direct visualisation of perinephric fat indicate renal collecting system injury. Perforation of the renal pelvis may necessitate immediate cessation of the surgical procedure and adequate drainage through ureteric stent, nephrostomy tube, or percutaneous drain. Use of isotonic solutions for irrigation, fluoroscopic guidance, and continuous or open irrigation system can minimise this type of complication [39].

The anesthesiologist should remain vigilant and cautious to detect electrolyte imbalance and features of volume overload, which is easier to detect in patients under RA. It may manifest as irritability and discomfort followed by altered hemodynamics and ECG changes [35]. Under GA, hemodynamic changes indicate possible volume overload and should be promptly managed by restriction of intravenous fluids and diuretics. Monitoring of serum electrolytes and blood gases should be done both intra- and postoperatively.

Renal collecting system obstruction may occur rarely as a result of ureteric avulsion or stricture, leading to nephrocutaneous fistula, hydrocalyx, and hydronephrosis [40, 41]. Prolonged operative time, extended nephrostomy tube drainage, and large stone burden are some of the predisposing factors.

Renal dysfunction following PCNL is very rare and may occur secondary to other operative complications. Intraoperative or postoperative bleeding and subsequent requirement for angioembolization may compromise renal perfusion and lead to renal parenchymal infarction. Transient rise in serum creatinine may occur in 1% of patients and those who had an uneventful intra- and postoperative course exhibit <1% renal parenchymal damage [7].

Postoperative fevers may occur transiently in 30% of patients undergoing PCNL while sepsis may develop in 3% of cases. According to Korets and colleagues, 2011, 9.8% of cases of PCNL developed severe infection preceded by clinical features of systemic inflammatory response syndrome (SIRS). Univariate analysis revealed that female patients with multiple punctures, stone burden >10 $cm^2$, struvite calculi, positive pelvic urine, and stone cultures were at risk for development of SIRS while multivariate analysis identified a total stone load >10 $cm^2$, positive pelvic urine or stone cultures, and multiple pelvic punctures as potential risk factors [7, 42]. Since the reports of the cultures collected intraoperatively are not immediately available in the postoperative period, it becomes difficult to guide appropriate antibiotic therapy [42]. In another study by Margel et al., 2006, 25% of patients who had positive stone cultures had negative voided urine culture preoperatively [43]. The appropriate management of post-PCNL sepsis becomes difficult in this scenario as the correct antibiotic therapy may not be followed. Around 30% of the patients who develop features of SIRS require ICU care, with morbidity and mortality being high [42].

With a high index of suspicion for sepsis, broad spectrum antibiotics should be considered within one hour of admission to ICU and if required, mechanical ventilation with lung protective strategy should be considered. Inotropic support should be initiated in case of persistent hypotension (MAP < 65 mmHg). Urine output, mixed venous saturation, blood gases, and other routine parameters should be monitored. Once the patient's condition is stabilized and sepsis is under control, gradual weaning-off from inotropes and ventilatory support should be considered.

Death following PCNL is very rare and incidence ranges between 0.1 and 0.7%, occurring secondary to complications like pulmonary embolism, myocardial infarction, and sepsis [6, 44].

## 6. Conclusion and Recommendation

Though PCNL is a routinely performed, minimal access surgery, yet it may have many devastating and life threatening complications. It is safe to conduct the procedure under GA for complicated or prolonged procedures. RA is preferred only when the surgical team has a high degree of expertise and the procedure is uncomplicated. The anesthesiologist must be familiar with the various complications and their appropriate management. Effective communication between the surgical and anesthesia teams is desirable to formulate the correct perioperative management plan for every patient.

## Competing Interests

The authors declare that they have no competing interests.

## References

[1] I. Fernstorm and B. Johansson, "Percutaneous pyelolithotomy. A new extraction technique," *Scandinavian Journal of Urology and Nephrology*, vol. 10, pp. 257–259, 1976.

[2] M. Goh and J. S. Wolf Jr., "Almost totally tubeless percutaneous nephrolithotomy: further evolution of the technique," *Journal of Endourology*, vol. 13, no. 3, pp. 177–180, 1999.

[3] M. M. Said, Z. M. Sonbul, M. Kenawaym, and M. M. Atallah, "Spinal and interpleural bupivacaine for percutaneous nephrolithotomy," *Middle East Journal of Anesthesiology*, vol. 11, pp. 259–264, 1991.

[4] S. V. Jackman, S. P. Hedican, C. A. Peters, and S. G. Docimo, "Percutaneous nephrolithotomy in infants and preschool age children: experience with a new technique," *Urology*, vol. 52, no. 4, pp. 697–701, 1998.

[5] V. Romero, H. Akpinar, and D. G. Assimos, "Kidney stones: a global picture of prevalence, incidence and associated risk factors," *Reviews in Urology*, vol. 12, pp. e86–e96, 2010.

[6] T. S. Shin, H. J. Cho, S.-H. Hong, J. Y. Lee, S. W. Kim, and T.-K. Hwang, "Complications of percutaneous nephrolithotomy classified by the modified Clavien grading system: a single center's experience over 16 years," *Korean Journal of Urology*, vol. 52, no. 11, pp. 769–775, 2011.

[7] E. Taylor, J. Miller, T. Chi, and M. L. Stoller, "Complications associated with percutaneous nephrolithotomy," *Translational Andrology and Urology*, vol. 1, no. 4, pp. 223–228, 2012.

[8] G. Sunana, G. Rahul, M. Nandita, M. Arti, V. Siddarth, and M. Rajesh, "Per cutaneous nephrolithotomy under spinal anesthesia and the efficacy of adding adjuvant clonidine to intrathecal hyperbaric bupivacaine: a comparative study," *The Internet Journal of Anaesthesiology*, vol. 33, no. 1, 2014.

[9] J. de la Rosette, D. Assimos, M. Desai et al., "The clinical research office of the endourological society percutaneous nephrolithotomy global study: indications, complications, and outcomes in 5803 patients," *Journal of Endourology*, vol. 25, no. 1, pp. 11–17, 2011.

[10] P.-A. Clavien, J. R. Sanabria, and S. M. Strasberg, "Proposed classification of complications of surgery with examples of utility in cholecystectomy," *Surgery*, vol. 111, no. 5, pp. 518–526, 1992.

[11] D. Dindo, N. Demartines, and P.-A. Clavien, "Classification of surgical complications: a new proposal with evaluation in a cohort of 6336 patients and results of a survey," *Annals of Surgery*, vol. 240, no. 2, pp. 205–213, 2004.

[12] A. Tefekli, M. A. Karadag, K. Tepeler et al., "Classification of percutaneous nephrolithotomy complications using the modified Clavien Grading System: Looking for a Standard," *European Urology*, vol. 53, no. 1, pp. 184–190, 2008.

[13] V. Ballestrazzi, C. Zboralski, P. Smith-Morel et al., "Importance of suspended peridural anesthesia in percutaneous nephrolithotomy. Apropos of 112 patients in the urology service of the Regional Hospital Center of Lille," *Cahiers d'Anesthésiologie*, vol. 36, no. 2, pp. 85–88, 1988.

[14] R. Sari, M. Dursum, and A. Pirale, "A comparison of levobupivacaine versus racemic bupivacaine in PCNL with spinal anaesthesia," *European Journal of Anaesthesia*, vol. 27, pp. 130–132, 2010.

[15] B. Borzouei, S. Habibollah, and M. Bahar, "Results of Percutaneous Nephrolithotomy under spinal anaesthesia," *World Academy of Science, Engineering and Technology*, vol. 6, pp. 5–20, 2012.

[16] S. Mehrabi and K. K. Shirazi, "Results and complications of spinal anaesthesia in PCNL," *The Journal of Urology*, vol. 7, pp. 22–25, 2010.

[17] B. Kuzgunbay, T. Turunc, S. Akin, P. Ergenoglu, A. Aribogan, and H. Ozkardes, "Percutaneous nephrolithotomy under general versus combined spinal-epidural anesthesia," *Journal of Endourology*, vol. 23, no. 11, pp. 1835–1838, 2009.

[18] M. M. Atallah, A. A. Shorrab, Y. M. Abdel Mageed, and A. D. Demian, "Low-dose bupivacaine spinal anaesthesia for percutaneous nephrolithotomy: the suitability and impact of adding intrathecal fentanyl," *Acta Anaesthesiologica Scandinavica*, vol. 50, no. 7, pp. 798–803, 2006.

[19] T. Tangpaitoon, C. Nisoog, and B. Lojanapiwat, "Efficacy and safety of percutaneous nephrolithotomy (PCNL): a prospective and randomized study comparing regional epidural anesthesia with general anesthesia," *International Brazilian Journal of Urology*, vol. 38, no. 4, pp. 504–511, 2012.

[20] H. E. S. Moawad and A. S. El Hefnawy, "Spinal vs. general anesthesia for percutaneous nephrolithotomy: a prospective randomized trial," *Egyptian Journal of Anaesthesia*, vol. 31, no. 1, pp. 71–75, 2015.

[21] V. Singh, R. J. Sinha, S. N. Sankhwar, and A. Malik, "A prospective randomized study comparing percutaneous nephrolithotomy under combined spinal-epidural anesthesia with percutaneous nephrolithotomy under general anesthesia," *Urologia Internationalis*, vol. 87, no. 3, pp. 293–298, 2011.

[22] M. K. Moslemi, S. H. Mousavi-Bahar, and M. Abedinzadeh, "The feasibility of regional anesthesia in the percutaneous nephrolithotomy with supracostal approach and its comparison with general anesthesia," *Urolithiasis*, vol. 41, no. 1, pp. 53–57, 2013.

[23] T. Cicek, U. Gonulalan, R. Dogan et al., "Spinal anesthesia is an efficient and safe anesthetic method for percutaneous nephrolithotomy," *Urology*, vol. 83, no. 1, pp. 50–55, 2014.

[24] A. Taylor Jr., "Quantitation of renal function with static imaging agents," *Seminars in Nuclear Medicine*, vol. 12, no. 4, pp. 330–344, 1982.

[25] A. Shaban, A. Kodera, M. N. El Ghoneimy, T. Z. Orban, K. Mursi, and A. Hegazy, "Safety and efficacy of supracostal access in percutaneous renal surgery," *Journal of Endourology*, vol. 22, no. 1, pp. 29–34, 2008.

[26] M. A. Bjurlin, T. O'Grady, R. Kim, M. D. Jordan, S. M. Goble, and C. M. P. Hollowell, "Is routine postoperative chest radiography needed after percutaneous nephrolithotomy?" *Urology*, vol. 79, no. 4, pp. 791–795, 2012.

[27] G. M. Preminger, D. G. Assimos, J. E. Lingeman et al., "Chapter 1. AUA guideline on management of staghorn calculi: diagnosis and treatment recommendations," *The Journal of Urology*, vol. 173, no. 6, pp. 1991–2000, 2005.

[28] R. Munver, F. C. Delvecchio, G. E. Newman, and G. M. Preminger, "Critical analysis of supracostal access for percutaneous renal surgery," *The Journal of Urology*, vol. 166, no. 4, pp. 1242–1246, 2001.

[29] K. D. Hopper and W. F. Yakes, "The posterior intercostal approach for percutaneous renal procedures: risk of puncturing the lung, spleen, and liver as determined by CT," *American Journal of Roentgenology*, vol. 154, no. 1, pp. 115–117, 1990.

[30] H. Öztürk, "Gastrointestinal system complications in percutaneous nephrolithotomy: a systematic review," *Journal of Endourology*, vol. 28, no. 11, pp. 1256–1267, 2014.

[31] S. H. Mousavi-Bahar, S. Mehrabi, and M. K. Moslemi, "Percutaneous nephrolithotomy complications in 671 consecutive patients: a single-center experience," *Urology Journal*, vol. 8, no. 4, pp. 271–276, 2008.

[32] M. Sartelli, "A focus on intra-abdominal infections," *World Journal of Emergency Surgery*, vol. 5, article 9, 2010.

[33] A. R. El-Nahas, A. A. Shokeir, A. M. El-Assmy et al., "Colonic perforation during percutaneous nephrolithotomy: a study of risk factors," *Urology*, vol. 67, no. 5, pp. 937–941, 2006.

[34] M. S. Michel, L. Trojan, and J. J. Rassweiler, "Complications in percutaneous nephrolithotomy," *European Urology*, vol. 51, no. 4, pp. 899–906, 2007.

[35] A. R. El-Nahas, A. A. Shokeir, A. M. El-Assmy et al., "Post-percutaneous nephrolithotomy extensive hemorrhage: a study of risk factors," *Journal of Urology*, vol. 177, no. 2, pp. 576–579, 2007.

[36] A. Srivastava, K. J. Singh, A. Suri et al., "Vascular complications after percutaneous nephrolithotomy: are there any predictive factors?" *Urology*, vol. 66, no. 1, pp. 38–40, 2005.

[37] Y. Wang, Y. Wang, F. Jiang et al., "Post-percutaneous nephrolithotomy septic shock and severe hemorrhage: a study of risk factors," *Urologia Internationalis*, vol. 88, no. 3, pp. 307–310, 2012.

[38] R. Kukreja, M. Desai, S. Patel, S. Bapat, and M. Desai, "Factors affecting blood loss during percutaneous nephrolithotomy: prospective study," *Journal of Endourology*, vol. 18, no. 8, pp. 715–722, 2004.

[39] A. Skolarikos and J. de la Rosette, "Prevention and treatment of complications following percutaneous nephrolithotomy," *Current Opinion in Urology*, vol. 18, no. 2, pp. 229–234, 2008.

[40] J. W. Segura, D. E. Patterson, A. J. LeRoy et al., "Percutaneous removal of kidney stones: review of 1,000 cases," *Journal of Urology*, vol. 134, no. 6, pp. 1077–1081, 1985.

[41] J. K. Parsons, T. W. Jarrett, V. Lancini, and L. R. Kavoussi, "Infundibular stenosis after percutaneous nephrolithotomy," *The Journal of Urology*, vol. 167, no. 1, pp. 35–38, 2002.

[42] R. Korets, J. A. Graversen, M. Kates, A. C. Mues, and M. Gupta, "Post-percutaneous nephrolithotomy systemic inflammatory response: a prospective analysis of preoperative urine, renal pelvic urine and stone cultures," *The Journal of Urology*, vol. 186, no. 5, pp. 1899–1903, 2011.

[43] D. Margel, Y. Ehrlich, N. Brown, D. Lask, P. M. Livne, and D. A. Lifshitz, "Clinical implication of routine stone culture in percutaneous nephrolithotomy-a prospective study," *Urology*, vol. 67, no. 1, pp. 26–29, 2006.

[44] M. Aron, R. Yadav, R. Goel et al., "Multi-tract percutaneous nephrolithotomy for large complete staghorn calculi," *Urologia Internationalis*, vol. 75, no. 4, pp. 327–332, 2005.

# 25

# Injectable Anesthesia for Mice: Combined Effects of Dexmedetomidine, Tiletamine-Zolazepam, and Butorphanol

**Laura A. Cagle,[1] Lisa M. Franzi,[1] Steven E. Epstein,[2] Philip H. Kass,[3] Jerold A. Last,[1] and Nicholas J. Kenyon[1]**

[1]*Division of Pulmonary, Critical Care, and Sleep Medicine, School of Medicine, University of California, Davis, CA, USA*
[2]*Department of Surgical and Radiological Sciences, School of Veterinary Medicine, University of California, Davis, CA, USA*
[3]*Department of Population Health and Reproduction, School of Veterinary Medicine, University of California, Davis, CA, USA*

Correspondence should be addressed to Laura A. Cagle; lacagle@ucdavis.edu

Academic Editor: Ronald G. Pearl

Anesthetic protocols for murine models are varied within the literature and medetomidine has been implicated in the development of urethral plugs in male mice. Our objective was to evaluate the combination of butorphanol, dexmedetomidine, and tiletamine-zolazepam. A secondary objective was to identify which class of agent was associated with urethral obstructions in male mice. BALB/c male ($n = 13$) and female ($n = 23$) mice were assigned to dexmedetomidine and tiletamine-zolazepam with or without butorphanol or to single agent dexmedetomidine or tiletamine-zolazepam. Anesthesia was achieved in 58% (14/24) of mice without butorphanol and in 100% (24/24) of mice with butorphanol. The combination of dexmedetomidine (0.2 mg/kg), tiletamine-zolazepam (40 mg/kg), and butorphanol (3 mg/kg) resulted in an induction and anesthetic duration of 12 and 143 minutes, respectively. Urethral obstructions occurred in 66% (25/38) of trials in male mice that received dexmedetomidine with a mortality rate of 38% (5/13). Tiletamine-zolazepam, when used alone, resulted in a 0% (0/21) incidence of urethral obstructions. Combination use of dexmedetomidine, tiletamine-zolazepam, and butorphanol results in a longer and more reliable duration of anesthesia than the use of dexmedetomidine and tiletamine-zolazepam alone. Dexmedetomidine is not recommended for use in nonterminal procedures in male mice due to the high incidence of urethral obstructions and resultant high mortality rate.

## 1. Introduction

Optimized injectable and inhalational anesthetic protocols for hours-long anesthesia are essential for laboratory animal research. Many laboratories do not have the ability to use inhalational vapor anesthesia, necessitating the use of injectable anesthetics. Researchers have utilized a wide array of injectable anesthetic protocols including the use of barbiturates, ketamine, or xylazine with varying success [1–9].

The use of dexmedetomidine in conjunction with tiletamine-zolazepam with or without the addition of an opioid as an anesthetic protocol has yet to be evaluated in a mouse model. An opioid receptor agonist can be added to an anesthetic regimen to reduce the dosing of other agents or prolong the duration of anesthesia in some species [10], but we do not know whether this is true in a murine model. Urethral obstructions using medetomidine (combination of levomedetomidine and dexmedetomidine isomer) in combination with ketamine have been documented in male mice [11, 12]. The occurrence of urethral obstructions with the use of medetomidine and ketamine is presumed to be due to the use of medetomidine, as ketamine-xylazine anesthesia has not been associated with this adverse effect [12].

The purpose of this study was to determine whether the addition of an opioid would prolong the anesthetic effects of the combination of dexmedetomidine and tiletamine-zolazepam (Telazol®). A secondary objective was to establish a reliable anesthetic protocol for use in mice by determining appropriate drug dosages. A tertiary objective of this study was to determine which anesthetic agent was associated with urethral obstructions in male mice.

TABLE 1: Anesthetic combinations of dexmedetomidine and tiletamine-zolazepam with or without butorphanol. BALB/c female mice were assigned with the intent for six mice in each group, but, due to the high mortality associated with the use of tiletamine-zolazepam above 50 mg/kg, groups were reduced. Dexmedetomidine and tiletamine-zolazepam were given IP and butorphanol was given SC.

| Dexmedetomidine (mg/kg) Tiletamine-zolazepam (mg/kg) ($n$) | | | Dexmedetomidine (mg/kg) Tiletamine-zolazepam (mg/kg) Butorphanol (3 mg/kg) ($n$) | | |
|---|---|---|---|---|---|
| 0.4<br>20<br>($n$ = 6) | 0.4<br>40<br>($n$ = 6) | 0.4<br>60<br>($n$ = 3) | 0.2<br>10<br>($n$ = 6) | 0.2<br>20<br>($n$ = 6) | 0.2<br>40<br>($n$ = 6) |
| 0.6<br>20<br>($n$ = 6) | 0.6<br>40<br>($n$ = 6) | 0.6<br>60<br>($n$ = 3) | 0.4<br>10<br>($n$ = 6) | 0.4<br>20<br>($n$ = 6) | 0.4<br>40<br>($n$ = 6) |
| 0.8<br>20<br>($n$ = 6) | 0.8<br>40<br>($n$ = 5) | 0.8<br>60<br>($n$ = 2) | 0.6<br>10<br>($n$ = 6) | 0.6<br>20<br>($n$ = 6) | 0.6<br>40<br>($n$ = 6) |

## 2. Animals

Specific pathogen-free BALB/c mice ($n$ = 36), 14–25 grams, 4–16-week-old males and females, were obtained from Jackson Laboratory (Bar Harbor, ME) and allowed to acclimatize for one week prior to study enrollment. Animals were housed in plastic cages over autoclaved bedding in a HEPA-filtered laminar flow cage rack on a 12-hour light/dark cycle. All mice were allowed free access to water and a standard diet (Purina Rodent Chow). Procedures with the mice were performed in accordance with an approved IACUC protocol. Mice were routinely screened and cared for by the veterinary staff of the Animal Resource Service at the University of California, Davis, in AAALAC-accredited facilities.

## 3. Materials and Methods

*3.1. Anesthetic Protocols.* Females ($n$ = 23) were assigned to receive combinations of dexmedetomidine and tiletamine-zolazepam (DTZ) or combinations of dexmedetomidine, tiletamine-zolazepam, and butorphanol (DTZB) as shown in Table 1. Mice were not assigned to the same dosage group more than once. Dosages in the DTZ group started at 0.4 mg/kg and 20 mg/kg and increased to 0.8 mg/kg and 60 mg/kg, respectively. Dosages in the DTZB group started at 0.2 mg/kg, 10 mg/kg, and 3 mg/kg and increased to 0.6 mg/kg, 40 mg/kg, and 3 mg/kg, respectively. Dexmedetomidine and tiletamine-zolazepam were administered intraperitoneally (IP) while butorphanol was administered via a subcutaneous (SC) injection.

Male mice ($n$ = 13) were assigned to groups receiving dexmedetomidine and tiletamine-zolazepam ($n$ = 7), dexmedetomidine ($n$ = 2), or tiletamine-zolazepam ($n$ = 4). Mice were not assigned to the same dosage group more than once. Dexmedetomidine-only animals received dosages ranging from 0.025 to 0.6 mg/kg, while the tiletamine-zolazepam-only groups received dosages ranging from 10 to 80 mg/kg. Combination groups of dexmedetomidine and tiletamine-zolazepam received 0.2 to 0.8 mg/kg and 0 to 50 mg/kg, respectively. Mice were given at least 48 hours between injections and each mouse received multiple injections over a four-week period.

*3.2. Anesthetic Monitoring and Recovery.* Mice were placed on warming pads and monitored continuously, with assessment of heart rate, respiratory rate, response to noxious stimulation, movement, and ambulation every 15 minutes. Heart and respiratory rates were determined by auscultation. Response to noxious stimulation was determined by a negative toe pinch response. Urinary bladder palpation and expression, if needed, were performed every 15 minutes in the male mice and every 60 minutes in the female mice. Urethral plugs, if noted in the distal urethra, were manually extracted. Induction time, anesthetic duration, heart rate, respiratory rate, and the time for return of movement, ambulation, and righting ability were recorded. Induction time was defined, for the purpose of this paper, as the time from anesthetic injection to an absent response to noxious stimulation. Anesthetic duration was defined as the period of time without a response to noxious stimulation after anesthetic induction with survival to anesthetic recovery. Anesthetic recovery was defined as the time for movement, ambulation, and righting ability to return from the initial injection; we used this definition to keep consistency amongst groups that did not result in an anesthetic level. Mice were given at least 48 hours of recovery between injections. Mice were euthanized at the end of the study period with an intraperitoneal overdose of pentobarbital.

*3.3. Statistics.* Data were analyzed using GraphPad Prism version 6 (San Diego, CA) and Stata/IC 13.1 (College Station, TX). Mice were grouped based on anesthetic drug combinations (DTZ and DTZB) and then subgrouped based on drug dosages. Mixed-effects logistic regression was used to evaluate the effects of anesthetic drug doses on the ability to induce an acceptable level of anesthesia; results are presented as odds ratios and 95% confidence intervals (95% CI). Mixed-effects linear regression was used to compare the effects of anesthetic drug dosages on anesthetic induction, duration, and

TABLE 2: Trials with dexmedetomidine and tiletamine-zolazepam (DTZ). Dexmedetomidine and tiletamine-zolazepam were administered IP and butorphanol was administered at 3 mg/kg SC. Data is reported in marginal means and standard error.

| | Anesthetic duration (minutes) | Recovery time (minutes) | Anesthesia achieved (%) | Heart rate (bpm) | Respiratory rate (bpm) |
|---|---|---|---|---|---|
| Dexmedetomidine 0.4 mg/kg | | | | | |
| Tiletamine-zolazepam | | | | | |
| 20 mg/kg | 63 (±22) | 279 (±25) | 50% (3/6) | 187 (±14) | 128 (±3) |
| 40 mg/kg | 67 (±22) | 240 (±25) | 33% (2/6) | 222 (±14) | 136 (±3) |
| 60 mg/kg | 77 (±22) | 240 (±25) | 33% (1/3) | 227 (±20) | 135 (±4) |
| Dexmedetomidine 0.6 mg/kg | | | | | |
| Tiletamine-zolazepam | | | | | |
| 20 mg/kg | 23 (±16) | 222 (±17) | 67% (4/6) | 229 (±14) | 134 (±3) |
| 40 mg/kg | 73 (±13) | 265 (±16) | 100% (6/6) | 209 (±14) | 132 (±3) |
| 60 mg/kg | 47 (±22) | 243 (±25) | 67% (2/3) | 193 (±20) | 130 (±4) |
| Dexmedetomidine 0.8 mg/kg | | | | | |
| Tiletamine-zolazepam | | | | | |
| 20 mg/kg | 58 (±18) | 253 (±20) | 50% (3/6) | 254 (±14) | 145 (±3) |
| 40 mg/kg | 48 (±18) | 286 (±35) | 40% (2/5) | 207 (±16) | 130 (±3) |
| 60 mg/kg | 175 (±31) | 404 (±35) | 50% (1/2) | 233 (±25) | 125 (±5) |

recovery time, as well as their effects on heart and respiratory rates; results are reported as predicted marginal means and standard errors. Cox proportional hazards regression with robust variance estimation to account for replicate measurements in individuals was used to determine whether the rate of induction varied depending on the anesthetic drug administered; results are reported as hazard ratios (HR) and 95% confidence intervals (95% CI). $p$ values $< 0.05$ were considered statistically significant.

## 4. Results

*4.1. Outcomes and Anesthetic Monitoring in Female Mice.* Female mice ($n = 23$) were assigned to the DTZ and DTZB groups with the intent for six mice in each group, although, due to the high mortality associated with the use of tiletamine-zolazepam above 50 mg/kg, numbers in each group were adjusted. Anesthetic trials for the female mice amounted to 43 in the DTZ group and 54 in the DTZB group, resulting in an average of 4 anesthetic trials per mouse, and data are reported in Tables 2 and 3.

Use of dexmedetomidine and tiletamine-zolazepam (DTZ) achieved anesthesia in 58% (25/43) of the anesthetic trials; there were three reported fatalities within this group (dexmedetomidine 0.6 mg/kg and 0.8 mg/kg with tiletamine-zolazepam 40 mg/kg). A strong association with acceptable induction was noted with increasing the dosage of dexmedetomidine from 0.4 mg/kg to 0.6 mg/kg (OR: 10.5, 95% CI: 1.4–80.8, $p = 0.024$), but the higher dosage of 0.8 mg/kg compared to 0.4 mg/kg was not significantly improved (OR: 2.1, 95% CI: 0.4–12.1, $p = 0.40$).

Anesthetic duration varied from 15 minutes to 165 minutes. Anesthetic duration was not significantly altered by increased dosages of dexmedetomidine and tiletamine-zolazepam. Heart rate was significantly elevated with increased dosages of dexmedetomidine from 0.4 to 0.6 mg/kg (187 to 229 bpm, $p = 0.041$) and from 0.6 to 0.8 mg/kg (229 to 254 bpm, $p = 0.001$). Respiratory rate significantly increased (128 to 145 breaths per minute) with increasing dosages of dexmedetomidine in the tiletamine-zolazepam 20 mg/kg group ($p < 0.001$). However, significant interactions were noted for heart rate and respiratory rate with various dosages of dexmedetomidine and tiletamine-zolazepam. At tiletamine-zolazepam dosages greater than 20 mg/kg, increasing the dosages of dexmedetomidine resulted in a decreasing trend in the respiratory rate.

Use of dexmedetomidine, tiletamine-zolazepam, and butorphanol (DTZB) resulted in an anesthetic occurrence of 91% (48/54) in all groups and 100% (36/36) at dexmedetomidine dosages of 0.2 to 0.6 mg/kg and tiletamine-zolazepam 20 to 40 mg/kg. One fatality was reported at dexmedetomidine 0.6 mg/kg, tiletamine-zolazepam 20 mg/kg, and butorphanol 3 mg/kg. Anesthetic duration ranged from 0 to 270 minutes. Induction time ranged from 0 to 69 minutes and recovery time ranged from 75 minutes to 425 minutes. No significant changes in heart rate or respiratory rate were noted with increasing the dosage of either dexmedetomidine or tiletamine-zolazepam within these groups. Anesthetic duration and recovery time were increased with higher dosages of dexmedetomidine and tiletamine-zolazepam (Table 3). The rate of induction was significantly decreased with increased dosages of tiletamine-zolazepam from 10 to 20 mg/kg (HR = 2.2, 95% CI = 1.6–3.0, $p < 0.001$) and from 20 to 40 mg/kg (HR = 4.6, 95% CI = 2.1–10.1, $p < 0.001$).

Dexmedetomidine and tiletamine-zolazepam at dosages of 0.4 to 0.6 mg/kg and 20 to 40 mg/kg, respectively, were

TABLE 3: Trials with dexmedetomidine, tiletamine-zolazepam, and butorphanol (DTZB). Dexmedetomidine and tiletamine-zolazepam were administered IP and butorphanol was administered at 3 mg/kg SC. Data is reported in marginal means and standard error.

| | Anesthetic duration (minutes) | Recovery time (minutes) | Anesthesia achieved (%) | Heart rate (bpm) | Respiratory rate (bpm) |
|---|---|---|---|---|---|
| Dexmedetomidine 0.2 mg/kg | | | | | |
| Tiletamine-zolazepam | | | | | |
| 10 mg/kg | 28 (±21) | 105 (±16) | 50% (3/6) | 188 (±12) | 132 (±4) |
| 20 mg/kg | 73 (±16) | 168 (±16) | 100% (6/6) | 191 (±12) | 137 (±4) |
| 40 mg/kg | 143 (±16) | 217 (±16) | 100% (6/6) | 198 (±12) | 137 (±4) |
| Dexmedetomidine 0.4 mg/kg | | | | | |
| Tiletamine-zolazepam | | | | | |
| 10 mg/kg | 90 (±18) | 161 (±16) | 33% (2/6) | 199 (±12) | 129 (±4) |
| 20 mg/kg | 110 (±16) | 224 (±16) | 100% (6/6) | 202 (±12) | 134 (±4) |
| 40 mg/kg | 163 (±16) | 273 (±16) | 100% (6/6) | 209 (±12) | 134 (±4) |
| Dexmedetomidine 0.6 mg/kg | | | | | |
| Tiletamine-zolazepam | | | | | |
| 10 mg/kg | 80 (±16) | 213 (±16) | 100% (6/6) | 195 (±12) | 131 (±4) |
| 20 mg/kg | 195 (17) | 276 (±17) | 100% (6/6) | 198 (±12) | 136 (±4) |
| 40 mg/kg | 216 (±16) | 325 (±16) | 100% (6/6) | 205 (±12) | 136 (±4) |

compared to the same dosages with the addition of butorphanol at 3 mg/kg SC. Anesthesia was achieved in 58% (14/24) of mice without butorphanol and in 100% (24/24) of mice that received butorphanol. Induction time ranged from 16 to 90 minutes without butorphanol and 8 to 51 minutes with butorphanol. The rate of induction was significantly decreased with the addition of butorphanol (HR = 4.2, 95% CI = 1.8–9.8, $p = 0.001$). Direct statistical comparison between the groups with butorphanol and without butorphanol was unable to be evaluated, as all animals that received butorphanol achieved anesthesia. The odds ratio of dexmedetomidine at 0.4 mg/kg compared to 0.6 mg/kg for resulting in induction of anesthesia was 42.3 (95% CI: 1.0–1855, $p = 0.052$). Anesthetic duration ranged from 15 to 150 minutes without butorphanol and from 60 to 270 minutes with butorphanol. Recovery time ranged from 125 to 318 minutes without butorphanol and from 124 to 425 minutes with butorphanol.

*4.2. Outcomes and Adverse Effects in Male Mice.* Male mice ($n = 7$) had a total of 27 anesthetic trials in the DTZ group. The two male mice ($n = 2$) receiving only dexmedetomidine had a total of 12 anesthetic trials and male mice ($n = 4$) receiving only tiletamine-zolazepam had a total of 21 anesthetic trials.

The incidence of urethral obstructions was 66% (25/38) in male mice that received dexmedetomidine. Use of dexmedetomidine alone resulted in a 67% (8/12) incidence of urethral plugs. When used in combination with tiletamine-zolazepam, dexmedetomidine resulted in a 65% (17/26) incidence of urethral plugs. Tiletamine-zolazepam, when used alone, resulted in a 0% (0/21) incidence of urethral obstructions.

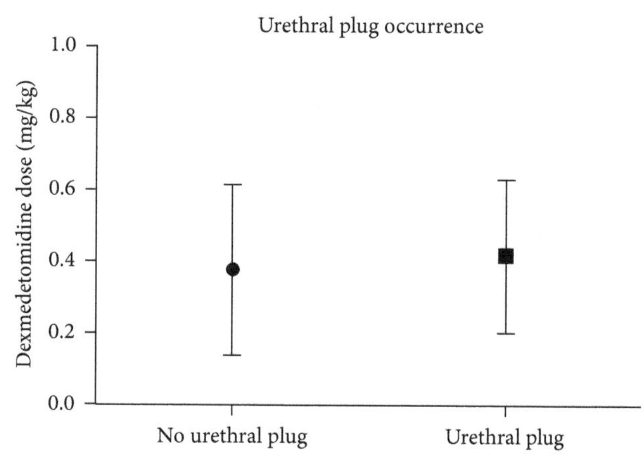


FIGURE 1: Seminal coagulum plugs occurred at dosages ranging from 0.05 to 0.8 mg/kg. No significant differences were noted in the occurrence of a urethral plug based on the dosage of dexmedetomidine ($p = 0.61$). Data are presented as the mean ± SEM.

The mean dosages of dexmedetomidine were 0.38 mg/kg in the no urethral plug group and 0.42 mg/kg in the urethral plug group, respectively. Increasing the dosage of dexmedetomidine was not associated with an increased occurrence of urethral plugs as shown in Figure 1. Seminal coagulum plugs varied in size from 2 mm to 8 mm. Necropsy confirmed the presence of eosinophilic homogenous proteinaceous material within the urinary bladder and the proximal urethra in one mouse as shown in Figure 2. No bacteria or inflammatory cells were noted within the plug, or within a seminal plug submitted separately from a second mouse.

TABLE 4: Recommended dosages of dexmedetomidine, tiletamine-zolazepam, and butorphanol. Dosages recommended for use were determined based on anesthetic duration, induction, and recovery time, as well as safety, as measured by mortality. Increased dosages of dexmedetomidine and tiletamine-zolazepam resulted in an increasing trend of anesthetic duration and recovery times. Dexmedetomidine and tiletamine-zolazepam were administered IP and butorphanol was administered in all above listed trials at 3 mg/kg SC. Data are reported in predicted marginal means and standard error.

| | Anesthetic duration (minutes) | Recovery time (minutes) | Anesthesia achieved (%) | Heart rate (bpm) | Respiratory rate (bpm) |
|---|---|---|---|---|---|
| Dexmedetomidine 0.2 mg/kg | | | | | |
| Tiletamine-zolazepam 20 mg/kg | 73 (±16) | 168 (±16) | 100% (6/6) | 191 (±12) | 137 (±4) |
| Tiletamine-zolazepam 40 mg/kg | 143 (±16) | 217 (±16) | 100% (6/6) | 198 (±12) | 137 (±4) |
| Dexmedetomidine 0.4 mg/kg | | | | | |
| Tiletamine-zolazepam 20 mg/kg | 110 (±16) | 224 (±16) | 100% (6/6) | 202 (±12) | 134 (±4) |
| Tiletamine-zolazepam 40 mg/kg | 163 (±16) | 273 (±16) | 100% (6/6) | 209 (±12) | 134 (±4) |

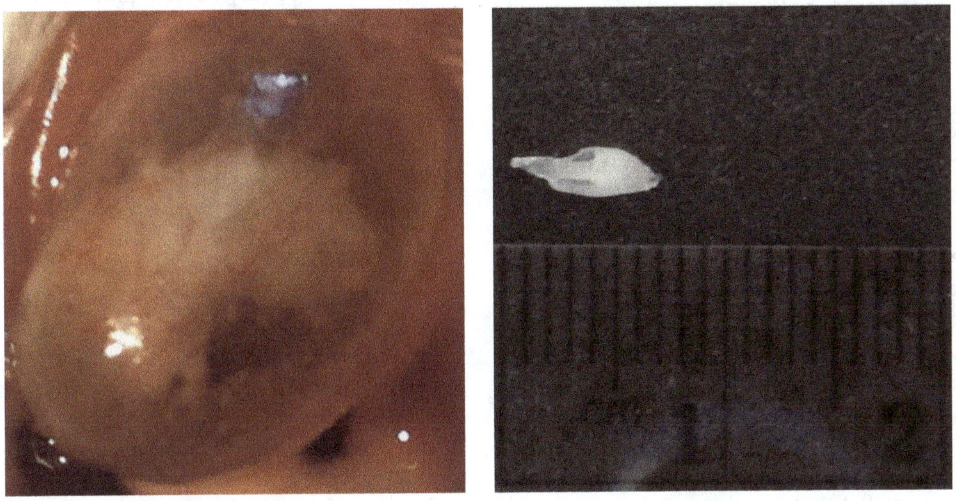

(a) (b)

FIGURE 2: Urinary bladder with homogenous proteinaceous material within it (a) and seminal coagulum plug pulled from the urethra in a male mouse (b).

*4.3. Mortality.* Mortality due to anesthetic complications was 17.4% (4/23) in female mice and 15.4% (2/13) in male mice, resulting in an overall mortality rate from anesthetic complications of 16.7% (6/36) in males and females. Mortality rates, when calculated per anesthetic trial, gave an overall anesthetic mortality of 4.8% (6/124) in all anesthetic trials. Mortality increased with tiletamine-zolazepam at dosages of 50 mg/kg ($n = 1$) and 80 mg/kg ($n = 1$) as well as combinations of dexmedetomidine and tiletamine-zolazepam at 0.6 mg/kg and 40 mg/kg ($n = 1$) and 0.8 mg/kg and 40 mg/kg ($n = 2$) and dexmedetomidine 0.6 mg/kg, tiletamine-zolazepam 20 mg/kg, and butorphanol 3 mg/kg ($n = 1$). The mortality rate due to urethral obstructions was 38% (5/13). Recommended dosages are reported in Table 4 and the drugs used at these dosages had a 0% (0/36) mortality rate. Use of tiletamine-zolazepam at dosages of 40 mg/kg resulted in a 0% (0/36) mortality rate when used in combination with dexmedetomidine at dosages less than or equal to 0.4 mg/kg.

## 5. Discussion

Dexmedetomidine and tiletamine-zolazepam, when used in combination, provided inconsistent levels of anesthesia. The addition of an opioid such as butorphanol resulted in adequate to excellent levels of anesthesia at appropriate dosages. Sedation of male mice with dexmedetomidine resulted in a 66% incidence of urethral obstructions and a 38% mortality rate due to urethral obstructions.

Use of dexmedetomidine and tiletamine-zolazepam was poor at inducing a reliable plane of anesthesia and increased dosages resulted in a higher mortality rate. Induction was faster when the dosage of dexmedetomidine was increased from 0.4 to 0.6 mg/kg, but a ceiling affect was reached at dosages above 0.6 mg/kg. Anesthetic duration was not significantly altered by increased dosages of dexmedetomidine or tiletamine-zolazepam, suggesting that a ceiling effect was reached with these two anesthetic drugs with no benefit of increasing dosages above 0.6 mg/kg of dexmedetomidine or 40 mg/kg of tiletamine-zolazepam. Without the addition of an opioid, the combination of dexmedetomidine and tiletamine-zolazepam cannot be recommended as an anesthetic protocol. This was an unexpected occurrence as the dissociative anesthetic (tiletamine-zolazepam) is thought to be a reliable anesthetic drug in multiple mammalian species. We theorize that in BALB/c mice the combination of these two drugs creates a narrow therapeutic index with the toxic dose in some individuals being lower than the anesthetic dose.

The addition of butorphanol resulted in a 100% (36/36) occurrence of anesthesia at dosages of 0.2 to 0.6 mg/kg of dexmedetomidine and 20 to 40 mg/kg of tiletamine-zolazepam, indicating that the addition of an opioid resulted in a consistent plane of anesthesia at this dose range. Induction time was significantly decreased with increasing dosages of tiletamine-zolazepam, whereas anesthetic duration and recovery time were significantly increased with increased dosages of dexmedetomidine and tiletamine-zolazepam. Direct comparison of the addition of butorphanol was achieved at dexmedetomidine dosages of 0.4 to 0.6 mg/kg with tiletamine-zolazepam dosages of 20 to 40 mg/kg, respectively. Anesthesia was achieved in all groups with the addition of butorphanol and only 58% (14/24) of groups without butorphanol, indicating the need for an opioid to achieve a reliable plane of anesthesia. This is likely due to the addition of a drug with sedative effects at a different receptor site (kappa agonist) potentiating the effect of dexmedetomidine and tiletamine-zolazepam thereby lowering the amount needed for anesthesia to below the toxic dose. Recommended dosages of dexmedetomidine, tiletamine-zolazepam, and butorphanol for use in BALB/c mice are expressed in Table 4. Although the stated dosages resulted in 0% mortality and no complications upon recovery, it is recommended that supplemental oxygen and fluids for hemodynamic support be used to offset the adverse effects of these drugs.

Adverse effects of anesthetic regimens are major concerns, with the most commonly reported adverse effects being respiratory depression and hypoxia [13]. Respiratory depression occurred with tiletamine-zolazepam dosages above 20 mg/kg as dosages of dexmedetomidine were increased, supporting the use of supplemental oxygen with this anesthetic combination. Results appear consistent with other pilot studies in our lab and a previous study involving the use of dexmedetomidine in animals [13].

The occurrence of urethral obstructions appears to be associated with the use of dexmedetomidine, as urethral obstructions occurred in 67% of male mice that received only dexmedetomidine in contrast with 0% of the male mice that received only tiletamine-zolazepam. The incidence of urethral plugs does not appear to be dose related as no significant differences were noted between the individual dosages. Necropsy and analysis of the urethral plug confirmed that the plug was composed of proteinaceous debris; however, the etiology for the development of the urethral plug remains unknown. Seminal plugs have been discovered in male mice postmortem, but, to our knowledge, the etiology of these plugs is also unknown. Urethral obstructions due to seminal coagulum plugs have been reported with the use of medetomidine and ketamine in male mice (C57BL/6 and mixed genetic mice) [12]. Wells et al. discovered that the morbidity and mortality rates were significantly higher ($p < 0.001$) in the group treated with medetomidine-ketamine than in the xylazine-ketamine group [12]. None of the male mice anesthetized with ketamine-xylazine developed urethral obstructions, which suggests that the urethral obstructions were related to the use of medetomidine in this study [12].

As this and previous studies show an association of urethral plugs due to the use of an alpha$_2$ agonist, it is reasonable to make the assumption that this is due to effects at either the alpha$_1$ or the alpha$_2$ receptor. Dexmedetomidine at higher concentrations has been reported to have dual alpha$_2$ agonist and alpha$_1$ adrenergic antagonist effects [14] while xylazine, a different alpha$_2$ agonist which has higher receptor affinity for the alpha$_1$ receptor, has not been associated with seminal coagulum plugs [12]. Given that the incidence of urethral obstructions in this study is not dose dependent with dexmedetomidine, this would lead us to believe that the alpha$_1$ receptor cannot be the only receptor involved. Given this, the cause of the obstruction is likely multifactorial with the alpha$_2$ adrenergic effects of dexmedetomidine resulting in a decreased ability to void the urinary bladder and the alpha$_1$ adrenergic effects causing urethral sphincter tightening [15]. At this time, the role of seminal coagulum plugs in this obstructive process is unclear.

Several limitations of this study need mentioning. Due to the experimental design of this study with mice receiving multiple dosages of drugs and our inability to measure drug levels during these experiments, there may have been an additive effect of repeat anesthetic dosages that affected the results although there was a washout period. Groups of mice receiving either dexmedetomidine ($n = 2$) or tiletamine-zolazepam ($n = 4$) alone were small. Increasing the number of mice within each group and therefore the statistical power may have altered the results. Mortality due to anesthetic complications was suspected, but not confirmed, as necropsy was not performed on each of these mice. Only BALB/c mice were studied with these drug combinations; it is likely that the anesthetic duration and recovery times will be altered in mice of different strains. Dosages were lowered from the dexmedetomidine and tiletamine-zolazepam group compared to the dexmedetomidine, tiletamine-zolazepam, and butorphanol group, which limited our ability to directly compare results between these groups. Thus, only a direct comparison of four dosages instead of nine dosages was performed.

In conclusion, the combination use of dexmedetomidine, tiletamine-zolazepam, and butorphanol results in a longer and more reliable duration of anesthesia than the use of dexmedetomidine and tiletamine-zolazepam alone. Research into alternative anesthetic protocols for nonterminal procedures in male mice is needed due to the occurence of urethral obstructions with the use of dexmedetomidine.

## Abbreviations

DTZ: Dexmedetomidine and tiletamine-zolazepam anesthesia group

DTZB: Dexmedetomidine, tiletamine-zolazepam, and butorphanol anesthesia group
IACUC: Institutional Animal Care and Use Committee
AAALAC: Association for Assessment and Accreditation of Laboratory Animal Care.

## Competing Interests

The authors declare that there are no competing interests regarding the publication of this paper.

## Acknowledgments

This work was performed at the Department of Pulmonary, Critical Care, and Sleep Medicine, School of Medicine, University of California, Davis. This study was supported by NIH/NHLBI R01 HL105573 and NIH/NHLBI T32 HL007013. This study was presented at the American Thoracic Society Symposium 2013, American Journal of Respiratory and Critical Care Medicine, Vol. 187, Meeting Abstracts, 2013.

## References

[1] H. C. Alves, A. M. Valentim, I. A. S. Olsson, and L. M. Antunes, "Intraperitoneal anaesthesia with propofol, medetomidine and fentanyl in mice," *Laboratory Animals*, vol. 43, no. 1, pp. 27–33, 2009.

[2] M. Arras, P. Autenried, A. Rettich, D. Spaeni, and T. Rülicke, "Optimization of intraperitoneal injection anesthesia in mice: drugs, dosages, adverse effects, and anesthesia depth," *Comparative Medicine*, vol. 51, no. 5, pp. 443–456, 2001.

[3] W. M. Burnside, P. A. Flecknell, A. I. Cameron, and A. A. Thomas, "A comparison of medetomidine and its active enantiomer dexmedetomidine when administered with ketamine in mice," *BMC Veterinary Research*, vol. 9, article 48, 2013.

[4] S. Gargiulo, A. Greco, M. Gramanzini et al., "Mice anesthesia, analgesia, and care, Part I: anesthetic considerations in preclinical research," *ILAR journal*, vol. 53, no. 1, pp. E55–E69, 2012.

[5] S. Gargiulo, A. Greco, M. Gramanzini et al., "Mice anesthesia, analgesia, and care, Part II: anesthetic considerations in preclinical imaging studies," *ILAR Journal*, vol. 53, no. 1, pp. E70–E81, 2012.

[6] S. He, C. Atkinson, F. Qiao, X. Chen, and S. Tomlinson, "Ketamine-xylazine-acepromazine compared with isoflurane for anesthesia during liver transplantation in rodents," *Journal of the American Association for Laboratory Animal Science*, vol. 49, no. 1, pp. 45–51, 2010.

[7] J. M. Izer, T. L. Whitcomb, and R. P. Wilson, "Atipamezole reverses ketamine-dexmedetomidine anesthesia without altering the antinociceptive effects of butorphanol and buprenorphine in female C57BL/6J mice," *Journal of the American Association for Laboratory Animal Science*, vol. 53, no. 6, pp. 675–683, 2014.

[8] B. J. A. Janssen, T. De Celle, J. J. M. Debets, A. E. Brouns, M. F. Callahan, and T. L. Smith, "Effects of anesthetics on systemic hemodynamics in mice," *American Journal of Physiology—Heart and Circulatory Physiology*, vol. 287, no. 4, pp. H1618–H1624, 2004.

[9] S. Wenger, "Anesthesia and analgesia in rabbits and rodents," *Journal of Exotic Pet Medicine*, vol. 21, no. 1, pp. 7–16, 2012.

[10] D. M. Dickerson, "Acute pain management," *Anesthesiology Clinics*, vol. 32, no. 2, pp. 495–504, 2014.

[11] M. D. Sinclair, "A review of the physiological effects of $\alpha_2$-agonists related to the clinical use of medetomidine in small animal practice," *Canadian Veterinary Journal*, vol. 44, no. 11, pp. 885–897, 2003.

[12] S. Wells, C. Trower, T. A. Hough, M. Stewart, and M. T. Cheeseman, "Urethral obstruction by seminal coagulum is associated with medetomidine-ketamine anesthesia in male mice on C57BL/6J and mixed genetic backgrounds," *Journal of the American Association for Laboratory Animal Science*, vol. 48, no. 3, pp. 296–299, 2009.

[13] J. C. H. Ko, L. A. Abbo, A. B. Weil, B. M. Johnson, and M. Payton, "A comparison of anesthetic and cardiorespiratory effects of tiletamine-zolazepam-butorphanol and tiletamine-zolazepam-butorphanol-medetomidine in cats," *Veterinary Therapeutics*, vol. 8, no. 3, pp. 164–176, 2007.

[14] J. Hamasaki, I. Tsuneyoshi, R. Katai, T. Hidaka, W. A. Boyle, and Y. Kanmura, "Dual $\alpha$2-adrenergic agonist and $\alpha$1-adrenergic antagonist actions of dexmedetomidine on human isolated endothelium-denuded gastroepiploic arteries," *Anesthesia and Analgesia*, vol. 94, no. 6, pp. 1434–1440, 2002.

[15] T. Streng, R. Santti, and K.-E. Andersson, "Voiding effects mediated by $\alpha$2-adrenoceptors in the anaesthetized male rat," *BJU International*, vol. 106, no. 10, pp. 1546–1549, 2010.

# 26

# The Influence of Differences in Solvents and Concentration on the Efficacy of Propofol at Induction of Anesthesia

**Yukako Obata,[1] Yushi U. Adachi,[2] Katsumi Suzuki,[3] Taiga Itagaki,[4] Hiromi Kato,[1] Maiko Satomoto,[5] and Yoshiki Nakajima[1]**

[1]*Department of Intensive Care Unit, Hamamatsu University School of Medicine, 1-20-1 Handayama, Higashi-ku, Hamamatsu, Shizuoka 4313192, Japan*
[2]*Department of Intensive Care Medicine, Tokyo Medical and Dental University Medical Hospital, Tokyo, Japan*
[3]*Department of Anesthesia, Enshu Hospital, Hamamatsu, Japan*
[4]*Pulmonary and Critical Care Medicine, Massachusetts General Hospital, Boston, USA*
[5]*Department of Anesthesiology, Graduate School of Medical and Dental Sciences, Tokyo Medical and Dental University, Japan*

Correspondence should be addressed to Yushi U. Adachi; yuadachi.ccm@tmd.ac.jp

Academic Editor: Michael R. Frass

*Background.* Propofol is a popular intravenous anesthetic and varieties of formulations were produced from different laboratories. The present study compared efficacy of propofol of different laboratories and different concentrations (1 and 2%) during induction of anesthesia. *Methods.* Seventy-five scheduled surgical patients were randomly allocated into three groups. The patients of group D1 received AstraZeneca Diprivan 1% (Osaka, Japan) at a rate of 40 mg kg$^{-1}$ h$^{-1}$. Group M1 was given 1% Maruishi (Maruishi Pharmaceutical, Osaka, Japan) and group M2 was given 2% formulation at the same rate of propofol. Achieving hypnosis was defined as failure to open their eyes in response to a verbal command and the venous blood sample was withdrawn. *Results.* The hypnotic doses of M2 were significantly larger (D1: 91.4±30.9, M1: 90.7±26.7, and M2: 118.4±40.2 mg, resp. (mean ± SD). $p < 0.005$). Age and gender were selected as statistically significant covariates using general linear model-ANOVA. The blood concentration showed no significant difference among the groups (3.73 ± 2.34, 4.10 ± 3.04, and 4.70 ± 2.12 $\mu$g mL$^{-1}$, resp.). *Conclusion.* The required dose of propofol was different among the formulations; however, the serum concentration showed no significant difference. This trial is registered with UMIN Clinical Trial Registry: UMIN000019925.

## 1. Introduction

Propofol is a popular intravenous anesthetic [1] and is widely administered to patients not only for managing anesthesia but also for maintaining adequate level of sedation in Intensive Care Unit [2]. The pharmacodynamics of propofol was modified by plenty of physiological factors [3–6].

Propofol is a highly lipophilic agent and is distributed as micellized fluid composed of propofol and soybeans oil. Nowadays, varieties of formulations are produced from different laboratories. Calvo et al. [7] reported that the pharmacokinetics and pharmacodynamics of propofol were not equal among the formulations. The five products were studied for determining each pharmacological property; however, the concentration of propofol and the composition of soybeans oil were almost the same.

The aim of the present study was to compare the efficacy of propofol of different laboratories (differences in solvents) and concentrations (1% versus 2%) during the induction of anesthesia in clinical settings.

## 2. Materials and Methods

A prospective double-blind control study was conducted after obtaining approval from the Institutional Review Board of Hamamatsu University School of Medicine (Registration number: 20-22, Ethics Committee of Medicine). All interventional procedures, including written informed consent from the participants, conformed to the study protocols.

TABLE 1: Patients' demographic data and the results.

| | Diprivan 1% | 1% propofol Maruishi | 2% propofol Maruishi |
|---|---|---|---|
| Age (yr) | 60.4 ± 18.4 | 60.1 ± 17.7 | 55.1 ± 18.6 |
| Sex (m/f) | 11/14 | 14/11 | 10/15 |
| Body height (cm) | 157 ± 8.9 | 161 ± 8.9 | 161 ± 8.2 |
| Body weight (kg) | 58.6 ± 11.3 | 56.7 ± 8.8 | 60.5 ± 11.0 |
| Hypnotic dose (mg) | 91.4 ± 30.9 | 90.7 ± 26.7 | 118.4 ± 40.2 |
| Hypnotic dose/body weight ($mg\,kg^{-1}$) | 1.54 ± 0.34 | 1.59 ± 0.31 | 1.95 ± 0.55* |
| The serum concentration of propofol ($\mu g\,mL^{-1}$) | 3.73 ± 2.34 | 4.10 ± 3.04 | 4.7 ± 2.12 |

Data are expressed as mean ± SD. $^*p < 0.05$.

Seventy-five scheduled surgical patients, ASA physical states I and II without any severe cardiovascular, respiratory, liver, and renal complications, were enrolled into the study. The sample size was determined as both effect size and statistical power are 0.8. The patients received no premedication on the day of surgery.

In the operating room, standard ECG, noninvasive blood pressure, and pulse oximetry were monitored and recorded. The intravenous infusion catheter was placed on the back of hand. The participants were randomly allocated into three groups using an envelope method. After preoxygenation using face mask, the patients of group D1 received Diprivan (1%, AstraZeneca) at a rate of 40 $mg\,kg^{-1}\,h^{-1}$ [3]. Patients of group M1 were given 1% Maruishi (Maruishi Pharmaceutical) and of group M2 were given 2% Maruishi at the same rate of propofol. The carrier fluid was infused at a rate of 300 $mL\,h^{-1}$. Achieving hypnosis was defined as failure to open their eyes in response to a verbal command with light stimuli (tactile) by an anesthesiologist in charge and 3 mL of venous blood sample was simultaneously withdrawn at the cubitalis vein of upper extremities. After confirming the hypnosis, the infusion rate of propofol was reduced to 10 $mg\,kg^{-1}\,h^{-1}$, and 0.1 to 0.2 mg of fentanyl and 5 to 10 mg of vecuronium were subsequently administered for orotracheal intubation.

The venous sample was centrifuged and the serum was stored at −40°C until analysis. The other day, the serum concentration of propofol ($C_p$) was determined using an HPLC with a fluorescence detector [3, 6].

The required dose of propofol for hypnosis and $C_p$ were analyzed using general linear model-ANOVA using patients' background parameters including age and gender as covariates. A $p$ value less than 0.05 was considered as significant and subsequent post hoc analysis was applied using Newman-Keuls multiple comparison test. All calculations were performed using statistical software (NCSS2000, NCSS, LLC, Kaysville, UT).

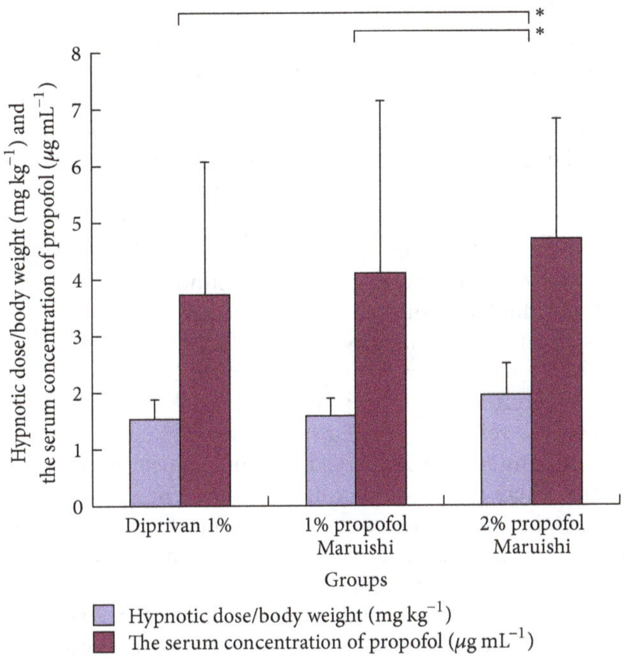


FIGURE 1: The results of the hypnotic dose of propofol and the serum concentration of propofol. The results were expressed as mean ± SD. $^*p < 0.05$ between the groups.

## 3. Results

All patients completed the study. There was no significant difference in the patients' characteristics among the groups (Table 1). The hypnotic doses of groups D1 and M1 showed no significant difference (statistical power = 0.80), whereas the dose of group M2 was significantly larger (91.4 ± 30.9, 90.7 ± 26.7, and 118.4 ± 40.2, resp. (mean ± SD). $p < 0.005$, Table 1, Figure 1). Age (−0.66 ± 0.19 mg a year (regression coefficient and SE), $p < 0.002$) and gender (−28.6 ± 6.9 mg, $p < 0.03$) were selected as statistically significant covariates for the general linear model for the dose of propofol. Elderly and female patients included potential factors decreasing the required dose of propofol for achieving hypnosis in the current study population. $C_p$ showed no significant difference among the groups (3.73 ± 2.34, 4.10 ± 3.04, and 4.70 ± 2.12 $\mu g\,mL^{-1}$, resp. (mean ± SD)). The age and gender were not correlative with $C_p$ in all 75 patients.

## 4. Discussion

The results of current investigation demonstrated that the efficacy of propofol was distinctive not by the difference of solvents (long-chain triglycerides (Diprivan) versus long- and medium-chain triglycerides (Maruishi)) but by the difference of concentration. Higher concentration of propofol compound showed lower efficacy for achieving hypnosis. Although age and gender were selected as significant determinant factors for propofol induction dose, $C_p$ was independent of the parameters.

The pharmacodynamics between blood and brain might depend on the concentration of free propofol in aqueous phase [8, 9]. There is a possibility that the differences of solvent would modify the efficacy of propofol [7, 10]. We use generic or copy formulations of propofol and the equivalency or dissimilarity among the products becomes a worrisome subject; however, the detailed information was limited [11]. The identity of the distributed formulations should be secured. If there is an apparent difference between the drugs, physicians are required to modify the dose of drugs and the timing of administration. We preliminary studied the efficacy of propofol in the institute during the induction of anesthesia [3] and reported the independent physiological factors on the hypnotic dose of propofol. The infusion method [3] was considered as showing high sensitivity, and the current study investigated a slight difference using the same manner.

There is no clear explanation for the results concerning the effect of the concentration. In the preliminary and laboratory animal experiments, we found opposite results that the diluted propofol showed greater potency [12]. In clinical settings, variability of the effect of propofol might absolutely depend on pathophysiological backgrounds [13] and the difference of formulations might be negligible. Indeed, the results of current study showed that the patient's age and gender were confirmed as significant covariates of the results. There is a possibility that the difference of efficacy of formulation might be a sequel of the interferences between these physiological factors and other unknown properties, not of the concentration of propofol.

Recently, water soluble propofol has been developed [14, 15]. Anesthesiologists will have much more options for induction of anesthesia and for maintenance of adequate sedation, and the further investigations for evaluating the properties of each formulation are absolutely required.

## Key Messages

Anesthesiologists will have much more options for intravenous anesthetics, and the further investigations for evaluating the properties of each formulation are absolutely required.

## Disclosure

Part of the results was presented in Annual Meeting of American Society of Anesthesiologists, in 2009, at Orland, Florida, USA. The presentations of the results including the current paper were in accordance with the study protocol approved by Institutional Review Board, Hamamatsu University School of Medicine. The investigational data sets have no connections to the participants by unidentified recording procedures in the institute. Yushi U. Adachi is principal investigator of the current study at Intensive Care Unit of Hamamatsu University School of Medicine during the clinical trials.

## Conflict of Interests

All authors have no conflict of interests.

## Authors' Contribution

Yukako Obata is chief investigator of the study as an anesthesiologist. Yushi U. Adachi is principal investigator of the study, receiving the approval from IRB as a principal responsible physician, collecting and analyzing the data, and writing the paper. Adachi worked in the Intensive Care Unit of Hamamatsu University School of Medicine, from August 2005 to January 2010. Katsumi Suzuki is investigator of the study, revising the paper. Suzuki worked in the Intensive Care Unit of Hamamatsu University School of Medicine, from April 2006 to March 2010. Taiga Itagaki is investigator of the study, revising the paper. Itagaki worked in the Intensive Care Unit of Hamamatsu University School of Medicine, from April 2006 to March 2012. Hiromi Kato is investigator of the study, revising the paper. Kato worked in the Intensive Care Unit of Hamamatsu University School of Medicine, from April 2007 to March 2009. Maiko Satomoto is supervisor of the study and the coresponsible physician of the study. Yoshiki Nakajima is supervisor of the study and the coresponsible physician of the study, concurrent Director of Intensive Care Unit of Hamamatsu University School of Medicine.

## References

[1] E. I. Eger, P. F. White, and M. S. Bogetz, "Clinical and economic factors important to anaesthetic choice for day-case surgery," *PharmacoEconomics*, vol. 17, no. 3, pp. 245–262, 2000.

[2] K. McKeage and C. M. Perry, "Propofol: a review of its use in intensive care sedation of adults," *CNS Drugs*, vol. 17, no. 4, pp. 235–272, 2003.

[3] Y. U. Adachi, K. Watanabe, H. Higuchi, and T. Satoh, "The determinants of propofol induction of anesthesia dose," *Anesthesia and Analgesia*, vol. 92, no. 3, pp. 656–661, 2001.

[4] M. Kodaka, J. W. Johansen, and P. S. Sebel, "The influence of gender on loss of consciousness with sevoflurane or propofol," *Anesthesia & Analgesia*, vol. 101, no. 2, pp. 377–381, 2005.

[5] M. White, G. N. C. Kenny, and S. Schraag, "Use of target controlled infusion to derive age and gender covariates for propofol clearance," *Clinical Pharmacokinetics*, vol. 47, no. 2, pp. 119–127, 2008.

[6] Y. U. Adachi, M. Satomoto, H. Higuchi, and K. Watanabe, "Rapid fluid infusion therapy decreases the plasma concentration of continuously infused propofol," *Acta Anaesthesiologica Scandinavica*, vol. 49, no. 3, pp. 331–336, 2005.

[7] R. Calvo, S. Telletxea, N. Leal et al., "Influence of formulation on propofol pharmacokinetics and pharmacodynamics in anesthetized patients," *Acta Anaesthesiologica Scandinavica*, vol. 48, no. 8, pp. 1038–1048, 2004.

[8] M. K. Zamacona, E. Suárez, E. García, C. Aguirre, and R. Calvo, "The significance of lipoproteins in serum binding variations of propofol," *Anesthesia & Analgesia*, vol. 87, no. 5, pp. 1147–1151, 1998.

[9] M. Schicher, M. Polsinger, A. Hermetter, R. Prassl, and A. Zimmer, "In vitro release of propofol and binding capacity with regard to plasma constituents," *European Journal of Pharmaceutics and Biopharmaceutics*, vol. 70, no. 3, pp. 882–888, 2008.

[10] A. W. Doenicke, M. F. Roizen, J. Rau et al., "Pharmacokinetics and pharmacodynamics of propofol in a new solvent," *Anesthesia and Analgesia*, vol. 85, no. 6, pp. 1399–1403, 1997.

[11] H. Ihmsen, C. Jeleazcov, J. Schüttler, H. Schwilden, and F. Bremer, "Pharmacodynamics of two different propofol formulations," *Anaesthesist*, vol. 55, no. 6, pp. 635–642, 2006.

[12] Y. U. Adachi, A. Numaguchi, and N. Matsuda, "Not only bupivacaine but also propofol is sinking in lipid?" *Journal of Anesthesia*, vol. 28, no. 3, p. 476, 2014.

[13] T. Kazama, K. Ikeda, K. Morita et al., "Investigation of effective anesthesia induction doses using a wide range of infusion rates with undiluted and diluted propofol," *Anesthesiology*, vol. 92, no. 4, pp. 1017–1028, 2000.

[14] B. Mahajan, S. Kaushal, and R. Mahajan, "Fospropofol," *Journal of Pharmacology and Pharmacotherapeutics*, vol. 3, no. 3, pp. 293–296, 2012.

[15] F. Ravenelle, P. Vachon, A. E. Rigby-Jones et al., "Anaesthetic effects of propofol polymeric micelle: a novel water soluble propofol formulation," *British Journal of Anaesthesia*, vol. 101, no. 2, pp. 186–193, 2008.

27

# Leakage Characteristics of Dual-Cannula Fenestrated Tracheostomy Tubes during Positive Pressure Ventilation

**Thomas Berlet**[1] **and Mathias Marchon**[2]

[1]*Department of Intensive Care Medicine, Inselspital-Bern University Hospital, 3010 Bern, Switzerland*
[2]*Department of Anaesthesiology and Pain Therapy, Inselspital-Bern University Hospital, 3010 Bern, Switzerland*

Correspondence should be addressed to Thomas Berlet; thomas.berlet@hospital-lingen.de

Academic Editor: Michael R. Frass

This study compared the leakage characteristics of different types of dual-cannula fenestrated tracheostomy tubes during positive pressure ventilation. Fenestrated Portex® Blue Line Ultra®, TRACOE® twist, or Rüsch® Traceofix® tracheostomy tubes equipped with nonfenestrated inner cannulas were tested in a tracheostomy-lung simulator. Transfenestration pressures and transfenestration leakage rates were measured during positive pressure ventilation. The impact of different ventilation modes, airway pressures, temperatures, and simulated static lung compliance settings on leakage characteristics was assessed. We observed substantial differences in transfenestration pressures and transfenestration leakage rates. The leakage rates of the best performing tubes were <3.5% of the delivered minute volume. At body temperature, the leakage rates of these tracheostomy tubes were <1%. The tracheal tube design was the main factor that determined the leakage characteristics. Careful tracheostomy tube selection permits the use of fenestrated tracheostomy tubes in patients receiving positive pressure ventilation immediately after stoma formation and minimises the risk of complications caused by transfenestration gas leakage, for example, subcutaneous emphysema.

## 1. Introduction

Percutaneous dilatational tracheostomy (PDT) is frequently performed in the intensive care unit [1]. Common indications for PDT are a prolonged duration of and gradual weaning from mechanical ventilation, protection of the tracheobronchial tree in patients at risk for aspiration, and the requirement to frequently access the respiratory tract for diagnostic or therapeutic purposes [2].

As soon as the need for high-level respiratory support subsides, trials of spontaneous breathing are usually introduced. During the rehabilitation phase the initial configuration of a tightly sealed tracheostomy tube during positive pressure ventilation is changed to cuff deflation during episodes of spontaneous breathing [3]. Here, the use of a fenestrated tracheostomy tube in combination with a fenestrated inner cannula is advantageous, because the work of breathing is minimised by the low airflow resistance afforded by these tubes [4, 5]. Even more importantly, swallowing, communication, postural stabilisation, and weight-bearing ability are better supported by dual-cannula fenestrated tracheostomy tubes, particularly when a speaking valve is mounted [6–9].

Following the publication of reports of subcutaneous emphysema and pneumothorax developing in connection with the use of dual-cannula fenestrated tracheostomy tubes for PDT, many authors advised against the use of these types of tubes in patients who require positive pressure ventilation [1, 10–12].

We hypothesised that the risk of surgical emphysema formation is related to the degree of air leakage through the fenestrations. We therefore performed a bench study to quantify and compare the leakage characteristics of different types of commonly used dual-cannula fenestrated tracheostomy tubes under varying conditions. A pseudotrachea was used to study ex vivo the performance of tracheostomy tubes.

TABLE 1: Types and specifications of tracheostomy tubes tested.

| Type | Manufacturer | Size | Inner cannula Internal diameter | Outer cannula Outer diameter |
|---|---|---|---|---|
| Portex Blue Line Ultra | Smith Medical, Grasbrunn, Germany | 8 | 6.5 mm | 11.9 mm |
| TRACOE twist | Tracoe Medical, Nieder-Olm, Germany | 8 | 8.0 mm | 11.4 mm |
| Rüsch Traceofix | Teleflex, Kernen, Germany | 8.5 | 7.0 mm | 10.3 mm |

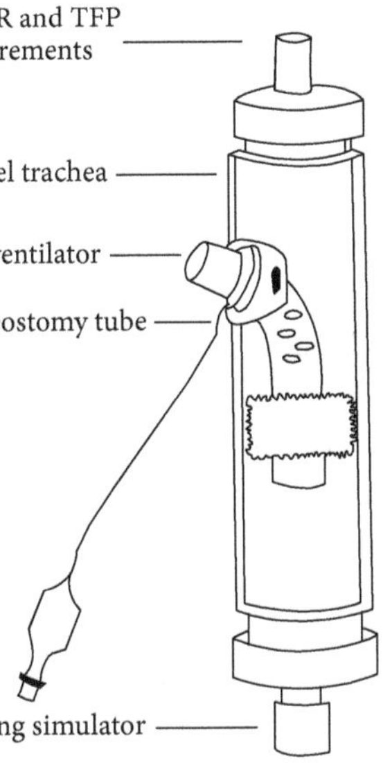


FIGURE 1: Schematic drawing of tracheostomy simulator with a fenestrated tracheostomy tube sited. TFLR: transfenestration leakage rate; TFP: transfenestration pressure.

Our aim was to derive recommendations regarding the safe use of fenestrated tracheostomy tubes immediately after tracheostomy formation.

## 2. Materials and Methods

We built a tracheostomy simulator comprising a polyethylene tube that represented the trachea (length, 20 cm; internal diameter, 25 mm). A 10 mm side hole was fashioned at one-third the length of the tubing; it represented the tracheostomy (Figure 1). Different types of fenestrated tracheostomy tubes with nonfenestrated inner cannulas were studied (Table 1).

A tracheostomy tube to be tested was inserted through the tracheostomy, and the cuff was inflated. A seal was fashioned around the tracheostomy insertion site using rubber washers and putty. Leak testing was performed prior to each experiment to ascertain the leak tightness of both the tracheostomy tube cuff within the trachea and the insertion site of the tracheostomy tube. The trachea simulator was then placed upright into a laboratory stand. The lower ("bronchial") portion of the artificial trachea was connected to a single compartment lung simulator (LS-122; Medishield, Harlow, Essex, UK), and the upper ("pharyngeal") portion of the artificial trachea was connected to a 2.3-l anaesthesia breathing bag so that any gas escaping through the fenestrations of the tracheostomy tube could be collected. Polyvinylchloride fittings and nonexpandable polyethylene tubing were used for all connections. A SERVO-i® ventilator (Maquet, Rastatt, Germany) was connected to the tracheostomy tube. The ventilator and lung simulator compliance settings were varied as described in Table 2.

TABLE 2: Ventilator and lung simulator compliance settings.

| Variable | Settings |
|---|---|
| Ventilation mode | Volume-controlled<br>Pressure-controlled |
| Ventilator rate (breaths·min$^{-1}$) | 15 |
| Tidal volume (mL) | 450 ± 5% |
| Inspiration : expiration ratio | 1 : 2 |
| Positive end-expiratory pressure (mbar) | 3, 6, 9, 12 |
| Lung simulator compliance (mL·mbar$^{-1}$) | 20, 50 |
| Lung simulator resistance (mbar·mL$^{-1}$·sec$^{-1}$) | 5 |

Experiments were run at either 21° ± 1°C or 37° ± 1°C. For the latter experimental runs, a polyethylene hood was fashioned to encase the laboratory stand holding the tracheostomy simulator. Preheated air, generated by a Bair Hugger® temperature management device (3M, Rüschlikon, Switzerland), was fed into the hood. The temperature of the tracheostomy simulator was continuously monitored with a digital thermometer (TFA®; Conrad Electronic SE, Hirschau, Germany).

Two types of measurements were obtained for each combination of ventilator and lung simulator settings and temperatures. The first measurement was the transfenestration pressure (TFP): the pharyngeal end of the trachea was occluded by clamping the connecting tubing, and the build-up of pressure in the space above the tracheostomy tube was measured with a digital manometer (PCE-P01; PCE Instruments, Meschede, Germany) until a steady state was reached. The second measurement was the transfenestration leak rate (TFLR) (minute ventilation fraction). Prior to each experimental run, the anaesthesia bag was thoroughly emptied and gas escaping through the fenestrations of the tracheostomy tube was collected into the anaesthesia breathing bag for 1–3 min, depending on the magnitude of the leakage. The volume of the collected gas was measured using the water displacement method. To distinguish between the amount of gas leaking through the fenestration and the amount of gas leaking through the connection site of the inner and outer cannula, the difference between the inspiratory and expiratory minute volumes measured by the ventilator and the TFLR was calculated. All experiments were run in duplicate. Measurements were repeated if corresponding pressure

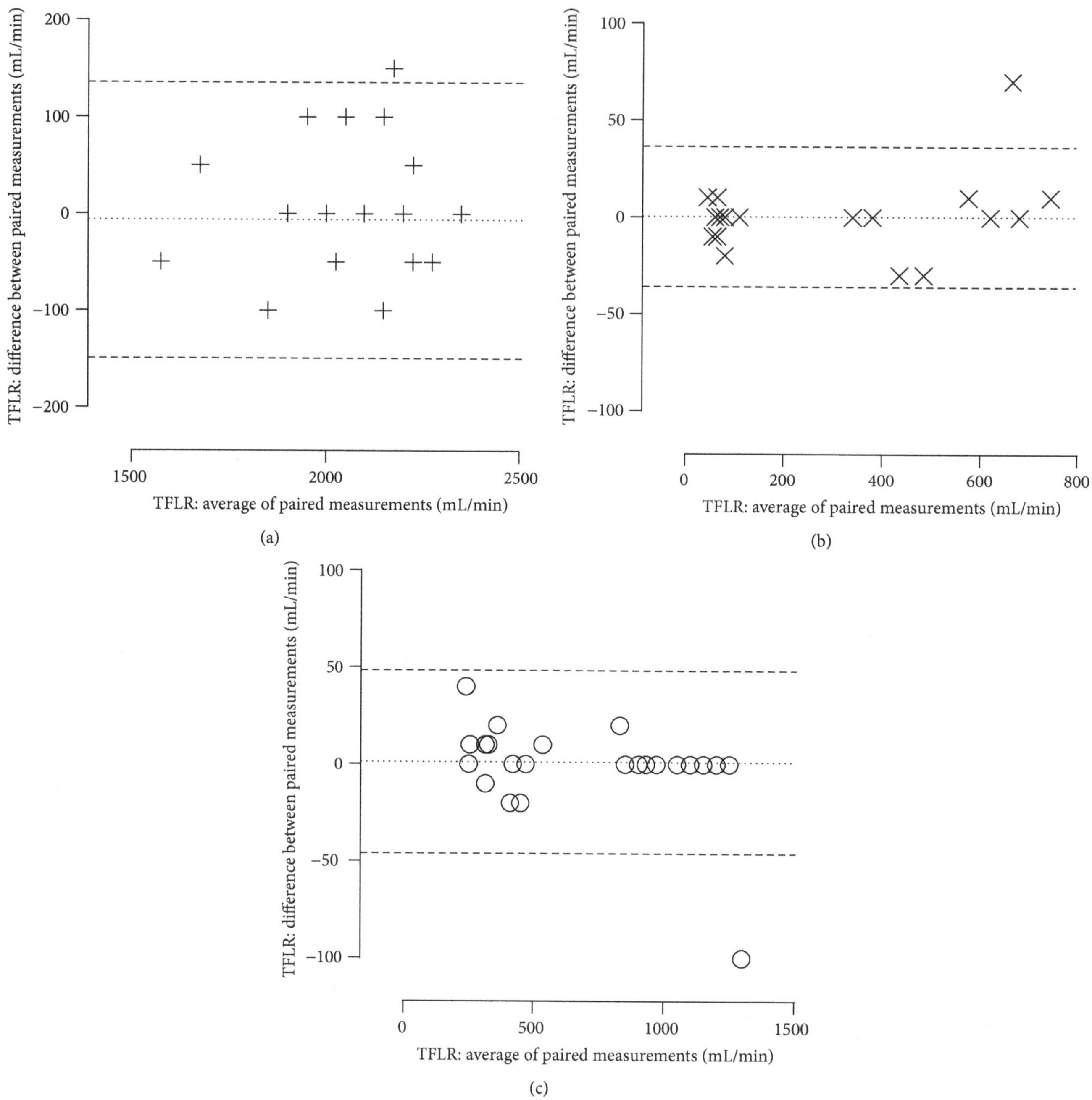


FIGURE 2: Bland-Altman plot of paired transfenestration leakage rates of Portex Blue Line Ultra (+), TRACOE twist (×), or Rüsch Traceofix (O) tracheostomy tubes. TFLR: transfenestration leakage rate.

measurements differed by >5% or volume measurements differed by >5% and >10 mL·min$^{-1}$.

Statistical analysis was performed using the StatPlus® 8 software package (AnalystSoft Inc., Alexandria, VA, USA). Data are presented as individual measurements. The Mann-Whitney test was used for comparisons of nonnormally distributed continuous data, and the Wilcoxon matched-pairs test was used for comparisons of nonnormally distributed paired data. Spearman's rank order correlation coefficient was used to assess the relationships between continuous variables. All tests of statistical significance were two-sided. *P* values of <0.05 were considered statistically significant.

## 3. Results

The reliability of the experimental setup as assessed by the Bland-Altman method is depicted in Figures 2(a)–2(c). One hundred and thirty-six of 144 paired TFLR measurements differed by no more than 5% or 10 mL·min$^{-1}$.

Differences in TFLR and TFP were observed between different types of tracheostomy tubes exposed to identical

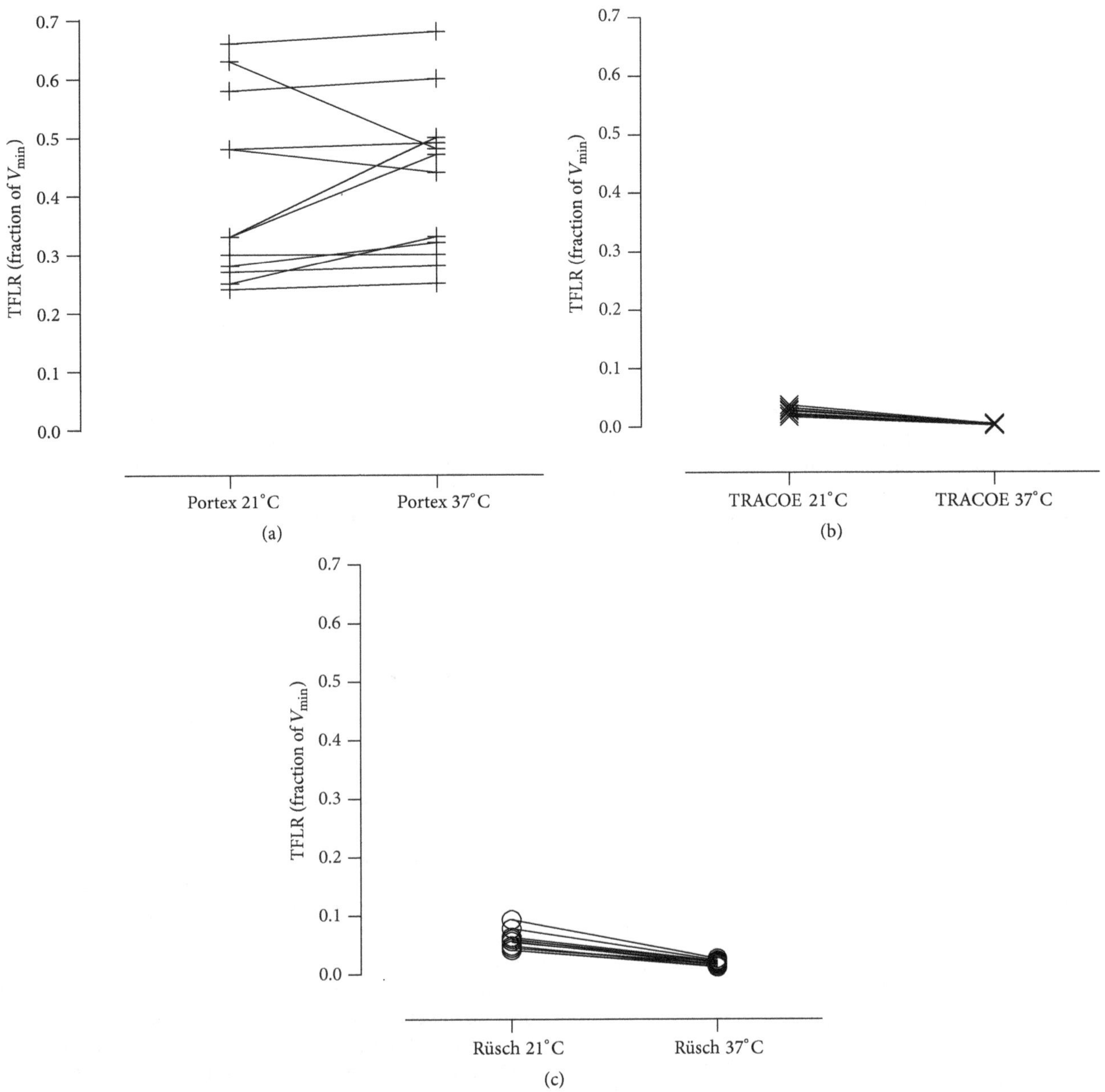


FIGURE 3: Transfenestration leakage rates of Portex Blue Line Ultra (+), TRACOE twist (×), or Rüsch Traceofix (O) tracheostomy tubes. Measurements were performed at 21 ± 1°C or 37 ± 1°C. TFLR: transfenestration leakage rate; $V_{min}$: minute ventilation.

experimental conditions. Additionally, variations in TFLR and TFP were observed for each tracheostomy tube as the experimental conditions were modified.

TFLR ranged from 0.2% to 67.6% of minute ventilation, and TFP ranged from 1 to 16 mbar across the entire range of investigated combinations of types of tracheostomy tubes, temperatures, ventilation modes, and compliance settings.

Figures 3(a)–3(c) illustrate the variations in TFLR at different temperature settings. Raising the temperature of the experimental setup from 21°C ± 1°C to 37°C ± 1°C resulted in no statistically significant changes in TFLR when using the Portex Blue Line Ultra tracheostomy tubes ($P = 0.403$). In contrast, TFLR decreased significantly when using the TRACOE twist and Rüsch Traceofix tubes ($P = 0.0022$).

Because tracheostomy tube's performance at body temperature is relevant to clinical practice, the following results refer to experiments that were performed at 37 ± 1°C.

Figure 4 illustrates the relationship between the mean airway pressure and TFP. The correlation coefficient was 0.98 for the Rüsch Traceofix tubes, 0.99 for the TRACOE twist tubes, and 1.0 for the Portex Blue Line Ultra tubes.

Figure 5 illustrates the relationship between the mean airway pressure and TFLR. The correlation coefficient was 0.89 for the TRACOE twist tubes, 0.98 for the Portex Blue Line Ultra tubes, and 0.99 for the Rüsch Traceofix tubes.

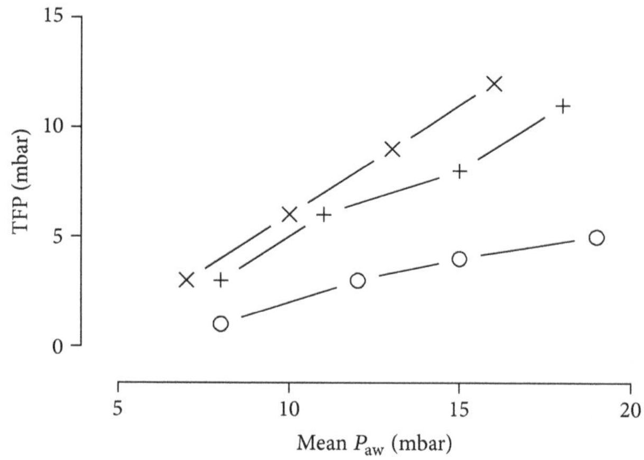


FIGURE 4: Transfenestration pressures of Portex Blue Line Ultra (+), TRACOE twist (×), or Rüsch Traceofix (○) tracheostomy tubes plotted against increase in mean airway pressures. Measurements were obtained in volume-controlled ventilation (ventilator rate: 15 breaths·min$^{-1}$, tidal volume: 450 mL) at 37 ± 1°C. Lung simulator compliance: 20 mL·mbar$^{-1}$. TFP: transfenestration pressure; $P_{aw}$: mean airway pressure.

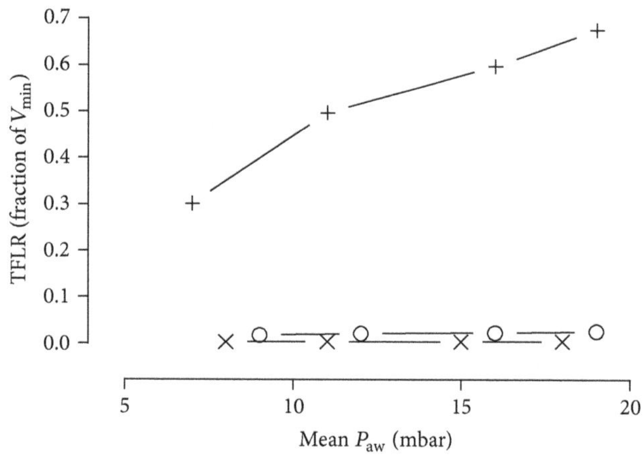


FIGURE 5: Transfenestration leakage rates of Portex Blue Line Ultra (+), TRACOE twist (×), or Rüsch Traceofix (○) tracheostomy tubes plotted against increase in mean airway pressures. Measurements were obtained in volume-controlled ventilation (ventilator rate: 15 breaths·min$^{-1}$, tidal volume: 450 mL) at 37 ± 1°C. Lung simulator compliance: 20 mL·mbar$^{-1}$. TFLR: transfenestration leakage rate; $P_{aw}$: mean airway pressure; $V_{min}$: minute ventilation.

By comparing the ratio of TFLR to the difference in the inspiratory and expiratory minute volume as measured by the ventilator, an additional source of leakage at the interface of the inner and outer cannulas was identified in the TRACOE twist tube (Figure 6).

Switching from the volume-controlled ventilation mode to the pressure-controlled ventilation mode resulted in no statistically significant variation in TFP or TFLR for any make of tracheostomy tube.

Changes in static compliance did not significantly alter TFP or TFLR for any make of tracheostomy tube.

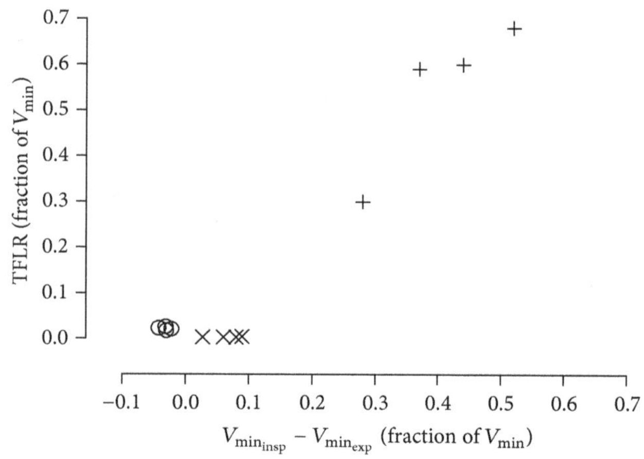


FIGURE 6: Loss of delivered minute volume of Portex Blue Line Ultra (+), TRACOE twist (×), or Rüsch Traceofix (○) tracheostomy tubes plotted against transfenestration leakage rate measured at PEEP settings of 3, 6, 9, and 12 mbar. Measurements were obtained in volume-controlled ventilation (ventilator rate: 15 breaths·min$^{-1}$, tidal volume: 450 mL) at 37 ± 1°C. Lung simulator compliance: 20 mL·mbar$^{-1}$. TFLR: transfenestration leakage rate; $V_{min_{insp}}$: inspiratory minute ventilation; $V_{min_{exp}}$: expiratory minute ventilation.

## 4. Discussion

In this study, the sources and degree of leakage of different types of tracheostomy tubes during positive pressure ventilation, the impact of the tube design, and the variability of tracheostomy tube's performance at different temperatures were investigated for the first time.

We found substantial variations in TFLR and TFP for different types of fenestrated tracheostomy tubes when used in combination with nonfenestrated inner cannulas. The leakage rates of the best performing tubes did not exceed 3.5% of the delivered minute volume. When tested at body temperature, the leakage rates of these tracheostomy tubes dropped even further to <1%. The tracheal tube design was the main factor that determined the leakage characteristics. Two features of the cannula design were found to be associated with the lowest TFLR and TFP: connection of the ventilator catheter mount to the inner cannula and a tightly sealed interface of the inner and outer cannulas. The Blue Line Ultra tracheostomy tube is designed to connect to the ventilator catheter mount via the outer cannula; it yielded the highest TFLR and TFP. The TRACOE twist tube had low TFLR but a significant degree of leakage at the interface of the inner and outer cannulas. The Rüsch Traceofix tracheostomy tube had low TFLR and TFP and a tight seal at the cannula interface. The ventilation mode and lung compliance had little impact on the leakage characteristics.

The cause of subcutaneous emphysema after PDT and insertion of dual-cannula fenestrated tracheostomy tubes is the tracking of air between the nonfenestrated inner cannula and the fenestrated outer cannula with subsequent leakage through the fenestrations [10, 12]. If the air cannot escape through the glottis or the tracheostomy wound, it tracks into the soft tissue of the neck, particularly if the fenestrations abut the subcutaneous tissue.

Mostert and Stuart [10] gave the first report of a patient who developed subcutaneous emphysema while being mechanically ventilated through a newly inserted fenestrated Portex Blue Line Ultra tracheostomy tube. Following the publication of that case report, the manufacturer issued a warning to confirm the correct position of the fenestration after the procedure. A review of the tracheostomy tube's design implicated in the critical incident was envisaged; however, the design of the Portex Blue Line Ultra tracheostomy tube with regard to the position of the fenestrations appears to have since remained unchanged.

Fikkers et al. [12] presented a review of the literature on emphysema and pneumothorax after percutaneous tracheostomy. Sixty-six cases of pneumothorax or subcutaneous emphysema were identified; two of these (3%) were caused by extraluminal misplacement of the fenestrations of the tracheotomy tubes. These authors performed a bench study using a fenestrated Shiley tracheostomy tube fitted with a nonfenestrated inner tube. The leakage rate, as detected by the difference between the inspiratory and expiratory tidal volumes during pressure-controlled ventilation, reached 2780 mL·min$^{-1}$. The authors also measured the size of the gap between the inner circumference of the outer cannula and the outer circumference of the inner cannula at 0.14 mm. In the present study, comparable leakage rates were found in the Blue Line Ultra tracheostomy tube.

Orme and Welham [11] reported a case of subcutaneous emphysema that occurred with the use of a fenestrated Portex Blue Line Ultra tracheostomy tube with a nonfenestrated inner cannula. Two faults contributed to the emphysema formation: malpositioning of the fenestrations of the tracheostomy tube and undetected partial detachment of the inner cannula. These problems caused the surrounding tissues to be fully exposed to the pressure generated by the ventilator. The authors called for discontinuation of the use of fenestrated cannulas early after tracheostomy. Their report corroborates our findings of the significance of the tightness of the seal at the interface between the inner and outer cannulas.

In 2008, the UK Intensive Care Society [13] recommended against the use of fenestrated tracheostomy tubes early after stoma formation. This advice was carried forward to the current version of the guidelines [1]. Powell et al. [14] conducted a survey of the use of nonfenestrated versus fenestrated tracheostomy tubes in UK intensive care units. Eight of eight units that used fenestrated tracheostomy tubes reported the occurrence of surgical emphysema in any of their patients. The authors interpreted this as a powerful indicator of the frequent causation of subcutaneous emphysema by the use of fenestrated tubes.

Weaning from mechanical ventilation and from the tracheostomy itself is a challenging, often drawn out task, particularly after long-term ventilator support. The ability to communicate verbally is an important step towards reestablishing patient autonomy and quality of life [7, 15, 16]. Cuff deflation of the tracheostomy tube is performed not only to facilitate spontaneous breathing and promote swallowing but also, and arguably more importantly, to enable communication.

During spontaneous breathing through a tracheostomy tube, airflow resistance should be decreased to minimise the work of breathing [4]. In this scenario, the use of a fenestrated tracheostomy tube is preferable to the use of a nonfenestrated tube [5]. Communication is aided by the use of a fenestrated tube [2]. If a speaking valve is attached, its tolerance can be increased by the additional airflow through the fenestrations of the tracheostomy tube [3]. Engaging vocal cord function improves postural stability and weight-bearing ability. This is best achieved with a cuff-deflated fenestrated tracheostomy tube used in combination with a speaking valve [9]. However, care must be taken not to negate the benefits of reduced airflow resistance of fenestrated tracheostomy tubes by malpositioning of the fenestrations [17].

Abandoning the use of fenestrated tracheostomy tubes reduces both the speed and the efficiency of the rehabilitation process, because the advantages of these types of tubes will be unavailable until a change of tracheostomy tube. This can only be safely performed several days after the initial procedure; it requires resources and carries certain risks [17].

Our work provides insight into the benefits of using particular types of fenestrated tracheostomy tubes and can be used in the selection of a suitable tracheostomy tube. In devising a pseudotrachea we built on the experience reported by Hussey and Bishop of the use of a model trachea to study tracheostomy tube's performance [5]. We believe that our experimental setup offered sufficient fidelity to serve as a surrogate for an in vivo tracheostomy scenario.

Our study could be criticised for not including the entire range of commercially available tracheostomy tubes. Because we aimed to explore not only the implication of the tube design but also the impact of temperature, ventilator settings, and lung compliance, we made a conscious decision to limit the scope of the study to a selection of widely used tracheostomy tubes.

The thermal behaviour of plastic materials provides a possible explanation for our observation of a significant improvement in leakage rates when tracheostomy tubes were tested at body temperature. Tracheostomy tubes are made from polyvinylchloride or polyurethane, and inner tubes are made from polypropylene. These materials are thermoplastics: they expand and become more pliable as temperature rises [18]. Temperature-dependent expansion of both the outer cannula and inner cannula will narrow the gap between these two components, thus reducing the potential of air tracking toward the fenestration. The increase in pliability may have a synergistic effect: the pressure exerted by the inflated cuff may push the outer cannula further toward the inner cannula, thus further narrowing the gap between the two. As a result of the overall reduction in space available for air leakage, the gas flow will diminish, significantly reducing TFP and particularly TFLR.

Little is known about the impact of the thermoplastic characteristics of the various plastic materials used on tracheostomy tube performance [19]. Further research should be performed to explore this aspect in more detail with the aim of further optimisation of the design of fenestrated tracheostomy tubes.

## 5. Conclusion

Transfenestration gas leakage of fenestrated tracheostomy tubes is highly variable when these tubes are used in combination with nonfenestrated inner cannulas and exposed to positive pressure ventilation. In vitro leakage testing enables the identification of fenestrated tracheostomy tubes that are suitable for immediate use after stoma formation in patients expected to benefit from early trials of spontaneous breathing and rehabilitation of swallowing, communication, and mobilisation.

## Competing Interests

The authors declare that there are no competing interests regarding the publication of this paper.

## Acknowledgments

The authors are indebted to Professor Jukka Takala, chairman of the Department of Intensive Care Medicine at Inselspital, for providing the opportunity to conduct this investigational project.

## References

[1] Intensive Care Society, "Standards for the care of adult patients with a temporary tracheostomy," 2014, http://www.ics.ac.uk/ics-homepage/guidelines-and-standards/.

[2] H. G. W. Paw and A. R. Bodenham, "Indications and timing of tracheostomy," in *Percutaneous Tracheostomy. A Practical Handbook*, pp. 21–28, Cambridge University Press, Cambridge, UK, 2004.

[3] C. Russell, "Tracheostomy tubes," in *Tracheostomy. A Multiprofessional Handbook*, pp. 85–114, Cambridge University Press, Cambridge, UK, 2004.

[4] B. Beard and F. J. Monaco, "Tracheostomy discontinuation: impact of tube selection on resistance during tube occlusion," *Respiratory Care*, vol. 38, no. 3, pp. 267–270, 1993.

[5] J. D. Hussey and M. J. Bishop, "Pressures required to move gas through the native airway in the presence of a fenestrated vs a nonfenestrated tracheostomy tube," *Chest*, vol. 110, no. 2, pp. 494–497, 1996.

[6] A.-L. Sutt, P. Cornwell, D. Mullany, T. Kinneally, and J. F. Fraser, "The use of tracheostomy speaking valves in mechanically ventilated patients results in improved communication and does not prolong ventilation time in cardiothoracic intensive care unit patients," *Journal of Critical Care*, vol. 30, no. 3, pp. 491–494, 2015.

[7] D. R. Hess, "Facilitating speech in the patient with a tracheostomy," *Respiratory Care*, vol. 50, no. 4, pp. 519–525, 2005.

[8] H. G. W. Paw and A. R. Bodenham, "Aftercare, decannulation and follow-up," in *Percutaneous Tracheostomy. A Practical Handbook*, pp. 121–130, Cambridge University Press, Cambridge, UK, 2004.

[9] M. Massery, M. Hagins, R. Stafford, V. Moerchen, and P. W. Hodges, "Effect of airway control by glottal structures on postural stability," *Journal of Applied Physiology*, vol. 115, no. 4, pp. 483–490, 2013.

[10] M. J. Mostert and H. Stuart, "Subcutaneous emphysema caused by a fenestrated tracheostomy tube," *Anaesthesia*, vol. 56, no. 2, pp. 183–197, 2001.

[11] R. M. L. Orme and K. L. Welham, "Subcutaneous emphysema after percutaneous tracheostomy—time to dispense with fenestrated tubes?" *Anaesthesia*, vol. 61, no. 9, pp. 911–91, 2006.

[12] B. G. Fikkers, J. A. van Veen, J. G. Kooloos et al., "Emphysema and pneumothorax after percutaneous tracheostomy: case reports and an anatomic study," *Chest*, vol. 125, no. 5, pp. 1805–1814, 2004.

[13] Intensive Care Society, "Care of the adult patient with a temporarytracheostomy," 2008.

[14] H. R. F. Powell, S. Hanna-Jumma, J. M. Philpott, and D. Higgins, "National survey of fenestrated versus non-fenestrated tracheostomy tube use and the incidence of surgical emphysema in UK adult intensive care units," *Journal of the Intensive Care Society*, vol. 12, no. 1, pp. 25–28, 2011.

[15] V. Pandian, C. P. Smith, T. Kling Cole et al., "Optimizing communication in mechanically ventilated patients," *Journal of Medical Speech-Language Pathology*, vol. 21, pp. 309–318, 2014.

[16] A. L. Freeman-Sanderson, L. Togher, M. R. Elkins, and P. R. Phipps, "Return of voice for ventilated tracheostomy patients in ICU: a randomized controlled trial of early-targeted intervention," *Critical Care Medicine*, 2016.

[17] D. R. Hess and N. P. Altobelli, "Tracheostomy tubes," *Respiratory Care*, vol. 59, no. 6, pp. 956–973, 2014.

[18] Engineer's Handbook, "Plastic thermal expansion coefficients," 2010, http://www.engineershandbook.com/Tables/plasticthermalexp.htm.

[19] S. Maguire, F. Haury, and K. Jew, "An in vitro comparison of tracheostomy tube cuffs," *Medical Devices: Evidence and Research*, vol. 8, pp. 185–192, 2015.

# 28

# Length of Stay in Ambulatory Surgical Oncology Patients at High Risk for Sleep Apnea as Predicted by STOP-BANG Questionnaire

**Diwakar D. Balachandran,[1] Saadia A. Faiz,[1] Mike Hernandez,[2] Alicia M. Kowalski,[3] Lara Bashoura,[1] Farzin Goravanchi,[3] Sujith V. Cherian,[4] Elizabeth Rebello,[3] Spencer S. Kee,[3] and Katy E. French[3]**

[1] *Department of Pulmonary Medicine, The University of Texas MD Anderson Cancer Center, Houston, TX, USA*
[2] *Department of Biostatistics, The University of Texas MD Anderson Cancer Center, Houston, TX, USA*
[3] *Department of Anesthesia and Perioperative Medicine, The University of Texas MD Anderson Cancer Center, Houston, TX, USA*
[4] *Divisions of Pulmonary, Critical Care and Sleep Medicine, The University of Texas Health Science Center at Houston, Houston, TX, USA*

Correspondence should be addressed to Diwakar D. Balachandran; dbalachandran@mdanderson.org

Academic Editor: Enrico Camporesi

*Background.* The STOP-BANG questionnaire has been used to identify surgical patients at risk for undiagnosed obstructive sleep apnea (OSA) by classifying patients as low risk (LR) if STOP-BANG score < 3 or high risk (HR) if STOP-BANG score ≥ 3. Few studies have examined whether postoperative complications are increased in HR patients and none have been described in oncologic patients. *Objective.* This retrospective study examined if HR patients experience increased complications evidenced by an increased length of stay (LOS) in the postanesthesia care unit (PACU). *Methods.* We retrospectively measured LOS and the frequency of oxygen desaturation (<93%) in cancer patients who were given the STOP-BANG questionnaire prior to cystoscopy for urologic disease in an ambulatory surgery center. *Results.* The majority of patients in our study were men (77.7%), over the age of 50 (90.1%), and had BMI < 30 kg/m$^2$ (88.4%). STOP-BANG results were obtained on 404 patients. Cumulative incidence of the time to discharge between HR and the LR groups was plotted. By 8 hours, LR patients showed a higher cumulative probability of being discharged early (80% versus 74%, $P = 0.008$). *Conclusions.* Urologic oncology patients at HR for OSA based on the STOP-BANG questionnaire were less likely to be discharged early from the PACU compared to LR patients.

## 1. Introduction

Obstructive sleep apnea (OSA) is characterized by repetitive episodes of apnea or reduced inspiratory airflow due to upper airway obstruction, resulting in increased respiratory effort, oxyhemoglobin desaturation, and frequent neuronal arousals during sleep. General anesthesia and perioperative analgesia may often exacerbate this pathophysiology; thus, OSA patients may suffer from postoperative respiratory, cardiovascular, and neurological complications [1–6]. OSA can further complicate perioperative care by impacting recovery time and increasing hospital length of stay (LOS). Surprisingly, up to 70% of patients undergoing surgery may have undiagnosed OSA, thus increasing the need to develop strategies to identify patients at risk [7, 8].

The STOP-BANG is a simple patient-administered questionnaire developed by Chung and associates with screen for OSA in the perioperative setting, and it has a high sensitivity for detecting OSA in this setting [9]. The STOP-BANG consists of 8 items producing a numerical score that can be used to classify patients as low risk (LR, score < 3), intermediate risk (IR, score of 3 or 4), and high risk (HR, score ≥ 5) for OSA. Several studies have demonstrated that patients with higher preoperative STOP-BANG scores have increased postoperative complications, including increased difficulty with intubations and unanticipated critical care admissions [10–12].

Although the American Society of Anesthesiologists (ASA) and the Society for Ambulatory Anesthesia have issued guidelines for the perioperative management of OSA, standardized data addressing the appropriate duration and setting for monitoring patients undergoing ambulatory procedures is lacking [13–15]. Furthermore, the optimal management strategy for mitigating the risk of complications in patients with OSA remains unclear. No previous study has examined the incidence and risk of perioperative OSA in an oncologic population. The purpose of our study was to use the STOP-BANG questionnaire to classify patients as LR or HR for OSA and determine if HR patients were less likely to be discharged early from the PACU when compared to LR patients.

## 2. Methods

This study is a retrospective review of the medical records of 1666 consecutive patients with urologic cancer who underwent cystoscopy in the ambulatory surgical center at University of Texas MD Anderson Cancer Center in Houston, Texas, from March 2013 to February 2015. The study was conducted with the approval of our institution's institutional review board. Due to the retrospective nature of this study and adherence to the established standard of care, a waiver of informed consent was obtained.

Patients and clinical characteristics included basic demographics: (i) age, (ii) sex, and (iii) body mass index (BMI). The STOP-BANG questionnaire was administered to 404 patients as part of the standard of care while in the perioperative anesthesia assessment center to determine risk of OSA. The STOP-BANG survey consists of the following 8 items: (i) loud snoring; (ii) being tired, fatigued, or sleepy; (iii) observed stop of breathing; (iv) high blood pressure; (v) body mass index (BMI) > $35\,kg/m^2$; (vi) age older than 50; (vii) neck size > 17 inches (40 cm); and (viii) male gender. Patients were assigned a value of "1" if the response was affirmative with each item and a "0" if negative. STOP-BANG scores range from 0 to 8. We utilized a dichotomous framework with HR patients defined as those with a STOP-Bang score ≥ 3 and LR patients defined as those with a STOP-Bang score < 3 [9]. Complete STOP-BANG scores were acquired on 404 patients. If a patient had more than one cystoscopy during the course of the study period, the STOP-BANG score and other parameters were gathered from the first procedure.

Medical information from the time spent in the postanesthesia care unit (PACU) was obtained from an integrated perioperative electronic medical record (PICIS, Westfield, MA). Parameters recorded while in the PACU included the following: (i) vital signs during observation, (ii) time of admission to PACU, (iii) time of discharge from PACU, and (iv) procedure time. Length of stay (LOS) was defined as the duration of time in PACU, and it was calculated as the time from admission to the PACU to the time the patient met established discharge criteria such as adequate pain control, voiding, and tolerance of oral intake. All patients were kept for a minimum of 2 hours in the PACU. Oxygen desaturation was defined as oxygen saturation less than 93% with or without supplemental oxygen for 10 seconds, as recorded by pulse oximetry.

*2.1. Statistical Analysis.* Descriptive statistics were used to summarize patients' demographic and clinical characteristics by LR and HR status established by the STOP-BANG questionnaire. Histograms, box plots, and one-way scatter plots were used to visually assess the distributions of continuous characteristics of interest. Independent samples $t$-tests, or Wilcoxon rank-sum tests if more appropriate, were used to compare continuous characteristics between the LR and HR patients. In cases where the data was categorical, comparisons were made using Chi-square tests. Our primary hypothesis was that HR patients would have longer discharge times relative to LR patients. Cumulative incidence plots were generated to illustrate the cumulative probability of patient discharge at any time during the postoperative follow-up period. The distributions of discharge times were compared between HR and LR patients using a log-rank test. Secondary aims included the assessment of LOS and more frequent episodes of oxygen desaturation where a correlation coefficient was estimated. All statistical tests were two-sided, and a $P$ value < 0.05 was used to signify statistical significance. All analyses were performed using Stata version 12.0 (Stata, College Station, TX).

## 3. Results

Four hundred and four consecutive cancer patients provided complete information to obtain a STOP-BANG score. Patient characteristics are summarized in Table 1. The majority of patients surveyed were men (77.7%), over 50 years of age (90.1%), and had BMI < $30\,kg/m^2$ (88.4%). Anesthesia duration between the two groups was similar with a mean of 63 minutes in the LR group and 61.3 minutes in the HR group ($P = 0.560$, Table 2).

The patients were categorized into HR and LR categories on the basis of the patients' STOP-BANG scores (Table 2). The average PACU LOS, procedure time, and frequency of oxygen saturation <93% during the PACU stay are also shown in Table 2 for both the HR and LR categories. Overall, the mean PACU LOS was 372.4 minutes. Figure 1 shows the cumulative incidence plots which illustrate the time to discharge between HR and the LR groups. By 8 hours, LR patients showed a higher cumulative probability of being discharged early (80% versus 74%, $P = 0.008$). The separation of the curves does not persist beyond 20 hours, although, by then, most patients were discharged. All patients were discharged home, and there were no patients admitted overnight. Figure 2 demonstrates that the mean duration of anesthesia in LR and HR patients was similar.

Oxygen desaturation was examined as a potential etiology for increased LOS (Figure 3), but there was no statistical difference in the frequency of oxygen desaturation between the LR and HR groups ($P = 0.131$). However, there was a statistically significant positive correlation between LOS and frequency of oxygen desaturation ($r = 0.30$, $P < 0.001$).

TABLE 1: Patient characteristics.

| | $N = 404^*$ | Percentage |
|---|---|---|
| BMI (kg/m²) | | |
| Mean ± SD | 28.5 ± 5.7 | |
| Median (min to max) | 27.3 (16.5 to 51) | |
| Neck circumference (cm) | | |
| Mean ± SD | 39.8 ± 4.6 | |
| Median (min to max) | 40 (28 to 54) | |
| PACU LOS (minutes) | | |
| Mean ± SD | 372.4 ± 433.0 | |
| Median (min to max) | 137.5 (39 to 1667) | |
| Procedure time (minutes) | | |
| Mean ± SD | 61.7 ± 24.2 | |
| Median (min to max) | 55 (26 to 256) | |
| Oxygen saturation below 93% (count) | | |
| Mean ± SD | 3.7 ± 3.8 | |
| Median (min to max) | 2 (1 to 18) | |
| STOP-BANG items | | |
| Snoring | | |
| No | 305 | 75.5 |
| Yes | 99 | 24.5 |
| Tiredness | | |
| No | 227 | 56.2 |
| Yes | 177 | 43.8 |
| Observed apneas | | |
| No | 361 | 89.4 |
| Yes | 43 | 10.6 |
| High blood pressure | | |
| No | 169 | 41.8 |
| Yes | 235 | 58.2 |
| BMI > 35 kg/m² | | |
| No | 357 | 88.4 |
| Yes | 47 | 11.6 |
| Age > 50 years | | |
| No | 40 | 9.9 |
| Yes | 364 | 90.1 |
| Neck > 40 cm | | |
| No | 234 | 57.9 |
| Yes | 170 | 42.1 |
| Gender | | |
| Female | 90 | 22.3 |
| Male | 314 | 77.7 |
| STOP-BANG criteria | | |
| Low risk (<3) | 100 | 24.8 |
| High risk (≥3) | 304 | 75.2 |

TABLE 1: Continued.

| | $N = 404^*$ | Percentage |
|---|---|---|
| Bicarbonate ≥ 28 mmol/L | | |
| No | 194 | 48 |
| Yes | 210 | 52 |

BMI, body mass index; SD, standard deviation; PACU, postanesthesia care unit. *404 patients provided complete STOP-BANG information to derive a total score.

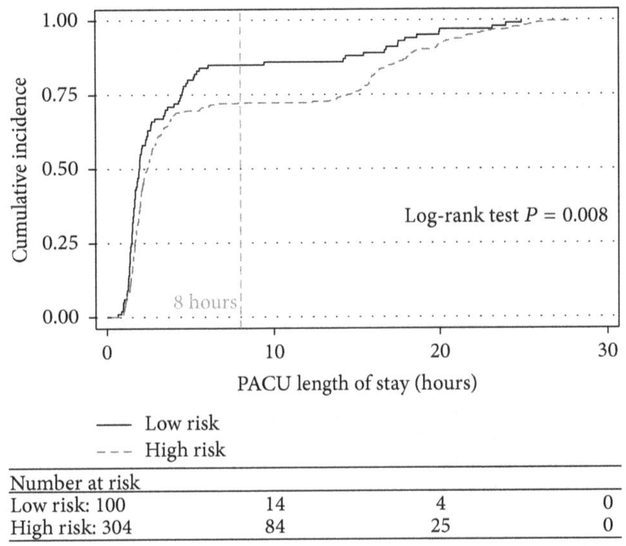


FIGURE 1: Cumulative incidence of discharge over time in the PACU.

## 4. Discussion

Our study demonstrates a longer LOS for those stratified as HR patients based on the STOP-BANG questionnaire in an ambulatory oncologic setting. Although more frequent oxygen desaturations were not observed, an increased time to discharge between the LR and HR groups was noted. Our data further corroborates other published works using this screening tool for postoperative outcome in general surgery patients. It is the first study to utilize the STOP-BANG and assess outcomes in a purely oncologic and ambulatory population.

Many oncologic patients require general anesthesia and surgery multiple times throughout the treatment of their cancer. Although little is known about the clinical impact of OSA in surgical oncology patients, undiagnosed OSA in the perioperative setting has been shown to have more complications, especially cardiac or respiratory in origin [16]. The nature of anesthesia places patients with sleep apnea at higher risk due to multiple factors including medications (sedation, analgesics), alterations in upper airway patency, and positioning [17]. The supine position required in many surgeries may create dead space thus reducing lung volumes and oxygen saturations. Atelectasis as a result of pain induced splinting or sedation may further contribute to hypoventilation and respiratory insufficiency [18]. Sedation, neuromuscular blockade, and postsurgical opioid pain

TABLE 2: Patient characteristics based on STOP-BANG questionnaire.

| | STOP-BANG < 3 (LR) $N = 100$ | STOP-BANG STOP-BANG ≥ 3 (HR) $N = 304$ | $P$ value |
|---|---|---|---|
| BMI (kg/m$^2$) | | | |
| Mean ± SD | 25.7 ± 3.9 | 29.4 ± 5.9 | — |
| Median (min to max) | 25.4 (18.4 to 36.8) | 28 (16.5 to 51) | |
| Neck circumference (cm) | | | |
| Mean ± SD | 36.0 ± 3.3 | 41.1 ± 4.2 | — |
| Median (min to max) | 36 (28 to 46) | 41 (29 to 54) | |
| PACU LOS (minutes) | | | |
| Mean ± SD | 278.6 ± 358.6 | 403.2 ± 451.1 | —# |
| Median (min to max) | 117.5 (39 to 1492) | 146 (44 to 1667) | |
| Anesthesia duration (minutes) | | | |
| Mean ± SD | 63.0 ± 32.1 | 61.3 ± 20.9 | 0.560* |
| Median (min to max) | 52 (30 to 256) | 55.5 (26 to 147) | 0.277** |
| Oxygen sat below 93% (count) | | | |
| Mean ± SD | 2.7 ± 2.6 | 3.9 ± 3.9 | 0.131* |
| Median (min to max) | 2 (1 to 12) | 3 (1 to 18) | |

LR, low risk; HR, high risk; SD, standard deviation.
—: BMI and neck circumference were used to create the STOP-BANG score.
#$P$ value is not provided; PACU LOS has a bimodal distribution.
*$P$ value is based on independent samples $t$-test.
**$P$ value is based on Wilcoxon rank-sum test.

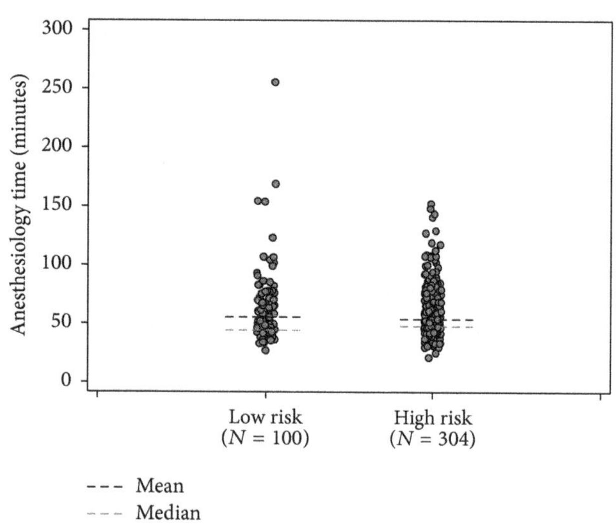


FIGURE 2: Procedure time by low and high risk patients based on STOP-BANG questionnaire.

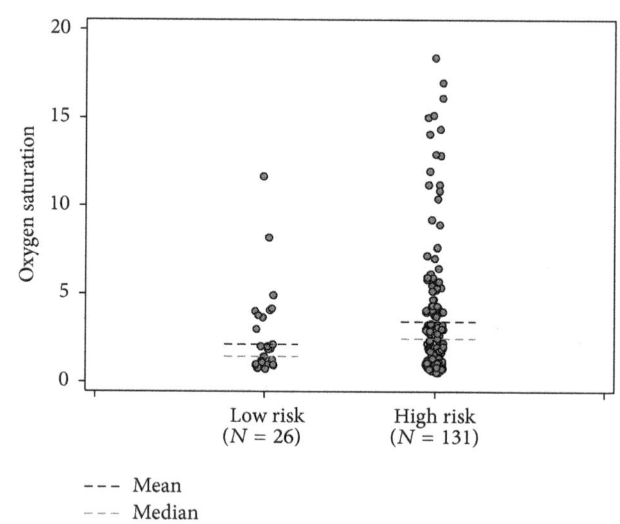


FIGURE 3: Oxygen saturation by low and high risk patients based on STOP-BANG questionnaire.

medications decrease arousal and may elicit sleep apnea symptoms postoperatively by decreasing neuromuscular tone in the upper airway [19, 20]. Finally, sleep fragmentation after surgery can reduce rapid eye movement (REM) sleep stage, immediately postoperatively, following which REM sleep rebound can occur. REM sleep rebound is associated with muscle atonia and may promote sleep apnea and cardiac dysrhythmia days after surgery [7, 21]. We did not observe any new onset atrial fibrillation, ICU admissions, or respiratory distress in our cohort, and we suspect the selection of an ambulatory population with short procedure times likely influenced the lack of these complications. In general, however, complications related to OSA in the perioperative setting may result in longer length of stay and consequent increased resource utilization.

The application of the STOP-BANG questionnaire in an oncologic setting is novel. Intuitively, one may question the use of this tool since most assume that cancer patients will be fatigued or tired, thus potentially reducing the specificity of the survey. Interestingly, in our study, only 43.8% of cancer patients affirmed feeling "tired." It is unclear if that fatigue is due to undiagnosed OSA or cancer, but regardless the nonuniform response shows promise for this tool in surgical cancer patients. Given the success of this tool in the perioperative setting, the application to our cancer population seems logical. It is important to recognize however that the use of the STOP-BANG or any screening tools to diagnose sleep apnea and predict outcomes has limitations, for OSA shares common symptoms with many other diseases, thus lowering their specificity [22]. The score, itself, contains elements such as obesity, age, hypertension, gender, and fatigue. Each of these factors might be associated with increased postoperative stay, regardless of the presence or absence of OSA. Disentangling these contributors to sleep apnea from the disease itself, therefore, is challenging [23]. Finally, the discovery of an early discharge in LR patients despite short procedure duration in an outpatient setting further demonstrates the potential robustness of the STOP-BANG questionnaire. Our study establishes areas of application for the STOP-BANG questionnaire in cancer patients.

Our study has limitations inherent to most retrospective studies. We tried to use an adequate sample size and had controls for many of the variables. An electronic medical record and an integrated perioperative medical record were used so loss of patient data was marginal. The procedures for each patient, including the anesthetic agents, process of care, monitoring, and standardized criteria for discharge from the PACU, were the same. Although discharge criteria were standardized, variability due to factors, related to the delivery of care and unrelated to the risk for sleep apnea, such as patient transportation needs, nursing shift changes, and provider implementation, may have affected LOS. We attempted to minimize this variability by evaluating a large number of consecutive patients. All our patients were ambulatory and procedure times were similar and brief, so there may be selection bias since these procedures were not extensive or prolonged. In our study, the difference in time to discharge did not persist beyond 20 hours, although, by then, most patients were discharged. This finding may signify that factors other than risk for sleep apnea may be responsible for prolonged time to discharge from the PACU for some patients. Expansion of our study to include the nonambulatory setting and longer surgery times may identify patients at increased risk of respiratory or cardiovascular complications. Evaluation of these patients may also magnify the difference found between the HR and LR groups.

Our findings support the recommendations of the ASA guidelines, which call for more intensive monitoring of patients with OSA [13]. Further delineation of the patient population and surgical procedures which are less prone to complications and lower risk, respectively, may help guide escalation of care for OSA. This would be especially beneficial for anesthesiologists, given the advent of the Affordable Care Act. As in other medical specialties, anesthesiologists will be asked to focus on cost containment by increasing the number of procedures performed in the ambulatory setting, without compromising patient safety. Alternatively, monitoring for complications beyond the PACU may also be considered, for it is known that the effects of anesthesia on respiratory and sleep patterns reach their peak approximately 72 hours postoperatively [24]. Further prospective studies in the oncologic population undergoing longer and more complex surgeries in hospitalized patients with the STOP-BANG score could also better define the role of this screening tool and correlate with more intensive and prolonged monitoring.

To date, this study represents the largest group of cancer patients screened preoperatively with the validated STOP-BANG. This study demonstrates that cancer patients undergoing a relatively minor procedure with less known cardiorespiratory morbidity may benefit from screening for OSA with the STOP-BANG questionnaire. Knowing the average duration of LOS for HR patients may assist healthcare providers in selecting an appropriate duration of monitoring. If the LOS is higher for ambulatory patients with suspected OSA, then guidelines that recommend an increase in the duration of observation are justifiable and worth the increased resources that such monitoring entails. Systematically designed studies to better define which patient may undergo higher risk surgery in ambulatory centers safely are needed. The potential role for the STOP-BANG survey in cancer patients may be greater than previously anticipated.

## Competing Interests

The authors declare that there is no conflict of interests regarding the publication of this paper.

## Acknowledgments

This research is supported in part by the National Institutes of Health through MD Anderson's Cancer Center Support Grant (CA016672).

## References

[1] R. W. Riley, N. B. Powell, C. Guilleminault, R. Pelayo, R. J. Troell, and K. K. Li, "Obstructive sleep apnea surgery: risk management and complications," *Otolaryngology—Head and Neck Surgery*, vol. 117, no. 6, pp. 648–652, 1997.

[2] D. J. Cullen, "Obstructive sleep apnea and postoperative analgesia—a potentially dangerous combination," *Journal of Clinical Anesthesia*, vol. 13, no. 2, pp. 83–85, 2001.

[3] N. N. Boushra, "Anaesthetic management of patients with sleep apnoea syndrome," *Canadian Journal of Anaesthesia*, vol. 43, no. 6, pp. 599–616, 1996.

[4] S. S. Jain and R. Dhand, "Perioperative treatment of patients with obstructive sleep apnea," *Current Opinion in Pulmonary Medicine*, vol. 10, no. 6, pp. 482–488, 2004.

[5] D. Hwang, N. Shakir, B. Limann et al., "Association of sleep-disordered breathing with postoperative complications," *Chest*, vol. 133, no. 5, pp. 1128–1134, 2008.

[6] B. Mokhlesi, M. D. Hovda, B. Vekhter, V. M. Arora, F. Chung, and D. O. Meltzer, "Sleep-disordered breathing and postoperative outcomes after elective surgery: analysis of the nationwide inpatient sample," *Chest*, vol. 144, no. 3, pp. 903–914, 2013.

[7] F. Chung, P. Liao, B. Yegneswaran, C. M. Shapiro, and W. Kang, "Postoperative changes in sleep-disordered breathing and sleep architecture in patients with obstructive sleep apnea," *Anesthesiology*, vol. 120, no. 2, pp. 287–298, 2014.

[8] M. Singh, P. Liao, S. Kobah, D. N. Wijeysundera, C. Shapiro, and F. Chung, "Proportion of surgical patients with undiagnosed obstructive sleep apnoea," *British Journal of Anaesthesia*, vol. 110, no. 4, pp. 629–636, 2013.

[9] F. Chung, B. Yegneswaran, P. Liao et al., "STOP questionnaire: a tool to screen patients for obstructive sleep apnea," *Anesthesiology*, vol. 108, no. 5, pp. 812–821, 2008.

[10] R. M. Corso, F. Petrini, M. Buccioli et al., "Clinical utility of preoperative screening with stop-bang questionnaire in elective surgery," *Minerva Anestesiologica*, vol. 80, no. 8, pp. 877–884, 2014.

[11] P. Chia, E. Seet, J. D. Macachor, U. S. Iyer, and D. Wu, "The association of pre-operative STOP-BANG scores with postoperative critical care admission," *Anaesthesia*, vol. 68, no. 9, pp. 950–952, 2013.

[12] E. M. Lockhart, M. D. Willingham, A. B. Abdallah et al., "Obstructive sleep apnea screening and postoperative mortality in a large surgical cohort," *Sleep Medicine*, vol. 14, no. 5, pp. 407–415, 2013.

[13] American Society of Anesthesiologists Task Force on Perioperative Management of Patients with Obstructive Sleep Apnea, "Practice guidelines for the perioperative management of patients with obstructive sleep apnea: an updated report by the American Society of Anesthesiologists Task Force on Perioperative Management of patients with obstructive sleep apnea," *Anesthesiology*, vol. 120, no. 2, pp. 268–268, 2014.

[14] G. P. Joshi, S. P. Ankichetty, T. J. Gan, and F. Chung, "Society for ambulatory anesthesia consensus statement on preoperative selection of adult patients with obstructive sleep apnea scheduled for ambulatory surgery," *Anesthesia & Analgesia*, vol. 115, no. 5, pp. 1060–1068, 2012.

[15] S. G. Memtsoudis, M. C. Besculides, and M. Mazumdar, "A rude awakening—the perioperative sleep apnea epidemic," *The New England Journal of Medicine*, vol. 368, no. 25, pp. 2352–2353, 2013.

[16] T. S. Vasu, K. Doghramji, R. Cavallazzi et al., "Obstructive sleep apnea syndrome and postoperative complications: clinical use of the STOP-BANG questionnaire," *Archives of Otolaryngology—Head & Neck Surgery*, vol. 136, no. 10, pp. 1020–1024, 2010.

[17] P. R. Eastwood, I. Szollosi, P. R. Platt, and D. R. Hillman, "Comparison of upper airway collapse during general anaesthesia and sleep," *The Lancet*, vol. 359, no. 9313, pp. 1207–1209, 2002.

[18] J. Porhomayon, N. D. Nader, K. B. Leissner, and A. A. El-Solh, "Respiratory perioperative management of patients with obstructive sleep apnea," *Journal of Intensive Care Medicine*, vol. 29, no. 3, pp. 145–153, 2014.

[19] J. R. Norton, D. S. Ward, S. Karan et al., "Differences between midazolam and propofol sedation on upper airway collapsibility using dynamic negative airway pressure," *Anesthesiology*, vol. 104, no. 6, pp. 1155–1164, 2006.

[20] M. Eikermann, F. M. Vogt, F. Herbstreit et al., "The predisposition to inspiratory upper airway collapse during partial neuromuscular blockade," *American Journal of Respiratory and Critical Care Medicine*, vol. 175, no. 1, pp. 9–15, 2007.

[21] T. S. Vasu, R. Grewal, and K. Doghramji, "Obstructive sleep apnea syndrome and perioperative complications: a systematic review of the literature," *Journal of Clinical Sleep Medicine*, vol. 8, no. 2, pp. 199–207, 2012.

[22] F. Chung, H. R. Abdullah, and P. Liao, "Stop-bang questionnaire: a practical approach to screen for obstructive sleep apnea," *Chest*, vol. 149, no. 3, pp. 631–638, 2016.

[23] P. Gokay, S. Tastan, and M. E. Orhan, "Is there a difference between the STOP-BANG and the Berlin Obstructive Sleep Apnoea Syndrome questionnaires for determining respiratory complications during the perioperative period?" *Journal of Clinical Nursing*, vol. 25, no. 9-10, pp. 1238–1252, 2016.

[24] R. Kaw, J. Golish, S. Ghamande, R. Burgess, N. Foldvary, and E. Walker, "Incremental risk of obstructive sleep apnea on cardiac surgical outcomes," *The Journal of Cardiovascular Surgery*, vol. 47, no. 6, pp. 683–689, 2006.

# 29

# Effects of Tibetan Music on Neuroendocrine and Autonomic Functions in Patients Waiting for Surgery

**Antonella Cotoia,[1] Floriana Dibello,[1] Fiorenzo Moscatelli,[2] Alberto Sciusco,[3] Pietro Polito,[4] Alberto Modolo,[5] Crescenzio Gallo,[2] Giuseppe Cibelli,[2] and Gilda Cinnella[1]**

[1]*Department of Anesthesia, Intensive Care, and Pain Therapy, University of Foggia, Policlinico "OO. Riuniti", Foggia, Italy*
[2]*Department of Clinical and Experimental Medicine, University of Foggia, Policlinico "OO. Riuniti", Foggia, Italy*
[3]*Department of Intensive Care and Anaesthesia, North Bristol NHS Trust, Bristol, UK*
[4]*Department of Blood Transfusion Medicine, ASS 5 Friuli Occidentale, Pordenone, Italy*
[5]*Naturopathy, A.N.E.A. Academy, Prato, Italy*

Correspondence should be addressed to Antonella Cotoia; antonella.cotoia@unifg.it

Academic Editor: Enrico Camporesi

*Background.* The aim of this study was to investigate the effects of listening to Tibetan music on anxiety and endocrine, autonomic, cognitive responses in patients waiting for urologic surgery. *Methods.* Sixty patients waiting for surgery were enrolled to the study. They were randomized in music (M) and control (C) groups. The M group listened to a low-frequency Tibetan music for 30 min ($T_0$–$T_{30}$) through headphones, and the C group wore headphones with no sound. The State Trait Anxiety Inventory Questionnaire (STAI) Y-1 was administered at $T_0$ and $T_{30}$. Normalized low (LFnu) and high frequencies (HFnu) of heart rate variability, LF/HF ratio, and galvanic skin response (GRS) data were analyzed at $T_0$, $T_{10}$, $T_{20}$, $T_{30}$, and $T_{35}$. The salivary $\alpha$-amylase (sAA) samples were collected at $T_0$, $T_{35}$, and $T_{45}$. *Results.* In the M group, the STAI Y-1 score decreased at $T_{30}$ versus baseline ($p < 0.001$), sAA levels decreased at $T_{35}$ versus $T_0$ ($p = 0.004$), and GSR remained unchanged. In the C group, the STAI Y-1 score remained unchanged, sAA level increased at $T_{35}$ versus $T_0$ ($p < 0.001$), and GSR slightly increased at $T_{35}$ versus baseline ($p = 0.359$). LFnu was lower, and HFnu was significantly higher ($T_{10}$–$T_{30}$) in M versus C group. Mean LF/HF ratio slightly reduced in the M group. *Conclusions.* Our results suggest that preoperative listening to relaxing Tibetan music might be a useful strategy to manage preoperative anxiety.

## 1. Introduction

Preoperative anxiety is an emotional state characterized by feelings of tension, fear, nervousness, and apprehension which is common in patients waiting for surgery [1, 2]. The experience of anxiety and psychological stress before surgery is a complex phenomenon that comprises both physiological and psychological components and might require preoperative treatment [3].

The physiological response to stress involves the activation of the hypothalamic-pituitary-adrenal axis and the autonomic nervous system (ANS) through modulation of its branches, sympathetic and parasympathetic [4, 5], which can be evaluated by biochemical and physiological measurements, including salivary alpha-amylase (sAA) levels, heart rate variability (HRV), and galvanic skin response (GSR) [6–9].

Music is attracting increasing interest as a nonpharmaceutical therapeutic alternative for the treatment of preoperative anxiety in adult patients. Previous investigations found that music was effective in reducing the perceived levels of psychological stress and the need for additional analgesic doses [10, 11]. Other studies focused on physiological anxiolytic effects of music in the clinical setting [12, 13]. However, a clear understanding has not yet emerged regarding which genre of music is most beneficial to patients [14]. The perception of music as relaxing may vary in each patient, and the selection of the preferred music is suggested [15]. The most common notion is that the self-chosen music involves patient's mind with something familiar and restful, focusing the patient's attention away from negative stimuli to something pleasant and encouraging [11, 14]. Some music therapists prefer classical music for relaxation because the musical pieces are consistent [16]. Conversely, a study showed that melodies with elements of natural sound had positive effects in relation to patient's discomfort and pain [17].

We hypothesized that a relaxing music with low frequency has itself an effect on anxiety levels where it is listened for the first time and it is not self-selected. The aim of this study was to investigate the cognitive and emotional responses of listening to Tibetan relaxing music preoperatively and its effects on the endocrine system and ANS, in patients waiting for urologic surgery.

## 2. Materials and Methods

This prospective randomized, double-blinded study was performed in the Urologic Department of University Hospital of Foggia, Italy, from April 2017 to June 2017. Ethical approval for this study (Ethical Committee N° 5/CE/2016) was provided by the Ethical Committee of the University Hospital of Foggia on 14 February 2016. Consecutive patients between 45 and 65 years, undergoing elective major urologic surgery, and with American Society of Anesthesiologists (ASA) physical status of class II-III, were considered for enrollment. Prior to data collection, the purpose of this study was carefully explained and written informed consent was obtained from each participant, according to the Declaration of Helsinki.

The sound of Tibetan Bowls, invented and played by Alberto Modolo, was found in a range from 0 to 1 kHz by the time-frequency analysis (Mathematica software, Version 11.0, Wolfram Research Inc.) via short-time Fourier transform (Supplementary Material S1).

Patients playing any musical instrument, smokers, having hearing impairment, endocrine disorders, any known psychiatric or neurologic disorders, or taking any medication affecting ANS were excluded.

*2.1. Measures.* Quantitative measurements of anxiety in both physiological and psychological aspects were included.

*2.1.1. State Trait Anxiety Inventory Questionnaire (STAI).* The STAI consists in 40 items to measure the presence and severity of preoperative anxiety (STAI Y-1) and generalized propensity to be anxious (STAI Y-2). Total score obtained from each STAI range from 20 to 80, and the higher score indicates greater anxiety [18, 19]. A cut point of 39-40 has been suggested to detect clinically significant symptoms for the STAI scales [20, 21].

*2.1.2. Amsterdam Preoperative Anxiety and Information Scale (APAIS).* The APAIS is a 6-item questionnaire created to identify anxious patients (4 items to investigate on fear of anesthesia and the surgical procedure) and their need for information (2 items) [22].

The measurement for each item is rated on a 5-point Likert scale, where point 1 matches 'not at all' and point 5 represents the 'extremely anxiety' (total range 6–30).

The cutoff score for the anxiety scale was ≥10 for the whole sample [23].

*2.1.3. Heart Rate Variability (HRV).* Heart rate variability (HRV) is the physiological phenomenon of variation in the time interval between heartbeats, and it can be measured with frequency analysis of the ECG. Low frequency (LF, 0.04–0.15 Hz) reflects the combination of sympathetic and parasympathetic ANS modulation; high frequency (HF, 0.15–0.40 Hz) is a measure of vagal modulation on the heart; the LF/HF ratio is used, not without some controversy, to quantify the degree of sympathovagal balance [24].

The patients' HRV was measured with the Faros device (eMotion Faros 90°, Mega Electronics Ltd, Finland) whose sensor, placed on the right midclavicular line, was attached to the cable connected to the ECG electrode placed on the lower left abdomen within the rib cage frame. After recording was over, the data were transferred to computer, and we used Kubios HRV software (Kubios HRV, Version 2.2, http://kubios.uef.fi) to perform the HRV analysis. The powers of LF and HF bands in normalized units were considered for the data analysis (LFnu and HFnu) [25].

*2.1.4. Galvanic Skin Response (GSR).* We also monitored the emotional state by GSR, which originates from the autonomic activation of sweat glands in the skin. An increase in the stress level will cause sweat and a decreased skin resistance, resulting in measurable increased skin conductance by the balance of positive and negative ions in the secreted fluid.

The GSR parameters were measured using the SenseWear Pro Armband™ (Version 3.0, Body Media, Inc., PA, USA), which was worn on the right arm over the triceps muscle at the midpoint between the acromion and olecranon processes, as recommended by the manufacturer [26].

*2.1.5. Salivary Alpha-Amylase (sAA) Kinetic Enzyme Assay.* We measured the sAA levels whose secretion was controlled by the autonomic nervous signals.

Salivary samples were collected with special sampling tubes (Salivette, Sarstedt, Numbrecht, Germany), and sAA were assayed by Salimetrics® $\alpha$-Amylase Kinetic Enzyme Assay Kit following the standard guidelines outlined in the manual provided by the manufacturer Salimetrics Inc. [27].

*2.2. Procedure.* Sampling was performed between 8 : 00 and 11 : 00 am in a quiet room of the urologic ward before arrival in the operating room. Patients were randomized via

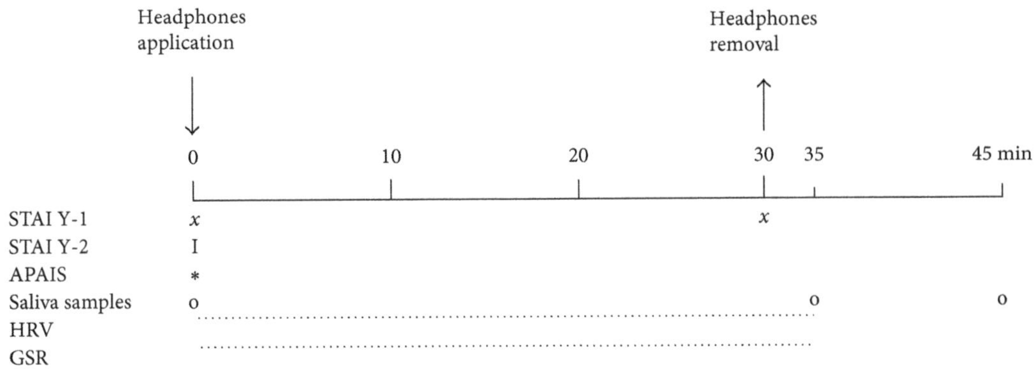


Figure 1: Timeline of the study procedure: State Trait Anxiety Inventory Questionnaire (STAI); Amsterdam Preoperative Anxiety and Information Scale (APAIS); heart rate variability (HRV); galvanic skin response (GSR).

computer-generated assignment to 2 groups: the music group (M) and the control group (C).

No sedatives were given in any groups. The M group listened to the Tibetan soundtrack for 30 min through headphones that covered the whole ear so that no external noise could interfere; the C group wore headphones for 30 min with no sound.

Before the application of the headphones ($T_0$), we collected STAI Y-1 and STAI Y-2 scores, APAIS questionnaires score, and sAA samples.

After removal of the headphones ($T_{30}$), we collected STAI Y-1 score.

Additionally, sAA samples were obtained at 5 min and 15 min after the headphones removal ($T_{35}$ and $T_{45}$).

The HRV and GSR data were analyzed at $T_0$, $T_{10}$, $T_{20}$, $T_{30}$, and $T_{35}$ (Figure 1).

*2.3. Statistical Analysis.* On the basis of previous investigations, a sample size of 22 subjects per group was able to detect a normalized LF decrease of 8.5% in stress-induced students after listening music for 20 min (assuming $\alpha = 0.05$ and power = 0.95) [28]. This number was increased to 30 per group to allow for a 35% patients dropout rate.

The normality of distribution was assessed by Shapiro-Wilkinson test. Since we found all of the data normally distributed, the data were expressed as mean ± SD. Data were analyzed using one-ways ANOVA and repeated measurement analysis of variance. The Bonferroni multiple comparison test was performed to identify significant differences among measures. Differences between the groups at each time point were examined post hoc using independent sample $t$-test. A paired sample $t$-test was used to detect changes within the groups. A value of $p < 0.05$ was considered statistically significant. Statistical analysis was performed by Statistical Package for the Social Sciences (SPSS Inc., Chicago, IL) Version 15.0 for Windows.

## 3. Results

The enrollment flow diagram is reported in Figure 2. 60 out of 65 candidates for enrollment were included in the study and were randomly divided into two groups: 30 patients (15 males and 15 females) in the "Music group" (M) and 30 patients (15 males and 15 females) in the "Control group" (C).

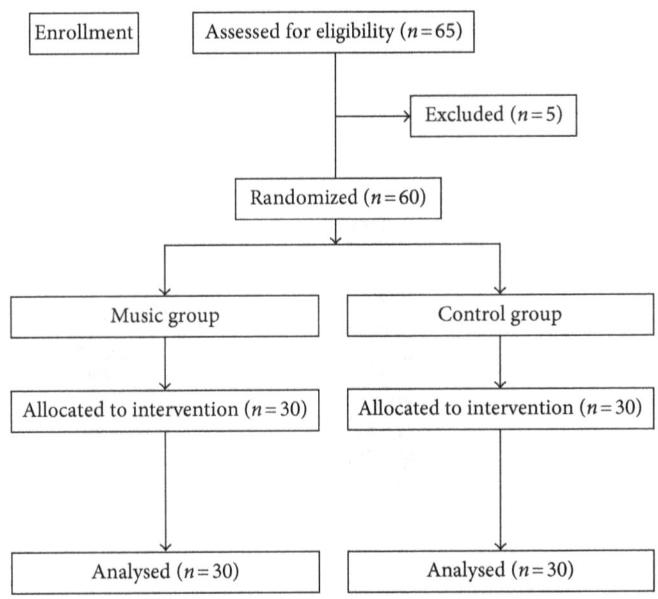


Figure 2: Flowchart of patients' enrollment.

There were no differences between the two groups as regards for age, sex, ASA, and types of surgical procedures performed (Table 1).

*3.1. Psychological Tests.* The baseline STAI Y-1, STAI Y-2, and APAIS scores were similar in both groups (Table 1). The STAI Y-1 score decreased at $T_{30}$ versus baseline only in the M group (39.13 ± 6.7 versus 60.2 ± 8.2, $p < 0.001$), while it remained unchanged in the C group (60.3 ± 9 versus 61.6 ± 9, $p = 0.178$). Intergroup analysis showed a difference in M versus C groups at $T_{30}$ ($p < 0.001$) (Figure 3).

*3.2. Analysis of Salivary α-Amylase.* Baseline sAA was similar in both groups (M versus C groups: 30.3 ± 11 U/ml versus 24.8 ± 6 U/ml, $p = 0.083$). In the M group, the sAA markedly decreased at $T_{35}$ ($T_{35}$ versus $T_0$, $p = 0.004$; M versus C groups 18.5 ± 7 U/ml versus 28.3 ± 7 U/ml, $p < 0.001$) and

Table 1: Demographic and psychological tests.

| | Music group | Control group | $p$ value |
|---|---|---|---|
| Age (years) | 55.1 ± 8.9 | 58.2 ± 7.7 | 0.096 |
| *Sex* | | | |
| Males/females | 15/15 | 15/15 | 1 |
| ASA II/III | 21/9 | 19/11 | 0.6 |
| *Urologic surgery* | | | 0.08 |
| RRP | 10 | 8 | |
| PCNL | 14 | 8 | |
| Others | 6 | 14 | |
| STAI Y-1 $T_0$ | 60.2 ± 8 | 61.6 ± 9 | 0.25 |
| STAI Y-2 $T_0$ | 38.9 ± 9 | 35.9 ± 9 | 0.10 |
| APAIS $T_0$ | 21.2 ± 5 | 20.7 ± 4 | 0.34 |

Data are expressed as mean ± SD. RRP = radical retropubic prostatectomy; PCNL = percutaneous nephrolithotomy; STAI = State Trait Anxiety Inventory Questionnaire; APAIS = Amsterdam Preoperative Anxiety and Information Scale.

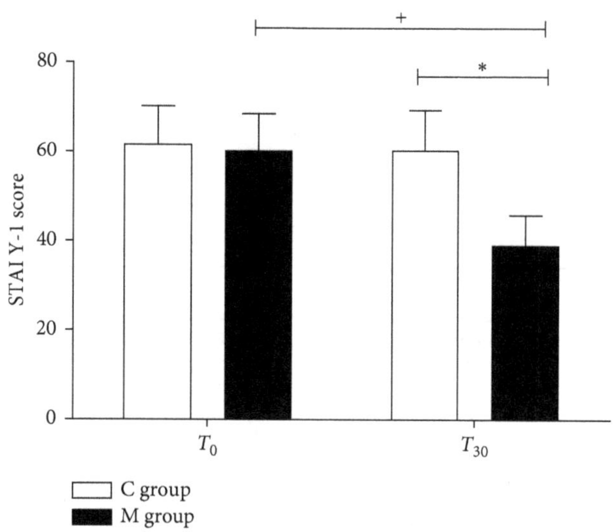


Figure 3: State Trait Anxiety Inventory Questionnaire score. State Trait Anxiety Inventory Questionnaire (STAI Y-1) score in the music group (M group) and control group (C group) at $T_0$ and $T_{30}$. Data are presented as mean ± SD; $^{+,*}p < 0.001$.

slightly increased at $T_{45}$ ($T_{45}$ versus $T_0$, $p = 0.5$; M versus C groups 26.5 ± 11 U/ml versus 27.3 ± 9 U/ml, $p = 0.810$). Conversely, in the C group, the sAA level increased at $T_{35}$ ($T_{35}$ versus $T_0$: $p < 0.001$) and slightly decreased at $T_{45}$ ($T_{45}$ versus $T_0$: $p = 0.292$) (Figure 4).

*3.3. Analysis of Galvanic Skin Response.* Baseline GSR was similar in M and C groups (0.076 ± 0.061 $\mu$S versus 0.04 ± 0.051 $\mu$S, resp., $p = 0.122$). GSR remained unchanged throughout the study period in the M group, while it slightly increased in the C group ($T_{35}$ versus baseline, $p = 0.359$).

Intergroup analysis showed a difference between M and C groups at $T_{30}$ (0.064 ± 0.043 $\mu$S versus 0.127 ± 0.123 $\mu$S, $p = 0.031$) and $T_{35}$ (0.068 ± 0.044 $\mu$S versus 0.155 ± 0.189 $\mu$S, resp., $p = 0.045$) (Figure 5).

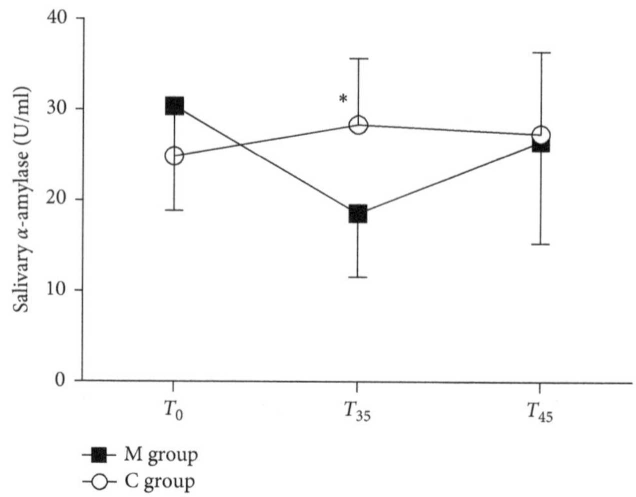


Figure 4: Salivary $\alpha$-amylase levels (U/ml). Salivary $\alpha$-amylase levels (U/ml) in the music group (M group) and control group (C group) at $T_0$, $T_{35}$, and $T_{45}$. Data are presented as mean ± SD. $^*p < 0.001$.

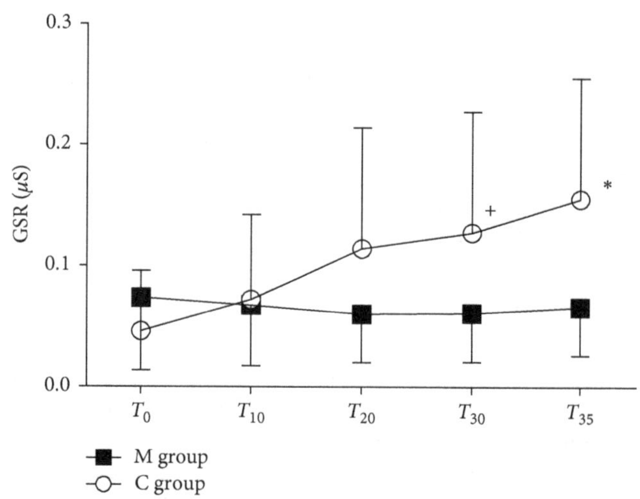


Figure 5: Galvanic skin response. Galvanic skin response ($\mu$S) in the music group (M group) and control group (C group) at different time point. Data are presented as mean ± SD. $^+p = 0.031$ and $^*p < 0.045$.

*3.4. Analysis of Heart Rate Variability.* Baseline LFnu, HFnu, and LF/HF ratio showed similar values in M and C groups (LFnu: 69 ± 16 versus 64 ± 20, resp., $p = 0.813$; HFnu: 30 ± 16 versus 35 ± 20, $p = 0.376$; LF/HF ratio: $p = 0.908$). On $T_{10}$, $T_{20}$, and $T_{30}$, LFnu decreased and HFnu increased in the M group versus C group (LFnu and HFnu $p = 0.042$, $p = 0.007$, and $p = 0.021$ at $T_{10}$, $T_{20}$, and $T_{30}$, resp.) (Figures 6(a) and 6(b)).

In the M group, LFnu progressively reduced during the observation time, especially at $T_{20}$ and $T_{30}$ versus $T_0$ ($p = 0.025$ and $p = 0.045$, resp.) and returned to baseline at $T_{35}$; HFnu significantly increased at $T_{20}$ and $T_{30}$ versus $T_0$ ($p = 0.025$ and $p = 0.045$, resp.). In the C group, LFnu and HFnu trends remained constant during the study (Figures 6(a) and 6(b)).

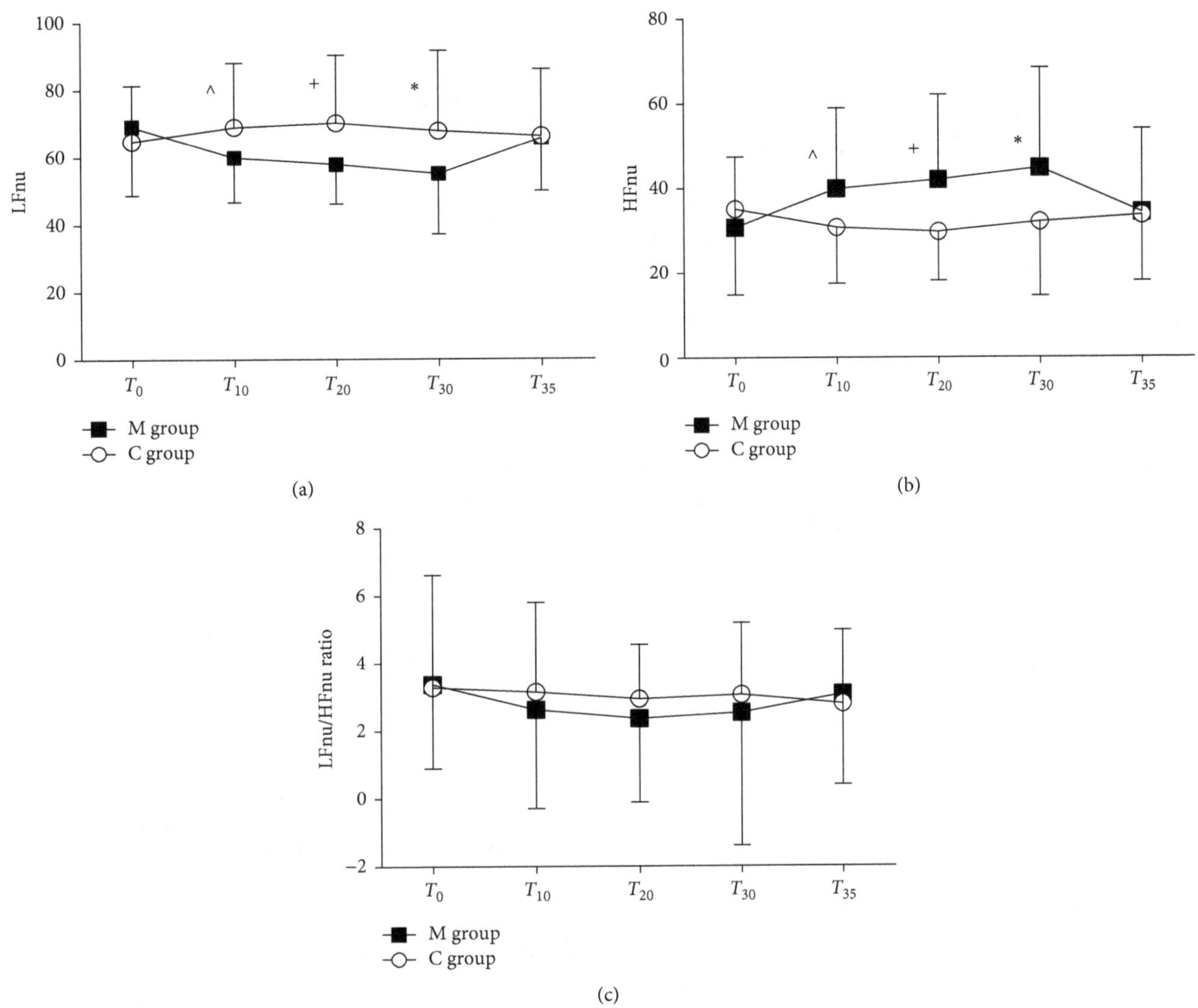


FIGURE 6: Heart rate variability. (a) Normalized low frequency (LFnu), (b) normalized high frequency (HFnu), and (c) LF/HF ratio in the music group (M group) and control group (C group) at each time point. Data are presented as mean ± SD. $^{\wedge}p = 0.042$, $^{+}p = 0.007$, and $^{*}p = 0.021$.

Mean LF/HF ratio slightly reduced in the M group but not significantly during the time as compared to the C group (Figure 6(c)).

## 4. Discussion

The main results of our study are that, in the group listening to Tibetan music preoperatively, a marked improvement of all anxiety measurements was observed: (a) STAI Y-1 score of anxiety reduced, (b) salivary $\alpha$-amylase levels reduced, (c) GSR trend was constant, and (d) LFnu reduced and HFnu increased during the study period.

To our knowledge, this is the first study examining the effect of Tibetan music on preoperative anxiety, by simultaneous evaluation of the cognitive-emotional, the endocrine, and the autonomic responses by physiological and psychological tests.

Recently, it was demonstrated that allowing patients to listen to the classical or selected favorite music is effective in alleviating acute stress caused by an acute-short term stress factor especially in hospitalized patients and in patients waiting for surgery [15, 28–31]. Furthermore, providing a choice of music was considered a critical factor in lowering anxiety, promoting relaxation, and pain relief [15].

Tibetan music is different from traditional music and classical harmony played by string, flute, or piano, which are usually recommended as therapeutic music [32]. In our study, we used music composed with low frequencies, a constant sonority, and a regular rhythm which may help the relaxation and meditation [33]. The present data showed that subjective anxiety level, as measured by the STAI test, decreased only in patients listening to Tibetan music. Interestingly, this finding was similar to those studies using preferred relaxing music or classical music [12], especially if we consider the Yilmaz et al. investigation showing a lower STAI score in the patients who chose their preferred music versus premedicated patients with midazolam [10].

A series of studies found a correlation between psychological behavior and sAA, assessing the reliability of sAA as an easy to use and noninvasive sympathetic biomarker for stress evaluation [34, 35].

Similarly, we showed that the sAA levels decreased at $T_{35}$ only in patients listening to Tibetan music. Conversely, no sound in the control group increased the sAA levels, suggesting a stressful condition. Interestingly, the impact of various musical genres has important implications in the autonomic response. Nater et al. showed an increased secretion of sAA in men listening to heavy metal music [36].

One explanation might be that the sAA response to stress is complex, since both branches of the ANS are involved in maintaining the oral homeostasis depending upon saliva and its content of proteins. Whereas sAA is secreted from the salivary glands under sympathetic activity, the parasympathetic impulses stimulate the saliva secretion [37].

The focus on the physiological monitoring of anxiety is indicative of the medical concern about the impact of stress on safe anesthesia. Although galvanic skin monitoring has long been considered a measure of physiological and mental stress, a recent Cochrane review showed only one study that analyzed the skin conductivity variations in preoperative anxiety [38]. The authors concluded that anxiety reduction in the patient-selected music group was not reflected in the GSR [39].

Accordingly, we observed a constant GSR trend in the M group.

More recent evidence suggests that HRV is gaining recognition as a measure of cardiac parasympathetic activity and, therefore, an indicator of a relaxation response other than a sensitive indicator of autonomic dysfunction such as in alcoholics, diabetic or cardiopathic patients [40–43]. Previous studies, supported by a recent meta-analysis, revealed that the activation of the ANS in anxiety disorders, can lead to an increase in LF and decrease in HF [12, 38, 44].

Although there is ongoing debate as to interpret HRV [24, 39], there is a large consensus that LF power is modulated by baroreflexes with a combination of sympathetic and parasympathetic activity, whereas HF reflects primary parasympathetic activity [45–47]. LF/HF ratio has a more difficult interpretation, since its use in evaluating the sympathovagal balance has been recently questioned. Many researchers have regarded the notion of sympathovagal balance as merely simplification of a relationship which appears to be more complex than was previously thought. [24, 45].

In this study, normalization of LF and HF has been applied in an attempt to better quantify modulation of the parasympathetic and sympathetic branches of the ANS [40, 48].

Our HRV results appeared consistent with the other cognitive and endocrine results: over the course of the study, an evident decrease in LFnu and an increase in HFnu were observed only in the M group. Furthermore, it is difficult to compare our findings with the classical or preferred music studies regarding to the frequency range due to the scarce information available in the literature [32, 49]. Tibetan music had immediate effects and seems contingent on listening timing which could represent a limit for longer time interval between preoperative preparation and surgery. However, we chose headphones to deliver the music according to the literature, although Lee et al. demonstrated that broadcast is also effective [12, 14]. These overall findings indicate that Tibetan music reduced preoperative stress and may be considered a good strategy for patients waiting for surgery without premedications [12].

Another limit is that the C group had to wear headphones with no sound in order to reduce methodological bias [38, 39]. Even though the severity of self-reported anxiety remained unchanged in this group, we cannot simply exclude that wearing headphones with no sound could have had some effect on their stress level.

Therefore, future studies need to investigate the anxiolytic effect of Tibetan music in perioperative setting by physiological and psychological tools, especially in patients needing emergency surgery.

In conclusion, by combining cognitive and somatic data with endocrine and autonomic response, our results suggest that listening to Tibetan music could help patients to manage preoperative anxiety. The implementation of music in the perianesthesia setting is a noninvasive intervention, easy to administer, and should be considered for clinical practice.

## Abbreviations

ANS: Autonomic nervous system
sAA: Salivary alpha-amylase
HRV: Heart rate variability
GSR: Galvanic skin response
ASA: American Society of Anesthesiologists (ASA)
STAI: State Trait Anxiety Inventory Questionnaire.

## Conflicts of Interest

The authors declare that they have no conflicts of interest.

## Acknowledgments

A special thanks are due to S. Intenso, MD, and M. A. P. Ciliberti for their assistance in coconducting the study.

## References

[1] N. H. Badner, W. R. Nielson, S. Munk, C. Kwiatkowska, and A. W. Gelb, "Preoperative anxiety : detection and contributing factors," *Canadian Journal of Anaesthesia*, vol. 37, no. 4, pp. 444–447, 1990.

[2] T. Leinonen and H. Leino-Kilpi, "Research in peri-operative nursing care," *Journal of Clinical Nursing*, vol. 8, no. 2, pp. 123–138, 1999.

[3] L. W. Morris and W. B. Engle, "Assessing various coping strategies and their effects on test performance and anxiety," *Journal of Clinical Psychology*, vol. 37, no. 1, pp. 165–171, 1981.

[4] C. Kirschbaum and D. H. Hellhammer, "Salivary cortisol in psychoneuroendocrine research: recent developments and applications," *Psychoneuroendocrinology*, vol. 19, no. 4, pp. 313–333, 1994.

[5] W. S. Gozansky, J. S. Lynn, M. L. Laudenslager, and W. M. Kohrt, "Salivary cortisol determined by enzyme immunoassay is preferable to serum total cortisol for assessment of dynamic hypothalamic-pituitary-adrenal axis activity," *Clinical Endocrinology*, vol. 63, no. 3, pp. 336–341, 2005.

[6] D. S. Goldstein, "Catecholamines and stress," *Endocrine Regulations*, vol. 37, pp. 69–80, 2003.

[7] E. P. Davis and D. A. Granger, "Developmental differences in infant salivary alpha-amylase and cortisol responses to stress," *Psychoneuroendocrinology*, vol. 34, no. 6, pp. 795–804, 2009.

[8] Task force of the European Society of Cardiology and the North American Society of Pacing and Electrophysiology, "Heart rate variability: standards of measurement, physiological interpretation, and clinical use," *Circulation*, vol. 93, no. 5, pp. 1043–1065, 1996.

[9] W. D. Fenz and S. Epstein, "Gradients of physiological arousal in parachutists as a function of an approaching jump," *Psychosomatic Medicine*, vol. 29, no. 1, pp. 33–51, 1967.

[10] E. Yilmaz, S. Ozcan, M. Basar, H. Basar, E. Batislam, and M. Ferhat, "Music decreases anxiety and provides sedation in extracorporeal shock wave lithotripsy," *Urology*, vol. 61, no. 2, pp. 282–286, 2003.

[11] A. M. Beccaloni, "The medicine of music: a systematic approach for adoption into perianesthesia practice," *Journal of PeriAnesthesia Nursing*, vol. 26, no. 5, pp. 323–330, 2011.

[12] K. C. Lee, Y. H. Chao, J. J. Yiin, P. Y. Chiang, and Y. F. Chao, "Effectiveness of different music-playing devices for reducing preoperative anxiety: a clinical control study," *International Journal of Nursing Studies*, vol. 48, no. 10, pp. 1180–1187, 2011.

[13] Y. Z. Tan, S. Ozdemir, A. Temiz, and F. Celik, "The effect of relaxing music on heart rate and heart rate variability during ECG GATED-myocardial perfusion scintigraphy," *Complementary Therapies in Clinical Practice*, vol. 21, no. 2, pp. 137–140, 2015.

[14] U. Nilsson, "The anxiety- and pain-reducing effects of music interventions: a systematic review," *AORN Journal*, vol. 87, no. 4, pp. 780–807, 2008.

[15] L. A. Mitchell and R. A. R. Macdonald, "An experimental investigation of the effects of preferred and relaxing music listening on pain perception," *Journal of Music Therapy*, vol. 43, no. 4, pp. 295–316, 2006.

[16] L. Bunt, B. Stige, and A. Storr, "Music therapy: an art beyond words," *BMJ*, vol. 308, no. 6937, pp. 1175-1176, 2014.

[17] A. C. Fredriksson, L. Hellstrom, and U. Nilsson, "Patients' perception of music versus ordinary sound in a post-anaesthesia care unit: a randomised crossover trial," *Intensive and Critical Care Nursing*, vol. 25, no. 4, pp. 208–213, 2009.

[18] C. Spielberger, *Manual for the State-Trait Anxiety Inventory (STAI)*, Consulting Psychologists Press, Palo Alto, CA, USA, 1983.

[19] C. D. Spielberger, R. L. Gorsuch, P. R. Lushene, P. R. Vsagg, and A. G. Jacobs, *Manual for the State-Trait Anxiety Inventory (Form Y) (self-Evaluation Questionnaire)*, Consulting Psychologists Press, Palo Alto, CA, USA, 1983.

[20] L. J. Julian, "Measures of anxiety: state-trait anxiety inventory (STAI), beck anxiety inventory (BAI), and hospital anxiety and depression scale-anxiety (HADS-A)," *Arthritis Care and Research*, vol. 63, no. S11, pp. 467–472, 2011.

[21] P. Vitasari, M. N. A. Wahab, T. Herawan, A. Othman, and S. K. Sinnadurai, "Re-test of state trait anxiety inventory (STAI) among engineering students in Malaysia: reliability and validity tests," *Procedia-Social and Behavioral Sciences*, vol. 15, pp. 3843–3848, 2011.

[22] N. Moerman and H. Oosting, "The amsterdam preoperative anxiety and information scale (APAIS)," *Anesthesia and Analgesia*, vol. 82, no. 3, pp. 445–451, 1996.

[23] S. Goebel, L. Kaup, and H. M. Mehdorn, "Measuring preoperative anxiety in patients with intracranial tumors: the Amsterdam preoperative anxiety and information scale," *Journal of Neurosurgical Anesthesiology*, vol. 23, no. 4, pp. 297–303, 2011.

[24] W. Von Rosenberg, T. Chanwimalueang, T. Adjei, U. Jaffer, V. Goverdovsky, and D. P. Mandic, "Resolving ambiguities in the LF/HF ratio: LF-HF scatter plots for the categorization of mental and physical stress from HRV," *Frontiers in Physiology*, vol. 8, pp. 1-12, 2017.

[25] M. P. Tarvainen, J. P. Niskanen, J. A. Lipponen, P. O. Ranta-aho, and P. A. Karjalainen, "Kubios HRV-heart rate variability analysis software," *Computer Methods and Programs in Biomedicine*, vol. 113, no. 1, pp. 210–220, 2014.

[26] D. Andre, R. Pelletier, J. Farringdon et al., *The Development of the SenseWear® armband, a Revolutionary Energy Assessment Device to Assess Physical Activity and Lifestyle*, BodyMedia, Pittsburgh, PA, USA, 2006.

[27] S. A. Kinetic and R. Assay, *Technical Bulletin Running Multiple Amylase Strips*, Salimetrics, State College, PA, USA, 2012.

[28] K. S. Lee, H. C. Jeong, J. E. Yim, and M. Y. Jeon, "Effects of music therapy on the cardiovascular and autonomic nervous system in stress-induced university students: a randomized controlled trial," *Journal of Alternative and Complementary Medicine*, vol. 22, no. 1, pp. 59–65, 2015.

[29] J. Kushnir, A. Friedman, M. EhrenFeld, and T. Kushnir, "Coping with preoperative anxiety in cesarean section: physiological, cognitive, and emotional effects of listening to favorite music," *Birth*, vol. 39, no. 2, pp. 121–127, 2012.

[30] S. M. Wang, L. Kulkarni, J. Dolev, and Z. N. Kain, "Music and preoperative anxiety: a randomized, controlled study," *Anesthesia and Analgesia*, vol. 94, no. 6, pp. 1489–1494, 2002.

[31] J. Hole, M. Hirsch, E. Ball, and C. Meads, "Music as an aid for postoperative recovery in adults: a systematic review and meta-analysis," *The Lancet*, vol. 386, no. 10004, pp. 1659–1671, 2015.

[32] M. F. Cunningham, B. Monson, and M. Bookbinder, "Introducing a music program in the perioperative area," *AORN Journal*, vol. 66, no. 4, pp. 674–682, 1997.

[33] C. Pereira, "Frequencies of the buddhist meditative chant," *International Journal of Science and Research (IJSR)*, vol. 5, no. 4, pp. 761–766, 2016.

[34] Y. Noto, T. Sato, M. Kudo, K. Kurata, and K. Hirota, "The relationship between salivary biomarkers and state-trait anxiety inventory score under mental arithmetic stress: a pilot study," *Anesthesia and Analgesia*, vol. 101, pp. 1873–1876, 2005.

[35] M. R. Rashkova, L. S. Ribagin, and N. G. Toneva, "Correlation between salivary alpha-amylase and stress-related anxiety," *Folia Medica*, vol. 54, no. 2, pp. 46–51, 2012.

[36] U. M. Nater, E. Abbruzzese, M. Krebs, and U. Ehlert, "Sex differences in emotional and psychophysiological responses to musical stimuli," *International Journal of Psychophysiology*, vol. 62, no. 2, pp. 300–308, 2006.

[37] G. B. Proctor and G. H. Carpenter, "Regulation of salivary gland function by autonomic nerves," *Autonomic Neuroscience*, vol. 133, no. 1, pp. 3–18, 2007.

[38] J. Bradt, C. Dileo, and M. Shim, "Music interventions for preoperative anxiety (review)," *Cochrane Database of Systematic Reviews*, vol. 6, p. CD006908, 2013.

[39] J. Guo and J. Wang, "Study on individual music intervention to reduce preoperative anxiety on patients undergoing

laparoscopic surgery," *Chinese Journal of Nursing*, vol. 40, pp. 485–488, 2005.

[40] R. E. Kleiger, P. K. Stein, and J. T. Bigger, "Heart rate variability: measurement and clinical utility," *Annals of Noninvasive Electrocardiology*, vol. 10, no. 1, pp. 88–101, 2005.

[41] S. C. Malpas, E. A. Whiteside, and T. J. Maling, "Heart rate variability and cardiac autonomic function in men with chronic alcohol dependence," *Heart*, vol. 65, no. 2, pp. 84–88, 1991.

[42] S. C. Malpas and T. J. B. Maling, "Heart-rate variability and cardiac autonomic function in diabetes," *Diabetes*, vol. 39, no. 10, pp. 1177–1181, 1990.

[43] M. M. Wolf, G. A. Varigos, D. Hunt, and J. G. Sloman, "Sinus arrhythmia in acute myocardial infarction," *Medical Journal of Australia*, vol. 2, pp. 52-53, 1978.

[44] J. A. Chalmers, D. S. Quintana, M. J.-A. Abbott, and A. H. Kemp, "Anxiety disorders are associated with reduced heart rate variability: a meta-analysis," *Frontiers in Psychiatry*, vol. 5, p. 80, 2014.

[45] M. L. Appel, R. D. Berger, J. P. Saul, J. M. Smith, and R. J. Cohen, "Beat to beat variability in cardiovascular variables: noise or music?," *Journal of the American College of Cardiology*, vol. 14, no. 5, pp. 1139–1148, 1989.

[46] G. E. Billman and J. P. Dujardin, "Dynamic changes in cardiac vagal tone as measured by time-series analysis," *American Journal of Physiology-Heart and Circulatory Physiology*, vol. 258, no. 3, pp. H896–H902, 1990.

[47] R. Furlan, S. Guzzetti, W. Crivellaro et al., "Continuous 24-hour assessment of the neural regulation of systemic arterial pressure and RR variabilities in ambulant subjects," *Circulation*, vol. 81, no. 2, pp. 537–547, 1990.

[48] R. L. Burr, "Interpretation of normalized spectral heart rate variability indices in sleep research: a critical review," *Sleep*, vol. 30, no. 7, pp. 913–919, 2007.

[49] M. V. Thoma, R. La Marca, R. Brönnimann, L. Finkel, U. Ehlert, and U. M. Nater, "The effect of music on the human stress response," *PLoS One*, vol. 8, no. 8, article e70156, 2013.

30

# A New Look at Trigger Point Injections

**Clara S. M. Wong and Steven H. S. Wong**

*Department of Anaesthesiology, Queen Elizabeth Hospital, 30 Gascoigne Road, Kowloon, Hong Kong*

Correspondence should be addressed to Steven H. S. Wong, wonghss@ha.org.hk

Academic Editor: Andrea Trescot

Trigger point injections are commonly practised pain interventional techniques. However, there is still lack of objective diagnostic criteria for trigger points. The mechanisms of action of trigger point injection remain obscure and its efficacy remains heterogeneous. The advent of ultrasound technology in the noninvasive real-time imaging of soft tissues sheds new light on visualization of trigger points, explaining the effect of trigger point injection by blockade of peripheral nerves, and minimizing the complications of blind injection.

## 1. Introduction

Myofascial pain syndrome is a common, painful musculoskeletal disorder characterized by the presence of trigger points. They have been implicated in patients with headache, neck pain, low back pain, and various other musculoskeletal and systemic disorders [1–4]. The prevalence of myofascial trigger points among patients complaining of pain anywhere in the body ranged from 30% to 93% [5]. Although the most important strategy in treatment of myofascial pain syndrome is to identify the etiological lesion that causes the activation of trigger points and to treat the underlying pathology [6], trigger point injections are still commonly practised pain interventional technique for symptomatic relief.

Despite the popularity of trigger point injections, the pathophysiology of myofascial trigger points remains unclear. Localization of a trigger point is often based on the physician's examination. However, such physical examination is often unreliable. Lack of objective clinical measurements has also been a barrier for critically evaluating the efficacy of the therapeutic methods.

Ultrasound is used extensively for noninvasive real-time imaging of soft tissues including muscle, nerve, tendon, fascia, and blood vessels. With the advent of portable ultrasound technology, ultrasound is now commonly employed in the field of regional analgesia. In this paper, we will look at the potential application of ultrasound in trigger point injections.

## 2. Diagnosis of Trigger Points

Physician's sense of feel and patient expressions of pain upon palpation are the most commonly used method to localize a trigger point. The most common physical finding is palpation of a hypersensitive bundle or nodule of muscle fibre of harder than normal consistency. The palpation will elicit pain over the palpated muscle and/or cause radiation of pain towards the zone of reference in addition to a twitch response [7].

In myofascial pain syndrome, trigger points have been classified into active or latent. In an active trigger point, there is an area of tenderness at rest or on palpation, a taut band of muscle, a local twitch response, and referred pain elicited by firm compression similar to the patient's complaint. Latent trigger points are more commonly seen. They may display hypersensitivity and exhibit all the characteristics of an active trigger point except that it is not associated with spontaneous pain [7].

Trigger points have also been further classified into key or satellite. An active key trigger point in one muscle can induce an active satellite trigger point in another muscle. Inactivation of the key trigger point often also inactivates its satellite trigger point without treatment of the satellite trigger point itself [7].

The diagnosis of trigger points depends very much on the subjective experience of the physician. Pressure algometry has been used to quantify the sensitivity of trigger points.

A hand-held pressure meter with a $1\,cm^2$ rubber disc attached to a force gauge calibrated up to 10 kg is applied over a trigger point to measure its pain threshold [8]. However, this method is not commonly employed clinically, and there have not been any imaging criteria for the diagnosis of trigger points.

## 3. Pathophysiology of Trigger Points

Trigger points are defined as palpable, tense bands of skeletal muscle fibres. They can produce both local and referred pain when compressed.

The local pain could be explained by the tissue ischemia resulting from prolonged muscle contraction with accumulation of acids and chemicals such as serotonin, histamine, kinins, and prostaglandins [9]. These changes are fed into a cycle of increasing motor or sympathetic activity and can lead to increased pain. A painful event can sustain itself once a cycle is established even after the initial stimulus has been removed [10].

The pathogenesis of trigger points is probably related to sensitized sensory nerve fibres (nociceptors) associated with dysfunctional endplates [11]. In fact, endplate noise was found to be significantly more prevalent in myofascial trigger points than in sites that were outside of a trigger point but still within the endplate zone [12].

Studies have found that development of trigger points is dependent on an integrative mechanism in the spinal cord. When the input from nociceptors in an original receptive field persists (pain from an active trigger point), central sensitization in the spinal cord may develop, and the receptive field corresponding to the original dorsal horn neuron may be expanded (referred pain). Through this mechanism, new "satellite trigger points" may develop in the referred zone of the original trigger point [11].

## 4. Mechanisms of Action of Trigger Point Injections

Noninvasive measures for treatment of trigger points include spray and stretch, transcutaneous electrical stimulation, physical therapy, and massage. Invasive treatments include injections with local anaesthetics, corticosteroids, or botulinum toxin, or dry needling [13–18].

Hong reported that with either lidocaine injection or dry needling of trigger points, the patients experienced almost complete relief of pain immediately after injection if local twitch responses were elicited. On the other hand, they experienced only minimal relief if no such response occurred during injection. Hong has suggested that nociceptors (free nerve endings) are encountered and blocked during trigger point injection if local twitch response can be elicited [19].

The mechanism of action of trigger point injections is thought to be disruption of the trigger points by the mechanical effect of the needle or the chemical effect of the agents injected, resulting in relaxation and lengthening of the muscle fibre. The effect of the injectate may include local vasodilation, dilution, and removal of the accumulated nociceptive substrates. Botulinum toxin A has been used to block acetylcholine release from the motor nerve ending and subsequently relieve the taut band [6].

While the relief of local pain could easily be explained by the relaxation of the muscle fibre, the relief of referred pain could not be explained without attributing it to a peripheral nerve blockade. However, little has been said in the literature regarding the mechanism of trigger point injection in this respect.

## 5. Could the Application of Ultrasound Solve the Mystery of Trigger Points?

*5.1. Direct Visualization of Trigger Points.* As mentioned above, the most common physical finding of a trigger point is palpation of a hypersensitive bundle or nodule of muscle fibre of harder than normal consistency. Attempts to confirm the presence of myofascial trigger points using imaging have been demonstrated by magnetic resonance elastography [20]. For ultrasound, earlier studies have failed to find any correlation between physical findings and diagnostic ultrasound [21]. This may be attributed to poorer quality of ultrasound imaging in earlier dates.

Recently, Sikdar et al. have tried to use ultrasound to visualize and characterize trigger points. They found that trigger points appeared as focal, hypoechoic regions of elliptical shape, with a size of 0.16 cm [22]. This is promising as ultrasound can provide a more objective diagnosis of trigger point. Even if visualization of individual trigger point is difficult due to the small size, some advocate the use of ultrasound to guide proper needle placement in muscle tissue and to avoid adipose or nonmusculature structures during trigger point injections [23].

*5.2. Injection of Peripheral Nerves.* Trigger point injections have been implicated in patients with headache, low back pain, and various other musculoskeletal and systemic disorders. Some of these injections may involve injectate deposition directly to the nerves supplying the region. Indeed, entrapment, compression, or irritation of the sensory nerves of local regions has been implicated in various conditions.

*5.2.1. Greater Occipital Nerve.* Entrapment of the greater occipital nerve is often implicated as the cause of cervicogenic headache, and the characteristic occipital headache can be reproduced by finger pressure over the corresponding occipital nerve over the occipital ridge [3, 24–26]. This referral pattern of pain coincides with that of the properties of a trigger point, and it could explain the mechanism of referred pain for trigger points.

Simons has considered that the effect of greater occipital nerve injection is due to the release of the entrapment by relaxation of semispinalis muscle [7]. However, injection of local anaesthetics with or without steroid over the occipital nerve has been found to result in alleviation of occipital headache [27]. In migraine headaches, local injection of local anaesthetics or botulinum toxin type A to the greater occipital nerve has been demonstrated to provide relief of the condition [24].

There are several techniques of ultrasound-guided blockade of greater occipital nerve. The classical distal block technique involves placing the transducer at the superior nuchal line, while for the new proximal approach, the transducer is placed at the level of C2, and the greater occipital nerve lies superficial to the obliquus capitis inferior muscle [28, 29].

*5.2.2. Abdominal Cutaneous Nerve.* Kuan et al. showed that local injection of anaesthetics or steroid can treat some patients with lower abdominal pain presenting with trigger points in the abdomen, thus avoiding diagnostic laparoscopy and medications [30].

Trigger points over the abdominal wall may in fact be entrapped cutaneous nerves. Peripheral nerve entrapment (e.g., ilioinguinal-iliohypogastric nerves, thoracic lateral cutaneous nerve) has been suggested to cause lower abdominal pain [31, 32].

Ultrasound-guided blocks for ilioinguinal and iliohypogastric nerves have been practised widely in anaesthesia [33–35]. Recently, ultrasound-guided transversus abdominis plane (TAP) block is also commonly used to provide postoperative pain relief for patients undergoing laparotomy [35–38].

By placing the ultrasound probe about 5 cm cranial to the anterior superior iliac spine, the ilioinguinal and iliohypogastric nerves can be found between the transverse abdominal and the internal oblique muscle [39]. For TAP block, the transducer can be placed in a transverse plane between the iliac crest and the anterior axillary line. Local anaesthetics can be deposited between the transversus abdominis muscle and the internal oblique muscle [40].

*5.2.3. Dorsal Ramus of Spinal Nerve.* Low back pain is a common chronic pain syndrome; however, in most cases, a specific diagnosis cannot be established. Trigger point injections have been found to relieve myofascial low back pains. However, there has been lack of evidence in the literature to support its efficacy. This could be attributed to the heterogeneity in the diagnosis and technique of localization of trigger points in low back pain. Most of the studies employed subjective localization of trigger points, and the techniques of localization and injection of trigger points were not well described.

Miyakoshi et al. demonstrated that CT-guided total dorsal ramus block was effective in the treatment of chronic low back pain in a group of patients with overlapping facet syndrome with myofascial syndrome with pain originating from myofascial structure, facet joint, or both [41]. They demonstrated that a single injection of a larger volume of local anaesthetics over the conventional target point for medial branch block, which was the junction of the L5 superior articular process and the transverse process, was effective to block the medial, intermediate, and lateral branches of the lumbar dorsal ramus, with significantly better pain reduction compared to conventional trigger point injection. The findings in this study shed light to the possibility of relief of myofascial pain syndrome by a single nerve injection. It may explain the poor results of pure intramuscular injections in controlled studies, in contrast to the better results with uncontrolled studies and case reports, in which some of the results may be attributable to accidental nerve injection using the conventional blind injection techniques.

For ultrasound-guided medial branch block, the transducer is first placed longitudinally to find the respective transverse process and localize the lumbar level. Then the transducer can be rotated into a transverse plane to delineate the transverse process and the superior articular process of the adjacent facet joint. The bottom of the groove between the lateral surface of the superior articular process and the cephalad margin of the respective transverse process was defined as the target site [42].

Ultrasound-guided technique may be adapted to perform injection of the lower back, targeting at the dorsal rami of the lumbar spinal nerves to increase the efficacy of injection.

*5.2.4. Lumbar Plexus.* There have been case reports on the use of trigger point injection for treatment of pain that was remote from the site of trigger points. Interestingly, Iguchi et al. used trigger point injection for the amelioration of renal colic. In their paper, they described the injection technique as follows. Trigger points were located over the paraspinal region at around L3 level. A long needle (23-gauge 6 cm) was inserted deep into the trigger points, and 5–10 mL of 1% lignocaine was injected [43]. Such injection was in fact into the psoas muscle, and the effect could be attributed to a lumbar plexus block.

Lumbar plexus block with ultrasound guidance has been described. A curved transducer can be placed in the transverse plane at L2–L4 level for the lumbar plexus block. This transverse view should show the psoas muscle without the transverse process. The target of the needle tip is within the posterior 1/3 of the psoas muscle bulk [40].

*5.2.5. Pudendal Nerve.* Langford et al. reported the effective use of levator ani trigger point injection in the treatment of chronic pelvic pain. Trigger points were identified by manual intravaginal palpation, and the trigger points were injected with a large volume (up to about 20 mL) of a mixture of local anesthetics and depot steroid. The effect of such injection might in fact be caused by the concomitant pudendal nerve block [44].

Pudendal nerve blockade with ultrasound guidance can be performed via the transgluteal approach. The probe is placed transverse to the posterior superior iliac spine and moved caudally until the piriformis muscle is seen. The probe is then moved further caudad to identify the ischial spine, in which the pudendal nerve will be seen lying medial to the pudendal artery [29].

## 6. Other Advantages of Ultrasound in Trigger Point Injections

Trigger point injections are commonly performed in clinics as an outpatient procedure. Serious complications, although of rare occurrence, have been reported (e.g., pneumothorax, haematoma, intravascular injection of local anaesthetics, and intrathecal injections) [45]. Direct visualization of surrounding soft tissues and important structures can reduce the risk of such complications. Moreover, ultrasound allows real-time imaging of the spread of the injectate around the relevant structures and increases the success rate of injection.

## 7. Future Directions

The nonspecific diagnosis and lack of objective clinical measurements for trigger points mean that the evidence for the effectiveness of trigger point injection remains heterogenous. There is so far no strong evidence for the effectiveness of trigger point injections, and many physicians consider trigger point injections a little more than, if not equivalent to, placebo effects.

With the advancement of ultrasound technology, the quality of scans for soft tissues and musculature has improved dramatically. Future studies may focus on more objective diagnostic criteria of trigger points using ultrasound imaging. For the technique of trigger point injections, real-time visualization of trigger points, relaxation of locally contracting muscles, and visualization of surrounding tissues or important structures may improve the outcome and minimize complications of such treatments.

Moreover, efficacy of some of the trigger point injections traditionally performed may be related to some kind of peripheral nerve blocks, the implication which is yet to be explored.

## References

[1] S. C. Han and P. Harrison, "Myofascial pain syndrome and trigger-point management," *Regional Anesthesia*, vol. 22, no. 1, pp. 89–101, 1997.

[2] T. A. Garvey, M. R. Marks, and S. W. Wiesel, "A prospective, randomized, double-blind evaluation of trigger-point injection therapy for low-back pain," *Spine*, vol. 14, no. 9, pp. 962–964, 1989.

[3] A. Ashkenazi, A. Blumenfeld, U. Napchan et al., "Peripheral nerve blocks and trigger point injections in headache management—a systematic review and suggestions for future research," *Headache*, vol. 50, no. 6, pp. 943–952, 2010.

[4] C. Bron, A. de Gast, J. Dommerholt, B. Stegenga, M. Wensing, and R. A.B. Oostendorp, "Treatment of myofascial trigger points in patients with chronic shoulder pain: a randomized, controlled trial," *BMC Medicine*, vol. 9, 2011.

[5] D. G. Simons, "Clinical and etiological update of myofascial pain from trigger points," *Journal of Musculoskeletal Pain*, vol. 4, no. 1-2, pp. 93–121, 1996.

[6] C. Hong, "Myofascial Pain Therapy," *Regional Musculoskeletal Pain*, vol. 12, no. 3, pp. 37–43, 2004.

[7] D. Simons, J. Travell, and L. Simons, *Travell & Simons' Myofascial Pain and Dysfunction: The Trigger Point Manual*, Williams & Wilkins, Baltimore, Md, USA, 2nd edition, 1999.

[8] J. L. Reeves, B. Jaeger, and S. B. Graff-Radford, "Reliability of the pressure algometer as a measure of myofascial trigger point sensitivity," *Pain*, vol. 24, no. 3, pp. 313–321, 1986.

[9] J. Travel and S. H. Rinzler, "The myofascial genesis of pain," *Postgraduate Medicine*, vol. 11, no. 5, pp. 425–434, 1952.

[10] A. Sola and J. Bonica, "Myofascial pain syndromes," in *Bonica's Management of Pain*, J. Loeser et al., Ed., Lippincott Williams & Wilkins, Philadelphia, Pa, USA, 3rd edition, 2001.

[11] C. Z. Hong and D. G. Simons, "Pathophysiologic and electrophysiologic mechanisms of myofascial trigger points," *Archives of Physical Medicine and Rehabilitation*, vol. 79, no. 7, pp. 863–872, 1998.

[12] D. G. Simons, C. Z. Hong, and L. S. Simons, "Endplate potentials are common to midfiber myofacial trigger points," *American Journal of Physical Medicine and Rehabilitation*, vol. 81, no. 3, pp. 212–222, 2002.

[13] H. Iwama and Y. Akama, "The superiority of water-diluted 0.25% to neat 1% lidocaine for trigger-point injections in myofascial pain syndrome: a prospective randomized, double-blinded trial," *Anesthesia and Analgesia*, vol. 91, no. 2, pp. 408–409, 2000.

[14] H. Iwama, S. Ohmori, T. Kaneko, and K. Watanabe, "Water-diluted local anesthetic for trigger-point injection in chronic myofascial pain syndrome: evaluation of types of local anesthetic and concentrations in water," *Regional Anesthesia and Pain Medicine*, vol. 26, no. 4, pp. 333–336, 2001.

[15] J. Borg-Stein and D. Simons, "Focused review: myofascial pain," *Archives of Physical Medicine and Rehabilitation*, vol. 83, no. 3, supplement 1, pp. S40–S49, 2002.

[16] C. L. Graboski, D. Shaun Gray, and R. S. Burnham, "Botulinum toxin A versus bupivacaine trigger point injections for the treatment of myofascial pain syndrome: a randomised double blind crossover study," *Pain*, vol. 118, no. 1-2, pp. 170–175, 2005.

[17] K. Y. Ho and K. H. Tan, "Botulinum toxin A for myofascial trigger point injection: a qualitative systematic review," *European Journal of Pain*, vol. 11, no. 5, pp. 519–527, 2007.

[18] C. T. Tsai, L. F. Hsieh, T. S. Kuan, M. J. Kao, L. W. Chou, and C. Z. Hong, "Remote effects of dry needling on the irritability of the myofascial trigger point in the upper trapezius muscle," *American Journal of Physical Medicine and Rehabilitation*, vol. 89, no. 2, pp. 133–140, 2010.

[19] C. Z. Hong, "Lidocaine injection versus dry needling to myofascial trigger point: the importance of the local twitch response," *American Journal of Physical Medicine and Rehabilitation*, vol. 73, no. 4, pp. 256–263, 1994.

[20] D. G. Simons, "New views of myofascial trigger points: etiology and diagnosis," *Archives of Physical Medicine and Rehabilitation*, vol. 89, no. 1, pp. 157–159, 2008.

[21] J. Lewis and P. Tehan, "A blinded pilot study investigating the use of diagnostic ultrasound for detecting active myofascial trigger points," *Pain*, vol. 79, no. 1, pp. 39–44, 1999.

[22] S. Sikdar, J. P. Shah, T. Gebreab et al., "Novel applications of ultrasound technology to visualize and characterize myofascial trigger points and surrounding soft tissue," *Archives of Physical Medicine and Rehabilitation*, vol. 90, no. 11, pp. 1829–1838, 2009.

[23] K. P. Botwin, K. Sharma, R. Saliba, and B. C. Patel, "Ultrasound-guided trigger point injections in the cervicothoracic musculature: a new and unreported technique," *Pain Physician*, vol. 11, no. 6, pp. 885–889, 2008.

[24] J. E. Janis, D. A. Hatef, E. M. Reece, P. D. McCluskey, T. A. Schaub, and B. Guyuron, "Neurovascular compression of the greater occipital nerve: implications for migraine headaches," *Plastic and Reconstructive Surgery*, vol. 126, no. 6, pp. 1996–2001, 2010.

[25] A. Blumenfeld and A. Ashkenazi, "Nerve blocks, trigger point injections and headache," *Headache*, vol. 50, no. 6, pp. 953–954, 2010.

[26] A. Blumenfeld, A. Ashkenazi, B. Grosberg et al., "Patterns of use of peripheral nerve blocks and trigger point injections among headache practitioners in the USA: results of the American headache society interventional procedure survey (AHS-IPS)," *Headache*, vol. 50, no. 6, pp. 937–942, 2010.
[27] A. Ashkenazi and W. B. Young, "The effects of greater occipital nerve block and trigger point injection on brush allodynia and pain in migraine," *Headache*, vol. 45, no. 4, pp. 350–354, 2005.
[28] M. Greher, B. Moriggl, M. Curatolo, L. Kirchmair, and U. Eichenberger, "Sonographic visualization and ultrasound-guided blockade of the greater occipital nerve: a comparison of two selective techniques confirmed by anatomical dissection," *British Journal of Anaesthesia*, vol. 104, no. 5, pp. 637–642, 2010.
[29] S. Narouze, Ed., *Atlas of Ultrasound-Guided Procedures in Interventional Pain Management*, Springer, New York, NY, USA, 2011.
[30] L. C. Kuan, Y. T. Li, F. M. Chen, C. J. Tseng, S. F. Wu, and T. C. Kuo, "Efficacy of treating abdominal wall pain by local injection," *Taiwanese Journal of Obstetrics and Gynecology*, vol. 45, no. 3, pp. 239–243, 2006.
[31] J. L. Whiteside, M. D. Barber, M. D. Walters, T. Falcone, and A. Morse, "Anatomy of ilioinguinal and iliohypogastric nerves in relation to trocar placement and low transverse incisions," *American Journal of Obstetrics and Gynecology*, vol. 189, no. 6, pp. 1574–1578, 2003.
[32] R. Peleg, J. Gohar, M. Koretz, and A. Peleg, "Abdominal wall pain in pregnant women caused by thoracic lateral cutaneous nerve entrapment," *European Journal of Obstetrics Gynecology*, vol. 74, no. 2, pp. 169–171, 1997.
[33] S. L. Lim, S. Ng, and G. M. Tan, "Ilioinguinal and iliohypogastric nerve block revisited: single shot versus double shot technique for hernia repair in children," *Paediatric Anaesthesia*, vol. 12, no. 3, pp. 255–260, 2002.
[34] F. Oriola, Y. Toque, A. Mary, O. Gagneur, S. Beloucif, and H. Dupont, "Bilateral ilioinguinal nerve block decreases morphine consumption in female patients undergoing nonlaparoscopic gynecologic surgery," *Anesthesia and Analgesia*, vol. 104, no. 3, pp. 731–734, 2007.
[35] C. Aveline, H. Le Hetet, A. Le Roux et al., "Comparison between ultrasound-guided transversus abdominis plane and conventional ilioinguinal/iliohypogastric nerve blocks for day-case open inguinal hernia repair," *British Journal of Anaesthesia*, vol. 106, no. 3, pp. 380–386, 2011.
[36] J. Chiono, N. Bernard, S. Bringuier et al., "The ultrasound-guided transversus abdominis plane block for anterior iliac crest bone graft postoperative pain relief: a prospective descriptive study," *Regional Anesthesia and Pain Medicine*, vol. 35, no. 6, pp. 520–524, 2010.
[37] J. M. Baaj, R. A. Alsatli, H. A. Majaj, Z. A. Babay, and A. K. Thallaj, "Efficacy of ultrasound-guided transversus abdominis plane (TAP) block for post-cesarean section delivery analgesia—a double-blind, placebo-controlled, randomized study," *Middle East Journal of Anesthesiology*, vol. 20, no. 6, pp. 821–826, 2010.
[38] Y. S. Ra, C. H. Kim, G. Y. Lee, and J. I. Han, "The analgesic effect of the ultrasound-guided transverse abdominis plane block after laparoscopic cholecystectomy," *Korean Journal of Anesthesiology*, vol. 58, no. 4, pp. 362–368, 2010.
[39] U. Eichenberger, M. Greher, L. Kirchmair, M. Curatolo, and B. Moriggl, "Ultrasound-guided blocks of the ilioinguinal and iliohypogastric nerve: accuracy of a selective new technique confirmed by anatomical dissection," *British Journal of Anaesthesia*, vol. 97, no. 2, pp. 238–243, 2006.
[40] V. Chan, S. Abbas, R. Brull, B. Moriggl, and A. Perlas, *Ultrasound Imaging for Regional Anesthesia—A Practical Guide*, Vincent Chan, 3rd edition, 2010.
[41] N. Miyakoshi, Y. Shimada, Y. Kasukawa, H. Saito, H. Kodama, and E. Itoi, "Total dorsal ramus block for the treatment of chronic low back pain: a preliminary study," *Joint Bone Spine*, vol. 74, no. 3, pp. 270–274, 2007.
[42] M. Greher, L. Kirchmair, B. Enna et al., "Ultrasound-guided lumbar facet nerve block: accuracy of a new technique confirmed by computed tomography," *Anesthesiology*, vol. 101, no. 5, pp. 1195–1200, 2004.
[43] M. Iguchi, Y. Katoh, H. Koike, T. Hayashi, and M. Nakamura, "Randomized trial of trigger point injection for renal colic," *International Journal of Urology*, vol. 9, no. 9, pp. 475–479, 2002.
[44] C. F. Langford, S. U. Nagy, and G. M. Ghoniem, "Levator ani trigger point injections: an underutilized treatment for chronic pelvic pain," *Neurourology and Urodynamics*, vol. 26, no. 1, pp. 59–62, 2007.
[45] L. S. Nelson and R. S. Hoffman, "Intrathecal injection: unusual complication of trigger-point injection therapy," *Annals of Emergency Medicine*, vol. 32, no. 4, pp. 506–508, 1998.

# 31

# Bicarbonates for the Prevention of Postoperative Renal Failure in Endovascular Aortic Aneurysm Repair

**Véronique Brulotte,[1,2] François A. Leblond,[3] Stéphane Elkouri,[4] Éric Thérasse,[5] Vincent Pichette,[3,6] and Pierre Beaulieu[1,6]**

[1] *Anesthesiology Department, University of Montreal Hospital Centre, 3840 St. Urbain Street, Montréal, QC, Canada H2W 1T8*
[2] *Department of Anesthesiology, Maisonneuve-Rosemont Hospital, 5415 Boulevard de l'Assomption, Montréal, QC, Canada H1T 2M4*
[3] *Nephrology Department and Guy-Bernier Research Centre, Maisonneuve-Rosemont Hospital, Canada*
[4] *Vascular Surgery Department, University of Montreal Hospital Centre, 3840 St. Urbain Street, Montréal, QC, Canada H2W 1T8*
[5] *Radiology Department, University of Montreal Hospital Centre, 3840 St. Urbain Street, Montréal, QC, Canada H2W 1T8*
[6] *Department of Pharmacology, University of Montreal, 3840 St. Urbain Street, Montréal, QC, Canada H2W 1T8*

Correspondence should be addressed to Véronique Brulotte; verobrulotte@hotmail.com

Academic Editor: Peter Andrews

*Purpose.* Contrast-induced nephropathy (CIN) can contribute to acute kidney injury (AKI) in patients undergoing endovascular aortic aneurysm surgery. We evaluated the incidence of AKI together with the evolution of early biomarkers of renal injury in patients receiving bicarbonates or NaCl 0.9%. *Methods.* This study involved endovascular aortic aneurysm surgery patients. Group A ($n = 17$) received bicarbonates 3 mL/kg/h for 1 h before the procedure and then 1 mL/kg/h until 6 h after surgery, whereas group B ($n = 17$) received NaCl 0.9% using the same protocol. Biomarkers of renal injury from urine (interleukin-18 (IL-18), neutrophil gelatinase-associated lipocalin (NGAL), N-acetyl-$\beta$-D-glucosaminidase (NAG), and kidney injury molecule 1 (KIM-1)) and blood (NGAL, cystatin C) were measured at baseline and 3, 24, and 48 h postoperatively. *Results.* AKI occurred in 1 patient (2.9%), in the bicarbonates group. IL-18, NAG, NGAL, and KIM-1 significantly rose in both groups after the surgery. There was a greater rise in NGAL and IL-18 after 3 h in the bicarbonates versus NaCl 0.9% group: 1115% versus 240% increase ($P = 0.03$) and 338% increase versus 1.4% decrease ($P = 0.01$). *Conclusions.* Despite significant elevation in biomarkers of renal injury, we demonstrated a low rate of AKI following endovascular aortic surgery.

## 1. Introduction

The endovascular approach for the repair of aortic aneurysm is an interesting alternative to the open repair approach because of its associated reduced 30-day morbidity and mortality. This approach, however, carries its own risks such as renal complications [1–5].

Renal complications occur with variable incidence, ranging from 5.5 to 20% [3–6]. They may be caused by ischemic or embolic events but can also be secondary to the large amounts of contrast media used to guide prosthesis placement. This complication is known as contrast-induced nephropathy (CIN). Indeed, the volume of contrast media used in vascular surgery is important, ranging from 130 to 260 mL [1, 3, 4, 6, 7].

Many strategies have been developed in an attempt to prevent CIN. Among these, an intravenous volume expansion that covers the pre-, per- and postcontrast media exposure is the only established way [8–13]. N-acetylcysteine (NAC) administration has been suggested because of its low cost, safety, and possible benefit in patients with chronic renal failure [14–19], although its efficacy is controversial [14].

What type of infusion to use to achieve intravenous volume expansion is not known [14–29]. By its ability to alkalinize renal tubular fluid and reduce the formation of free radicals, sodium bicarbonate could reduce the incidence of CIN and prevent a potential acute kidney injury (AKI) from contrast media. Its potential protective effect has been shown by many authors, but it has not been found consistently [20–29]. Furthermore, these studies have only included patients undergoing radiologic or coronary angiographic procedures and have never been evaluated in the perioperative context.

Furthermore, serum creatinine is typically used for the diagnosis of AKI, but it is an insensitive and unreliable biomarker during acute changes in kidney function [30]. More sensitive markers of renal injury, such as urinary interleukin-18 (IL-18), neutrophil gelatinase-associated lipocalin (NGAL), N-acetyl-$\beta$-D-glucosaminidase (NAG), kidney injury molecule 1 (KIM-1) blood NGAL, and cystatin C, have been studied, and their evolution has been linked to the subsequent development of AKI [30–39].

The incidence of renal complications during endovascular aortic aneurysm repair varies in a fourfold proportion and furthermore may be modified by the hydration protocol used; therefore, their real incidence is not known. The primary goal of this pilot study was to evaluate the true incidence of AKI in this population of patients and to compare the evolution of numerous early biomarkers of renal injury before and after contrast media exposure in patients receiving either sodium bicarbonate or sodium chloride for intravascular volume expansion during endovascular aortic aneurysm repair.

## 2. Materials and Methods

This is a prospective randomized controlled pilot study (controlled-trials.com ISRCTN39325111) that took place between March 2009 and March 2011. The incidence of postoperative AKI, defined by an elevation in serum creatinine beyond 50% of baseline within 48 h (acute kidney injury network [40]), was evaluated. Furthermore, different early biomarkers of renal injury were measured following contrast media exposure, such as neutrophil gelatinase-associated lipocalin (NGAL), N-acetyl-$\beta$-D-glucosaminidase (NAG), interleukin-18 (IL-18), cystatin C (cysC), and kidney injury molecule-1 (KIM-1). The need for dialysis and mortality within 30 days of the surgery was also recorded.

*2.1. Enrolment.* The study protocol was approved by our local ethic committees (Maisonneuve-Rosemont Hospital, Montreal QC, Canada, no.: CER 09073 and CHUM, Montreal, QC, Canada, no.: HD 08.110). Over a two-year period, patients ranging from 18 to 85 years of age, and presenting for elective endovascular aortic repair, were approached by a member of the research team at Montréal Hôtel-Dieu (CHUM) and Maisonneuve-Rosemont hospitals (Quebec, Canada). Exclusion criteria included patient refusal, exposure to contrast media within 14 days prior to surgery, acute renal failure on the day of surgery, defined as serum creatinine 50% above normal patient values, patients who were renal transplant recipients, and patients on dialysis for chronic renal failure. All patients signed a written informed consent.

*2.2. Randomization.* Patients were randomly assigned based on a computer-generated list. Patients in group A were assigned to receive an infusion of sodium bicarbonate, whereas patients in group B received a sodium chloride (NaCl 0.9%) infusion. All patients received NAC. The randomization list was generated by the pharmacy which then supplied both solutions in an unidentifiable infusion bag to a blinded member of the research team.

*2.3. Perioperative Fluid and Drug Administrations.* Immediately after arriving in the operating room, study participants received their first dose of NAC, which was administered as an intravenous (i.v.) bolus over 15 minutes. This method is slightly different from the most common practice, however, can be used, and its efficacy has been demonstrated, particularly when patients cannot be prepared because of urgent procedure or lack of time [17]. The infusion consisted of NAC 150 mg/kg diluted in 500 mL NaCl 0.9%. Further doses of NAC (1200 mg PO twice a day) began in the evening after the surgery and continued for a total of three doses.

At the induction of general or spinal anesthesia, approximately 1 h before the contrast media was introduced, the study infusion were administered according to a protocol that is, used in most studies on bicarbonates for CIN prevention [20, 23, 26]: patients received a bolus of 3 mL/kg over 1 h of either sodium bicarbonate 150 MEq/L or sodium chloride 0.9%. This infusion was then continued at the rate of 1 mL/kg/h for a total of 6 h after the end of surgery.

The attending anesthesiologist, who was blinded to patient group, was instructed to give crystalloids (Lactated Ringer), colloids (6% hydroxyethyl starch (HES) 130/0.4) or blood products according to clinical judgement to cover for insensible and blood losses. The contrast media administered to the patients were iodixanol (Visipaque, Amersham Health, UK), a nonionic iso-osmolar opacifying agent. Mannitol and furosemide use was not permitted. Diuretics were routinely withheld on the day of surgery. Nonsteroidal anti-inflammatory agents use was prohibited during the entire perioperative period.

*2.4. Data Recording.* Information on demographics and comorbid conditions was obtained from the patients and their medical records. CIN risk score was then calculated for each patient. This risk score, as developed by Mehran et al. [41] for patients undergoing coronary angiography, is widely used to estimate individual patient's risk of CIN.

Detailed medication history was recorded. Recorded procedural data included the occurrence of intraoperative hypotension, which was defined as systolic blood pressure below 100 mm Hg for at least 30 minutes or necessitating the use of vasopressors to be maintained above 100 mm Hg, blood losses, total volume of crystalloids, colloids, blood products, and total volume of contrast media administered.

Samples were collected to evaluate the evolution of the following biomarkers: urinary NGAL, IL-18, NAG, KIM-1 serum NGAL, and cysC. Urinary and blood specimens were collected after the induction of anesthesia and 3 h, 24 h, and

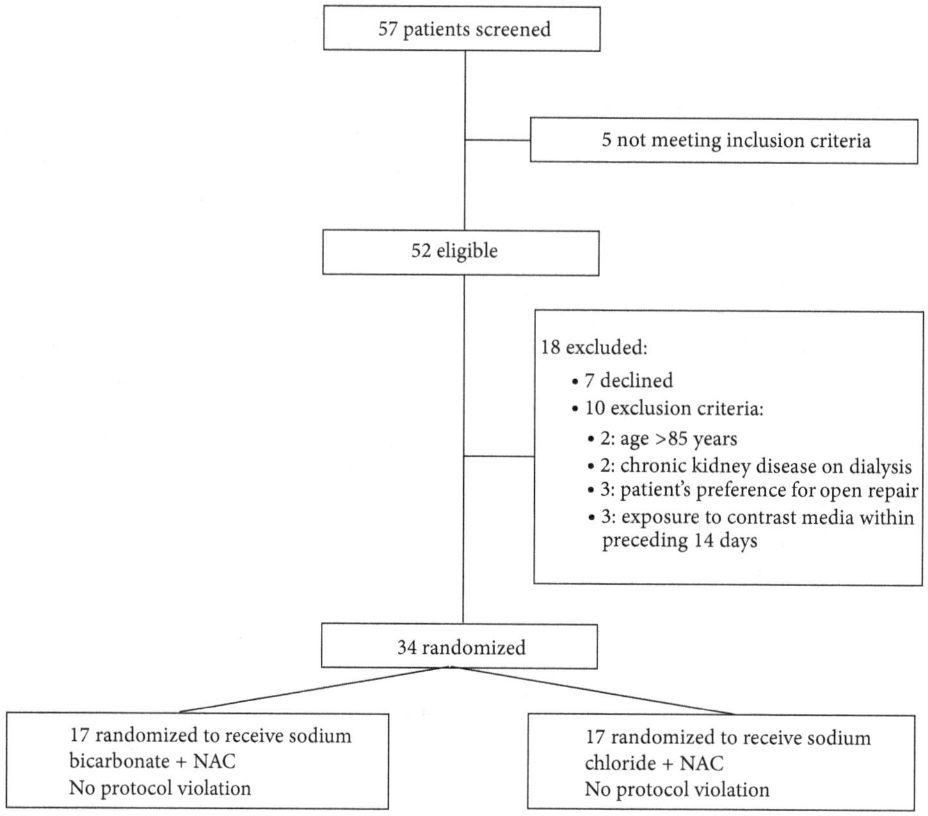


NAC: N-acetylcysteine

FIGURE 1

48 h after exposure to contrast media. Serum creatinine was collected at the same time points.

Samples were kept frozen at −80°C up to the time of the analysis. NGAL in serum and urine was assayed using Rapid ELISA kit from Antibody Shop A/S (Gentofte, Denmark). IL-18 was measured in urine by using quantitative ELISA assay from Medical & Biological Laboratories Co. Ltd. (Naka-ku Nagoya, Japan). KIM-1 and cystatin C were measured using Quantikine Human TIM-1/KIM-1/HAVCR and Quantikine Human cystatin C ELISA kit, respectively, from R&D Systems (Minneapolis, USA). Urinary NAG activity was assayed manually using NAG assay from BioQuant (San Diego, USA). Creatinine was measured on Architect C16000, Abbott Diagnostics (Mississauga, Canada).

*2.5. Statistical Analysis.* Data were collected using Microsoft Excel and were analyzed using IBM SPSS Statistics 19. All continuous variables were first analyzed with a one sample Kolmogorov Smirnov test to determine normality. Demographic and perioperative continuous and categorical data were analyzed using Student's $t$- and chi-squared tests, respectively. Kruskal-Wallis and Mann-Whitney $U$ tests were used to analyze ordinal and nonnormally distributed continuous data.

According to each study group, the incidence of postoperative AKI was analyzed as a categorical data with a Fisher's exact test. Serum and urinary levels for each of the biomarkers were compared to their baseline levels by calculating the percentage of change that was analyzed with a Student's $t$-test. Comparison between study groups for the percent change in each biomarker at each time point was analyzed with a Student's $t$-test. A $P$ value $< 0.05$ was considered statistically significant.

## 3. Results

*3.1. Patient Population and Baseline Characteristics.* From March 2009 to March 2011, 57 eligible patients were asked to participate in the research project. Of these, six were not randomized because the planned surgery also included vascular procedures on vessels other than the aorta (femoral angioplasty (3) and iliac stenting (3)). Seven patients refused to participate, and ten patients were excluded: age >85 years old (2), chronic kidney failure on dialysis (2), patient preference for an open repair (3), and exposure to contrast media in the last 14 days (3). A total of 34 patients were included, 17 randomized to group sodium bicarbonate and 17 to group sodium chloride (Figure 1). All patients received the assigned infusion, and there was no protocol violation.

Demographic, clinical, angiographic, and hemodynamic characteristics were comparable between study groups (Table 1). The mean age for the full cohort was 73.8 (6.3)

Table 1: Demographic subject characteristics.

| | Sodium bicarbonate $N = 17$ | Sodium chloride $N = 17$ |
|---|---|---|
| Age (yr) | 71.9 (6.1) | 75.6 (6.0) |
| Sex (male) | 14/17 | 14/17 |
| Weight (kg) | 80.5 (14.2) | 80.6 (12.1) |
| Aneurysm | | |
| Thoracic | 0/17 | 1/17 |
| Infrarenal | 17/17 | 16/17 |
| CIN risk score[a] | 4.5 (3.8) | 5.8 (4.1) |
| Diabetes | 2/17 (12) | 2/17 (12) |
| Intraoperative hypotension | 3/17 (18) | 3/17 (18) |
| CHF[b] | 1/17 (6) | 0/17 |
| Age >75 | 6/17 (35) | 9/17 (53) |
| Anemia | 4/17 (24) | 4/17 (24) |
| Chronic renal failure | 0/17 | 4/17 (24) |
| Contrast volume (mL) | 140.1 (70.7) | 159.5 (50.7) |
| Baseline creatinine($\mu$mol/L) | 82.1 (14.5) | 96.5 (41.8) |
| Medication[c] | | |
| ACE inhibitors | 6/17 (35) | 5/17 (29) |
| Aminoglycosides | 0/17 | 0/17 |
| Diuretics | 3/17 (17) | 4/17 (24) |
| Vancomycin[b] | 4/17 (24) | 4/17 (24) |
| Duration[d] (min)[†] | 105.0 (30) | 117.0 (31) |
| Days to discharge[†] | 2.0 (1) | 2.0 (1) |
| Perioperative fluids | | |
| Ringer lactate (mL) | 1767.6 (544.6) | 1561.8 (536.1) |

Values are reported as means (standard deviation) and as proportions (%).
[†]Values expressed as median (interquartile range).
ACE: angiotensin-converting enzyme; CHF: congestive heart failure; CIN: contrast-induced nephropathy; IABP: intra-aortic balloon pump.
[a]As defined by Mehran et al. [41]. See Appendix 1 for details; [b]defined by a NYHA class > III/IV and/or history of pulmonary edema; [c]received on the day of surgery; [d]duration from skin incision to complete wound closure.

Table 2: Baseline values for creatinine, cystatin C, serum, and urinary NGAL, IL-18, NAG, and KIM-1 according to study group.

| | Bicarbonates | Sodium chloride |
|---|---|---|
| Serum | | |
| Creatinine ($\mu$mol/L) | 82.1 (14.5) | 96.5 (41.8) |
| Cystatin C (ng/mL)[†] | 886.80 (172.1) | 866.10 (383.40) |
| NGAL (ng/ml) | 112.02 (36.67) | 110.99 (46.86) |
| Urinary | | |
| NGAL (ng/$\mu$mol creatinine)[†] | 0.90 (3.10) | 1.80 (2.75) |
| IL-18 (pg/$\mu$mol creatinine) | 8.45 (5.60) | 10.67 (7.97) |
| NAG (IU/mmol creatinine)[†] | 0.60 (1.19) | 0.54 (2.0) |
| KIM-1 (ng/$\mu$mol creatinine) | 0.175 (0.132) | 0.186 (0.145) |

Values are expressed as means (standard deviation).
[†]Values expressed as median (interquartile range).
IL-18: interleukin-18; KIM-1: kidney injury molecule-1; NAG: N-acetyl-$\beta$-D-glucosaminidase; NGAL: neutrophil gelatinase-associated lipocalin.

years old, and 83% was men. The Mehran risk score for developing CIN was 5.1 and was comparable between groups. This risk score predicted a 7.5% risk of CIN [41]. Contrast media volume administered, perioperative crystalloids and colloids, and surgery duration were all comparable between the two groups. IABP was not used. One patient in the sodium chloride group received 1 unit of packed red blood cells ($P = 0.31$). Baseline levels for creatinine, cysC, serum and urinary NGAL, IL-18, NAG, and KIM-1 were comparable between groups (Table 2).

Overall, postoperative AKI, as defined by a 50% increase in serum creatinine at 48 h, occurred in 2.9% (1/34) of the patients. AKI occurred in 1 patient in the sodium bicarbonate group (5.9%), compared to no patient in the sodium chloride group (0%): difference 5.9%, 95% CI of −5.3% to 17.1%, $P = 0.50$. No patient required dialysis, but one died within 30 days after the procedure. This patient was in the sodium bicarbonate group, and he was the one who developed postoperative AKI.

Overall, most biomarkers of renal injury and cysC increased from baseline after exposure to contrast media, with this change being statistically significant only for urinary IL-18 at 24 and 48 h, NAG, and KIM-1 (Table 3). Conversely, serum creatinine levels significantly decreased compared to baseline in both groups after surgery and did not return to normal levels after 48 h. Baseline urinary pH was comparable between groups, but urine pH measurements after the procedure confirmed urine alkalinization in the sodium bicarbonate group ($P = 0.03$).

There was a significantly greater rise in urinary NGAL and IL-18 after 3 h in the bicarbonate versus sodium chloride group: 1115% versus 240% increase ($P = 0.03$) and 338% increase versus 1.4% decrease ($P = 0.01$), respectively. This difference was not found at other time points.

As early as 3 h after exposure to contrast media, the patient who developed postoperative AKI had significantly higher values of creatinine and urinary IL-18, NAG, and NGAL compared to those who did not develop postoperative AKI. This difference persisted after 24 and 48 h (Table 4). This patient received a higher volume of contrast media, had a longer surgery, and received more colloids and crystalloids, but the baseline risk score was comparable to that of the other patients (Table 5).

## 4. Discussion

The rate of postoperative AKI in this two-year study was 2.9%, which is lower than expected using Mehran risk score, lower than what is reported after endovascular aortic surgery [3, 5] and lower than what is found in most recent studies on CIN prevention using bicarbonates (mean incidence 10.8–11.8%) [28, 42]. This is probably because these studies mostly included patients with baseline chronic kidney disease, which represents a higher risk population [20–22, 25, 26]. We included both patients with normal and decreased kidney function in order to recruit all eligible patients. Most of

Table 3: Mean difference from baseline of various biomarkers before and after (3, 24, and 48 hours) surgery, regardless of study group.

| | Mean difference from baseline (%) | 95% CI for difference | $P$ value |
|---|---|---|---|
| Serum | | | |
| NGAL | | | |
| Δ3 h | 3.2 | −6.4 to 12.8 | 0.51 |
| Δ24 h | 12.1 | −0.6 to 24.8 | 0.06 |
| Δ48 h | 18.9 | −10.4 to 48.1 | 0.19 |
| cysC | | | |
| Δ3 h | −6.5 | −15.1 to 2.0 | 0.13 |
| Δ24 h | 2.0 | −6.2 to 10.2 | 0.62 |
| Δ48 h | 10.9 | −6.9 to 28.7 | 0.22 |
| Creatinine | | | |
| Δ3 h | −22.8 | −26.6 to −18.9 | <0.001 |
| Δ24 h | −12.9 | −18.7 to −7.1 | <0.001 |
| Δ48 h | −9.7 | −17.0 to −2.4 | 0.01 |
| Urinary | | | |
| IL-18 | | | |
| Δ3 h | 145.7 | −116.5 to 407.8 | 0.27 |
| Δ24 h | 328.9 | 95.3 to 562.6 | 0.01 |
| Δ48 h | 410.2 | 126.5 to 693.8 | 0.01 |
| NAG | | | |
| Δ3 h | 1294.0 | 422.6 to 2165.5 | 0.01 |
| Δ24 h | 775.9 | 328.6 to 1223.2 | <0.001 |
| Δ48 h | 1306.4 | 550.3 to 2062.6 | <0.001 |
| NGAL | | | |
| Δ3 h | 619.3 | −123.0 to 1361.5 | 0.10 |
| Δ24 h | 647.5 | 94.6 to 1200.4 | 0.02 |
| Δ48 h | 1641.7 | −430.4 to 3713.7 | 0.11 |
| KIM-1 | | | |
| Δ3 h | 20.8 | 3.2 to 38.3 | 0.02 |
| Δ24 h | 168.6 | 103.1 to 234.1 | <0.001 |
| Δ48 h | 246.4 | 149.6 to 343.2 | <0.001 |

Values expressed as mean percent change. CI: confidence interval.
cysC: cystatin C; IL-18: interleukin 18; KIM-1: kidney injury molecule 1; NAG: N-acetyl-$\beta$-D-glucosaminidase; NGAL: neutrophil gelatinase-associated lipocalin.

the studies on CIN prevention used a 25% elevation in creatinine to define the outcome. We evaluated the incidence of AKI, defined by a creatinine elevation >50%, because it is a recognized definition (AKI network) and because using an increase of 25% would have implied that a postoperative creatinine elevation can only be secondary to CIN. Although it is a very likely cause, given the large volume of contrast media injected near the renal arteries, we could not exclude an ischemic or embolic etiology. Using a 25% increase in creatinine as a definition would not have changed our results.

Another possible explanation of the lower rate of AKI may be the total amount of i.v. fluids received by the patients in this study (mean of 1665 mL on top of the hydration protocol).

Our results also show an increase in all biomarkers of renal injury following exposure to contrast media. This increase was significant for NAG and KIM-1 as early as 3 h after exposure, whereas it took 24 h for IL-18 and urinary NGAL to increase significantly. This can be attributed to their different kinetics [34, 39].

These biomarkers are produced by renal tubular cells and are highly specific for renal tubular injury [30–39]. This rise is very suggestive of kidney injury following contrast media exposure despite adequate hydration, although their significance in this study is not clear since it was not associated with a later rise in serum creatinine.

The low rate of AKI observed in this study could also be due to the fact that we stopped assessing creatinine 48 h postoperatively. Although creatinine typically starts to rise within the first 24 h in most cases of CIN [41], it is possible that a significant rise could occur later, as observed by Maioli et al. [43]. If they had limited their assessment to the first 48 h, they would have missed 30% of CIN-positive patients.

Furthermore, some of these biomarkers might be too sensitive, without being clinically relevant. Exposure to contrast media has caused an increase in urinary NAG excretion, without leading to AKI [37–39].

The rise in these biomarkers was higher in the bicarbonates group for urinary IL-18 and NGAL 3 h after exposure to contrast media. A greater rise in these specific biomarkers has shown to be an accurate predictor of CIN [32–34], and their elevation in this study could indicate possible harm from bicarbonates on the incidence of renal tubular injury after exposure to contrast media, although this remains speculative. Indeed, the one patient who developed postoperative AKI was in the bicarbonates group and had significantly higher levels of IL-18, NAG, and urinary NGAL 3 h after contrast media exposure. Therefore, the greater rise in these biomarkers in the bicarbonates group could be only a reflection of this patient's values.

This study could not confirm the role of the early biomarkers of renal injury on the prediction of postoperative AKI after endovascular aortic surgery. However, it would be interesting to measure their role in a larger, definitive trial evaluating the impact bicarbonates have on the incidence of postoperative AKI following endovascular aortic aneurysm repair. Given the very low incidence of postoperative AKI demonstrated in this trial, such a study would require 2850 patients per group to have the power of detecting a 30% difference between groups.

*4.1. Limitations.* This pilot study was limited by the small number of patients recruited and by the fact that we stopped assessing for serum creatinine after 48 h.

## 5. Conclusion

The results of this pilot study indicate a low rate of post-operative AKI following endovascular aortic surgery in a low risk population, despite significant elevation in early

TABLE 4: (a) Baseline values and (b) percent variation from baseline at 3, 24, and 72 hours postcontrast media exposure in the patient who developed AKI, as opposed to those who did not.

(a)

| | Serum | | | Urinary | | | |
|---|---|---|---|---|---|---|---|
| | Creatinine (μmol/L) | cysC (ng/mL) | NGAL (ng/mL) | IL-18 (pg/μmol creatinine) | NAG (IU/mmol creatinine) | NGAL (ng/μmol creatinine) | KIM-1 (ng/μmol creatinine) |
| Baseline | | | | | | | |
| AKI | 62 | 775.90 | 106.50 | 3.50 | 0.20 | 1.10 | 0.149 |
| No AKI | 90.1 | 830.47 | 111.61 | 9.92 | 1.38 | 6.49 | 0.182 |

Values expressed as means.
AKI: acute kidney injury; cysC: cystatin C; IL-18: interleukin 18; KIM-1: kidney injury molecule 1; NAG: N-acetyl-β-D-glucosaminidase; NGAL: neutrophil gelatinase-associated lipocalin.

(b)

| | Serum | | | Urinary | | | |
|---|---|---|---|---|---|---|---|
| | Creatinine (μmol/L) | cysC (ng/mL) | NGAL (ng/mL) | IL-18 (pg/μmol creatinine) | NAG (IU/mmol creatinine) | NGAL (ng/μmol creatinine) | KIM-1 (ng/μmol creatinine) |
| Δ3 h (%) | | | | | | | |
| AKI | 69.68 | 33.78 | 30.70 | 3854.28 | 11550.00 | 10700.00 | −34.23 |
| No AKI | −23.88 | −7.91 | 2.33 | 17.76 | 940.38 | 271.66 | 22.66 |
| Δ24 h (%) | | | | | | | |
| AKI | 66.13 | 3.45 | 87.61 | 1217.14 | 2150.00 | 7818.18 | 161.74 |
| No AKI | −15.31 | 1.99 | 9.51 | 298.28 | 728.48 | 400.23 | 168.85 |
| Δ48 h (%) | | | | | | | |
| AKI | 75.81 | 54.71 | 286.20 | 2282.86 | 3200.00 | 22281.82 | 296.64 |
| No AKI | −12.72 | 8.81 | 6.14 | 316.51 | 1211.74 | 658.79 | 243.75 |

Values expressed as mean percent change from baseline.
AKI: acute kidney injury; cysC: cystatin C; IL-18: interleukin 18; KIM-1: kidney injury molecule 1; NAG: N-acetyl-β-D-glucosaminidase; NGAL: neutrophil gelatinase-associated lipocalin.

TABLE 5: Baseline characteristics between the patient who developed AKI versus the patients who did not.

| | AKI | No AKI |
|---|---|---|
| Contrast volume (mL) | 300 | 145.3 (56.2) |
| Crystalloids (mL) | 3000 | 1624.2 (495.8) |
| Colloids (mL) | 1000 | 75.8 (220.8) |
| Urinary pH at 3 h | 8.0 | 6.7 (0.74) |
| Surgery duration (min) | 390 | 117.6 (41.7) |
| Mehran risk score [41] | 3 | 5.18 (3.9) |

Values expressed as mean (standard deviation).
AKI: acute kidney injury.

markers of renal injury. Their role in the prediction of postoperative AKI has not been substantiated in this study and should be evaluated in a much larger, definitive study determining the impact of bicarbonates on postoperative AKI after endovascular aortic surgery.

## Conflict of Interests

The authors declare that they have no conflict of interests.

## Funding

Maisonneuve-Rosemont Hospital Foundation through Nephrology research.

## References

[1] The EVAR trial participants, "Endovascular aneurysm repair versus open repair in patients with abdominal aortic aneurym (EVAR trial 1): randomised controlled trial," *The Lancet*, vol. 365, no. 9478, pp. 2179–2186, 2005.

[2] The EVAR trial participants, "Endovascular aneurysm repair and outcome in patients unfit for open repair of abdominal aortic aneurysm (EVAR trial 2): randomised controlled trial," *The Lancet*, vol. 365, no. 9478, pp. 2187–2192, 2005.

[3] M. L. Schermerhorn, A. J. O'Malley, A. Jhaveri, P. Cotterill, F. Pomposelli, and B. E. Landon, "Endovascular vs. open repair of abdominal aortic aneurysms in the medicare population," *The New England Journal of Medicine*, vol. 358, no. 5, pp. 464–474, 2008.

[4] S. S. Parmer and J. P. Carpenter, "Endovascular aneurysm repair with suprarenal vs infrarenal fixation: a study of renal effects," *Journal of Vascular Surgery*, vol. 43, no. 1, pp. 19–25, 2006.

[5] J. P. Carpenter, R. M. Fairman, C. F. Barker et al., "Endovascular AAA repair in patients with renal insufficiency: strategies for reducing adverse renal events," *Cardiovascular Surgery*, vol. 9, no. 6, pp. 559–564, 2001.

[6] J. Alsac, C. K. Zarins, M. A. Heikkinen et al., "The impact of aortic endografts on renal function," *Journal of Vascular Surgery*, vol. 41, no. 6, pp. 926–930, 2005.

[7] N. N. Moore, M. Lapsley, A. G. Norden et al., "Does N-acetylcysteine prevent contrast-induced nephropathy during endovascular AAA repair? A randomized controlled pilot study," *Journal of Endovascular Therapy*, vol. 13, no. 5, pp. 660–666, 2006.

[8] C. M. Erley, "Does hydration prevent radiocontrast-induced acute renal failure?" *Nephrology Dialysis Transplantation*, vol. 14, no. 5, pp. 1064–1066, 1999.

[9] C. Mueller, G. Buerkle, H. J. Buettner et al., "Prevention of contrast media-associated nephropathy: randomized comparison of 2 hydration regimens in 1620 patients undergoing coronary angioplasty," *Archives of Internal Medicine*, vol. 162, no. 3, pp. 329–336, 2002.

[10] H. S. Trivedi, H. Moore, S. Nasr et al., "A randomized prospective trial to assess the role of saline hydration on the development of contrast nephrotoxicity," *Nephron Clinical Practice*, vol. 93, no. 1, pp. C29–34, 2003.

[11] B. D. Bader, E. D. Berger, M. B. Heede et al., "What is the best hydration regimen to prevent contrast media-induced nephrotoxicity?" *Clinical Nephrology*, vol. 62, no. 1, pp. 1–7, 2004.

[12] S. Holt, "Radiocontrast media-induced renal injury: saline is effective in prevention," *Nephron Clinical Practice*, vol. 93, no. 1, pp. 5–6, 2003.

[13] C. Mueller, "Prevention of contrast-induced nephropathy with volume supplementation," *Kidney International*, no. 100, pp. S16–19, 2006.

[14] D. A. Gonzales, K. J. Norsworthy, S. J. Kern et al., "A meta-analysis of N-acetylcysteine in contrast-induced nephrotoxicity: unsupervised clustering to resolve heterogeneity," *BMC Medicine*, vol. 5, article 32, 2007.

[15] H. Trivedi, S. Daram, A. Szabo, A. L. Bartorelli, and G. Marenzi, "High-dose N-acetylcysteine for the Prevention of Contrast-induced Nephropathy," *The American Journal of Medicine*, vol. 122, no. 9, pp. 874–915, 2009.

[16] C. Briguori, A. Colombo, A. Violante et al., "Standard vs double dose of N-acetylcysteine to prevent contrast agent associated nephrotoxicity," *European Heart Journal*, vol. 25, no. 3, pp. 206–211, 2004.

[17] C. S. R. Baker, A. Wragg, S. Kumar, R. De Palma, L. R. I. Baker, and C. J. Knight, "A rapid protocol for the prevention of contrast-induced renal dysfunction: the RAPPID study," *Journal of the American College of Cardiology*, vol. 41, no. 12, pp. 2114–2118, 2003.

[18] A. M. Kelly, B. Dwamena, P. Cronin, S. J. Bernstein, and R. C. Carlos, "Meta-analysis: effectiveness of drugs for preventing contrast-induced nephropathy," *Annals of Internal Medicine*, vol. 148, no. 4, pp. 284–294, 2008.

[19] S. D. Weisbord and P. M. Palevsky, "Strategies for the prevention of contrast-induced acute kidney injury," *Current Opinion in Nephrology and Hypertension*, vol. 19, no. 6, pp. 539–549, 2010.

[20] G. J. Merten, W. P. Burgess, L. V. Gray et al., "Prevention of contrast-induced nephropathy with sodium bicarbonate: a randomized controlled trial," *Journal of the American Medical Association*, vol. 291, no. 19, pp. 2328–2334, 2004.

[21] C. Briguori, F. Airoldi, D. D'Andrea et al., "Renal insufficiency following contrast media administration trial (REMEDIAL): a randomized comparison of 3 preventive strategies," *Circulation*, vol. 115, pp. 1211–1217, 2007.

[22] H. Ueda, T. Yamada, M. Masuda et al., "Prevention of contrast-induced nephropathy by bolus injection of sodium bicarbonate in patients with chronic kidney disease undergoing emergent coronary procedures," *The American Journal of Cardiology*, vol. 107, no. 8, pp. 1163–1167, 2011.

[23] M. Motohiro, H. Kamihata, S. Tsujimoto et al., "A new protocol using sodium bicarbonate for the prevention of contrast-induced nephropathy in patients undergoing coronary angiography," *The American Journal of Cardiology*, vol. 107, no. 11, pp. 1604–1608, 2011.

[24] M. Pakfetrat, M. H. Nikoo, L. Malekmakan et al., "A comparison of sodium bicarbonate infusion versus normal saline infusion and its combination with oral acetazolamide for prevention of contrast-induced nephropathy: a randomized, double-blind trial," *International Urology and Nephrology*, vol. 41, no. 3, pp. 629–634, 2009.

[25] S. S. Brar, A. Y. Shen, M. B. Jorgensen et al., "Sodium bicarbonate vs sodium chloride for the prevention of contrast medium-induced nephropathy in patients undergoing coronary angiography: a randomized trial," *Journal of the American Medical Association*, vol. 300, no. 9, pp. 1038–1046, 2008.

[26] E. Adolph, B. Holdt-Lehmann, T. Chatterjee et al., "Renal insufficiency following radiocontrast exposure trial (REINFORCE): a randomized comparison of sodium bicarbonate versus sodium chloride hydration for the prevention of contrast-induced nephropathy," *Coronary Artery Disease*, vol. 19, no. 6, pp. 413–419, 2008.

[27] A. Vasheghani-Farahani, G. Sadigh, S. E. Kassaian et al., "Sodium bicarbonate plus isotonic saline versus saline for prevention of contrast-induced nephropathy in patients undergoing coronary angiography: a randomized controlled trial," *The American Journal of Kidney Diseases*, vol. 54, no. 4, pp. 610–618, 2009.

[28] S. Zoungas, T. Ninomiya, R. Huxley et al., "Systematic review: sodium bicarbonate treatment regimens for the prevention of contrast-induced nephropathy," *Annals of Internal Medicine*, vol. 151, no. 9, pp. 631–638, 2009.

[29] V. Kunadian, A. Zaman, I. Spyridopoulos, and W. Qiu, "Sodium bicarbonate for the prevention of contrast induced nephropathy: a meta-analysis of published clinical trials," *European Journal of Radiology*, vol. 79, no. 1, pp. 48–55, 2011.

[30] S. S. Soni, C. Ronco, N. Katz, and D. N. Cruz, "Early diagnosis of acute kidney injury: the promise of novel biomarkers," *Blood Purification*, vol. 28, no. 3, pp. 165–174, 2009.

[31] J. Mishra, M. A. Qing, A. Prada et al., "Identification of neutrophil gelatinase-associated lipocalin as a novel early urinary biomarker for ischemic renal injury," *Journal of the American Society of Nephrology*, vol. 14, no. 10, pp. 2534–2543, 2003.

[32] R. Hirsch, C. Dent, H. Pfriem et al., "NGAL is an early predictive biomarker of contrast-induced nephropathy in children," *Pediatric Nephrology*, vol. 22, no. 12, pp. 2089–2095, 2007.

[33] W. Ling, N. Zhaohui, H. Ben et al., "Urinary IL-18 and NGAL as early predictive biomarkers in contrast-induced nephropathy after coronary angiography," *Nephron Clinical Practice*, vol. 108, no. 3, pp. c176–c181, 2008.

[34] D. N. Cruz, C. Y. Goh, A. Haase-Fielitz, C. Ronco, and M. Haase, "Early biomarkers of renal injury," *Congestive Heart Failure*, vol. 16, no. 1, pp. S25–S31, 2010.

[35] J. Malyszko, H. Bachorzewska-Gajewska, B. Poniatowski, J. S. Malyszko, and S. Dobrzycki, "Urinary and serum biomarkers after cardiac catheterization in diabetic patients with stable angina and without severe chronic kidney disease," *Renal Failure*, vol. 31, no. 10, pp. 910–919, 2009.

[36] K. Sethi and L. H. Diamond, "Aminoglycoside nephrotoxicity and its predictability," *Nephron*, vol. 27, no. 4-5, pp. 265–270, 1981.

[37] G. Roche, B. Brugerolle, J. Straczek et al., "Value of the assay of 4 urinary enzyme activities in the diagnosis of the infectious or toxic (aminoglycosides) origin of a renal disease," *La Revue De MéDecine Interne*, vol. 4, pp. 327–334, 1983.

[38] H. G. Hartmann, H. E. Braedel, and G. A. Jutzler, "Detection of renal tubular lesions after abdominal aortography and selective renal arteriography by quantitative measurements of brush-border enzymes in the urine," *Nephron*, vol. 39, no. 2, pp. 95–101, 1985.

[39] J. Wethuyzen et al., "Urinary protein excretion following coronary angiography using a non-toxic radiocontrast agent," *Annals of Clinical Biochemistry*, vol. 33, pp. 349–351, 1996.

[40] R. L. Mehta, J. A. Kellum, S. V. Shah et al., "Acute Kidney Injury Network: report of an initiative to improve outcomes in acute kidney injury," *Critical Care*, vol. 11, no. 2, article R31, 2007.

[41] R. Mehran, E. D. Aymong, E. Nikolsky et al., "A simple risk score for prediction of contrast-induced nephropathy after percutaneous coronary intervention: development and initial validation," *Journal of the American College of Cardiology*, vol. 44, no. 7, pp. 1393–1399, 2004.

[42] P. Meier, D. T. Ko, A. Tamura, U. Tamhane, and H. S. Gurm, "Sodium bicarbonate-based hydration prevents contrast-induced nephropathy: a meta-analysis," *BMC Medicine*, vol. 7, article 23, 2009.

[43] M. Maioli, A. Toso, M. Leoncini et al., "Sodium bicarbonate versus saline for the prevention of contrast-induced nephropathy in patients with renal dysfunction undergoing Coronary angiography or intervention," *Journal of the American College of Cardiology*, vol. 52, no. 8, pp. 599–604, 2008.

# Arterial Blood Gas Analysis and the Outcome of Treatment in Tricyclic Antidepressants Poisoned Patients with Benzodiazepine Coingestion

**Ahmad Yaraghi,[1] Nastaran Eizadi-Mood,[2] Maryam Katani,[3] Shadi Farsaei,[4] Mahrang Hedaiaty,[3] Seyyed Mohammad Mahdy Mirhosseini,[3] Elham Beheshtian,[3] and Ali Mohammad Sabzghabaee[2]**

[1]*Department of Anesthesiology and Critical Care, School of Medicine, Isfahan University of Medical Sciences, Isfahan, Iran*
[2]*Isfahan Clinical Toxicology Research Center, Isfahan University of Medical Sciences, Isfahan, Iran*
[3]*Department of Clinical Toxicology, Noor and Ali Asghar (PBUH) University Hospital, Isfahan University of Medical Sciences, Isfahan, Iran*
[4]*Department of Clinical Pharmacy and Pharmacy Practice, School of Pharmacy and Pharmaceutical Sciences, Isfahan University of Medical Sciences, Isfahan, Iran*

Correspondence should be addressed to Ali Mohammad Sabzghabaee; sabzghaba@pharm.mui.ac.ir

Academic Editor: Uwe Rudolph

*Background.* Poisoning with tricyclic antidepressants (TCAs) is still a major concern for emergency physicians and intensivists. Concomitant ingestion of other psychoactive drugs especially benzodiazepines with TCAs may make this clinical situation more complex. This study aimed to compare the arterial blood gas (ABG) values and the outcome of treatment in patients with coingestion of TCA and benzodiazepine (TCA + BZD) poisoning and TCA poisoning alone. *Methods.* In this cross-sectional study which was carried out in a tertiary care university hospital in Iran, clinical and paraclinical characteristics of one hundred forty TCA only or TCA + BZD poisoned patients (aged 18–40 years) were evaluated. ABG analysis was done on admission in both groups. Outcomes were considered as survival with or without complication (e.g., intubation) and the frequency of TCA poisoning complications. *Results.* Arterial pH was significantly lower in TCA + BZD poisoning group compared with TCA only poisoning group ($7.34 \pm 0.08$ and $7.38 \pm 0.08$, resp.; $P = 0.02$). However, other complications such as seizure, and the need for the endotracheal intubation were not significantly different. All patients in both groups survived. *Conclusions.* Concomitant TCA plus BZD poisoning may make the poisoned patients prone to a lower arterial pH level on hospital admission which may potentially increases the risk of cardiovascular complications in TCA poisoning.

## 1. Introduction

Tricyclic antidepressant (TCA) overdose necessitating intensive care remains a major problem and an important critical cause of death due to poisoning around the world [1, 2]. Although new generation of antidepressants is introduced to the market with higher safety profile, physicians in many parts of the world including the Middle East still prescribe older antidepressant drugs including TCAs frequently. These agents have a narrow therapeutic index and regarding the mental condition of patients who take them, an increased prevalence of intentional and accidental overdoses is anticipated [3]. Unfortunately, these drugs alone or in concomitant with other agents including benzodiazepines (BZDs) have been abused for suicidal attempts [4].

Major complications of TCA poisoning involve cardiovascular and central nervous system (CNS) [5, 6]. The main theoretical mechanism of TCAs' cardiovascular toxicity is the inhibition of rapid sodium channels and an effective and practically used treatment for this condition is the administration of sodium bicarbonate [7]. With the rising of TCA poisoning, coingestion of BZDs with TCAs also became more prevalent in recent years, and in practice BZDs were reported to be the most common drugs accompanying cases of TCA overdose in Iran [8]. Coingestion of drugs could lead to different effects on severity and type of the complications, as well as the drug toxicokinetics and metabolism [9, 10]. In a previous study on overdosed patients coingested TCA plus BZD, it was observed that the cardiovascular complications and seizure were seen with less frequency in TCA-alone poisoned cases [10]. This study aimed to compare the arterial blood gas (ABG) values and hemodynamic parameters in patients with coingestion of TCA and benzodiazepine (TCA + BZD) poisoning and TCA poisoning alone. Moreover, patients' outcomes and complications in both groups were also evaluated and compared. To the best of our knowledge, there is not any similar report in the available medical literature.

## 2. Materials and Methods

This cross-sectional study was conducted in Noor and Ali Asghar (PBUH) University Hospital affiliated with Isfahan University of Medical Sciences during 2012-2013. This center which is the major referral medical center for poisoning emergencies for the central part of Iran is facilitated, staffed, and designed for the management of poisoned patients and approximately 400 poisoned patients are admitted to it monthly.

The target population for this study was defined as all symptomatic patients with intentional poisoning in the age range of 18–40 years, having solely TCA poisoning or concomitant coingestion of TCA plus BZD poisoning (TCA + BZD) and without a history of using any other drug in the past two weeks. Patients with a history or underlying disease of cardiovascular, kidney, liver, and chronic obstructive pulmonary diseases and those who had been receiving sodium bicarbonate in another health care center prior to the admission to our center were excluded. Discharge and death of patients before study were also considered as exclusion criteria.

The study protocol was approved by the institutional board of human studies at Isfahan University of Medical Sciences. In addition, after the study was accurately explained to each patient, informed consent was taken from them before their recruitment to this study. If the patient was not able or did not have the capacity for decision making, informed consent for inclusion to this study was taken from the patients' first degree family.

The sample size was estimated for a study power of 80% and a type I error of 5% and also by considering the mean clinically estimated effect size of TCA on ECG and ABG indices. In this regard, the sample size for each group was determined as 70 (total needed number of patients = 140).

On admission of each patient, a careful history was taken and physical examination was performed by a medical toxicologist. Moreover, ABG analysis and ECG were performed at the same time.

All patients underwent continuous heart and $O_2$ saturation monitoring during the time period of hospitalization. Any new complication which was developed during monitoring was recorded. Evaluation of cardiovascular symptoms was carried out according to the physical examination findings including vital signs (blood pressure, heart rate, and respiratory rate) and ECG. Moreover, central nervous system manifestations were evaluated according to neurological examinations and the consciousness level. Finally, outcomes were considered as the percent of survival with or without complication (intubation and mechanical ventilation) and cardiovascular or CNS problems regarding TCA poisoning.

For descriptive analysis of the data, continuous variables were expressed as mean ± SD and categorical data as percentage. Kolmogorov-Smirnov test was carried out to assess the normal distribution of continuous variables. Independent Student's $t$-test, chi-square test, and Fisher's exact test were used for statistical analysis of the results. Data processing was performed by SPSS statistical software (SPSS Inc., Chicago, IL, USA) version 20 and a two-tailed $P$ value less than 0.05 was considered to establish significance for all statistical tests.

## 3. Results

One hundred forty patients with intentional poisoning by oral ingestion of tablets were studied completely in two groups: TCA poisoning and concomitant ingestion of TCA plus BZD. Each group consisted of 70 patients and the estimated time that elapsed from their poison ingestion was not more than 6 hours. The distribution of gender was different between the two groups (Table 1). Whereas most of the patients were females in TCA group (58.6%), the number of males was higher in the TCA + BZD group ($P = 0.04$). The patients' mean age was not significantly different between groups (26.04 ± 7.6 and 28.97 ± 11.1 years in TCA and TCA + BZD groups, resp.; $P = 0.07$). Amitriptyline and nortriptyline were the most frequently abused drugs in both groups and diazepam and alprazolam were also the most frequently abused benzodiazepines in TCA + BZD group.

Levels of consciousness (awareness, confusion, stupor, and coma) were not significantly different in both groups at the time of admission ($P = 0.3$). Some patients experienced aspiration pneumonia but the groups were not significantly different in this regard ($P = 0.17$) (Table 2).

Comparing the cardiovascular indices obtained from the ECG on admission, the width of QRS complex was not significantly different in the two groups ($P = 0.67$). Statistical significance of the difference between the QT intervals of the patients in two groups was at the borderline ($P = 0.05$).

In addition, according to the pH value in the ABG analysis on admission, the mean pH level in patients with TCA poisoning was significantly higher than that in the patients with concomitant TCA plus BZD poisoning ($P = 0.02$) (Table 3). However, the need for endotracheal intubation was not significantly different in this respect ($P = 0.8$) and about 25% of patients in each group needed intubation. All patients in both groups were survived.

## 4. Discussion

Severe TCA poisoning is an important cause of death among the patients in poisoning emergency rooms around the world

Table 1: Demographic data of the studied patients in TCA only and TCA plus benzodiazepine ingestion groups.

| | TCA ($n = 70$) | TCA + BZD ($n = 70$) | $P$ value |
|---|---|---|---|
| Gender | | | |
| Male | 29 | 41 | 0.04* |
| Female | 41 | 29 | |
| Age (years) | 26.04 ± 7.6 | 28.97 ± 11.1 | 0.07** |
| Frequency and type of the abused TCA | | | |
| Amitriptyline | 25 | 31 | 0.058* |
| Nortriptyline | 29 | 25 | |
| Imipramine | 7 | 8 | |
| Clomipramine | 9 | 6 | |
| Smoking status | | | |
| Smokers | 17 | 22 | 0.34* |
| Nonsmokers | 53 | 48 | |
| Estimated TCA ingested amount (mg)*** | | | |
| <500 | 21 | 17 | 0.40* |
| 500–1000 | 30 | 38 | |
| >1000 | 19 | 15 | |

*Chi-square test; **independent $t$-test; ***according to patients' history; TCA: tricyclic antidepressant; BZD: benzodiazepine; results are presented as number of patients or mean ± SD where appropriate.

Table 2: Neurological, cardiovascular, and pulmonary characteristics of the studied patients at the time of admission and during hospitalization.

| Variables | TCA ($n = 70$) | TCA + BZD ($n = 70$) | $P$ value |
|---|---|---|---|
| Delirium | | | |
| Present | 23 (33) | 18 (26) | 0.11* |
| Absent | 47 (67) | 52 (74) | |
| Level of consciousness | | | |
| Alert | 11 (15.7) | 5 (7.1) | 0.30* |
| Lethargic | 35 (50) | 35 (50) | |
| Stupor | 12 (17.1) | 18 (25.7) | |
| Coma | 12 (17.1) | 12 (17.1) | |
| Seizure | | | |
| Present | 6 (8.6) | 8 (10.1) | 0.70* |
| Absent | 64 (91.4) | 62 (89.9) | |
| Cardiovascular variables | | | |
| Systolic blood pressure (mmHg) | 107.8 ± 17.4 | 111.6 ± 21.2 | 0.45** |
| Diastolic blood pressure (mmHg) | 71.4 ± 12.5 | 72 ± 12.9 | 0.97** |
| Pulse rate (/min) | 91.5 ± 25.9 | 86.7 ± 22.6 | 0.13** |
| QRS duration (msec) | 0.073 ± 0.02 | 0.072 ± 0.02 | 0.67** |
| QT interval (msec) | 0.35 ± 0.05 | 0.37 ± 0.06 | 0.05** |
| PR interval (msec) | 0.19 ± 0.03 | 0.19 ± 0.04 | 0.53** |
| Respiratory rate (/min) | 18.7 (8.9) | 17.9 (4.05) | 0.51** |
| Endotracheal intubation | | | |
| Performed | 17 (24.3) | 18 (25.7) | 0.08* |
| Not needed | 53 (75.7) | 52 (74.3) | |
| Aspiration pneumonia | | | |
| Occurred | 5 (7.4) | 10 (14.8) | 0.17* |
| Did not occur | 63 (92.6) | 58 (85.2) | |

*Chi-square test; **independent $t$-test; TCA, tricyclic antidepressant; BZD, benzodiazepine; data presented as number of patients (%) or mean ± SD where appropriate.

TABLE 3: Arterial blood gas values of the studied patients at the time of hospital admission.

| Variable | TCA ($n$ = 70) | TCA + BZD ($n$ = 70) | $P$ value* |
|---|---|---|---|
| pH | 7.38 ± 0.08 | 7.34 ± 0.08 | 0.02 |
| $O_2$ saturation | 73.62 ± 30.13 | 71.00 ± 35.88 | 0.1 |
| $P_aCO_2$ | 45.35 ± 6.04 | 39.00 ± 9.80 | 0.2 |
| $HCO_3^-$ | 22.39 ± 4.67 | 22.03 ± 7.27 | 0.5 |
| Base excess | 4.8 ± 1.26 | 8.25 ± 0.94 | 0.1 |

*Independent $t$-test; TCA: tricyclic antidepressant; BZD: benzodiazepine; data presented as mean± SD; $P_aCO_2$: arterial carbon dioxide pressure.

and also in our tertiary care poisoning medical center in Iran [11, 12]. Some factors that may underscore the reason of high mortality rate in TCA poisoning are easy availability of the drug for the depressed patients who are susceptible for suicide attempt and the severity of cardiovascular and CNS complications caused by these medications [13].

In the current study, arterial blood gas (ABG) parameters and TCA complications in patients with concomitant TCA and benzodiazepine (TCA + BZD) poisoning and TCA poisoning alone were measured and compared.

Liver cytochrome p450 iso-enzymes are responsible for TCA metabolism and its activity is age dependent. Therefore, patients' ages may have some effects on TCAs' levels and subsequently the manifestations of complications after poisoning [14]. However, in our study patients were not significantly different in terms of the average age (between groups) and age may not be a possible source of bias.

Our results showed that the decrease in consciousness level and seizures were not significantly different in the two groups. These results are somewhat different from similar recently published study which declared that seizure may be less in TCA plus BZD poisoned patients compared with patients intoxicated with TCA alone. BZDs have been used for controlling seizure caused by TCAs. Therefore, lower rate of seizure in previous study may be due to the higher amounts of BZD ingested and lower doses of ingested TCA [10]. It should be mentioned that the amounts of coingested BZDs were not reported in our previous study and also are not available for the current study to compare with each other. So, another clinical study is needed to evaluate the effect of BZDs' doses on the rate of TCAs induced seizure.

Moreover, because acidosis was somewhat compensated and the levels of consciousness were not significantly different in both groups, it was expected that the percent of patients who needed mechanical ventilation was nearly similar in both groups. Our results also show that the amount of coingested BZDs may not be sufficient enough to decrease the level of consciousness in patients with TCA poisoning which could justify the similar rate of seizure between both groups discussed above.

In the current study, vital signs and ECG indices in both groups were not significantly different on admission except for QT interval which is reported at the border line of statistical significance ($P$ = 0.05). The mechanism of cardiovascular toxicity caused by TCAs may be attributed to the rapid $Na^+$ channel blockade and slowing phase 0 of depolarization and impulse conduction in bundle of Hiss, the Purkinje fibers, and ventricular myocardium [15]. Moreover, rapid $Na^+$ channel blockade in heart is sensitive to arterial blood pH, and in this condition acidosis aggravates cardiovascular toxicity in TCA poisoning [10]. In our study according to the reported pH values in the ABG analysis of the patients on admission, the mean pH level in patients with TCA plus BZD poisoning was significantly lower than that in patients with TCA poisoning. This may justify the borderline statistical difference of the prolonged QT interval in patients with TCA plus BZD poisoning. Also, as blood pH value of the patients was increased, the cardiovascular complications and ECG changes appeared to be corrected [16].

Our study had some limitations. First of all, if we could have confirmatory serum levels of TCAs or at least a qualitative screening test in our patients, this could increase the reliability of our results. Secondly, we had samplings from one referral hospital and although this sampling was done in a systematic way it may lead to some concerns for the extrapolation of results. We also relied on the data provided by the patients or close relatives for the past medical history or concomitant drug use. This may have caused recall bias and is not in favor of reliability of our analysis but here in Isfahan we have not a comprehensive national medical recording system to confirm the medical and drug history of patients. Further investigations with confirmatory and screening measurement of TCA serum level and with a more diverse method of multicenter sampling of patients are recommended.

## 5. Conclusion

In conclusion, patients with concomitant TCA plus BZD poisoning may present with a lower pH level on admission and more blood acidity. Since the blood acidity may potentially increase the risk of cardiovascular complications in TCA poisoning, emergency physicians and the intensivists should be aware of these risks and conduct the prompt appropriate intervention for patient management.

## Conflict of Interests

The authors declare that there is no conflict of interest regarding the publication of this paper.

## Authors' Contribution

Ahmad Yaraghi, Nastaran Eizadi-Mood, and Ali Mohammad Sabzghabaee contributed in designing and conducting the study. Maryam Katani collected the data. Mahrang Hedaiaty, Seyyed Mohammad Mahdy Mirhosseini, and Elham Beheshtian helped in data analysis. Shadi Farsaei rechecked the statistical analysis and prepared the paper. All authors have assisted in preparation of the paper and have read and approved the content of the paper and are accountable for all aspects of the work.

## Acknowledgments

This study is the result of a Doctor of Medicine thesis project which was financially supported by the Vice Chancellery for Research and Technology of the Isfahan University of Medical Sciences. The authors would like to thank Dr. Farzad Gheshlaghi (forensic toxicologist) and Dr. Gholamreza Massoumi (anesthesiologist) for their kind cooperation during the study period. All of the personnel of the Emergency Department of Noor and Ali-Asghar (PBUH) University Hospital are also appreciated for their sincere help and support.

## References

[1] R. A. Mandour, "Antidepressants medications and the relative risk of suicide attempt," *Toxicology International*, vol. 19, no. 1, pp. 42–46, 2012.

[2] C. F. N. Koegelenberg, Z. J. Joubert, and E. M. Irusen, "Tricyclic antidepressant overdose necessitating ICU admission," *South African Medical Journal*, vol. 102, no. 5, pp. 293–294, 2012.

[3] E. Eliasson, J. D. Lindh, R. E. Malmström, O. Beck, and M.-L. Dahl, "Therapeutic drug monitoring for tomorrow," *European Journal of Clinical Pharmacology*, vol. 69, pp. 25–32, 2013.

[4] S. P. Kurtz, H. L. Surratt, M. A. Levi-Minzi, and A. Mooss, "Benzodiazepine dependence among multidrug users in the club scene," *Drug and Alcohol Dependence*, vol. 119, no. 1-2, pp. 99–105, 2011.

[5] B. S. Judge and L. L. Rentmeester, "Antidepressant overdose-induced Seizures," *Psychiatric Clinics of North America*, vol. 36, no. 2, pp. 245–260, 2013.

[6] F. Gheshlaghi, M. Mehrizi, A. Yaraghi, A. Sabzghabaee, F. Soltaninejad, and N. Eizadi-Mood, "ST-T segment changes in patients with tricyclic antidepressant poisoning," *Journal of Research in Pharmacy Practice*, vol. 2, no. 3, pp. 110–113, 2013.

[7] D. Müller and H. Desel, "Common causes of poisoning: etiology, diagnosis and treatment," *Deutsches Arzteblatt International*, vol. 110, no. 41, pp. 690–699, 2013.

[8] M. Islambulchilar, Z. Islambulchilar, and M. H. Kargar-Maher, "Acute adult poisoning cases admitted to a university hospital in Tabriz, Iran," *Human & Experimental Toxicology*, vol. 28, no. 4, pp. 185–190, 2009.

[9] S. M. R. Wille, S. G. Cooreman, H. M. Neels, and W. E. E. Lambert, "Relevant issues in the monitoring and the toxicology of antidepressants," *Critical Reviews in Clinical Laboratory Sciences*, vol. 45, no. 1, pp. 25–89, 2008.

[10] N. Eizadi-Mood, A. M. Sabzghabaee, M. Saghaei, F. Gheshlaghi, and B. Mohammad-Ebrahimi, "Benzodiazepines co-ingestion in reducing tricyclic antidepressant toxicity," *Medicinski Arhiv*, vol. 66, no. 1, pp. 49–52, 2012.

[11] T. M. Bosch, T. S. van der Werf, D. R. A. Uges et al., "Antidepressants self-poisoning and ICU admissions in a university hospital in The Netherlands," *Pharmacy World and Science*, vol. 22, no. 3, pp. 92–95, 2000.

[12] S. Dianat, M.-R. Zarei, H. Hassanian-Moghaddam, N. Rashidi-Ranjbar, R. Rahimian, and M. R. Rasouli, "Tricyclic antidepressants intoxication in Tehran, Iran: epidemiology and associated factors," *Human & Experimental Toxicology*, vol. 30, no. 4, pp. 283–288, 2011.

[13] K. Hawton, H. Bergen, S. Simkin et al., "Toxicity of antidepressants: rates of suicide relative to prescribing and non-fatal overdose," *British Journal of Psychiatry*, vol. 196, no. 5, pp. 354–358, 2010.

[14] S. F. Manzi and M. Shannon, "Drug interactions—a review," *Clinical Pediatric Emergency Medicine*, vol. 6, no. 2, pp. 93–102, 2005.

[15] A. Nada, G. A. Gintant, R. Kleiman et al., "The evaluation and management of drug effects on cardiac conduction (PR and QRS Intervals) in clinical development," *American Heart Journal*, vol. 165, no. 4, pp. 489–500, 2013.

[16] R. Body, T. Bartram, F. Azam, and K. Mackway-Jones, "Guidelines in Emergency Medicine Network (GEMNet): guideline for the management of tricyclic antidepressant overdose," *Emergency Medicine Journal*, vol. 28, no. 4, pp. 347–368, 2011.

# Lasting Developmental Effects of Neonatal Fentanyl Exposure in Preweanling Rats

**Dora Catré,[1,2] Maria Francelina Lopes,[1,3] and António Silvério Cabrita[1]**

[1] *Faculty of Medicine, University of Coimbra, 3004-504 Coimbra, Portugal*
[2] *Department of Anesthesiology, São Teotónio Hospital, EPE, 3504-509 Viseu, Portugal*
[3] *Pediatric Surgery Department, Pediatric Hospital, Centro Hospitalar e Universitário de Coimbra, EPE, 3000-602 Coimbra, Portugal*

Correspondence should be addressed to Maria Francelina Lopes, mfrancelina@yahoo.com

Academic Editor: Andrea Trescot

The present study aimed to determine whether neonatal treatment with fentanyl has lasting effects on stressed developing brain. Six-day-old rats were assigned to one of three groups (10 males/group): (1) fentanyl (incision+fentanyl), (2) saline (incision+0.9% saline), and (3) unoperated (unoperated sham). Pups with a plantar paw incision received repetitive subcutaneous injections of fentanyl or vehicle through postnatal days (PNDs) 6 to 8. A nonoperated sham group served as nonstressed control. Studies included assessment of development from PND 6 to PND 21 (growth indices and behavioral testing). Fentanyl administered twice daily for three days after surgical incision had no impact on early growth and development, as measured on PND 9, but showed a lasting impact on later growth, enhanced behavioral development, and lower anxiety, as measured through PNDs 10–21. While this does not completely support a benefit from such treatment, our findings may contribute to support the neonatal use of fentanyl, when indicated, even in premature newborns.

## 1. Introduction

Fentanyl, a potent $\mu$-opioid agonist, is a synthetic drug that has been widely used for pain management [1, 2] and as a general anesthetic for surgical procedures in pediatrics [3–5], namely in surgical neonatal intensive care units. In a previous study, fentanyl was identified as being within the 5 medications with the highest exposure rates in a pediatric intensive care unit [2].

Fentanyl is an appropriate medication that has rarely been linked to significant adverse effects on the central nervous system (CNS) or other systems, with proper monitoring [6]. However, concerning fentanyl use in pediatric critical care population, this is one of the many medications which are not properly tested for pediatric use [2].

It is well documented in clinics [7] and in experimental work [8, 9] that gradual increases of standard doses of fentanyl [7], illicit fentanyl abuse [10], drug interactions [11], or individual susceptibility may lead to severe neurotoxicity and death [10]. Animal studies have also reported adverse effects. Kofke et al. [8] evaluated the neuropathological effects of fentanyl in the brain and showed that it produces limbic system brain damage in rats and that the damage occurs over a broad range of doses. In another study, regarding fentanyl effects in rat brain ischemia, Kofke et al. [9] showed that fentanyl, in both high and low doses, can exacerbate incomplete forebrain ischemia in rats. Additionally, it is well known from the literature that large-dose opioids in rats produce hippocampal hypermetabolism, epileptiform activity, and neuropathologic lesions [12]. These doses in rats are comparable in potency to a large-dose regimen that might be used in humans [12].

The neonatal period is a time of rapid growth and development of the brain, and perturbations to the normal series of developmental events during this time can lead to adverse functional consequences that manifest later in life. Lack of data on the impact of fentanyl's repeated use during this vulnerable period of brain development raises special concern, as is well known that the developing CNS of the neonate is recognized as very sensitive to most anesthetics, in animal research studies.

Our study's primary goal was to further investigate the possibility that repeated administration of this opiate, in a window of developmental susceptibility, could have lasting impact on neurodevelopment. It was hypothesized that neonate rat pups, exposed to both postoperative and repetitive parenteral fentanyl, would show growth restriction and abnormal neurobehavioral functions. As postnatal growth and development are sensitive measures of central neurotoxicity and brain maturation, we assessed growth and development in the infant male rat after exposing a neonate rat model of postoperative pain to repeated administration of subcutaneous fentanyl during early postnatal life.

## 2. Materials and Methods

*2.1. Ethics Statement.* Animal protocols for this study were written in strict accordance with the recommendations in the European legislation and meet the standards of the National Institutes of Health, as set forth in the Guide for the Care and Use of Laboratory Animals [13]. These protocols were approved in advance by the Ethics Committee of the Faculty of Medicine of the University of Coimbra.

*2.2. Subjects.* For this experiment, the progeny (~12 per litter) of 9 multiparous Wistar rats (Charles River Laboratories, L'Arbresle Cedex, France) was used. Litters (3 per group) were assigned to the following groups: (1) fentanyl (incision + fentanyl, $n = 10$ males), (2) saline (incision + 0.9% saline control, $n = 10$ males), and (3) unoperated (unoperated sham control, $n = 10$ males). Lactating dams were maintained with their litters for 21 days, housed in polypropylene cages in a temperature-controlled environment (20–22°C) with a 12-hour light dark cycle and *ad libitum* access to water and pelleted rat chow.

*2.3. Procedures.* Figure 1 summarizes study tests and procedures timeframe.

Each litter was transferred together with the dam to a clean cage with fresh bedding on postnatal day 6 (PND 6). After baseline testing and weighing, rat pups received subcutaneously in the neck either the first dose of fentanyl (B|Braun Medical Lda. Barcarena, Portugal), 25 $\mu$g per kg body weight (0.1 mL per g weight of solution of fentanyl diluted to 0.25 $\mu$g/mL in 0.9% saline solution), or 0.9% saline solution, 0.1 mL per g body weight; this was immediately followed by creation of a deep plantar paw incision, as previously described [14]. Briefly, the plantar aspect of the right hindpaw was prepared in a sterile manner with a 10% povidone-iodine solution. Using a no. 11 surgical blade we performed a midline incision from the heel to the base of the toes under local anesthetic (ethyl chloride spray). The underlying flexor muscle was elevated and incised longitudinally. The skin incision was closed with nylon sutures (6/0). Equivalent subcutaneous doses of fentanyl, or 0.9% saline, were repeatedly given 8–12 hours apart from the first dose for three consecutive days, with a total of 6 doses (average total dose per animal: 135 $\mu$g/kg weight).

Any incidence of adverse effects (namely, respiratory depression) was recorded. Control sham animals underwent local anesthesia with skin preparation, but no incision.

On PND 9, at least eight hours after the last injection, assessment of growth and development was performed. Growth and physical development, such as teething, number of eyes open, was monitored daily through PND 6–21. The number of eyes open was scored; the observations for each item were coded as 0 (both eyes closed), 1 (1 eye open), and 2 (both eyes open).

Rats were assessed for motor and cognitive performance between postnatal days 18 and 21 through behavioral studies in the open-field, elevated plus maze, wire hanging maneuver, novel object recognition test of short-term memory and accelerating rotarod. Between test phases and animals, apparatus, and objects were thoroughly cleansed with 70% ethanol. Behavior experiments were recorded using a camera mounted above the testing apparatus and data were reviewed without knowledge of each rats' group.

Although every litter contained pups of both sexes, growth and behavioral results reported here include data collected only from males (10 per group).

Anesthetized rats were killed on PND 21.

*2.4. Early Outcome Assessment (Acute Effects of Fentanyl Exposure)*

*2.4.1. Righting Reflex.* This test took place on PND 6 (baseline information) and PND 9. It consists in the time in seconds required for a pup placed on its back to right itself (all 4 paws flat on the surface). The amount of time required for the pup to right itself on all 4 limbs was measured using a stopwatch, with a maximum of 30 seconds. This test, performed as previously described, assesses subcortical maturation [15].

*2.4.2. Negative Geotaxis.* This test took place on PND 6 (baseline information) and PND 9. It consists on the time in seconds required for a pup placed head down on a 25° incline to turn 180° and begin crawling up the slope. The cutoff time was 60 sec. The time spent for a turn of 180° upward was recorded using a stopwatch. If unsuccessful, each pup was given up to 3 trials. Each failed trial was recorded as value 61. Negative geotaxis, performed as previously described, is believed to test reflex development, motor skills and vestibular labyrinth, and cerebellar integration [15].

*2.4.3. Locomotor Activity.* This test took place on PND 6 (baseline information) and on PND 9, at least eight hours after the last fentanyl injection. Rat pups were individually placed in a circular hole (6 cm diameter/2 cm height), and locomotor activity was scored during 3 min as follows: 1: immobility and head down; 2: raises head up; 3: forepaws over borders; 4: climbs the borders.

*2.5. Later Outcomes Assessment*

*2.5.1. Behavior in the Open-Field Arena.* This test took place on PND 18 and was used with the aim of assessing locomotor activity. The test was performed as previously described [16], with slight modifications. Briefly, rats were placed

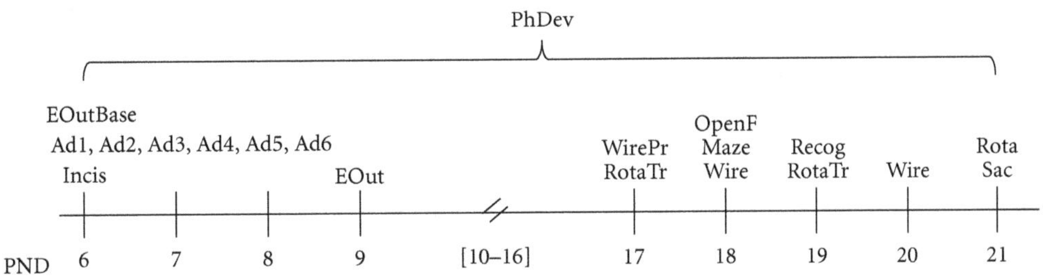


Figure 1: Study tests and procedures timeframe. PhDev: growth and physical development assessment (PND 6–21); EoutBase: baseline testing (righting reflex, negative geotaxis, and locomotor activity) (PND 6); EOut: early outcome assessment (PND 9); Adm: administration procedure, according to group (administration of fentanyl, administration of 0.9% saline solution, or manipulation) (PND 6–8); Incis: incision or manipulation, according to group (PND 6); WirePr: wire hanging maneuver pretest (PND 17); Wire: wire hanging maneuver test (PND 18 + 20); RotaTr: accelerating rotarod training (pretest) (PND 17 + 19); Rota: accelerating rotarod test (PND 21); OpenF: behavior in open-field arena (PND 18); Maze: elevated plus maze test (PND 18); Recog: novel object recognition test of short-term memory (PND 19); Sac: sacrifice (PND 21).

Table 1: Early outcomes.

| Measures | Groups | | | *P* |
|---|---|---|---|---|
| | Fentanyl | Saline | Unoperated | |
| Weight, mean (±SD), g: | | | | |
| PND 6 | 12 (±1) | 11 (±2) | 11 (±2) | >.05 |
| PND 9 | 18 (±2) | 16 (±3) | 16 (±2) | >.05 |
| Righting latency, median (IQR), sec: | | | | |
| PND 6 | 2 (1-2) | 2 (2-2) | 2 (2-2) | >.05 |
| PND 9 | 1 (1–1.3) | 1 (1-2) | 1 (1–1.3) | >.05 |
| Geotactic latency, median (IQR), sec: | | | | |
| PND 6 | 183 (152–183) | 29 (20–145) | 34 (12–48) | <.05* |
| PND 9 | 19 (13–27) | 23 (11–44) | 22 (12–48) | >.05 |
| Locomotor activity score, median (IQR): | | | | |
| PND 6 | 1 (1-2) | 2 (1–2.3) | 1 (1-2) | >.05 |
| PND 9 | 2 (1.8–3) | 3 (2-3) | 3 (2.8–3) | >.05 |

PND: postnatal day; IQR: interquartile range; *P*: significance for independent samples.
Locomotor activity scores: 1: immobility and head down; 2: raises head up; 3: forepaws over borders; 4: climbs the borders.
Fentanyl versus saline ($P = 0.005$) and fentanil versus unoperated ($P = 0.007$), both $^{*}P < .05$.

Table 2: Later Outcomes.

| Measures | Groups | | | *P* |
|---|---|---|---|---|
| | Fentanyl | Saline | Unoperated | |
| Weight PND 21, mean (±SD), g | 43 (±3)*§ | 36 (±6)* | 36 (±4)§ | *F versus S =.001; §F versus Un <.001; |
| Eye opening score, PND 14, median (IQR) | 2 (1-2) | 1 (0–2) | 0 (0–2) | NS |
| Open field, line crossing, mean (±SD) | 68 (±23) | 62 (±24) | 48 (±27) | NS |
| Latency time wire, median (IQR), sec: | | | | |
| PND 18 | 127 (20–183)* | 183 (183-183)* | 183 (162–183) | *F versus S =0.035 |
| PND 20 | 25 (15–98) | 75 (12–183) | 76 (9–183) | NS |
| Recognition index, mean (±SD) | 0.8 (±0.3)* | 0.6 ± (0.3)*§ | 0.8 (±0.2)§ | *F versus S =0.045; §Un versus S =0.025 |
| Time (%) spent open arms, median (IQR) | 18 (17–32)*§ | 7 (3–17)* | 10 (7–16)§ | *F versus S =0.034; §F versus Un =0.045 |
| Best latency time fall rod, mean (±SD), sec | 173 (±24)*§ | 123 (±73)* | 128 (±24)§ | *F versus S =0.022; §F versus Un =0.04 |

PND: postnatal day; IQR: interquartile range; *P*: significance for independent samples: NS: nonsignificant; F: Fentanyl; S: Saline; Un: Unoperated.

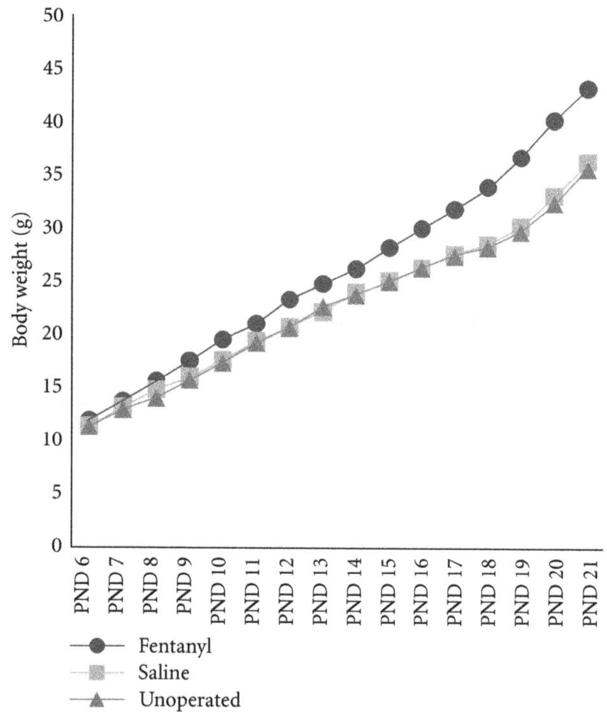


FIGURE 2: Growth curves representing mean body weight (g) through postnatal days (PNDs) 6–21. Fentanyl group showed enhanced weight gain compared to controls, after PND 12.

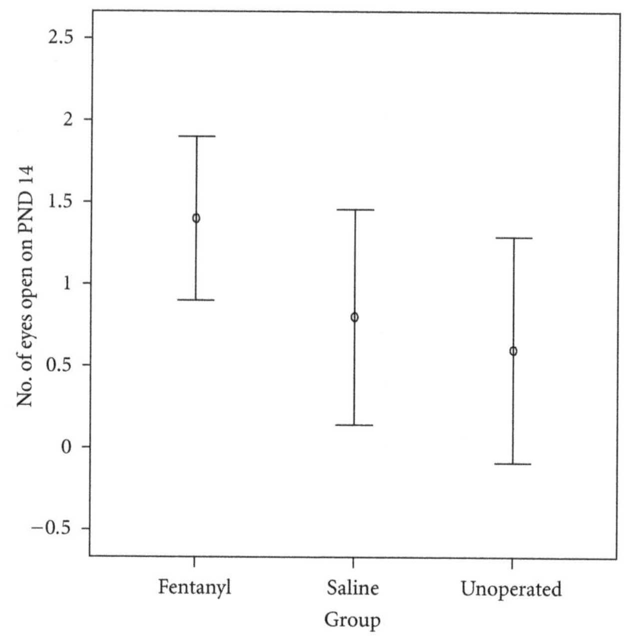


FIGURE 3: Number of eyes open on postnatal day (PND) 14. The number of eyes open was higher in the fentanyl group than in both the saline and unoperated groups ($P > 0.05$). Values represent mean and 95% confidence interval for mean.

individually in a transparent box (60 × 40 × 25 cm) with the floor divided into twelve identical areas in a dim room. Line crossings (with all four paws placed into an adjacent area) were recorded in a 5 min period.

In addition, the presence/absence of exploratory behaviors such as rearing (standing on hind legs), grooming (using paws or tongue to clean/scratch body), and corner-facing (standing or sitting with the face directed toward the corner of the box) was recorded.

*2.5.2. Anxiety-Like Behavior.* This test was performed on PND 18 to assess anxiety-like behavior as previously described [17], with slight modifications. Rats were placed in an elevated plus maze which consisted of a cross-shaped platform (height: 49.5 cm) with four arms (width: 10 cm; length: 110.5 cm), two of which were enclosed by walls 30.5 cm high. Each rat was placed into the central area facing an open arm and allowed to explore for 5 min. The percentage of time spent on the open arms and number of entries into the open arms were used as measures of anxiety-like behavior.

*2.5.3. Wire Hanging Maneuver.* Wire hanging maneuver assesses neuromuscular and locomotor development [16]. This test was conducted over 3 days (maneuvers performed on PNDs 18 and 20). Rats were allowed 1 pretest on PND 17. Normal pups suspended by the forelimbs from a horizontal wire supported between two platforms (15 cm above the table top) tend to support themselves with their hind limbs, preventing falling and aiding in progression along the wire to reach the platform [16]. A sponge at the base of the apparatus served as protection for the falling rats. Latency to reach one of the platforms from the wire was measured and recorded in seconds, with a cutoff time of 60 sec. Each unsuccessful trial was recorded as value 61, with a maximum of 3 trials allowed each day. Therefore, latency values may vary from 1 to 183 per test.

*2.5.4. Novel Object Recognition Test of Short-Term Memory.* This test, based on the natural tendency of rodents to investigate a novel object instead of a familiar one, was carried out as previously described [18]. On PND 19 each rat was allowed to move freely in an open-field box for 3 min, as habituation, followed by an exposition trial in which the rat was placed in the center of the box containing two identical objects (transparent white blocks) located in two adjacent corners. The cumulative time spent exploring each object was recorded during a 5 min period. Exploration was defined as actively touching or directly facing the object. One hour later the rats were tested for memory using the same procedure, except that one of the familiar objects was replaced with a novel different looking object. The time of exploration of each object ($t_n$ and $t_f$ for novel and familiar objects, resp.) was recorded for determination of the recognition index (RI): $\text{RI} = t_n/(t_n + t_f)$.

*2.5.5. Rotarod.* This test was performed as previously described [15], with slight modifications, to examine potential effects of fentanyl exposure on motor balance and coordination, using the accelerating rotarod (Rota Rod LI 8200; Letica

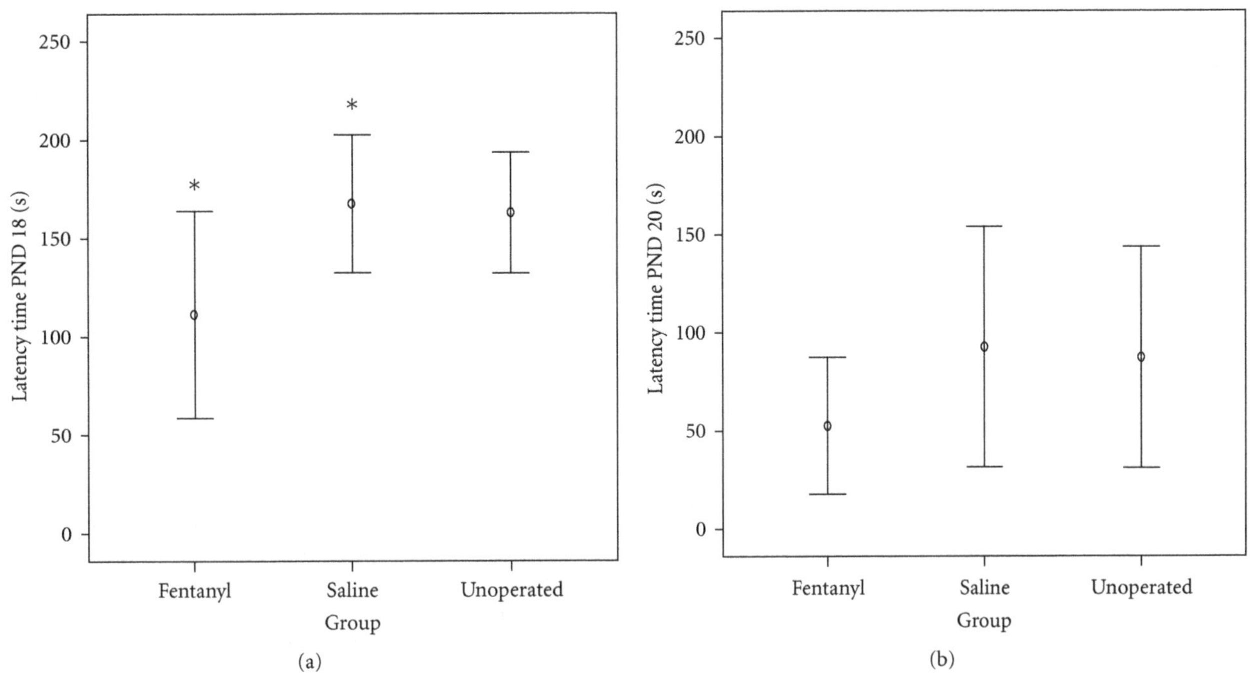


FIGURE 4: Latency times to complete the task of reaching the platform in the wire hanging maneuver on (a) postnatal day 18 and (b) postnatal day 20. Both on PND 18 and 20, rats in the fentanyl group were faster than controls, with statistical difference to the saline group ($*P = 0.035$) on PND 18. Values represent mean and 95% confidence interval for mean.

SA Scientific Instruments). The rotarod test was conducted over 3 days and consisted of 2 pretests which took place on PND 17 and 19 and a test performed on PND 21. In the 2 pretests, the rats underwent habituation and training, by placement on the still rod to acclimate, followed by training on the moving rotarod, beginning at a constant speed of 5–10–20 revolutions per minute (rpm) on a schedule of three 5-minute trials. This training was repeated under the same protocol on PND 19.

On PND 21 the rats were tested using the accelerating rotarod: the apparatus was set to accelerate linearly from 4 to 40 rpm over 300 seconds. The sessions consisted of three 5-minute trials. The latency to fall from the rotarod during a 300 sec trial was recorded. Each animal was given 3 trials, and the best latency of three trials was calculated for each animal.

*2.6. Statistics.* Statistical analysis was performed using SPSS statistical software package (version 17, SPSS, Inc., Chicago, Il). Normality of distribution was determined using Kolmogorov-Smirnov and Shapiro-Wilk tests. Comparisons were made using multigroup, one-way ANOVA to test for the significance of changes among the different groups, followed by the Least Significant Difference test to compare differences between groups. If the data were not normally distributed, the Kruskal-Wallis test (nonparametric ANOVA) was used, and, where differences were identified, pairwise comparisons were performed using Mann-Whitney $U$ test with appropriate correction by Holm-Bonferroni method. All differences were considered significant at $P < 0.05$. Values are expressed as means ± standard deviation (±SD) or as median and interquartile range (IQR): 25th and 75th percentiles, mean and 95% confidence interval for the mean (95% Cl), or number (percentage), as appropriate.

## 3. Results

*3.1. Early Outcomes.* There were no deaths. All animals reached PND 9. Table 1 summarizes the most relevant outcomes.

Baseline characteristics of the groups were equivalent. No significant ($P > 0.05$) intergroup differences were found in the baseline (PND 6) body weight, locomotor activity score, and righting reflex latency. However, rats in the fentanyl group showed significantly longer baseline geotactic responses than saline ($P = 0.005$) and unoperated rats ($P = 0.007$).

During the early period of the experiment, from PND 6 to PND 9, all rats increased body weight in a steady manner, showing no delay in physical development.

When compared to baseline results, outcomes of the fentanyl, saline and unoperated groups, recorded on PND 9, showed an improvement in all parameters, such as weight gain, enhancement of locomotor activity score, and reduced postural reflex latencies.

Comparison of the PND 9 results between fentanyl group and the controls did not show significant differences ($P > 0.05$) on righting reflex latency, negative geotactic latency, or locomotor activity score (Table 1).

*3.2. Later Outcomes.* Table 2 summarizes the most relevant outcomes.

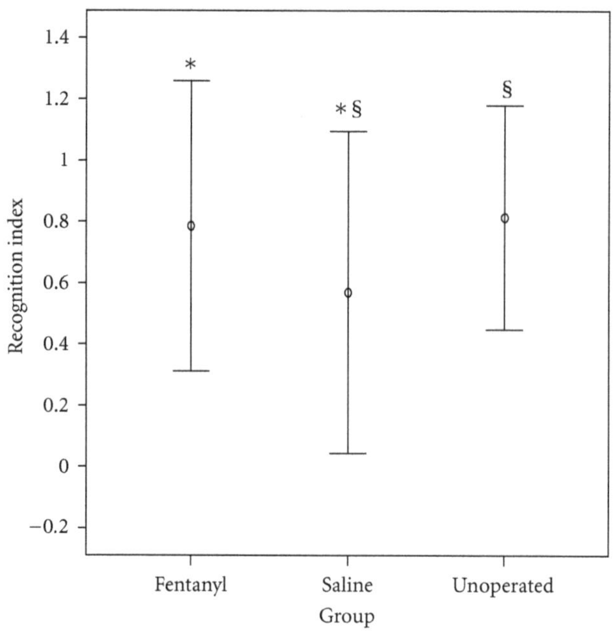


FIGURE 5: Object recognition test of short-term memory. Recognition index of novel object exploration is exploration time on new object/total exploration time (RI $= t_n/(t_n + t_f)$). The recognition index (RI) of a novel object in fentanyl group was not significantly different from that for the unoperated sham controls. However, a significant difference (*$P = 0.045$) was evidenced between the fentanyl group compared to the saline group, showing better cognitive function for the first group. A difference was also seen between the controls: unoperated sham rats displayed significantly (§$P = 0.025$) better short-term memory compared to saline-treated rats. Values are mean ± SD.

*3.2.1. Developmental and Growth Indices.* As expected, all animals reached the defined endpoint (PND 21).

All rats maintained weight gain throughout the study; however, fentanyl-treated rats weighed significantly more than saline-treated and unoperated controls, from PND 12 to PND 21 (Figure 2). The mean weights (±SD) for fentanyl, saline, and unoperated rats on PND 21 were 43 (±3) g, 36 (±6) g, and 36 (±4) g, respectively. Significant differences between fentanyl versus saline ($P = 0.001$) and fentanyl versus unoperated rats ($P < 0.001$) were seen. There was no significant difference between the control groups ($P > 0.05$).

Eyes started to open from PND 14. The median number of eyes open (scored as 0 or 1 or 2 eyes open) on this day was higher in fentanyl (2) than in saline (1) and unoperated groups (0), although without statistical significance ($P > 0.05$) (Table 2 and Figure 3).

*3.3. Behavior in the Open Field.* There were no observable intergroup differences on locomotor activity and exploratory profile. Although there was a trend for an increased mean number of line crossings in the fentanyl group (mean number: 68), compared to the saline (mean number: 62) or the unoperated ones (mean number: 48), the differences between groups were not statistically significant ($P > 0.05$), as seen in Table 2. Additionally, all rats showed a similar exploratory behavior profile, characterized by immediate beginning of locomotor activity (latency up to 20 sec) following the placement of the animal in the central area of the open field apparatus; they also showed similar profiles in the type of exploratory activity periods (with rearing and grooming behaviors) and preference for the corners exploration over that of the central area.

*3.3.1. Behavior during the Wire Hanging Maneuver.* On PND 17 (habituation trial) all rats failed the task of platform reaching.

The success in reaching the platform differed among groups both in PND 18 and PND 20. On PND 18, 60% of the rats in the fentanyl group, 10% in the saline group, and 20% in the unoperated sham group successfully completed the task of reaching the platform; these differences were statistically significant (data not shown). Moreover, rats in the fentanyl group were faster than controls. The median latency time to complete the task in fentanyl group (127 sec) was not significantly different from that in the unoperated sham group (183 sec); however we found a significantly ($P = 0.035$) shorter median latency time in the fentanyl group (127 sec) when compared to the saline group (183 sec), as seen in Table 2 and Figure 4.

On PND 20, while 100% of the rats in the fentanyl group completed the task successfully, only 60% in the saline and 70% in the unoperated sham groups were successful (data not shown). Again, median latency time to reach the platform was shorter ($P > 0.05$) in the fentanyl rats (25 sec) compared to saline (75 sec) or unoperated ones (76 sec), as seen in Table 2 and Figure 4.

*3.4. Effects of Neonatal Fentanyl Exposure on Novel Object Recognition Task of Short-Term Memory.* Cognitive performance in an object recognition task of short-term memory, performed on PND 19, evidenced no adverse lasting impact in preweanling rats after neonatal exposure to six doses of fentanyl (average total dose per animal: 135 $\mu$g/kg weight).

The mean recognition index (RI) of a novel object in fentanyl group (0.79) was not significantly different ($P > 0.05$) from that for the unoperated sham controls (0.8). However, a significant difference ($P = 0.045$) was found between the fentanyl group (0.8) compared to the saline group (0.6), showing better cognitive function for the first group. A significant difference was also seen between the controls; unoperated sham rats displayed significant ($P = 0.025$) better short-term memory (0.8) compared to saline-treated rats (0.6), as seen in Table 2 and Figure 5.

*3.5. Effects of Neonatal Fentanyl Exposure on Anxiety-Like Behavior.* Fentanyl-treated rats were significantly less anxious than the saline-treated rats ($P = 0.035$) or the unoperated ones ($P = 0.043$) in the elevated plus maze, as indicated by the increase in the median percent time spent in the open arms by the fentanyl-treated rats (18%, IQR 17–32), compared to the saline (7%, IQR 3–17) or to the

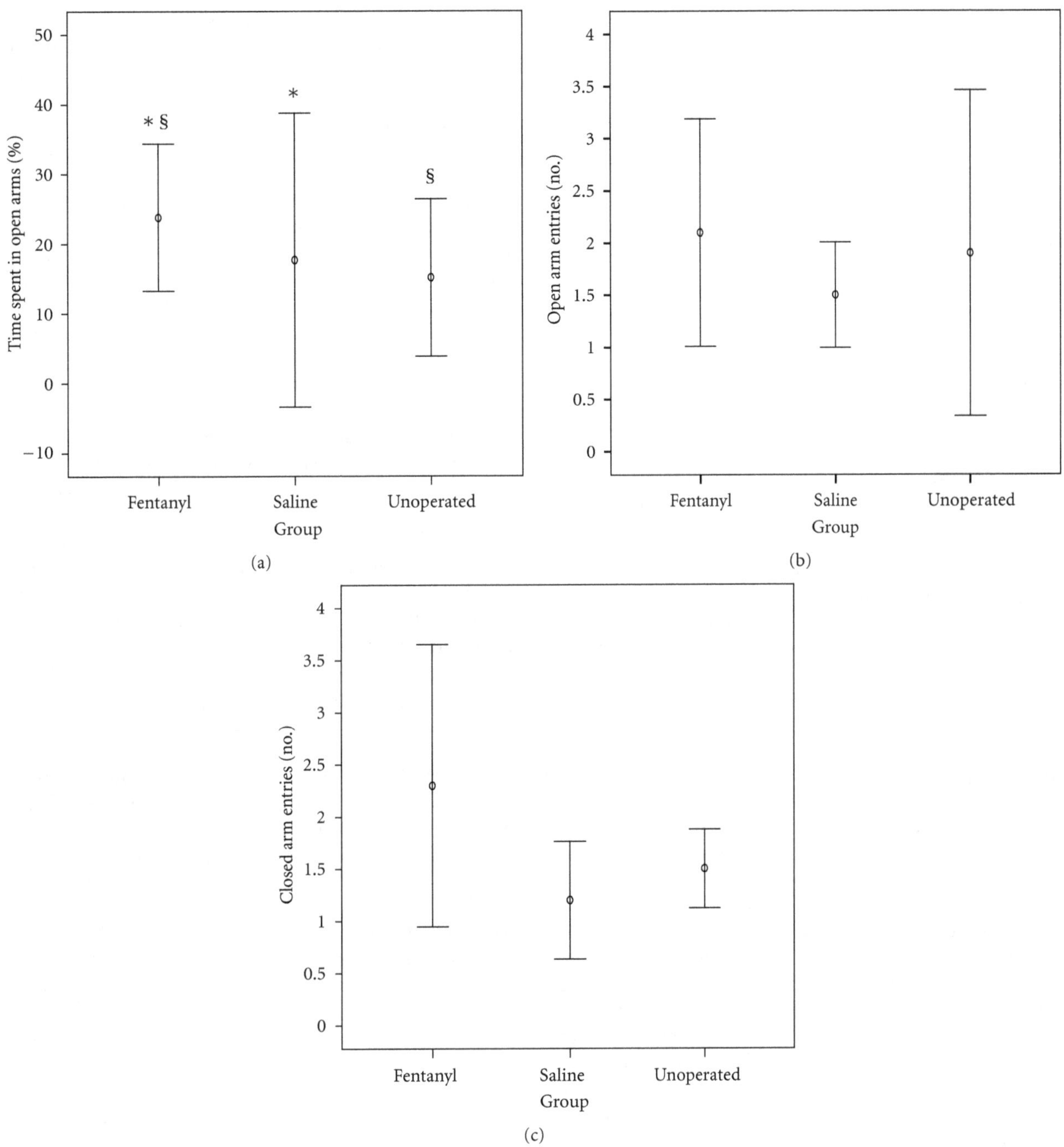


FIGURE 6: Performance in the elevated plus maze: (a) percent time in the open arms was significantly increased in fentanyl rats compared to saline rats ($^{*}P = 0.034$) or unoperated controls ($^{\S}P = 0.045$), suggesting that neonatal fentanyl exposure reduces some measures of anxiety-like behavior on the elevated plus maze; (b) and (c) represent the number of open arm and the number of closed arm entries, respectively, showing no significant differences between groups. Values represent mean and 95% confidence interval for mean.

unoperated sham controls (10%, IQR 7–16). However, there were no significant intergroup differences between open or closed arm entries (Table 2 and Figure 6).

*3.6. Effects on the Accelerating Rotarod.* The effects of fentanyl exposure on locomotor coordination and balance, as measured by the accelerating rotarod, are shown in Figure 7.

The best (largest) of the three fall latency values (mean ± SD) achieved per rat on PND 21 was used for data analysis. Mean latency to fall from the rod for fentanyl group was 173 sec, for saline group was 123 sec, and for unoperated sham rats was 128 sec. Rats treated with fentanyl spent significantly more time on rod, compared to rats treated with saline ($P = 0.022$) or unoperated sham rats ($P = 0.04$), as seen in Table 2 and Figure 7.

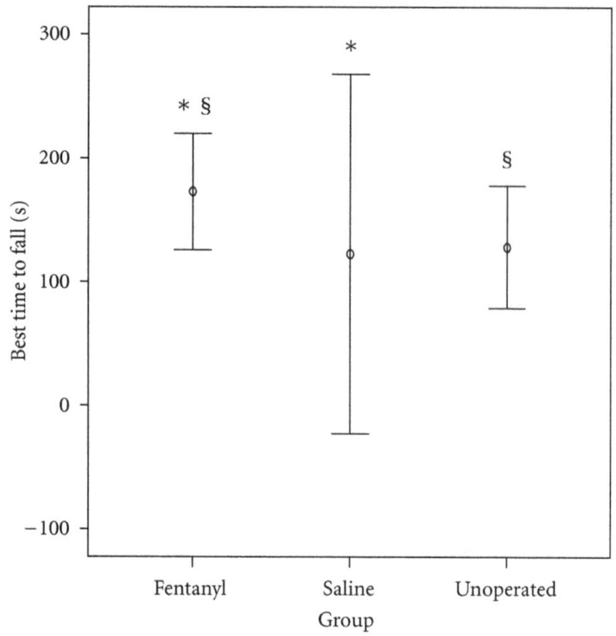


FIGURE 7: Best latency time to fall from the accelerating rotarod (speed 5–40 rpm). Rats administered fentanyl spent significantly more time on rod, compared to rats administered saline ($^*P = 0.022$) or unoperated sham rats ($^{\S}P = 0.040$). Values are mean ± SD.

## 4. Discussion

The present study was designed to assess whether exposure to repetitive injections of fentanyl during brain development influences later physical and neurological outcomes. Using a neonatal postoperative pain model, this study demonstrates, for the first time, lasting effects on growth and behavior of rat pups that underwent repeated fentanyl exposure during early postnatal life, when tested as later pre-weanling rats. The results showed that repeated fentanyl exposure of an immature stressed animal significantly interferes with growth, cognitive function, behavioral reactivity to stress, neuromuscular and locomotor development, and balance and coordination. All these outcomes (Table 2) suggest a neurological impact with possible consequences, either positive or negative, later in life.

To examine the role of fentanyl administration in the development of behaviors that occur following repeated exposure to this medication, both in immature CNS and pain settings, we combined two strategies: the model for the study of neonatal neurodevelopment (6-day-old rat pup) was combined with the postincisional pain of Brennan paw incision [14], as a model for neonatal neurodevelopmental and postoperative pain. Translation of developmental ages from rodents to humans continues to be debated. A review paper by Vidair [19], which discusses the adequacy of the postnatal rat to serve as a model for neurodevelopment in the postnatal human, concludes that the rat in the third postnatal week is the neurodevelopmental equivalent of the newborn human and that the two species share numerous pathways of postnatal neurodevelopment. Therefore, our neonatal rat model roughly corresponds to a human premature. Brennan's model of incisional pain [14] was chosen since it simulates the usual clinical setting involving critically ill prematures in neonatal intensive care units.

Premature newborns typically present a broad range of comorbidities which make them a complex group to study, given the many variables, painful/stressful procedures, and pharmacologic exposures involved. Therefore, experimental studies using animals allow us to exclude potential confounding variables. In our study we used a model without comorbidities in a postoperative pain and stress setting. Such a preclinical model, which leads to pain-related events that mirror the symptoms observed in patients undergoing surgery [20], gives us the opportunity to explore whether repetitive fentanyl exposure, early in neonates subject to painful stimuli, leads to later neurodevelopmental anomalies. The postoperative pain model we used was previously described by Brennan and coworkers [14]. This rat model consists of an incision of the plantar paw skin, with damage of the underlying muscle, which results in localized mechanical hypersensitivity that lasts 3–5 days. Further research by Brennan's group showed release of excitatory amino acids, such as glutamate and aspartate, activation of dorsal horn cells, and central sensitization [21].

Concerning protocol design, the dose of fentanyl used in this study, although at first sight much higher than the neonatal human recommended dose, was chosen according to the species known metabolism to relate to that typically encountered in clinical settings reflecting antinociceptive ED50 values for PND6 rats [22]. We assessed behavioral problems in our neonatal stressed model using a validated set of tests usually chosen for drug toxicity screening.

Among major findings in the present study, we highlight the significant enhancement of weight gain in fentanyl group compared to controls, as summarized in Table 2. Neither fentanyl nor control conditions had significant effects on normal early pup weight gain. In contrast, there were significant group differences in rat weights on PND 21. Rats in the fentanyl group weighed more than those in the saline and unoperated sham groups, with the difference becoming significant around PND 12 and expanding as the pups aged until weaning. These outcomes suggest that the effects of the early postnatal exposure were subtle but, nonetheless, predisposed the pups to abnormal weight gain. Many hypotheses are possible to explain this finding, namely, metabolic derangements, behavior anomalies related to eating disorders, or decreased physical activity. An important issue that can be raised is whether the weight change is transitory or if it can continue into adulthood.

Other major findings in the present study were behavioral changes induced by administration of fentanyl in our model. Somewhat surprisingly, the results point towards an overall apparently "positive" effect on neurodevelopment, instead of the expected negative one. This "positive" impact was evidenced by an apparent lack of significant acute toxic effects on early development. Moreover, later, in infant rats who were treated with fentanyl, we found enhancement of the recognition index of a novel object, lesser anxiety-like behavior, and better performances on the wire hanging maneuver and on the accelerating rotarod. Furthermore, there was a trend for sooner eye opening in this group, suggesting that the eye command center of CNS of rats in the fentanyl group ages earlier.

Interestingly, aversive stressful procedures performed in the current study, which should be associated with increased anxiety, seemed blunted by fentanyl treatment. In fact, fentanyl-treated rats were significantly less anxious than the saline and the unoperated rats in the elevated plus maze. This outcome is not clearly explained, but calmer subjects can probably better explain other outcomes found in this study, such as enhanced cognitive function, motor, and balance and coordination. It is possible that all these results are at least partially explained by a fentanyl impact on the development of central neuronal circuits, given the great plasticity of the CNS characteristic of the immature mammalian brain [23].

The effects of the impact of fentanyl on SNC are probably complex and multivariate with different possible mechanisms found in the literature, both potentially protective or detrimental, such as faster CNS myelination and enhanced neurogenesis by NeuroD activity level increase (a transcription factor essential for the development of the CNS) [24] eventually translating into enhanced performance or, on the other hand, cytotoxic lesion/blockade of the ventral hippocampus by N-methyl-D-aspartate (NMDA) receptor interference, manifesting as reduced anxiety [25]. It is well known from the literature that fentanyl modulates important cellular and molecular neuronal mechanisms, interfering not only in anatomically distributed neural network involved in generating states of anesthesia but also in mechanisms involved in hippocampus neurogenesis. In this setting, fentanyl may regulate the functions of the developing hippocampus, a region highly related to learning, memory, stress responses, and emotionality [25].

There is a growing body of evidence showing that drugs interfering in the SNC functions may cause pharmacologic neuroprotection or, on the opposite, detrimental effects, depending on the pathological conditions [19, 26–28]. Negative impact alerts are particularly alarming in the context of very ill preterm infants who usually present a multitude of physiological derangements and pathological pain conditions coupled with a very immature brain, therefore it is important to define safe indications and doses for the use of these drugs, such as fentanyl, in this stage.

In conclusion, the current study is the first to demonstrate that rat pups exposed to parenteral fentanyl in a painful context have lasting growth and behavioral changes. The study highlights behavioral changes that could potentially affect brain function either in a positive or negative manner. These results should serve as a basis for further research and should lead investigators to focus on specific pathways relevant to the changes in behavior we have shown. Our findings may contribute to support the neonatal use of fentanyl, when indicated, namely in postsurgical settings, even in premature newborns. However, extrapolating our data to a clinical setting must be done with caution, as with every animal study.

## Authors' Contribution

Dora Catré is responsible for design, intellectual and scientific content, and writing of the paper. Maria Francelina Lopes supervised all phases of the experimental study and writing of the paper. António Silvério Cabrita is responsible for collecting and processing of study information.

## References


[1] T. Lasky, F. R. Ernst, J. Greenspan, S. Wang, and L. Gonzalez, "Estimating pediatric inpatient medication use in the United States," *Pharmacoepidemiology and Drug Safety*, vol. 20, no. 1, pp. 76–82, 2011.

[2] B. Hsu and T. Brazelton, "Off-label medication use in an academic hospital pediatric critical care unit," *Wisconsin Medical Journal*, vol. 108, no. 7, pp. 343–348, 2009.

[3] A. N. Naguib, P. Winch, L. Schwartz et al., "Anesthetic management of the hybrid stage 1 procedure for hypoplastic left heart syndrome (HLHS)," *Paediatric Anaesthesia*, vol. 20, no. 1, pp. 38–46, 2010.

[4] J. D. Tobias, "Sedation and analgesia in the pediatric intensive care unit," *Pediatric Annals*, vol. 34, no. 8, pp. 636–645, 2005.

[5] J. G. Klamt, W. V. A. de Vicente, L. V. Garcia, and C. A. Ferreira, "Effects of dexmedetomidine-fentanyl infusion on blood pressure and heart rate during cardiac surgery in children," *Anesthesiology Research and Practice*, vol. 2010, Article ID 869049, 7 pages, 2010.

[6] M. Palot, H. Visseaux, and C. Botmans, "Conduction anesthesia and the newborn infant," *Cahiers d'Anesthesiologie*, vol. 43, no. 6, pp. 547–553, 1995.

[7] T. R. Okon and M. L. George, "Fentanyl-induced neurotoxicity and paradoxic pain," *Journal of Pain and Symptom Management*, vol. 35, no. 3, pp. 327–333, 2008.

[8] W. A. Kofke, R. H. Garman, R. L. Stiller, M. E. Rose, and R. Garman, "Opioid neurotoxicity: fentanyl dose-response effects in rats," *Anesthesia and Analgesia*, vol. 83, no. 6, pp. 1298–1306, 1996.

[9] W. A. Kofke, R. H. Garman, R. Garman, and M. E. Rose, "Opioid neurotoxicity: fentanyl-induced exacerbation of cerebral ischemia in rats," *Brain Research*, vol. 818, no. 2, pp. 326–334, 1999.

[10] J. E. Bailey, E. Campagna, and R. C. Dart, "RADARS System Poison Center Investigators. The underrecognized toll of prescription opioid abuse on young children," *Annals of Emergency Medicine*, vol. 53, no. 4, pp. 419–424, 2009.

[11] T. T. Levin, M. H. Bakr, and T. Nikolova, "Case report: delirium due to a diltiazem-fentanyl CYP3A4 drug interaction," *General Hospital Psychiatry*, vol. 32, no. 6, pp. 648.e9–648.e10, 2010.

[12] E. H. Sinz, W. A. Kofke, and R. H. Garman, "Phenytoin, midazolam, and naloxone protect against fentanyl-induced brain damage in rats," *Anesthesia and Analgesia*, vol. 91, no. 6, pp. 1443–1449, 2000.

[13] Institute of Laboratory Animal Research, Commission on Life Sciences, and National Research Council, *Guide for the Care and Use of Laboratory Animals*, The National Academies Press, Washington, DC, USA, 1996.

[14] T. J. Brennan, E. P. Vandermeulen, and G. F. Gebhart, "Characterization of a rat model of incisional pain," *Pain*, vol. 64, no. 3, pp. 493–501, 1996.

[15] K. Wallace, S. Veerisetty, I. Paul, W. May, J. J. Miguel-Hidalgo, and W. Bennett, "Prenatal infection decreases calbindin,

decreases purkinje cell volume and density and produces long-term motor deficits in Sprague-Dawley rats," *Developmental Neuroscience*, vol. 32, no. 4, pp. 302–312, 2010.

[16] L. W. Fan, R. F. Chen, H. J. Mitchell et al., "α-Phenyl-n-tert-butyl-nitrone attenuates lipopolysaccharide-induced brain injury and improves neurological reflexes and early sensorimotor behavioral performance in juvenile rats," *Journal of Neuroscience Research*, vol. 86, no. 16, pp. 3536–3547, 2008.

[17] Y. Silberman, O. J. Ariwodola, A. M. Chappell, J. T. Yorgason, and J. L. Weiner, "Lateral paracapsular GABAergic synapses in the basolateral amygdala contribute to the anxiolytic effects of β3 adrenoceptor activation," *Neuropsychopharmacology*, vol. 35, no. 9, pp. 1886–1896, 2010.

[18] J. A. Able, G. A. Gudelsky, C. V. Vorhees, and M. T. Williams, "3,4-Methylenedioxymethamphetamine in adult rats produces deficits in path integration and spatial reference memory," *Biological Psychiatry*, vol. 59, no. 12, pp. 1219–1226, 2006.

[19] C. A. Vidair, "Age dependence of organophosphate and carbamate neurotoxicity in the postnatal rat: extrapolation to the human," *Toxicology and Applied Pharmacology*, vol. 196, no. 2, pp. 287–302, 2004.

[20] T. J. Martin, N. L. Buechler, W. Kahn, J. C. Crews, and J. C. Eisenach, "Effects of laparotomy on spontaneous exploratory activity and conditioned operant responding in the rat: a model for postoperative pain," *Anesthesiology*, vol. 101, no. 1, pp. 191–203, 2004.

[21] P. K. Zahn, K. A. Sluka, and T. J. Brennan, "Excitatory amino acid release in the spinal cord caused by plantar incision in the rat," *Pain*, vol. 100, no. 1-2, pp. 65–76, 2002.

[22] S. R. Thornton and F. L. Smith, "Characterization of neonatal rat fentanyl tolerance and dependence," *Journal of Pharmacology and Experimental Therapeutics*, vol. 281, no. 1, pp. 514–521, 1997.

[23] S. Trojan, M. Langmeier, D. Maresová, J. Mourek, and J. Pokorný, "Plasticity of the brain in neuroontogenesis," *Prague Medical Report*, vol. 105, no. 2, pp. 97–110, 2004.

[24] H. Zheng, Y. Zeng, J. Chu, A. Y. Kam, H. H. Loh, and P. Y. Law, "Modulations of NeuroD activity contribute to the differential effects of morphine and fentanyl on dendritic spine stability," *Journal of Neuroscience*, vol. 30, no. 24, pp. 8102–8110, 2010.

[25] C. Barkus, S. B. McHugh, R. Sprengel, P. H. Seeburg, J. N. Rawlins, and D. M. Bannerman, "Hippocampal NMDA receptors and anxiety: at the interface between cognition and emotion," *European Journal of Pharmacology*, vol. 626, no. 1, pp. 49–56, 2010.

[26] V. Laudenbach, G. Calo, R. Guerrini et al., "Nociceptin/orphanin FQ exacerbates excitotoxic whitematter lesions in the murine neonatal brain," *Journal of Clinical Investigation*, vol. 107, no. 4, pp. 457–466, 2001.

[27] K. J. Anand, S. Garg, C. R. Rovnaghi, U. Narsinghani, A. T. Bhutta, and R. W. Hall, "Ketamine reduces the cell death following inflammatory pain in newborn rat brain," *Pediatric Research*, vol. 62, no. 3, pp. 283–290, 2007.

[28] S. R. Hays and J. K. Deshpande, "Newly postulated neurodevelopmental risks of pediatric anesthesia," *Current Neurology and Neuroscience Reports*, vol. 11, no. 2, pp. 205–210, 2011.

# Permissions

All chapters in this book were first published in JAR, by Hindawi Publishing Corporation; hereby published with permission under the Creative Commons Attribution License or equivalent. Every chapter published in this book has been scrutinized by our experts. Their significance has been extensively debated. The topics covered herein carry significant findings which will fuel the growth of the discipline. They may even be implemented as practical applications or may be referred to as a beginning point for another development.

The contributors of this book come from diverse backgrounds, making this book a truly international effort. This book will bring forth new frontiers with its revolutionizing research information and detailed analysis of the nascent developments around the world.

We would like to thank all the contributing authors for lending their expertise to make the book truly unique. They have played a crucial role in the development of this book. Without their invaluable contributions this book wouldn't have been possible. They have made vital efforts to compile up to date information on the varied aspects of this subject to make this book a valuable addition to the collection of many professionals and students.

This book was conceptualized with the vision of imparting up-to-date information and advanced data in this field. To ensure the same, a matchless editorial board was set up. Every individual on the board went through rigorous rounds of assessment to prove their worth. After which they invested a large part of their time researching and compiling the most relevant data for our readers.

The editorial board has been involved in producing this book since its inception. They have spent rigorous hours researching and exploring the diverse topics which have resulted in the successful publishing of this book. They have passed on their knowledge of decades through this book. To expedite this challenging task, the publisher supported the team at every step. A small team of assistant editors was also appointed to further simplify the editing procedure and attain best results for the readers.

Apart from the editorial board, the designing team has also invested a significant amount of their time in understanding the subject and creating the most relevant covers. They scrutinized every image to scout for the most suitable representation of the subject and create an appropriate cover for the book.

The publishing team has been an ardent support to the editorial, designing and production team. Their endless efforts to recruit the best for this project, has resulted in the accomplishment of this book. They are a veteran in the field of academics and their pool of knowledge is as vast as their experience in printing. Their expertise and guidance has proved useful at every step. Their uncompromising quality standards have made this book an exceptional effort. Their encouragement from time to time has been an inspiration for everyone.

The publisher and the editorial board hope that this book will prove to be a valuable piece of knowledge for researchers, students, practitioners and scholars across the globe.

# List of Contributors

**Ali Kord Valeshabad**
Department of Ophthalmology and Visual Sciences, University of Illinois at Chicago, IL 60612, USA

**Omid Nabavian, Hossein Vafainejad, Mehdi Rezaei, Hamed Darabi, Mohammad Koohkan, Poorya Golbinimofrad and Samira Jafari**
Department of Anaesthesiology, Tehran University of Medical Sciences, Tehran, Iran

**Keramat Nourijelyani**
Department of Epidemiology of Biostatistics, Tehran University of Medical Sciences, Tehran, Iran

**Hadi Kord**
Department of Dermatology, Golestan University of Medical Sciences, Gorgan 4934174515, Iran

**Reza Kord Valeshabad**
Zainaldin Martyr Research Center, Gorgan University of Agricultural Sciences and Natural Resources, Gorgan, Iran

**Ali Reza Feili**
Center for Cardiovascular Research, University of Illinois at Chicago, 835 S.Wolcott Avenue, Chicago, IL 60612, USA

**Denisa Madalina Anastase, Simona Cionac Florescu and Ana Maria Munteanu**
Department of Anesthesiology, Clinical Hospital of Orthopedy Foisor, Bulevardul Ferdinand, No. 35-37, 021382 Bucharest, Romania

**Traian Ursu and Cristian Ioan Stoica**
Department of Orthopedics, Foisor Clinical Orthopedics Hospital and "Carol Davila" University of Medicine and Pharmacy, 020022 Bucharest, Romania

**Robert E. Freundlich, Jessica W. Newman, Kevin K. Tremper, Sachin Kheterpal, Theodore J. Sanford Jr. and Alan R. Tait**
Department of Anesthesiology, University of Michigan Medical School, Ann Arbor, MI 48105, USA

**Jill M. Mhyre**
Department of Anesthesiology, University of Arkansas, Little Rock, AR 72205, USA

**Denise McCarthy and Gabriella Iohom**
Department of Anaesthesia and Intensive Care Medicine, Cork University Hospital, Cork, Ireland

**Emma J. Stodel**
Learning 4 Excellence, 749 Long Point Circle, Ottawa, ON, Canada K1T 4H5

**Anna Wyand, Simone Crooks, Stéphane Moffett and Michelle Chiu**
Department of Anesthesiology, The Ottawa Hospital, 1053 Carling Avenue, Ottawa, ON, Canada K1Y 4E9

**Christopher C. C. Hudson**
University of Ottawa Heart Institute, 40 Ruskin Street, Ottawa, ON, Canada K1Y 4W7

**Thomas Mencke, Amelie Zitzmann, Susann Machmueller, Martin Sauer and Gabriele Noeldge-Schomburg**
Department of Anesthesia and Intensive Care Medicine, University of Rostock, Schillingallee 35, 18057 Rostock, Germany

**Arne Boettcher, Hans-Wilhelm Pau and Steffen Dommerich**
Department of Otorhinolaryngology, University of Rostock, 18057 Rostock, Germany

**Shigeaki Otomo, Hajime Iwasaki, Kenichi Takahoko, Yoshiko Onodera, Tomoki Sasakawa, Takayuki Kunisawa and Hiroshi Iwasaki**
Department of Anesthesiology and Critical Care, Asahikawa Medical University, 2-1-1-1 Midorigaoka-higashi, Asahikawa, Hokkaido 078-8510, Japan

**Chi-Te Lin, Hsin-Ying Wang, Tzu-Yu Lin and June-Horng Lue**
Department of Anatomy and Cell Biology, College of Medicine, National Taiwan University, Taipei 10018, Taiwan

**Seu-Hwa Chen**
Department of Anatomy and Cell Biology, College of Medicine, National Taiwan University, Taipei 10018, Taiwan
Department of Anatomy, Taipei Medical College, Taipei 100, Taiwan

**Yi-Ju Tsai**
School of Medicine, College of Medicine, Fu Jen Catholic University, Taipei 24205, Taiwan

**Tracey Pons and Edward A. Shipton**
Department of Anaesthesia, University of Otago, Christchurch, Corner of Riccarton and Hagley Avenues, Christchurch 8042, New Zealand

**Jonathan Williman**
Department of Population Health, University of Otago, Christchurch, Corner of Riccarton and Hagley Avenues, Christchurch 8042, New Zealand

**Roger T. Mulder**
Department of Psychological Medicine, University of Otago, Christchurch, Corner of Riccarton and Hagley Avenues, Christchurch 8042, New Zealand

**Mario A. Inchiosa Jr.**
Departments of Pharmacology and Anesthesiology, New York Medical College, Basic Sciences Building, Valhalla, NY 10595, USA

**Fred Bulamba**
Department of Anaesthesia and Critical Care, Faculty of Health Sciences, Busitema University, Mbale, Uganda

**Andrew Kintu, Nodreen Ayupo, Charles Kojjo, Lameck Ssemogerere, Agnes Wabule and Arthur Kwizera**
Department of Anaesthesia and Critical Care, College of Health Sciences, Makerere University, Kampala, Uganda

**U. U. Johnson and L. N. Ebirim**
Department of Anaesthesiology, University of Port Harcourt Teaching Hospital, PMB 6173, Port Harcourt, Rivers State, Nigeria

**Yu Qi, Tokujiro Uchida, Mamoru Yamamoto, Yudai Yamamoto, Koji Kido, Hiroyuki Ito, Chieko Mitaka, and Koshi Makita**
Department of Anesthesiology, Tokyo Medical and Dental University, Graduate School of Medical and Dental Sciences, 1-5-45 Yushima, Bunkyo-ku, Tokyo 113-8519, Japan

**Nagara Ohno, Miho Asahara and Yoshitsugu Yamada**
Department of Anesthesiology, The University of Tokyo, Graduate School of Medicine, Tokyo, Japan

**Osamu Yamaguchi**
Department of Critical Care Medicine, Yokohama City University Medical Center, Kanagawa, Japan

**Makoto Tomita**
Clinical Research Center, Tokyo Medical and Dental University Hospital of Medicine, Tokyo, Japan

**Sangeeta Kumaraswami, Suryanarayana Pothula, Keshar Paul Kubal and Micah Alexander Burns**
Department of Anesthesiology, New York Medical College at Westchester Medical Center, 100 Woods Road, Macy Pavilion 2391, Valhalla, NY 10595, USA

**Mario Anthony Inchiosa Jr.**
Department of Pharmacology and Anesthesiology, New York Medical College at Westchester Medical Center, 100 Woods Road, Macy Pavilion 2391, Valhalla, NY 10595, USA

**Paul Picton**
Department of Anesthesiology, University of Michigan, Ann Arbor, MI, USA

**Olubukola O. Nafiu, Katari Carello and Anjana Lal**
Department of Anesthesiology, University of Michigan, Ann Arbor, MI, USA
Section of Pediatric Anesthesiology, University of Michigan, Ann Arbor, MI, USA

**John Magee**
Department of Surgery, University of Michigan, Ann Arbor, MI, USA

**Cattleya Thongrong and Pattramon Thaisiam**
Department of Anesthesiology, Faculty of Medicine, Khon Kaen University, Khon Kaen, Thailand

**Pornthep Kasemsiri**
Division of Skull Base Surgery, Department of Otorhinolaryngology, Faculty of Medicine, Khon Kaen University, Khon Kaen, Thailand

**Richard Mwase**
Uganda People's Defense Forces Directorate of Medical Services, Bombo Military Hospital, Bombo, Uganda

**Tonny Stone Luggya, Andrew Kintu, JoesphV. B. Tindimwebwa and Daniel Obua**
Department of Anesthesia, College of Health Sciences, Makerere University, Kampala, Uganda

**John Mark Kasumba**
Directorate of Surgical Services, Mulago Hospital, Kampala, Uganda

**Humphrey Wanzira**
Ministry of Health, Kampala, Uganda

**Cattleya Thongrong, Patitha Chullabodhi, Narin Plailaharn, Lumyai Sabangban and Thirada Jimarsa**
Department of Anesthesiology, Faculty of Medicine, Khon Kaen University, Khon Kaen, Thailand

**Pornthep Kasemsiri**
Division of Skull Base Surgery, Department of Otorhinolaryngology, Faculty of Medicine, Khon Kaen University, Khon Kaen, Thailand

**Amnat Kitkhuandee**
Division of Neurosurgery, Department of Surgery, Faculty of Medicine, Khon Kaen University, Khon Kaen, Thailand

**Sven Grauman and Jakob Boethius**
Department of Anaesthesia and Intensive Care, Östersund Hospital, Östersund, Sweden

**Joakim Johansson**
Department of Anaesthesia and Intensive Care, Östersund Hospital, Östersund, Sweden
Department of Surgical and Perioperative Sciences, Anesthesiology and Intensive Care, Unit of Research, Education and Development- Östersund, Umeå University, Umeå, Sweden

**Demeke Yilkal Fentie, Henos Enyew Ashagrie and Habtamu Getinet Kasahun**
Department of Anesthesia, School of Medicine, Gondar College of Medicine and Health Sciences, University of Gondar, Gondar, Ethiopia

**Luiz Eduardo de Paula Gomes Miziara, Luís Otávio Esteves, Luis Henrique Cangiani, Gil Fernando Ribeiro Grillo-Filho and Anderson Garcia Lima e Paula**
Department of Anesthesiology, Centro Médico Campinas, Rua Edilberto Luis Pereira da Silva 150, Campinas, SP, Brazil

**Ricardo Francisco Simoni**
Department of Anesthesiology, Centro Médico Campinas, Rua Edilberto Luis Pereira da Silva 150, Campinas, SP, Brazil
Department of Pharmacology, Universidade de Campinas (UNICAMP), Centro M´edico Campinas, Rua Edilberto Luis Pereira da Silva 150, 13083-190 Campinas, SP, Brazil

**Latha Naik, Neerja Bhardwaj and Indu Mohini Sen**
Department of Anaesthesia and Intensive Care Medicine, Postgraduate Institute of Medical Education and Research, Chandigarh 160012, India

**Rakesh V. Sondekoppam**
Department of Anesthesia and Perioperative Medicine, Schulich School of Medicine and Dentistry, Western University, London, ON, Canada N6A 5A5

**Vorasruang Thongsukh, Chanida Kositratana and Aree Jandonpai**
Department of Anesthesiology, Faculty of Medicine Ramathibodi Hospital, Mahidol University, Bangkok 10400, Thailand

**Indira Malik and Rachna Wadhwa**
Department of Anesthesiology and Critical Care, Dr. Baba Saheb Ambedkar Hospital, Rohini, Delhi 85, India

**Laura A. Cagle, Lisa M. Franzi, Jerold A. Last and Nicholas J. Kenyon**
Division of Pulmonary, Critical Care, and Sleep Medicine, School of Medicine, University of California, Davis, CA, USA

**Steven E. Epstein**
Department of Surgical and Radiological Sciences, School of Veterinary Medicine, University of California, Davis, CA, USA

**Philip H. Kass**
Department of Population Health and Reproduction, School of Veterinary Medicine, University of California, Davis, CA, USA

**Yukako Obata, Hiromi Kato and Yoshiki Nakajima**
Department of Intensive Care Unit, Hamamatsu University School of Medicine, 1-20-1 Handayama, Higashi-ku, Hamamatsu, Shizuoka 4313192, Japan

**Yushi U. Adachi**
Department of Intensive Care Medicine, Tokyo Medical and Dental University Medical Hospital, Tokyo, Japan

**Katsumi Suzuki**
Department of Anesthesia, Enshu Hospital, Hamamatsu, Japan

**Taiga Itagaki**
Pulmonary and Critical Care Medicine, Massachusetts General Hospital, Boston, USA

**Maiko Satomoto**
Department of Anesthesiology, Graduate School of Medical and Dental Sciences, Tokyo Medical and Dental University, Japan

**Thomas Berlet**
Department of Intensive Care Medicine, Inselspital-Bern University Hospital, 3010 Bern, Switzerland

**Mathias Marchon**
Department of Anaesthesiology and Pain Therapy, Inselspital-Bern University Hospital, 3010 Bern, Switzerland

**Diwakar D. Balachandran, Saadia A. Faiz and Lara Bashoura**
Department of Pulmonary Medicine, The University of Texas MD Anderson Cancer Center, Houston, TX, USA

**Mike Hernandez**
Department of Biostatistics, The University of Texas MD Anderson Cancer Center, Houston, TX, USA

**Alicia M. Kowalski, Farzin Goravanchi, Elizabeth Rebello, Spencer S. Kee and Katy E. French**
Department of Anesthesia and Perioperative Medicine, The University of Texas MD Anderson Cancer Center, Houston, TX, USA

**Sujith V. Cherian**
Divisions of Pulmonary, Critical Care and Sleep Medicine, The University of Texas Health Science Center at Houston, Houston, TX, USA

**Antonella Cotoia, Floriana Dibello and Gilda Cinnella**
Department of Anesthesia, Intensive Care, and Pain erapy, University of Foggia, Policlinico "OO. Riuniti", Foggia, Italy

**Fiorenzo Moscatelli, Crescenzio Gallo and Giuseppe Cibelli**
Department of Clinical and Experimental Medicine, University of Foggia, Policlinico "OO. Riuniti", Foggia, Italy

**Alberto Sciusco**
Department of Intensive Care and Anaesthesia, North Bristol NHS Trust, Bristol, UK

**Pietro Polito**
Department of Blood Transfusion Medicine, ASS 5 Friuli Occidentale, Pordenone, Italy

**Alberto Modolo**
Naturopathy, A.N.E.A. Academy, Prato, Italy

**Clara S. M. Wong and Steven H. S. Wong**
Department of Anaesthesiology, Queen Elizabeth Hospital, 30 Gascoigne Road, Kowloon, Hong Kong

**Véronique Brulotte**
Anesthesiology Department, University of Montreal Hospital Centre, 3840 St. Urbain Street, Montréal, QC, Canada H2W 1T8
Department of Anesthesiology, Maisonneuve-Rosemont Hospital, 5415 Boulevard de l'Assomption, Montréal, QC, Canada H1T 2M4

**Pierre Beaulieu**
Anesthesiology Department, University of Montreal Hospital Centre, 3840 St. Urbain Street, Montréal, QC, Canada H2W 1T8
Department of Pharmacology, University of Montreal, 3840 St. Urbain Street, Montréal, QC, Canada H2W 1T8

**François A. Leblond**
Nephrology Department and Guy-Bernier Research Centre, Maisonneuve-Rosemont Hospital, Canada

**Vincent Pichette**
Nephrology Department and Guy-Bernier Research Centre, Maisonneuve-Rosemont Hospital, Canada
Department of Pharmacology, University of Montreal, 3840 St. Urbain Street, Montr´eal, QC, Canada H2W 1T8

**Stéphane Elkouri**
Vascular Surgery Department, University of Montreal Hospital Centre, 3840 St. Urbain Street, Montréal, QC, Canada H2W 1T8

**Éric Thérasse**
Radiology Department, University of Montreal Hospital Centre, 3840 St. Urbain Street, Montréal, QC, Canada H2W 1T8

**Ahmad Yaraghi**
Department of Anesthesiology and Critical Care, School of Medicine, Isfahan University of Medical Sciences, Isfahan, Iran

**Nastaran Eizadi-Mood and Ali Mohammad Sabzghabaee**
Isfahan Clinical Toxicology Research Center, Isfahan University of Medical Sciences, Isfahan, Iran

**Maryam Katani, Mahrang Hedaiaty, Seyyed Mohammad Mahdy Mirhosseini and Elham Beheshtian**
Department of Clinical Toxicology, Noor and Ali Asghar (PBUH) University Hospital, Isfahan University of Medical Sciences, Isfahan, Iran

**Shadi Farsaei**
Department of Clinical Pharmacy and Pharmacy Practice, School of Pharmacy and Pharmaceutical Sciences, Isfahan University of Medical Sciences, Isfahan, Iran

**António Silvério Cabrita**
Faculty of Medicine, University of Coimbra, 3004-504 Coimbra, Portugal

**Dora Catré**
Faculty of Medicine, University of Coimbra, 3004-504 Coimbra, Portugal
Department of Anesthesiology, São Teotónio Hospital, EPE, 3504-509 Viseu, Portugal

**Maria Francelina Lopes**
Faculty of Medicine, University of Coimbra, 3004-504 Coimbra, Portugal
Pediatric Surgery Department, Pediatric Hospital, Centro Hospitalar e Universitário de Coimbra, EPE, 3000-602 Coimbra, Portugal

# Index

www.ingramcontent.com/pod-product-compliance
Lightning Source LLC
LaVergne TN
LVHW060525210926
848485LV00005B/1149